FINANCIAL MANAGEMENT OF HEALTH CARE ORGANIZATIONS

FINANCIAL MANAGEMENT OF HEALTH CARE ORGANIZATIONS

AN INTRODUCTION TO FUNDAMENTAL TOOLS, CONCEPTS, AND APPLICATIONS

Fourth Edition

William N. Zelman, Michael J. McCue, Noah D. Glick, and Marci S. Thomas

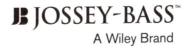

JOSSEY-BASS™

A Wiley Brand

Cover design by Jeff Puda

Cover image : © imagewerks | Getty

Published by Jossey-Bass

A Wiley Brand

One Montgomery Street, Suite 1200, San Francisco, CA 94104-4594—www.josseybass.com

Jossey-Bass books and products are available through most bookstores. To contact Jossey-Bass directly call our Customer Care Department within the U.S. at 800-956-7739, outside the U.S. at 317-572-3986, or fax 317-572-4002.

Wiley publishes in a variety of print and electronic formats and by print-on-demand. Some material included with standard print versions of this book may not be included in e-books or in print-on-demand. If this book refers to media such as a CD or DVD that is not included in the version you purchased, you may download this material at **http://booksupport.wiley.com**. For more information about Wiley products, visit **www.wiley.com**.

Library of Congress Cataloging-In-Publication Data

Zelman, William N., author.

Financial management of health care organizations : an introduction to fundamental tools, concepts, and applications / William N. Zelman, Michael J. McCue, Noah D. Glick, and Marci S. Thomas. – Fourth edition.

p. ; cm.

Includes bibliographical references and index.

ISBN 978-1-118-46656-8 (cloth) – ISBN 978-1-118-46659-9 (pdf) – ISBN 978-1-118-46658-2 (epub)

I. McCue, Michael J. (Michael Joseph), 1954- author. II. Glick, Noah D., author. III. Thomas, Marci S., 1953- author. IV. Title.

[DNLM: 1. Health Facility Administration–economics. 2. Financial Management, Hospital–methods. 3. Practice Management, Medical–economics. WX 157]

RA971.3

362.1068'1–dc23

2013025598

Printed in the United States of America

FOURTH EDITION

HB Printing 10 9 8 7 6 5 4 3 2

CONTENTS

To our families, for their love and patience

To our students and colleagues, for their invaluable

insights and feedback

This book offers an introduction to the most used tools and techniques of health care financial management. It contains numerous examples from a variety of providers, including health maintenance organizations, hospitals, physician practices, home health agencies, nursing units, surgical centers, and integrated health care systems. The book avoids complicated formulas and uses numerous spreadsheet examples so that these examples can be adapted to problems in the workplace. For those desiring to go beyond the fundamentals, many chapters offer additional information in appendices. Each chapter begins with a detailed outline and concludes with a detailed summary, followed by a set of questions and problems. Answers to the questions and problems are available for download to instructors at www.josseybass.com/go/zelman4e. Finally, a number of *perspectives* are included in every chapter. Perspectives—examples from the real world—are intended to provide additional insight into a topic. In some cases these are abstracted from professional journals and in other cases they are statements from practitioners—in their own words.

The book begins with an overview in Chapter One of some of the key factors affecting the financial management of health care organizations in today's environment. Chapters Two, Three, and Four focus on the financial statements of health care organizations. Chapter Two presents an introduction to these financial statements. Financial statements are (perhaps along with the budget) the most important financial documents of a health care organization, and the bulk of this chapter is designed to help readers understand these statements, how they are created, and how they link together.

Chapter Three provides an introduction to health care financial accounting. This chapter focuses on the relationship between the actions of health care providers and administrators and the financial condition of the organization, examining how the numbers on the financial statements are derived, the distinction between cash and accrual bases of accounting—and the importance of defining what is actually meant by *cost*. By the time students complete Chapters Two and Three, they will have been introduced to a large portion of the terms used in health care financial management.

Building on Chapters Two and Three, Chapter Four focuses on interpreting the financial statements of health care organizations. Three approaches to analyzing statements are presented: horizontal, vertical, and ratio analysis. Great care has been taken to show how the ratios are computed and how to summarize the results.

Chapter Five focuses on the management of working capital: current assets and current liabilities. This chapter emphasizes the importance of cash management and provides many practical techniques for managing the inflows and outflows of funds through an organization, including managing the billing and collections cycle and paying off short-term liabilities.

Chapter Six introduces one of the most important concepts in long-term decision making—the time value of money. Chapter Seven builds on this concept, incorporating it into the investment decision by presenting several techniques for analyzing investment decisions: the payback method, net present value, and internal rate of return. Examples are given for both not-for-profit and for-profit organizations.

Once an investment has been decided on, it is important to determine how this asset will be financed, and this is the focus of Chapter Eight. Whereas Chapter Five deals with issues of short-term financing, Chapter Eight focuses on long-term financing, with a particular emphasis on issuing bonds.

Chapters Nine through Twelve introduce topics typically covered in a managerial accounting course. Chapter Nine focuses on the concept of cost and on using cost information—including fixed cost, variable cost, and break-even analysis—for short-term decision making. In addition to covering the key concepts, this chapter offers a set of rules to guide decision makers in making financial decisions. Chapter Ten explores budget models and the budgeting process. Several budget models are introduced, including program, performance, and zero-based budgeting. The chapter ends with an example of how to prepare each of the five main budgets: statistics budget, revenue budget, expense budget, cash budget, and capital budget. It also includes examples for various types of payors, including those with flat fee and capitation plans.

Chapter Eleven deals with responsibility accounting. It discusses the different types of responsibility centers and focuses on performance measurement in general and budget variance analysis in particular. Chapter Twelve discusses methods used by health care providers to determine their costs, primarily focusing on the step-down method and activity-based costing. This book concludes with Chapter Thirteen, "Provider Payment Systems." This chapter, parts of which were combined with

Chapter Twelve in the first edition, describes the evolution of the payment system in the United States, especially under health reform, as well as the specifics of various approaches to managing care and paying providers.

Major Changes in the Fourth Edition

As noted below, the major changes from the third edition involve

- New sections to reflect changes in the health care environment
- Updated data used in examples
- Updated data used in problems
- New problems
- New perspectives

Chapter One: The Context of Health Care Financial Management

Changes to Chapter One, the introductory chapter, provide an updated and current view of today's health care setting. Much has happened in the industry with the advent of value-based payment systems, population-based approaches to care, and the Patient Protection and Affordable Care Act (ACA). Other new concepts include patient-centered medical homes and accountable care organizations (ACOs).

Enhancements include updated statistics in the chapter text and all the pertinent exhibits. All perspectives have been replaced with ones that look at more recent events.

Chapter Two: Health Care Financial Statements

Chapter Two has been updated to include recent changes in the literature issued by the Financial Accounting Standards Board (FASB). These changes address revenue recognition presentation of bad debt for many hospitals, increases in the level of charity care disclosure, and the guidance for self-insured risks. All perspectives and problems have been updated. There are also new key terms.

Chapter Three: Principles and Practices of Health Care Accounting

In Chapter Three, the perspectives have been replaced with four updated versions. Problems 11 through 20 have been changed and updated.

Chapter Four: Financial Statement Analysis

Chapter Four has been updated to include the latest hospital benchmark ratios from the *2013 Almanac of Hospital Financial and Operating Indicators* (a reference work from Optum Inc.).

This chapter also addresses the change mentioned previously to the reporting of bad debt expense. All chapter problems have been updated as well. In addition, ratio problems 11 through 25 have been revised to provide a better picture of what each ratio analyzed means, beyond its being above or below the relevant benchmark.

Chapter Five: Working Capital Management

Chapter Five has new sections on improving the revenue cycle management process and on fraud and abuse. All perspectives and problems have been revised and updated.

Chapter Six: The Time Value of Money

Chapter Six now includes perspectives illustrating time value of money concepts in use, as well as a new section that explains the effective rate function. In addition, all the problem sets have been updated.

Chapter Seven: The Investment Decision

Chapter Seven now offers an expanded discussion of how organizations measure the discount rate or cost of capital. This discussion also explains the weighted average cost of capital, which includes the cost of debt and the cost of equity. The key components of the capital asset pricing model, which is used to measure cost of equity, are presented as well. In addition, all perspectives have been updated, and problems have been changed and updated.

Chapter Eight: Capital Financing for Health Care Providers

Chapter Eight now includes revisions to the explanation of interest rate swaps and a new section on bank qualified private placement loans. All the problems on lease financing and bond valuation have been revised and updated.

Chapter Nine: Using Cost Information to Make Special Decisions

In Chapter Nine, the conceptual diagram and the related explanation for understanding breakeven have been substantially revised, and all perspectives have been replaced with updated versions. Most problems have updated figures, and three problems have been replaced with new ones. Also, a discussion of a new topic, physician practice valuation as it relates to the concept of breakeven, has been added as an appendix. This discussion also introduces the concepts of joint ventures and the value of downstream referrals.

Chapter Ten: Budgeting

Though the organization of Chapter Ten remains essentially the same, the basic model on which this chapter is based has been almost totally revised. The new model is a hospitalist practice that has only two services, a simplification from the previous edition. The discussion of supply chain operations and maximizing savings from evaluation of group purchasing organization discounts has been retained, but the supplies budget has been dropped. All perspectives have been replaced with updated versions. The problems have been revised to reflect the new content, though the general format is the same.

Chapter Eleven: Responsibility Accounting

The discussion of cost centers in Chapter Eleven has been modified slightly to recognize both service- and product-producing activities, and all perspectives and problem sets have been updated.

Chapter Twelve: Provider Cost-Finding Methods

The previous Chapter Twelve perspectives have been dropped, and two new ones have been added.

Chapter Thirteen: Provider Payment Systems

Chapter Thirteen has been updated to provide a discussion of evolving issues in provider payment. Among these issues are value-based purchasing, changes in payment for hospital readmissions and *never events*, and bundled payments. There is a more robust discussion on the mechanisms that Medicare uses to pay for hospital inpatient, hospital outpatient, and physician services. All perspectives have been replaced with updated versions. There are new key terms.

Glossary

The glossary has been completely updated, and includes each term defined in a chapter sidebar and each key term.

Web Pages and Additional Materials

The website for this book, including the instructor's manual and Excel spreadsheets, is located at www.josseybass.com/go/zelman4e. Comments about this book are invited and may be sent to publichealth @wiley.com.

ACKNOWLEDGMENTS

We attempt throughout this book to challenge and enlighten. Quantitative as well as qualitative issues are presented in an effort to help the reader better understand the wide range of issues considered under the topic *health care financial management.* We would like to thank the many students who over the past several years have pointed out errors, offered suggestions and improvements, and provided new ways to solve problems.

Our particular thanks go to Wafa Tarazi, Yurita Yakimin, Abdul Talib, Yen-Ju Lin, PhD, Tae Hyun Kim, PhD, and Julie Peterman, CFA, for their review of various chapters and problem sets. We also offer special thanks to Charles Walker, MBA, CPA, for his dedication and tireless efforts in reviewing the key chapters and problem sets of this book.

Proposal reviewers Steven D. Culler, Magdalene Figuccio, John Fuller, Kirk Harlow, Kelli Haynes, Robert Jeppesen, Charles Kachmarik, Eve Layman, David Lee, Cynthia Lerouge, Anne Macy, Michael Nowicki, William J. Oliver, Mustafa Z. Ounis, Theresa Parker, Kyle Peacock, Jen Porter, Patricia Poteat, Howard Rivenson, Judi Schack-Dugre, Robert Shapiro, Karen Shastri, Dean Smith, Sandie Soldwisch, Wendy Tietz, Bill Wakefield, and Steve Zuiderveen provided valuable feedback on the third edition and our fourth edition revision plan.

Most of all, we would like to thank our families for their encouragement and support and for their understanding during the countless hours we were not available to them.

The authors apologize for any errors or omissions in the above list and would be grateful for notifications to Michael McCue, at mccue@vcu.edu, of any corrections that should be incorporated in the next edition or reprint of this book and posted on the book's webpage.

The authors and the publisher gratefully acknowledge the copyright holders for permission to reproduce material in the perspectives throughout the book.

William N. Zelman is a full professor in the Department of Health Policy and Management, Gillings School of Public Health, University of North Carolina at Chapel Hill. He specializes in health care financial management, focusing on management-related issues, including organizational performance and cost management. He has served as director of the residential master's degree programs at UNC and is past chair of the Association of University Programs in Health Administration Task Force on Financial Management Education. He has authored or coauthored five books and numerous articles and has been an editorial board member or reviewer, or both, for a number of journals. He has extensive international experience, serving as a consultant to and presenting courses for academic, governmental, and other international organizations, primarily in South Asia and Central Europe.

Michael J. McCue is the R. Timothy Stack Professor of Health Care Administration in the Department of Health Administration at Virginia Commonwealth University in Richmond, Virginia. His research interests relate to corporate finance in the health care industry and the performance of hospitals, multihospital systems, and health plans. His previous research examines the determinants of hospital capital structure, the factors influencing hospitals' cash flow and cash on hand, and the evaluation of hospital bond ratings. His current research examines the effects of health reform on the financial performance of commercial health plans.

Noah D. Glick is currently a senior health care consultant for FTI Consulting in its corporate finance division, where he is engaged in physician strategy and health care analytics. Previously, he was administrative director for Rehabilitation Medical Associates and the South Shore Hospitalist Group outside Boston. Prior to that, he was a senior consultant for Integrated Healthcare Information Services in Waltham, Massachusetts, and a staff member in the Department of Decision Support at the University of North Carolina at Chapel Hill. He also taught simulation modeling in the master's in health administration program at UNC.

Marci S. Thomas is a clinical assistant professor in the Department of Health Policy and Management at the University of North Carolina at Chapel Hill, where she teaches health care consulting, strategy, and financial leadership. She is also a principal and director of quality control at Metcalf-Davis, CPAs. She consults with health care organizations, educational institutions, and other not-for-profit organizations and their boards on internal control, vulnerability to risk and fraud, strategic planning, and governance issues. She is a nationally recognized speaker on managing accounting issues in health care and related not-for-profit entities and on auditing these organizations. Thomas is a coeditor of and contributor to *Essentials of Physician Practice Management* (Jossey-Bass). Her book *Best of Boards: Sound Governance and Leadership for Nonprofit Organizations*, was published by the American Institute of CPAs (AICPA) in June 2011. She is a certified public accountant and a chartered global management accountant (CGMA).

FINANCIAL MANAGEMENT OF HEALTH
CARE ORGANIZATIONS

CHAPTER 1

THE CONTEXT OF HEALTH CARE FINANCIAL MANAGEMENT

Never before have health care professionals faced such complex issues and practical difficulties in trying to keep their organizations competitive and financially viable. With disruptive changes taking place in health care legislation and in payment, delivery, and social systems, health care professionals are faced with trying to meet their organizations' health-related missions in an environment of uncertainty and extreme cost pressures. These circumstances are stimulating high-performing provider organizations to focus on innovation to help lower costs and find creative ways to deliver services to a population whose members, while aging, are more informed and more demanding of a voice in their care and value for dollars spent than ever before.

The Patient Protection and Affordable Care Act (ACA) is the largest effort toward reform of the health care system since the advent of government entitlement programs in the 1960s. The goal of the ACA is to provide mechanisms to expand access to care, improve quality, and control costs.

But even before the enactment of the ACA in 2010, the Centers for Medicare and Medicaid Services (CMS) had articulated a vision for health care quality: "the right care for every person every time." CMS's stated objective is to promote safe, effective, timely, patient-centered, efficient, and equitable care.

CMS also needs to control the rising cost of care, which has become unsustainable. To accomplish its objectives CMS has been working to replace its old financing system, which basically rewarded the quantity of care, with value-based purchasing (VBP), a system that improves the linkage between payment and the quality of care. The

- Identify key elements that are driving changes in health care delivery.

- Identify key approaches to controlling health care costs and resulting ethical issues.

- Identify key changes in reimbursement mechanisms to providers.

Deficit Reduction Act of 2005 authorized CMS to develop a plan for VBP for Medicare hospital services beginning in fiscal year 2009. The ACA provided the implementation plan.

Many of these changes have been the source of controversy and lawsuits. Until President Obama's reelection in 2012, state governments as well as many providers faced uncertainty about whether the ACA provisions, even though found to be constitutional earlier in 2012, would be repealed. Some hesitated to move forward with implementation plans.

Regardless of whether or not all parties agree about the legislative outcome, the goal of the U.S. health care system remains to finance and deliver the highest possible quality to the most people at the lowest cost (Exhibit 1.1). But responses to today's challenges have resulted in a new business model that providers are embracing by controlling costs, developing new service offerings, and implementing new information technology, thereby creating added value (see Perspective 1.1 and Exhibit 1.2).

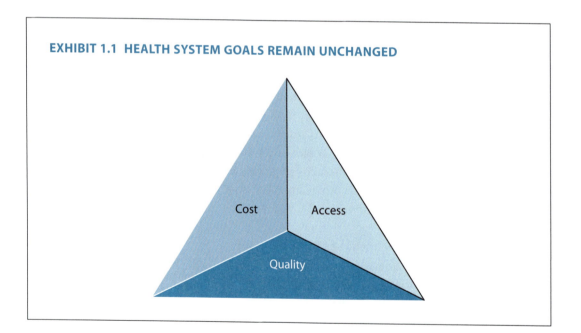

EXHIBIT 1.1 HEALTH SYSTEM GOALS REMAIN UNCHANGED

Cost

Access

Quality

To establish a context for the topics covered in this text, this chapter highlights key issues affecting health care organizations. It is organized into three sections: (1) changing methods of health care financing and delivery, (2) addressing the high cost of care, and (3) establishing value-based payment mechanisms. Without question the health care industry is under-

PERSPECTIVE 1.1 HEALTH CARE SYSTEM IN REFORM

No matter what their political view is, people generally agree that the financial platform on which the health care system rests cannot be sustained. There is a clear need to reduce the proportion of the gross domestic product (GDP) spent on health care. Since the 1960s, hospitals have experienced increases in utilization, accompanied by increases in payments from government as well as from commercial payors. Medicare market basket updates have increased an average of 3.2 percent annually since that time. Under Medicare's new payment model, utilization and reimbursement are expected to decline over time, limiting market basket and utilization increases to only 1.5 percent to 2 percent a year. In addition, the value-based payment structure will reward those organizations with better quality while penalizing those with poorer scores. Since Medicaid and commercial payors tend to follow Medicare models, this effect will be magnified.

Several disruptive trends are changing the competitive landscape. Where commercial and not-for-profit providers had distinct differences, now they are both heavily focused on cost, quality, market share, and how quickly they can get innovative products to market. For example, Duke University Health System, a not-for-profit health system, and LifePoint Hospitals, Inc., a commercial health system, formed a joint venture, Duke LifePoint Healthcare, to provide community hospitals and regional medical centers with innovative means of enhancing services, recruiting and retaining physicians, and developing new service lines. Insurers such as Humana and private equity groups have acquired health systems. Certain integrated health care organizations, such as the Mayo Clinic and Geisinger Health System, are directed by physicians. New technologies like mobile apps provide mid-level providers and consumers with the latest evidence-based guidance to aid in diagnosis and management of health issues. And hospitals are consolidating, taking the view that big is good, bigger is better, and biggest is better still.

Source: Adapted from K. Kaufman and M. E. Grube, The transformation of America's hospitals: economics drives a new business model, in Kaufman, Hall, & Associates, *Futurescan 2012: Healthcare Trends and Implications, 2012–2017* (Health Administration Press, 2011).

going rapid change (Exhibit 1.3). The providers who are open-minded and informed, embrace change, and look for effective solutions will be the ones who thrive in this uncertain environment.

Changing Methods of Health Care Financing and Delivery

The push toward health care reform began back in the early 1990s during the Clinton administration. However, it did not make significant inroads

EXHIBIT 1.2 KEY ELEMENTS OF HEALTH CARE BUSINESS MODEL CHANGE

	Old Medicare Business Model	New Post Reform Business Model
Value proposition	More market share, more patients, more services, more revenues	Best possible quality at the lowest price
Direction of price	Upward—Saks Fifth Avenue	Downward—Walmart
Cost environment	Cost management	Cost structure
Direction of utilization	Always up since 1966, growth industry	Flat/maybe down, mature industry
Relationship between hospital and doctors	Parallel play	Highly coordinated and integrated
Payment	Fee-for-service	Something else
System of care	Patient services	Patient/population management
Organizing for value creation	One patient at a time	Comprehensive health care for covered population
Importance of scale	Small and medium hospitals could survive	Big, bigger, biggest

Source: Kaufman, Hall, & Associates, published in *Futurescan 2012: Healthcare Trends and Implications, 2012–2017*, Society for Healthcare Strategy and Market Development of the American Hospital Association and the American College of Healthcare Executives.

until President Obama signed the ACA into law in early 2010, though the ACA is complex and has numerous provisions. The provisions that are expected to have the most significant impact on the delivery and financing of care are noted in the following list and discussed in the remainder of this chapter.[1]

- *Requirement that almost all individuals have insurance coverage.* This individual mandate lies at the heart of the legislation.

- *Requirement that states create insurance exchanges* where individuals and small businesses can obtain coverage. The ACA contains requirements for an essential benefits package and provides for changes to the tax law that include penalties for individuals who choose not to have insurance.

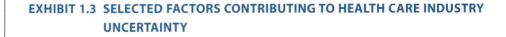

EXHIBIT 1.3 SELECTED FACTORS CONTRIBUTING TO HEALTH CARE INDUSTRY UNCERTAINTY

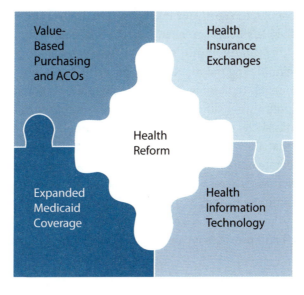

- *Provisions for expansion of Medicaid coverage to all eligible individuals under age sixty-five.* Since adults represent only 25 percent of those covered presently by Medicaid, this will be a significant expansion to include entire families. Federal funds will be made available for the expansion at a decreasing rate, down to 90 percent in 2020. This expansion is a state option and remains controversial as states realize that they will need to be equipped to shoulder the expense as the federal subsidies decrease.

- *Provisions for medical loss ratio and premium rate reviews for health plans.* Rebates will be paid to health plan enrollees by health plans that do not meet a required minimum level of spending on medical care.

- *Establishment of payment mechanisms for bundled payments and a value-based purchasing system* along with the restructuring of certain aspects of the Medicare payment system.

- *Provisions for providers organized as accountable care organizations (ACOs)* to share in cost savings that they achieve for the Medicare program.

Health Insurance Exchanges

Between 2001 and 2010, the number of uninsured rose from 36 million to 50 million people, before decreasing slightly (Exhibit 1.4). This rise is due to several factors, including (1) health insurance and out-of-pocket costs becoming too costly for many individuals, even when they are working; (2) individuals being screened out by insurance underwriters because of *pre-existing conditions*; (3) employers either scaling back employees' benefits or eliminating them altogether by hiring part-time workers; (4) state governments tightening Medicaid eligibility criteria; and (5) individuals voluntarily deciding not to purchase insurance for a variety of financial and nonfinancial reasons, including the assumption that they will not need care or that they will be taken care of by the "system" anyway. As a result, uncompensated care costs have doubled over the past decade (Exhibit 1.5), which has placed a tremendous burden on health care facilities, especially community hospitals.

The ACA authorizes a competitive insurance marketplace at the state level and provides for two types of exchanges, an individual exchange and

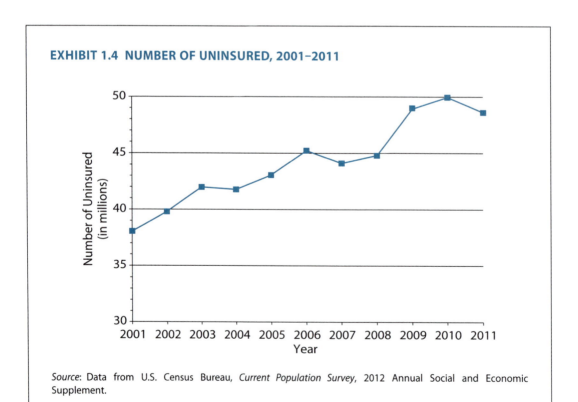

EXHIBIT 1.4 NUMBER OF UNINSURED, 2001–2011

Source: Data from U.S. Census Bureau, *Current Population Survey*, 2012 Annual Social and Economic Supplement.

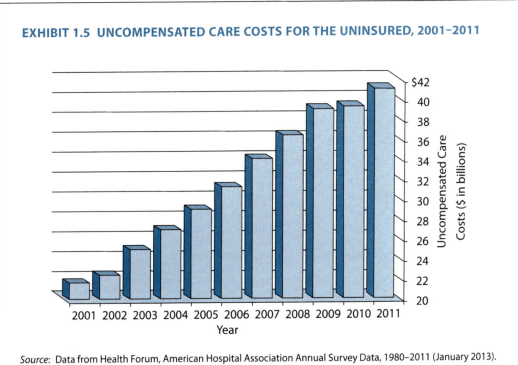

EXHIBIT 1.5 UNCOMPENSATED CARE COSTS FOR THE UNINSURED, 2001–2011

Source: Data from Health Forum, American Hospital Association Annual Survey Data, 1980–2011 (January 2013).

a small business exchange. The individual exchange provides a mechanism for implementing the individual mandate for those who either do not have access to health insurance through an employer plan or who are uninsured for other reasons. The small business exchange provides access for small businesses, enabling them to improve the quality of health insurance for their employees by pooling their buying power and providing multiple health insurance options.

States have the ability to choose whether they want to operate their exchanges themselves. For those that do not want to develop and manage their exchanges, the federal government will do it for them. These exchanges begin operation in 2014.

The ACA provides for a minimum benefits package; however, participants will be able to shop for health insurance from among an array of commercial health insurance products with varying levels of deductibles, coinsurance, and additional benefits over and above the minimum. The benefit packages are referred to as *bronze, silver, gold,* and *platinum,* depending on how much participants choose to pay.

Tax credits are available to low-income consumers, phasing out at 400 percent of the federal poverty level. In addition, consumers will not need to worry about denial of coverage because of any preexisting conditions they may have. The exchanges should promote transparency, to assist the participants in making an informed decision.

The health insurance exchanges, along with other ACA provisions, are expected to make coverage available to 32 million previously uninsured people by 2019. If this works as intended, it should reduce the amount of charity care currently being provided by providers, especially hospitals. However, because the rules providing for a tax penalty for individual non-compliance with the insurance mandate have some exceptions, it is possible that the benefit to providers will not be as effective as originally forecast.

Accountable Care Organizations

An ACO is a voluntary group of health care providers who come together to provide coordinated care to a patient population in order to improve quality and reduce costs by keeping patients healthy and by reducing unnecessary service duplication. This mechanism was initially created to serve Medicare beneficiaries but has now expanded into the non-Medicare population.

Participation is open to networks of primary care doctors, specialists, hospitals, and home health care services in which the network members agree to work together to better coordinate their patients' care. In June 2012, there were 221 ACOs in the United States. The majority were sponsored by hospital systems (118), followed by physician groups (70), insurers (29), and community-based organizations (4), and were located primarily in urban settings with relatively dense populations. By January 2013, there were more than 250 ACOs. As will be more fully discussed in Chapter Thirteen, ACOs are rewarded for reducing the cost of care while maintaining or improving quality under a variety of risk-based or risk-sharing mechanisms now being tested. Although certain medical groups, such as the Permanente Medical Group, Mayo Clinic, Intermountain Health Care, and Geisinger Health System, have shown positive correlations between practice organization and better performance, the ACO mechanism is too new to conclude that it will ultimately show the savings and quality improvements it was designed to achieve.[2]

Patient-Centered Medical Home

A partnership between primary care providers (PCPs), patients, and patients' families to deliver comprehensive care over the long term in a variety of settings.

Patient-Centered Medical Home

The *patient-centered medical home* (PCMH) is a partnership between primary care providers (PCPs), patients, and their families to deliver a coordinated and comprehensive range of services in the most appropriate settings. The PCP takes full responsibility for the overall care of the patient over an extended period of time, including preventive care, acute and chronic care, and end-of-life support. The PCMH is a patient-centered model using evidence-based medicine, care pathways, updated information technology, and voluntary reporting of performance results. In 2011, the National Commission on Quality Assurance created a program that recognizes providers as PCMHs on one of three levels, based on meeting certain administrative standards and achieving a degree of quality reporting. Practices with robust information technology, which includes electronic record keeping, electronic disease registries, internet communication with patients, and electronic prescribing, are the ones most likely to achieve level 3 status.

The PCMH is a good way for a primary care provider to distinguish itself as a quality practice. Until recently there has been little payment advantage associated with being a PCMH; however, programs run by various Blue Cross Blue Shield plans and other insurers are demonstrating that the concept pays off. For example, in late 2012, Horizon Blue Cross Blue Shield of New Jersey identified savings due to reduced emergency department use (26%) and reduced hospital readmissions (26%). At the same time, CMS announced that 500 practices with over 2,000 total physicians will participate in the comprehensive primary care initiative. WellPoint is expanding its program after announcing that it earned $2.50 to $4.50 for every dollar invested in its PMCH program.[3]

Addressing the High Cost of Care

Over the last decade health care costs have increased faster than has general inflation (Exhibit 1.6). The cost to keep people healthy has approximately doubled from 2001 to 2011 (Exhibit 1.7), although the average life expectancy of the general population has risen by only approximately five years since 1980. Even though the increases in the medical inflation rate are higher than those for the Consumer Price Index, the rate of growth has slowed, declining from approximately 5 percent at the turn of the century to 3.5 percent a decade later. However, looking ahead, forecasters are uncertain of what will happen. Certain factors tend to increase costs and others tend to lower them (see Exhibit 1.8).

Factors That Could Contribute to an Increase in Costs

- *The population is continuing to age.* As a person ages, the care he or she requires becomes significantly more costly. By the year 2035, 20

EXHIBIT 1.6 CONSUMER PRICE INDEX VERSUS MEDICAL CARE INFLATION, 2001–2012

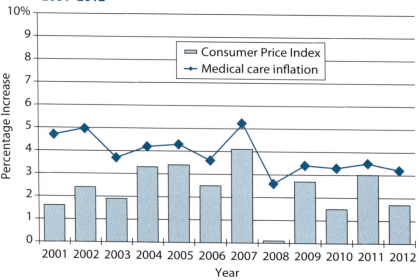

Source: Data from U.S. Labor Department, Bureau of Labor Statistics (January 2013).

EXHIBIT 1.7 ANNUAL HEALTH CARE EXPENDITURES IN THE UNITED STATES, 2001–2011

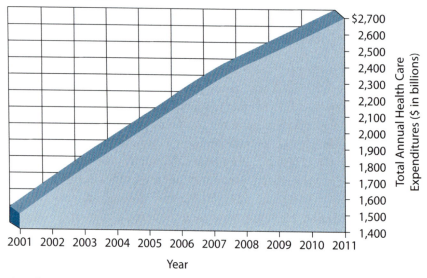

Source: Data from Centers for Medicare and Medicaid Services, Office of the Actuary, 2012.

EXHIBIT 1.8 FACTORS AFFECTING THE COST OF CARE

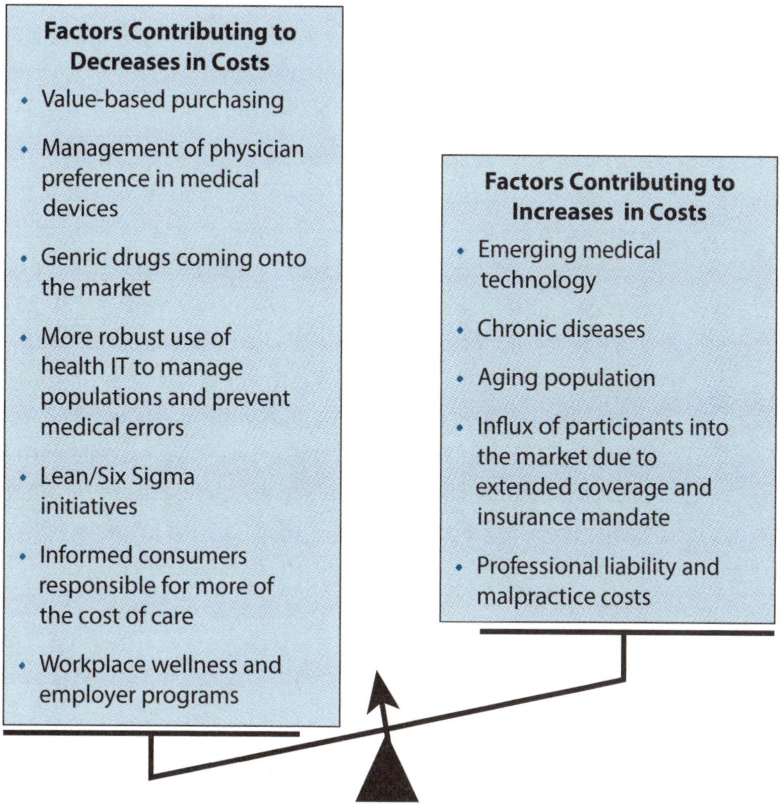

Factors Contributing to Decreases in Costs

- Value-based purchasing

- Management of physician preference in medical devices

- Genric drugs coming onto the market

- More robust use of health IT to manage populations and prevent medical errors

- Lean/Six Sigma initiatives

- Informed consumers responsible for more of the cost of care

- Workplace wellness and employer programs

Factors Contributing to Increases in Costs

- Emerging medical technology

- Chronic diseases

- Aging population

- Influx of participants into the market due to extended coverage and insurance mandate

- Professional liability and malpractice costs

percent of the population is expected to be sixty-five or older. However, research also supports the notion that the many baby boomers are demanding wellness and life enhancement services in order to be able to continue to work into their seventies or eighties, which may help. Nevertheless, as people live longer, their medical issues become more complex and costly.

- *New consumers will enter or reenter the marketplace.* Once fully implemented, the ACA will bring millions of newly insured people into the system. As they obtain services, their needs will likely raise total health care costs. The expectation is that receiving the appropriate care in the appropriate setting at the appropriate time will, in the end, reduce costs.

- *The medical technology industry continues to develop new systems.* Some of these advances, such as the positron-emission tomography (PET) scan, proton beam therapy for prostate cancer, and defibrillator implants, may improve outcomes for some patients, but not all. And more and more hospitals are performing robotic surgery, which may be highly effective. But all this use of advanced technology comes at a high cost.

- *Chronic disease contributes to the high cost of care.* Many chronic conditions, such as heart disease, are associated with the elderly, but long-term issues affect younger populations as well. A 2011 article in *Academic Pediatrics* stated that 43 percent of children have a chronic disease.[4] The top five chronic diseases reported in 2011 for adults were arthritis, cardiovascular disease, diabetes, asthma, and obesity,[5] and the effect and expense of chronic disease are compounded when multiple diseases are present. Chronic disease often requires costly drugs and monitoring over the span of a person's entire life. Higher rates of chronic disease also lead to higher rates of organ failure, and transplants have become one of the most expensive medical procedures. AIDS and mental health issues are also very costly chronic illnesses.

Factors That Could Contribute to a Decrease in Costs

- *Certain behaviors have begun to change, spurred in large part by employers who can no longer afford to pay for employee health care the way they have in the past.* Employers are shifting health care costs to their employees through changes in benefit plan design. Some larger companies offer workplace wellness centers, while others build wellness programs into insurance options that have incentives behind them. For example, to help reduce the cost of medical care associated with employees who smoke, are obese, or who have other unhealthy behaviors, some employers with self-funded health plans have raised the stakes by penalizing them unless they begin a behavior remediation program.

- *Employees faced with paying for a larger portion of their health care costs have become more informed and better consumers.* Consumers are demanding more price transparency and are comparing providers. Some go to alternate sites of care, such as a CVS/pharmacy retail clinic where they can see a nurse practitioner for a fraction of the cost of a traditional physician visit. Some are receiving cost reductions or bonuses to travel overseas where their health plans have negotiated lower rates for procedures that are especially expensive; this has become known as *medical tourism*.

- *Providers are using health information technology (IT) in a more robust way.* Providers are making large capital investments in technology to better understand costs, improve quality, reduce medical errors, and provide the information needed to participate in value-based purchasing initiatives. Both insurers and providers are working, oftentimes together, toward increased connectivity. Many are making use of population and disease management techniques to provide the appropriate level of care and enhance quality, which should continue to lower cost.

- *Pharmaceuticals are going off patent, creating opportunities for cost savings with generic drugs.*

- *Providers are embracing lean, Six Sigma and other techniques so that they can deliver better quality care with fewer resources.* The effects of these initiatives can be to streamline operational processes. For example, a project to improve the discharge process could result in freeing up beds to be used by other patients, thereby enhancing revenue. Other initiatives aimed at reducing medical errors and improving quality could also pay additional dividends on the reimbursement side of the equation.

- *Hospitals are overriding physician preferences in medical supplies.* Because medical supplies can amount to 40 percent of the cost of a procedure, the ability to achieve economies of scale by bulk purchases can have a significant impact on hospital costs. Many hospitals use the services of a group purchasing organization.

Information Technology

For the last several years providers have made significant investments in information technology, and perhaps the largest investment of time and resources in this area is the *electronic health record* (EHR). The HITECH Act (2009) was enacted with the goal of creating and expanding the current health care IT infrastructure, promoting electronic data exchange, and substantially and rapidly increasing EHR adoption to 90 percent for physicians and 70 percent for hospitals by 2019. The provisions of the act are intended to increase efficiency and reduce medical errors, at an expected savings to the government of billions of dollars. In addition, the HITECH Act substantially expanded HIPAA (Health Insurance Portability and Accountability Act of 1996) privacy and security rules and increased the penalties for HIPAA violations.

Medical Tourism
Travel to a foreign country to obtain normally expensive medical services at a steep discount. Even with a family member escorting the patient (and getting the added benefit of foreign travel), the total cost is typically less than it would be at home.

Electronic Health Record (EHR)
Also called an *electronic medical record* (EMR), this online version of patients' medical records can include patient demographics, insurance information, dictations and notes, medication and immunization histories, ancillary test results, and the like. Under strict security permissions, the information can be accessed either in-house or in private office settings.

Health Insurance Portability and Accountability Act (HIPAA)
A set of federal compliance regulations enacted in 1996 to ensure standardization of billing, privacy, and reporting practices as institutions convert to electronic systems.

The HITECH Act provides incentives for providers (hospitals, physicians, and other eligible providers) to achieve *meaningful use*. *Meaningful users* are those able to demonstrate that their EHR technology has been implemented in a manner that improves the quality of the health care they provide. This meaningful use includes, for example, e-prescribing, electronic exchange of health information, and submission of quality measures to CMS.

For achieving meaningful use, hospitals can receive up to $2 million, plus additional amounts calculated in accordance with each hospital's Medicare discharges. Medicaid permits up to six years of incentive payments. To achieve these incentives, a hospital must increase its use of comprehensive EHR systems from 10 percent to 55 percent by 2014.

Eligible physicians (a category that excludes physicians who are hospital based or in hospital-owned practices) and other eligible providers can receive incentive payments ranging up to $44,000 over five years under Medicare, or $63,750 over six years under Medicaid. Incentive payments are gradually reduced each year, ceasing in 2016.

Meaningful use is achieved in three stages. Stage 1 should have been achieved by 2012. Through July 2012, approximately 117,000 eligible professionals and 3,600 hospitals received some sort of incentive payment.

The stage 2 final rule, issued in 2012, requires hospitals, physicians, and other eligible providers to continue to increase interoperability among disparate forms of data, increase standardization of electronic formats, and demonstrate that they are relying on the EHR to improve patient care.

Stage 2 begins in 2014, and Medicare will impose penalties for not achieving meaningful use by 2015. A third and final stage of meaningful use is scheduled to begin in 2016.

Cost-Accounting Systems

Many hospital accounting systems have a strong billing and collections component but a weak cost-accounting system. This is due in large part to the fact that, historically, financial incentives were typically put in place to maximize reimbursement, not to control costs. Now that the environment has changed, providers have found it increasingly important to understand their costs at a more granular level. As a result there has been a major movement to separate cost-accounting systems from financial accounting systems and to move away from traditional allocation-based cost systems to activity-based cost systems (discussed in more depth in Chapter Twelve). Although this is an expensive endeavor, declining reimbursement is forcing hospitals to invest in more sophisticated cost-accounting systems.

Group Purchasing Organizations

With the rapid advances in computer hardware and software applications, many institutions have invested in information technologies in an effort to receive the most accurate information as quickly as possible. Most applications revolve around materials management, budgeting, accounts payable, payroll, patient registration, and human resource needs. An organization must track the flow of materials through its system and purchase supplies in the most cost-effective manner. Hospitals can keep funds longer and reduce inventory costs by incorporating *just-in-time* ordering techniques, and opportunity exists for cost savings by joining *group purchasing organizations* (GPOs) that can negotiate cost discounts through large volumes (discussed in more detail in Chapter Ten). When organizations can more accurately follow the flow of materials through the organization, they can better track costs and have better reporting and control over their budgets.

Reengineering or Redesigning

Health care organizations have been redesigning their work processes in order to achieve efficiencies and reduce cost. Common techniques include process analysis, layout redesign, work redesign, total quality management and care mapping, and layoffs of unnecessary personnel.

One such method that has gained widespread attention is Six Sigma, including the related concept of *lean thinking*, which offers a systematic approach to analysis and performance improvement. The five major components of the Six Sigma approach are define, measure, analyze, improve, and control (nicknamed DMAIC). Lean thinking breaks processes down into identifiable steps to ensure that each component is a value-added activity. A main tenet of lean thinking and Six Sigma is to reduce the variation in how activities are conducted, an important step toward quality improvement.

Mergers and Acquisitions

Mergers and acquisitions among health care organizations have increased significantly in response to health reform and especially since the passage of the ACA and the Health Care and Education Reconciliation Act of 2010. According to Levin Associates, there were 453 mergers and acquisitions in 2010, and Fierce Health Finance reported nearly 1,000 in 2011.[6] Health insurers and private equity firms are responsible for many of them.

From an accounting perspective, a *merger* requires that neither of the parties coming together has control. The two (or more) entities merge to start an entirely new entity with no step-up in basis of the assets. The new entity comes into being on the date of the merger. In an *acquisition*, there is a controlling party, and the assets and liabilities are marked to fair value. Acquisitions are more common than mergers in the health care industry. Health care systems are consolidating to be larger players in the market in order to

- Spread fixed technology and administrative costs over a larger revenue base.

- Strengthen market penetration.

- Gain better access to capital.

- Add new service lines.

- Obtain better contracts from commercial payors.

According to *Becker's Hospital Review*, although health systems acquire other health systems, transactions also exist whereby smaller community hospitals are acquired by larger systems. In addition, currently the biggest area of acquisition for community hospitals is in physician groups (see Perspective 1.2); such acquisitions were up 200 percent in 2011.[7]

Retail Health Care

Doctors' offices and hospitals are no longer the only settings where health care services are being provided. Given the tendency of consumers to use shopping malls, various retail outlets such as CVS/pharmacy and Walmart, which had already been providing pharmacy services for years, have expanded by offering basic preventive health care services in some of their stores. These *retail health care* outlets hire licensed professionals, such as nurse practitioners, to offer flu shots and provide remedies for minor ailments like a sore throat or the common cold. These sites of care are popular among the uninsured, students, and those who are simply in a hurry. The retailers also reap additional benefits by providing patients with convenient in-store purchase options for medications.

Retail Health Care
Walk-in medical services for basic preventive health care provided in a retail outlet, such as a pharmacy, by a licensed care provider.

Litigation

Unfortunately, the ACA falls short when it comes to *malpractice reform*. The legislation addresses medical liability in two ways:

PERSPECTIVE 1.2 LIFE IN THE "GAP"

In discussing accountable care organizations, economic futurist Ian Morrison refers to a hospital's "life in the gap." The "gap" is the period of time during which payments are still being made largely on a fee-for-service basis but health care organizations are being pressured to lower costs and improve quality. The question is how to prepare. Some hospitals and health systems have become pioneer accountable care organizations, while others have developed programs with commercial payors such as Cigna. Many are acquiring other health care organizations to become larger or are focusing on building relationships with physicians and community organizations.

Greater Baltimore Medical Center formed an ACO, the Greater Baltimore Health Alliance, which sought approval for Medicare's Shared Savings Program. It is the only ACO in Maryland with a hospital component and is working to increase the number of primary care access points it has in Maryland. The risk is that it may drive down utilization of services and then not be paid adequately for doing it.

The preparation for the future could involve a number of moves:

1. Drive out waste.

2. Implement new payment models, such as participating in CMS pilots like Pioneer ACOs or with insurers.

3. Collaborate with other health care providers such as physician practices, ambulatory centers, and rehab facilities. This will help when the organization later may need to be responsible for the continuum of care.

4. Partner with past competitors to combine resources, find creative ways to gain better operational effectiveness, and negotiate with payors.

5. Invest in primary care. By improving coordination of care with primary care practices and integrated health information systems, hospitals may be able to reduce unnecessary readmissions and utilization.

6. Develop health data analytics to assist in decision making. Hospitals can develop better ways to measure, track, analyze, and apply data to patient care.

7. Establish employee health programs, which may be a springboard toward beginning to prepare for population management, and which carry less risk. Hospitals can lower insurance costs for employees who perform certain wellness activities, such as going to a wellness center or having a nutrition consultation.

8. Begin a cultural revolution. The challenge is to develop a focus on the whole patient and wellness rather than on a single episode of care and sickness. This is a cultural shift as well as a financial one.

Source: Adapted from S. Rodak, Managing the transition to value-based reimbursement: 8 core strategies to mind the gap, *Becker's Hospital Review*, October 2, 2012, accessed November 25, 2012, from www .beckershospitalreview.com/strategic-planning/managing-the-transition-to-value-based-reimbursement-8 -core-strategies-to-mind-the-gap.html.

- Extension of federal malpractice protections to nonmedical personnel working in free clinics.

- Authorization of $50 million over five years for HHS to award demonstration project grants. These grants would be provided to states to develop, implement, institute, and evaluate alternatives to the present system used in the United States to resolve charges against physicians and other health care providers of wrongdoing to patients.

As the health care system moves closer to the practice of evidence-based medicine, certain demonstration projects could help to reduce health care errors by encouraging the collection and analysis of data on patient safety. But many believe that evidence-based medicine is not likely to do much.

Compliance

The process of abiding by governmental regulations, whether in the provision of care, billing, privacy, accounting standards, security, or any other regulated area.

Compliance

Providers spend a significant amount of time and expense on processes needed to comply with governmental regulations in such areas as the provision of care, billing, privacy, security, accounting standards, and the like. Examples of compliance requirements are

- HIPAA, the Health Insurance Portability and Accountability Act

- Health and safety regulations

- EMTALA, the Emergency Medical Treatment and Active Labor Act, also known as the patient anti-dumping law

- Billing, coding, and other standards designed to eliminate the following: charging for items or services not provided, providing medically unnecessary treatment, upcoding, diagnosis related group (DRG) creep, improperly providing outpatient services in connection with inpatient stays (in violation of the seventy-two-hour window rule), failure to follow teaching physician and resident requirements for teaching hospitals, duplicate billing, false cost reports, billing for discharge in lieu of transfer, failure to refund credit balances, providing hospital incentives that violate the anti-kickback statute, improper financial arrangements between hospitals and hospital-based physicians, and violations of the Stark physician self-referral law.

Recovery Audit Contractor (RAC) Program

A program created under the Medicare Modernization Act of 2003 to identify and recover improper Medicare payments to health care providers.

- Billing standards such as the move to ICD-10 (deferred to 2014), as discussed later in this chapter.

Recovery Audit Contractors

For over a decade now, significant media and public attention has been focused on the hospital industry due to ongoing investigations related to referrals. CMS's recovery audit contractor (RAC) program is designed to reduce overpayments (and underpayments) by addressing the root cause of provider billing errors. This program, which became permanent under the Tax Relief and Health Care Act of 2006, has been rolled out to all hospitals and to other targeted providers as well. In 2010, the RAC program was extended to Medicaid through the ACA.

RAC auditors are independent contractors hired by CMS to focus primarily on clinical documentation supporting billings under the Medicare program. They use proprietary software and systems in order to determine what areas to review, but they cannot simply randomly select claims or focus just on high-dollar claims. Instead, the purpose is to identify improper payments related to incorrect amounts, noncovered services (including services that may not be reasonable or necessary), incorrectly coded services, and duplicate services.

There are two types of reviews: automated and complex. The automated review requires no medical records. The complex review ensues when the automated review provides evidence of a high likelihood that the service received improper payment or that there is no Medicare policy, Medicare article, or Medicare-sanctioned coding guideline for the service provided. The RACs use medical literature and apply clinical judgment to make claims determinations, and a RAC can go on site to view or copy the medical records or request that the provider do so. When a RAC identifies an overpayment, it provides written notification requesting repayment in full. Providers can appeal within thirty days of the demand letter.

RACs are paid on a contingency basis: the more they find, the more they collect. As a result the provider community has had difficulties with the concept since the inception of the program, believing that RACs tend to focus on claims and services most likely to result in error to enhance their chances of payment.

Provider concern over the RACs has led to a significant increase for providers in personnel time, consulting fees, and new technologies to "scrub" claims prior to submission, not to mention the time it takes to research and defend claims identified by the RACs. The American Hospital Association believes that hospitals are experiencing a significant number of inappropriate denials, which has resulted in hundreds of unfair recoupment payments, with approximately 75 percent of the RACs' assessments being overturned by Medicare. Unfairly requested payments are returned to the hospitals.

The Medicare Audit Improvement Act of 2012 was designed to promote transparency and fairness in RAC reviews, and if passed, it would establish a penalty for a RAC's failure to follow the program requirements. It would also, among other things:

- Establish a consolidated limit for medical record requests.
- Require medical necessity audits to focus on widespread payment errors.
- Allow denied inpatient claims to be billed as outpatient claims when appropriate.
- Require physician review for Medicare denials.

Value-Based Payment Mechanisms

The introduction of Medicare and Medicaid in 1965 was in large part intended to guarantee health care coverage to the country's most vulnerable populations: the poor and the elderly. Unfortunately, many officials at the time failed to recognize that these "Great Society" programs would become the impetus for health care costs rising far beyond any costs ever predicted. The role of the federal government in health care has changed from being a small participant before the mid-1960s to being a major force in both setting amounts of payment and defining payment systems. Since that time numerous payment mechanisms have been used to compensate providers for services to patients. As more fully discussed in Chapter Thirteen, fee-for-service, flat fee, cost-based, and capitation reimbursement methodologies have been used for years by governmental and private payors, with varying degrees of success (see Exhibit 1.9).

EXHIBIT 1.9 PAYMENT SYSTEMS INTRODUCED BY MEDICARE SINCE THE 1960s

1960s	1980s–1990s
Fee-for-service (FFS) and cost-based reimbursement	Prospective payment (DRGs) Capitation and global payments
2000s	**2013**
Ambulatory payment classifications (APCs) and pay for performance (P4P) Pay for reporting (P4R)	Value-based payment Accountable care organizations Shared savings programs

Movement to a New DRG System

In 2008, CMS changed the way it paid hospitals. The new system, based on Medicare severity-adjusted diagnosis related groups (MS-DRGs), has 25 major disease categories, 745 diagnosis related groups, and 3 subclasses of complications and comorbidities. It is intended to more closely align reimbursement to patient severity of illness, which means that certain hospitals will earn more but many will earn less.

The purpose of the Deficit Reduction Act of 2005 was to reduce overall hospital costs by improving care, thus combining quality and cost control and improving equity. Under this act and in response to rising health care costs and knowing that the aging population would be consuming more health care services in the coming years, CMS began piloting new forms of reimbursement in 2005 with the objective of obtaining better quality care for patients at a lower cost. The value-based purchasing system was initially rolled out to hospitals for their inpatient services in demonstration projects, under the expectation that some sort of value-based system would improve quality and reduce costs. In this demonstration phase, the mechanisms being tried were referred to as *pay for performance*, or P4P.

Establishing Value-Based Purchasing

As more fully discussed in Chapter Thirteen, the ACA of 2010 established the inpatient Hospital Value-Based Purchasing Program, which became effective for discharges in late 2012. MS-DRGs form the basis of payments for this system, and providers are still reimbursed on this basis. However, the reimbursement is reduced in order to provide a pool of money to be used for value-based incentive payments.

The ACA requires that the total amount of value-based incentive payments available for distribution be equal to the total base operating DRG payments reduction, making this change budget neutral. Base operating payments represent payments for the health care services rendered. Hospitals also receive capital payments, which are not a part of this incentive calculation. The first incentive payments were based on hospital performance from mid-2011 to early 2012.

For high-performing hospitals, preparation for the new system has been expensive and challenging. Smaller hospitals oftentimes have found it next to impossible, forcing many of them into acquisitions by larger systems.

The federal government, of course, is not the only payor for hospital services, but its policies and reimbursement mechanisms for services

Value-Based Purchasing (VBP)
A payment methodology designed to provide incentives to providers for delivering quality health care at a lower cost. The financial rewards come from funds being withheld by the payor; these funds are then redistributed on providers' achievement of and improvement on specific performance measures, including patient satisfaction.

Shared Savings
A payment strategy that offers incentives for providers to reduce health care spending for a defined patient population; these incentives are a percentage of the net savings realized as a result of provider efforts.

Prospective Payment System (PPS)
The payment system used by Medicare to reimburse providers a predetermined amount. Several payment methods fall under the PPS umbrella,, including methods based on DRGs (for inpatient admissions), APCs (for outpatient visits), a resource-based relative value scale (RBRVS) (for professional services), and resource utilization groups (RUGs) (for skilled nursing home care). Use of DRGs was the first method that fell under this type of predetermined payment arrangement.

greatly influence the practices of other payors, including state governments and major insurance companies.

Although the initial push in value-based purchasing was toward inpatient services, demonstration projects and data collection have already started and will continue to be rolled out for other hospital services as well, and eventually to other providers over time. Additional VBP initiatives are being conducted in hospitals for services other than inpatient services and in physicians' offices, nursing homes, home health organizations, and dialysis facilities.

Even critical access hospitals that presently receive cost-based reimbursement, and other hospitals that are excluded from value-based purchasing owing to their low number of measures and cases, could at some point be subject to this legislation, given that demonstration projects, a precursor to implementation for these institutions, are already underway.

ICD-10

The World Health Organization's International Statistical Classification of Diseases and Related Health Problems (ICD) is a coding system for diseases that is used in the United States for health insurance claim reimbursement. Currently the United States uses the ninth version of the codes, which was developed in the 1970s. However, the ninth version has constraints in terms of structure and space limitations that hamper its ability to accommodate advances in medical knowledge and technology.

The tenth version, ICD-10, addresses these issues and also assists in morbidity and mortality data reporting, another important facet of what these codes were designed to do. The fact that the United States still uses ICD-9 while other countries are already using the more advanced version is also making it difficult to compare U.S. health information with information from other countries.

The final rule adopting ICD-10 as the U.S. standard was published in January 2009, with an original compliance date set for October 2013. This date was then pushed back by a full year because the government was concerned about the administrative burdens placed on providers in the midst of all of the other regulatory changes; however, health insurers, large hospitals, and large medical practices appear to have the majority of their planning complete. The American Health Information Management Association (AHIMA) has noted that the cost to the industry related to the delay is likely to be between $1 billion and $6.6 billion.[8] Nevertheless, there should also be some savings since earlier implementation could have resulted in health care providers and health plans having to process health care claims manually in order to be paid. In addition, small health care providers might have had to take out loans or apply for lines of credit in order to continue to provide health care in the face of delayed payments.

Once this standard is effective, entities covered under the Health Insurance Portability and Accountability Act of 1996 (HIPAA) will be required to use the ICD-10 diagnostic and procedure codes.

Key Point Pay for reporting is a precursor to value-based purchasing. Before the beginning of VBP, Medicare's Reporting Hospital Quality Data for Annual Payment Update (RHQDAPU) program, which is a pay-for-reporting (P4R) program, provided an incentive for hospitals to report on the care they provide to all adults, regardless of payor. Originally, hospitals reported on ten clinical performance measures to avoid a reduction in the Medicare annual payment update for inpatient services. In 2007, hospitals were required to report on twenty-one measures in order to receive their full payment update, or else face a penalty of 2 percent for failing to do so.

Summary

The health care administrator today and in the future will be faced with numerous complex issues to consider when making strategic and financial decisions. This is an exciting time to be in the health care field, and providers appear to be embracing a new business model. High-performing organizations will evaluate the possibilities of doing business a different way, focusing on populations instead of individuals, rightsizing the costs of the organization, focusing the necessary resources on the implementation of technology to ensure interoperability, and using data to manage costs and care. Through it all, the administrator must constantly maintain a high ethical standard in all decisions, not only for the obvious health and financial impacts but also for the myriad personal, professional, community, and societal implications.

The remainder of this book focuses on essential health care financial management topics such as how to analyze financial statements, manage internal funds, make sound business investments, borrow funds, analyze costs, and prepare a budget. It also provides in-depth analyses of the ways in which regulations and restrictions affect the operation of health care institutions. Although this knowledge is essential in the financial decision-making process, health care administrators always need to carefully weigh nonfinancial factors as well.

KEY TERMS

a. Accountable care organization (ACO)

b. Capitation

c. Care mapping

d. Compliance

e. Electronic health record (EHR)

f. Evidence-based medicine

g. Group purchasing organization (GPO)

h. Health insurance exchange

i. Health Insurance Portability and Accountability Act (HIPAA)

j. ICD-10

k. Malpractice reform

l. Medical tourism

m. Medicare severity-adjusted diagnosis related groups (MS-DRGs)

n. Patient-centered medical home

o. Patient Protection and Affordable Care Act (ACA)

p. Pay for performance (P4P)

q. Pay for reporting (P4R)

r. Prospective payment system (PPS)

s. Recovery audit contractor (RAC) program

t. Retail health care

u. Shared savings

v. Value-based purchasing (VBP)

REVIEW QUESTIONS

1. **Definitions**. Define the terms listed in the key terms list.

2. **Increased costs**. What are several factors that have led to increased health care costs?

3. **Cost control**. What are several of the efforts that have been attempted by payors to control costs?

4. **Malpractice reform**. What specific impacts will the provisions of the ACA have on malpractice reform?

5. **Information technology**. What is the trend of information technology usage in health care, and what effects are likely from that trend?

6. **Mergers and acquisitions**. What advantages do health care organizations seek to obtain by merging with each other or by acquiring or being acquired by another health care organization?

7. **Process techniques**. What are two or more techniques that health care organizations can implement to increase operational efficiency?

8. **Overall costs.** Which two factors may have the strongest tendency to increase health care costs? Which two may particularly decrease those costs? Why?

9. **The "gap."** Describe the "gap" that health care organizations are facing. What unique problems does it present? And what benefits?

Notes

1. The full text of the ACA can be found at www.kaiserhealthnews.org/final-health-reform-bill-patient-protection-and-affordable-care-act.aspx (last accessed June 9, 2013).

2. J. J. Crosson and L.A. Tollen, eds., *Partners in Heath: How Physicians and Hospitals Can Be Accountable Together* (San Francisco: Jossey-Bass, 2010).

3. R. S. Raskas, L. M. Latts, J. R. Hummel, D. Wenners, H. Levine, and S. R. Nussbaum, Early results show WellPoint's patient-centered medical home pilots have met some goals for costs, utilization, and quality, *Health Affairs*, 2012;31(9):2002–2009, doi: 10.1377/hlthaff.2012.0364.

4. C. D. Bethell, M. D. Kogan, B. B. Strickland, E. L. Schor, J. Robertson, and P. W. Newacheck, A national and state profile of leading health problems and health care quality for US children: key insurance disparities and across-state variations, *Academic Pediatrics*, 2011;11(3 Suppl):S22–33.

5. H.-Y. Chen, D. J. Baumgardner, and J. P. Rice, Health-related quality of life among adults with multiple chronic conditions in the United States, Behavioral Risk Factor Surveillance System, 2007, *Preventing Chronic Disease*, 2011; 8(1):A09, retrieved November 24, 2012, from www.cdc.gov/pcd/issues/2011/jan/09_0234.htm

6. Irving Levin Associates, Inc., Health care M&A accelerates in second quarter after passage of reform according to new report by Irving Levin Associates, Inc. (Press release), July 28, 2010, retrieved August 6, 2013, from www.levinassociates.com/pr2010/pr1007mamq2; R. Shinkman, Healthcare M&A finishes healthy in 2011, *FierceHealthFinance*, January 17, 2012, retrieved August 6, 2013, from www.fiercehealthfinance.com/story/healthcare-ma-finishes-healthy-2011/2012-01-17

7. 10 biggest hospital stories of 2011, *Becker's Hospital Review*, November/December 2011, retrieved August 6, 2013, from www.becker'shospitalreview.com/pdfs/hospital-review/Nov_Dec_2011_HR.pdf

8. C. Dimick, HHS announces ICD-10 delayed one year, *Journal of AHIMA*, August 24, 2012, retrieved August 6, 2013 from journal.ahima.org/2012/08/24/hhs-announces-icd-10-delayed-one-year

CHAPTER 2

HEALTH CARE FINANCIAL STATEMENTS

C reditors, investors, and governmental and community agencies often require considerable information
to make judgments about the financial performance of
health care entities. For instance, to decide whether to
lend money to an investor-owned[1] home health agency,
a lender may want to know how much debt the entity
already has, how much cash it has available, and how
much profit it is earning. Similarly, to make regulatory
decisions, a governmental agency may want to know how
much charity or uncompensated care is being provided or
what the profit margin is for a group of providers. It is
also important for creditors, investors, or grantors to be
able to make comparisons between health care entities.
For this reason generally accepted accounting principles,
whether promulgated by the Financial Accounting Standards Board (FASB) for commercial or not-for-profit
entities or by the Governmental Accounting Standards
Board (GASB) for governments, prescribe a standard set
of basic financial statements. Often these basic statements
are supplemented by additional statements and schedules.
Due to space constraints, this chapter discusses primarily
the statements and the health care–specific reporting
requirements set forth by the FASB. The basic financial
statements are shown in Exhibit 2.1.

The term *basic financial statement* applies to each of
the statements in Exhibit 2.1 *as well as* the notes to these
statements. The notes to the financial statements include
information about all the statements provided and explain
in more detail the significant elements. These notes are
placed after all the statements. GAAP requires certain
disclosure (footnote) information to be presented to give
readers of the financial statements a much clearer picture

LEARNING OBJECTIVES

- Identify the basic financial
  statements for investor-owned
  health care entities and not-for-
  profit entities.

- Identify and read the basic financial
  statements particular to not-for-
  profit, business-oriented health care
  entities: the balance sheet, the
  statement of operations, the
  statement of changes in net assets,
  and the statement of cash flows.

EXHIBIT 2.1 A COMPARISON OF FINANCIAL STATEMENTS FOR INVESTOR-OWNED AND NOT-FOR-PROFIT HEALTH CARE ENTITIES

Financial Statements Used by Investor-Owned Health Care Entities	Financial Statements Used by Not-for-Profit Health Care Entities
Balance sheet	Balance sheet
Statement of income and comprehensive income (combined statement) or two separate statements: a statement of income and a statement of comprehensive income	Statement of operations[a]
Statement of changes in stockholders' equity	Statement of changes in net assets[a]
Statement of cash flows	Statement of cash flows
Notes (footnotes) to the financial statements	Notes (footnotes) to the financial statements

[a]These are often combined, but since the combined statement is so large, it is often shown on two pages.

than they would have otherwise of the financial position and results of operations of the entity. Financial statements of health care entities are often audited due to financing or regulatory requirements, and it is the auditor's responsibility to evaluate the presentation of both the statements and the note disclosures. In this way similar entities can be compared, and users of the financial statements can make more informed decisions.

As shown in Perspectives 2.1 and 2.2, organizations' financial statements are of interest not only internally but also externally, to the outside parties that either invest in the organizations or fund them. Because health care entities can be investor-owned, not-for-profit, or governmental, the formats of their statements vary slightly, depending on the accounting principles particular to each business model. Nevertheless, because organizations often compete for the same funding, these formats are relatively consistent. The focus of this text is primarily not-for-profit, business-oriented health care entities, which are referred to hereafter as *not-for-profit health care entities.*

The Balance Sheet

The balance sheet of investor-owned entities presents a summary of the entity's *assets, liabilities,* and *stockholders' equity.* (Note that stockholders'

PERSPECTIVE 2.1 S&P: 2013 WILL TEST NOT-FOR-PROFIT HOSPITALS: HOSPITAL RATINGS WILL REMAIN STEADY THIS YEAR, AGENCY PREDICTS

Standard & Poor's Ratings Services (S&P) anticipates that its ratings for most U.S. not-for-profit health care providers will remain steady in 2013. This is, in part, due to a cushion that many of them have built over the last several years. S&P, however, expects credit quality trends in 2013 to be less favorable because of pressures that entities will face in 2013:

- Sequestration cuts and other Medicare cuts negotiated later this year
- Increased Affordable Care Act preparation
- Soft utilization trends
- New incentives and penalties for failing to meet value-based purchasing standards

Hospital management has been responsive to changes in the industry that have enabled hospitals to maintain positive credit rating metrics for the past two years even though pressures have been mounting. But 2013 will bring even more pressures, and hospitals are turning their strategic and operating priorities to health reform preparations.

Source: Adapted from The Advisory Board Company, S&P: 2013 will test not-for-profit hospitals, Daily Briefing, January 08, 2013, www.advisory.com/Daily-Briefing/2013/01/08/S-P-2013-will-test-not-for-profit-hospitals.

PERSPECTIVE 2.2 IRS TARGETS TAX-EXEMPT HOSPITALS: BOND INITIATIVES AND SCRUTINY OF COMMUNITY BENEFITS

The IRS has plans to begin an examination of tax-exempt bonds, including the hospital market this year, according to Bob Griffo, supervisory tax law specialist with the Internal Revenue Service (IRS), who spoke at an American Health Lawyers Association conference in January 2013. During the first year of the program, the IRS plans to examine between 20 to 40 tax-exempt hospitals. After that it will target 100 section 501(c)(3) tax-exempt entities outside the hospital industry. This announcement comes at a time when there have been increases in the number of examinations conducted by the IRS's Tax-Exempt Bond (TEB) Division as well as an increase in municipal bond disclosures from the Securities and Exchange Commission (SEC).

The IRS's TEB Division has found significant noncompliance in more than 30 percent of the bond issues it has examined since 2005, resulting in assessments to the entities involved from an average of approximately $873,000 in 2006 to in excess of $359,000 in 2010. The IRS is also launching an initiative to get entities to self-report violations and institute stronger internal controls to monitor compliance. To encourage self-monitoring by the borrowers, the IRS is sending out questionnaires to many issuers and asking whether they have adopted policies and procedures to ensure compliance with the tax-exempt bond rules. If an issuer provides answers that do not produce evidence that shows that steps have been taken to monitor compliance, then the IRS will use this to justify a full audit.

In addition, the IRS representative stated that the service will review the community benefit activities of 3,377 tax-exempt hospitals. The purpose of the review is to determine if they meet the requirements for tax exemption. The Affordable Care Act requires the IRS to review the community benefit activity of every hospital at least once every three years. The IRS will look at the hospital's Form 990 and Schedule H. These reviews are "stealth reviews," as hospitals will not be advised that they are under review and they will not know when these reviews begin or end.

These initiatives are likely cause for concern for the boards and management of tax-exempt and governmental hospitals, especially those with bond financing.

Source: Adapted from D. K. Anning, V. C. Gross, L. K. Mack, and T. J. Schenkelberg, IRS targeting 3,377 hospitals for community benefit review, November 13, 2012, www.jdsupra.com/legalnews/irs-targeting-3377-hospitals -for-commun-01576.

equity is also called *shareholders' equity*. In this text we will use the term *stockholders' equity*.) Similarly, the balance sheet of a not-for-profit health care entity presents a summary of the entity's assets, liabilities, and net assets (see Exhibit 2.2). (These terms and the relationship among them will be discussed in more detail shortly.) The balance sheet is similar to a snapshot of the entity, for it captures what the entity looks like *as of a particular point in time*, usually the last day of the accounting period (e.g., quarter or fiscal year). Exhibit 2.3 presents an illustration of a balance sheet and serves as an overview of this section of the chapter.

As shown in Exhibit 2.3, the balance sheet, like each of the other basic statements, contains a heading and then the body of the statement. The heading includes the name of the entity and the date (or point in time) of the balance sheet. The *entity name* is important because it provides the reader with the name of the specific entity (or group of entities) that is the subject matter of the statement. This is not as trivial as it might seem. A health care entity may produce financial statements that include information for more than one entity, depending on the degree of ownership, control, or economic interest or any combination of these circumstances. For example, a hospital may issue its own financial statements and also may have its financial data included with a parent's data. When information for more than one entity is being summarized, then the report is called

EXHIBIT 2.2 OVERVIEW OF MAIN BALANCE SHEET SECTIONS FOR INVESTOR-OWNED AND NOT-FOR-PROFIT HEALTH CARE ENTITIES AND RELATED NOTES

Heading	**Name of Investor-Owned Entity** **Balance Sheet** **Dates**	**Name of Not-for-Profit Entity** **Balance Sheet** **Dates**

Body	Assets
	    Current assets
	    Noncurrent assets
	 Total assets
	 Liabilities
	    Current liabilities
	    Noncurrent liabilities
	 Total liabilities
	 Stockholders' equity[a]
	    Common stock
	    Retained earnings
	
	 Total stockholders' equity
	 Total liabilities and stockholders' equity
		Assets
		    Current assets
		    Noncurrent assets
		 Total assets
		 Liabilities
		    Current liabilities
		    Noncurrent liabilities
		 Total liabilities
		 Net assets[a]
		    Unrestricted
		    Temporarily restricted
		    Permanently restricted
		 Total net assets
		 Total liabilities and net assets

Notes	Key pertinent information including • Accounting policies • Payment arrangements with third parties • Asset restrictions • Property and equipment • Long-term debt • Pension obligations	Key pertinent information including • Accounting policies • Payment arrangements with third parties • Asset restrictions • Property and equipment • Long-term debt • Pension obligations

[a]A major difference between the balance sheet of an investor-owned entity and a not-for-profit health care entity is in the owners' equity section. For an investor-owned organization, the section is organized to show the stockholders' ownership stake in the corporation. For a not-for-profit health care entity, the section is called *net assets* and is organized to show that a not-for-profit entity is not "owned" by any person. The net asset classes show the degree of donor restriction on the net assets.

EXHIBIT 2.3 ANNOTATED BALANCE SHEET FOR SAMPLE NOT-FOR-PROFIT HOSPITAL

The balance sheet provides a snapshot of the organization's assets, liabilities, and net assets at a particular point in time.

1 **Title.** The name of the organization, the name of the financial statement, and the date for which information is being provided.

2 **Assets.** The probable future economic benefits obtained or controlled by a particular entity as a result of past transactions or events. In many instances assets represent resources that the entity owns. Assets are recorded at their cost, unless donated. In the latter cases they are recorded at fair value at the date of donation.

3 **Current assets.** Assets that will be used or consumed within one year.

4 **Assets limited or restricted as to use, noncurrent portion.** Assets with limitations or restrictions (set by donors, funding sources, or the board) as to how they can be used.

5 **Noncurrent assets.** The resources of the entity that will be used or consumed over periods longer than one year.

6 **Liabilities.** The probable future sacrifices of economic benefits arising from present obligations of the entity to transfer assets or provide services to other entities in the future as a result of past transactions or events. Liabilities can be debts or other obligations; e.g., deferred revenue, which is an obligation to provide or deliver goods or services when payment has been received in advance.

7 **Current liabilities.** Financial obligations due within one year.

8 **Noncurrent liabilities.** The resources of the entity that will be used or consumed over periods longer than one year.

9 **Net assets (or equity).** The assets of an entity that remain after deducting its liabilities (also called *residual interest*). In a business enterprise the equity is the ownership interest. In a not-for-profit organization, which has no ownership interest, net assets is divided into three classes based on the presence or absence of donor-imposed restrictions—permanently restricted, temporarily restricted, and unrestricted net assets.

Dunhill Health System
Consolidated Balance Sheet
June 30, 2012
(in thousands)

Assets	
Current assets	
Cash and cash equivalents	$427,368
Investments	1,246,310
Assets limited or restricted as to use, current portion	15,780
Patient accounts receivable, net of allowance for doubtful accounts of $98.6 million	532,715
Estimated receivables from third-party payors	64,077
Other receivables	74,389
Inventories	75,450
Assets held for sale	
Prepaid expenses and other current assets	81,233
Total current assets	2,517,322
Assets limited or restricted as to use, noncurrent portion	
Held by trustees under bond indenture agreements	28,403
Self-insurance, benefit plans, and other	228,732
By Board for capital equipment	1,204,519
By donors	58,753
Total assets limited or restricted as to use, noncurrent portion	1,520,407
Property and equipment, net	2,301,768
Investments in unconsolidated affiliates	73,912
Goodwill	60,322
Intangible assets, net of accumulated amortization of $5.1 million	35,711
Other assets	70,588
Total assets	$6,580,030
Liabilities and net assets	
Current liabilities	
Commercial paper	$55,008
Short-term borrowings	511,301
Current portion of long-term debt	17,052
Accounts payable	182,390
Accrued expenses	145,688
Salaries, wages, and related liabilities	237,921
Estimated payables to third-party payors	146,092
Other current liabilities	72,377
Total current liabilities	1,367,829
Long-term debt, net of current portion	1,254,717
Self-insurance reserves	237,960
Accrued pension and retiree health costs	603,877
Other long-term liabilities	247,601
Total liabilities	3,711,984
Net assets	
Unrestricted net assets	2,761,115
Noncontrolling ownership interest in subsidiaries	11,413
Total unrestricted net assets	2,772,528
Temporarily restricted net assets	64,266
Total temporarily restricted net assets	64,266
Permanently restricted net assets	31,252
Total permanently restricted net assets	31,252
Total net assets	2,868,046
Total liabilities and net assets	$6,580,030

The accompanying notes are an integral part of the consolidated financial statements.

a *consolidated* or *combined* balance sheet, and the names of all the entities being summarized are stated in the notes. The Dunhill Health System financial statement used as an example throughout this chapter is a consolidated statement. Although a subsidiary may issue its own stand-alone financial statements, a parent may not do this because a provision of GAAP is that it must consolidate subsidiaries and other entities where required.

In the statement heading, below the name of the entity, the term *Balance Sheet* appears, to differentiate this document from the other financial statements. Finally, two years are shown. As mentioned earlier, the balance sheet reports what the entity looks like at a particular point in time, which is the last day of the accounting period (e.g., quarter, half-year, or fiscal year). Two dates are often shown so that the reader can compare two successive periods, although for nonpublic entities this is not required. Public companies are required to present two years of balance sheet information and three years of comparative information for the other statements.

Key Point The balance sheet reports the entity's assets, liabilities, and equity at a particular point in time, usually the last day of the accounting period (e.g., quarter or fiscal year). Many small health care entities prepare external facing statements only once a year, although internal statements are prepared more often. Others prepare statements once a quarter that summarize results at that point in time.

The three major sections making up the body of the not-for-profit entity's balance sheet are *assets*, *liabilities*, and *net assets* (Exhibits 2.2 and 2.3). The balance sheet derives its name from the fact that the assets always equal the sum of the liabilities plus the net assets. (Net assets is called *stockholders' equity* in investor-owned health care entities and *net assets* in not-for-profit health care entities. Hereafter, equity will be referred to as *stockholders' equity* for investor-owned health care entities.) The relationship among the three major sections of the balance sheet is expressed by the *basic accounting equation*:

$$\text{Assets} = \text{Liabilities} + \text{Net Assets}$$

In investor-owned entities, the equation becomes

$$\text{Assets} = \text{Liabilities} + \text{Stockholders' Equity}$$

Assets
The probable future economic benefits obtained or controlled by a particular entity as a result of past transactions or events. In many instances assets represent resources that the entity owns. Assets are recorded at their cost, unless donated. In these latter cases they are recorded at fair value at the date of donation.

Liabilities
The probable future sacrifices of economic benefits arising from present obligations of a particular entity to transfer assets or provide services to other entities in the future as a result of past transactions or events. Liabilities can be debts or other obligations: for example, deferred revenue, which is an obligation to provide or deliver goods or services when payment has been received in advance.

Net Assets (or Equity)
The assets of an entity that remain after deducting its liabilities (also called *residual interest*). In a business enterprise the equity is the ownership interest. In a not-for-profit entity, which has no ownership interest, net assets is divided into three classes based on the presence or absence of donor-imposed restrictions—permanently restricted, temporarily restricted, and unrestricted net assets.

In Exhibit 2.3, at June 30, 2012, the assets equal $6,580,030, and the liabilities plus the net assets also equal $6,580,030 ($3,711,984 plus $2,868,046), in thousands of dollars.

Basic Accounting Equation

Assets $=$ Liabilities $+$ Net Assets (or stockholders' equity).

Assets

The assets of an entity are the resources it owns. On the balance sheet the assets are divided into two categories, current assets and noncurrent assets. Exhibit 2.4 displays a *classified balance sheet*, one that presents current and noncurrent assets. Health care entities are required by GAAP to present a classified balance sheet, whereas other not-for-profit health care–related entities are not. There is an exception for continuing care retirement communities. They are permitted to sequence their accounts in liquidity order.

Current Assets

Current assets are assets that will be used or consumed within one year (Exhibit 2.4). They help to turn the capacity of the entity (i.e., buildings and equipment) into service. Examples of current assets are

- Cash and cash equivalents
- Investments (unless held for long-term purposes or held in an endowment fund)
- Assets limited as to use (current portion)
- Patient accounts receivable, net of allowance for doubtful accounts
- Inventories, prepaid expenses, and other similar assets

Liquidity refers to how quickly an asset can be turned into cash, and current assets are generally listed in liquidity order.

Because of their liquidity, current assets require special internal control procedures to ensure that they are handled appropriately and efficiently. For instance, a generally accepted internal control procedure in health care entities involves the segregation of duties. When duties are segregated, different people are involved in billing, receiving payments, and processing and recording payments, reconciling accounts receivable, calculating the allowance for doubtful accounts, and writing off receivables no longer

EXHIBIT 2.4 ASSET SECTION OF THE EXHIBIT 2.3 BALANCE SHEET, EMPHASIS ON CURRENT ASSETS

Dunhill Health System
Consolidated Balance Sheet
June 30, 2012
(in thousands)

Assets

Current assets	
Cash and cash equivalents	$427,368
Investments	1,246,310
Assets limited or restricted as to use, current portion	15,780
Patient accounts receivable, net of allowance for doubtful accounts of $98.6 million	532,715
Estimated receivables from third-party payors	64,077
Other receivables	74,389
Inventories	75,450
Assets held for sale	
Prepaid expenses and other current assets	81,233
Total current assets	2,517,322
Assets limited or restricted as to use, noncurrent portion	
Held by trustees under bond indenture agreements	28,403
Self-insurance, benefit plans and other	228,732
By Board for capital equipment	1,204,519
By donors	58,753
Total assets limited or restricted as to use, noncurrent portion	1,520,407
Property and equipment, net	2,301,768
Investments in unconsolidated affiliates	73,912
Goodwill	60,322
Intangible assets, net of accumulated amortization of $5.1 million	35,711
Other assets	70,588
Total assets	$6,580,030

Performance Indicator

The FASB requires not-for-profit health care entities to include a performance indicator in their statement of operations. The FASB defines it as an intermediate level that reports the results of operations. Note that *operations* includes both operating and nonoperating items. It is analogous to income from continuing operations or net income in an investor-owned entity.

Liquidity

A measure of how quickly an asset can be converted into cash.

considered collectible. In addition to the cash handling and processing controls, an entity should have monitoring controls, meaning that an independent party such as a supervisor or manager performs analytical procedures including a comparison of budget to actual, a period to period comparison, and an analysis of dollars per unit (such as patient day or procedure). Without segregation of duties, there is opportunity for error and fraud. Although larger entities are able to segregate duties fairly easily, smaller ones may not have the money to hire more personnel. This is when monitoring on a timely basis becomes more important.

The following sections discuss specific types of assets.

Cash and Cash Equivalents

Cash and cash equivalents are the most liquid current assets (and therefore listed first in Exhibit 2.4). This account is composed of actual money on hand as well as savings and checking accounts. Cash equivalents are short-term investments with an original maturity of three months or less. Examples are money market funds, certificates of deposits, and treasury securities with original maturities of three months or less. This asset group excludes cash that has restrictions or limitations regarding withdrawal or that is to be used for purposes other than current operations.

 Key Point   Cash (and cash equivalents) is the most liquid asset on the balance sheet.

Investments

The classification of investments depends on how long management intends to hold them and whether or not restrictions or other requirements are absent. Short-term investments often include certificates of deposit, commercial paper, and treasury bills (those with an original maturity of three months or less are included in cash and cash equivalents) and also marketable securities designated as trading securities. Short-term investments allow a health care facility to earn interest on idle cash and, at the same time, provide almost immediate access to cash for unexpected situations.

Investments held for long-term purposes such as endowment funds or those designated by the board for long-term use are not included in short-term investments.

Health care entities frequently invest in alternative investments, such as venture funds and other partnerships or derivative instruments. They may also have investments in other entities as business ventures. These are considered investments when the ownership is less than 50 percent, and the other entities' financial statements are not required to be consolidated with the investing entity's due to control. Health care entities may use the equity method to account for investments where the investor has significant influence but not control. Investments other than equity method investments are required to be marked to fair value, with the unrealized gains and losses included in other comprehensive income when investor owned, or below the performance indicator when not-for-profit. Marketable securities are discussed in greater detail in Chapter Five.

Assets Limited as to Use

The cash and short-term investments listed in the current assets section of the balance sheet are generally available for management to use to carry out its responsibilities. In addition, a health care entity may have other cash, marketable securities, or other current assets that can be used only under special conditions. For example, in taking out a loan, a health care entity may agree to set aside an amount of funds equal to six months' worth of loan payments. Assets limited as to use may be current or noncurrent or have both current and noncurrent portions (as in Exhibit 2.4), depending on how soon they may be liquidated. The assets limited as to use for Dunhill Health System are $15,780 (current portion) and $1,520,407 (noncurrent portion) (in thousands) in 2012.

Patient Accounts Receivable, Net of Allowance for Doubtful Accounts

Gross patient accounts receivable is the amount owed the health care entity at full charges. However, many payors, such as Medicaid, insurance companies, large employers, and managed care entities, are given discounts, called *contractual allowances*. After subtracting contractual allowances and *charity care discounts* from gross patient accounts receivable, what remains is the patient accounts receivable that the provider has a legal right to collect.

A reserve or allowance is deducted from patient accounts receivable on the balance sheet. It represents an estimate of how much of the entity's patient accounts receivable are not likely to be collectable. This estimate is called the *allowance for doubtful accounts.*

Assuming that Dunhill's gross patient accounts receivable were $735,819, discounts and contractual allowances were $104,504, and allowance for doubtful accounts was $98,600, then patient accounts receivable, net of the allowance for doubtful accounts, would be $532,715 (in thousands), as shown in Exhibit 2.5.

Charity Care Discounts
Discounts from gross patient accounts receivable given to patients who cannot pay their bills and who meet the entity's charity care policy.

EXHIBIT 2.5 CALCULATION OF PATIENT ACCOUNTS RECEIVABLE, NET OF ESTIMATED UNCOLLECTIBLES

Account Title	Amount (in thousands)	Explanation
Gross patient accounts receivable	$735,819	The amount owed to the organization, based on full charges. This amount is not reported on financial statements; because of the discounts and allowances, it does not represent how much the health care organization is really owed.
– Discounts and allowances	–104,504	Includes discounts given to third parties (large-scale purchasers of health care services) and discounts for charity care.
Patient accounts receivable	631,315	Gross charges less discounts and allowances.
– Allowance for uncollectibles	–98,600	An estimate of how much of patient accounts receivable will likely *not* be collectible.
Patient accounts receivable, net of estimated uncollectibles	$532,715	The amount expected to be collected.

Inventories, Prepaid Expenses, and Other Current Assets

Prepaid expenses and other current assets are presented together in the Dunhill financial statements (Exhibit 2.4), because of their relatively small size. In some entities *inventories and prepaid expenses* may be grouped together with other assets under the title *other current assets*. Inventories include the day-to-day supplies used by the entity in the provision of health care services, including food, drugs, office supplies, and medical supplies. A common mistake is to confuse supplies and equipment. *Supplies* refers to small-dollar items that will be used up or fully consumed within one year or less, such as pharmaceuticals and office supplies. *Equipment* refers to more expensive items that will be used over a longer period, such as buildings and radiology equipment. These are capitalized and depreciated. *Prepaid expenses* include items the health care entity has paid for in advance, such as rent and insurance. Although they are not tangible, they are still assets in the form of rights that the entity has purchased. For instance, by paying its rent in advance, the entity has a right to use a building for a specified period. When supplies and prepaid expenses are relatively large amounts, they may be broken out and reported separately rather than grouped together.

Key Point Supplies are sometimes called *inventory*.

Noncurrent Assets

Whereas current assets will be used or consumed within one year, noncurrent assets will be used or consumed over periods longer than one year (see Exhibit 2.6). Noncurrent assets are relatively costly items that allow the entity to deliver service over time. Whereas current assets require special management attention because of their liquidity and transportability, noncurrent assets require special attention because of their cost and the extensive time it takes to plan, acquire, and manage them. Examples of noncurrent assets are

• Assets limited as to use (noncurrent portion)

• Property and equipment, net

• Goodwill

• Other assets

Key Point The terms *noncurrent* and *long-term* are often used interchangeably.

Assets Limited as to Use

Assets limited as to use are assets whose use is limited by contracts or agreements with outside parties other than donors or grantors (assets such as proceeds of debt issues, funds deposited with a trustee, self-insurance funding arrangements, and statutory reserve requirements). The term also includes assets with limitations placed on them by the entity's board of directors or trustees. As is illustrated in Exhibit 2.6, Dunhill identifies the

EXHIBIT 2.6   ASSET SECTION OF THE EXHIBIT 2.3 BALANCE SHEET, EMPHASIS ON NONCURRENT ASSETS

Dunhill Health System
Consolidated Balance Sheet
June 30, 2012
(in thousands)

Assets

Current assets

Cash and cash equivalents	$427,368
Investments	1,246,310
Assets limited or restricted as to use, current portion	15,780
Patient accounts receivable, net of allowance for doubtful accounts of $98.6 million	532,715
Estimated receivables from third-party payors	64,077
Other receivables	74,389
Inventories	75,450
Assets held for sale	
Prepaid expenses and other current assets	81,233
Total current assets	2,517,322
Assets limited or restricted as to use, noncurrent portion	
Held by trustees under bond indenture agreements	28,403
Self-insurance, benefit plans and other	228,732
By Board for capital equipment	1,204,519
By donors	58,753
Total assets limited or restricted as to use, noncurrent portion	1,520,407
Property and equipment, net	2,301,768
Investments in unconsolidated affiliates	73,912
Goodwill	60,322
Intangible assets, net of accumulated amortization of $5.1 million	35,711
Other assets	70,588
Total assets	$6,580,030

assets limited as to use on the face of the balance sheet. However, these items may also be separately presented and not identified with the caption "assets limited as to use." When the term is used and the items are not separately identified on the face of the statements, they are then described in the notes.

In the case of Dunhill Health System in 2012, this category contains several items: the bond trustee is holding $28,403 under Dunhill's bond indenture agreements, $1,204,519 has been set aside by the board to purchase capital equipment, and $228,732 has been set aside to pay for Dunhill's employee insurance claims under its self-insured benefit plan. In addition, Dunhill combines its assets limited as to use with those that are restricted as to use, so the amount restricted to long-term purposes by donors is $58,753 (in thousands). Notice that the *current* portion of assets limited as to use (see the section emphasized in Exhibit 2.4) consists of the amounts in these accounts that are converted to cash in the current year. The current portion is not broken out in the same way as the noncurrent portion is.

Noncurrent Assets
The resources of the entity that will be used or consumed over periods longer than one year.

Investments

Most health care entities invest excess funds. Investments in marketable securities that are held by a not-for-profit entity are carried at fair value. This means that in every period, the value of those investments that have not been sold will be adjusted to the amount for which they could currently be sold. While this used to be called *market value*, the world of investments has become so volatile and complicated that the accounting literature now calls it *fair value*, defining it as "the price that would be received to sell an asset or paid to transfer a liability in an orderly transaction between market participants at the measurement date."

Although complete discussion of fair value is beyond the scope of this text, the important concept is that the fair value is an *exit value*, or how much one could expect to receive for the asset. A marketable security is one with a readily determinable fair value. Hospital systems, in particular, will also invest in complex instruments where the value cannot be readily determined by going to an investment pricing service. In those cases the fair value is the result of an estimate by the investment manager (of the hedge fund, limited partnership, etc.), which should be evaluated by management.

Investments held by an investor-owned health care entity are carried at fair value when they are considered *trading* or *available for sale* securities. The investment is considered *trading* when the intent is to sell (or trade) it. The investment is considered available for sale when it is not held for trading. The difference between the two lies in the placement of the unrealized gains and losses. When the securities are considered trading, the unrealized gains and losses go through operations. When they are not trading, they are shown in other comprehensive income. When there are investments in debt securities that will be held to maturity, then they are carried at amortized cost. Not-for-profit entities such as charities and social service organizations are not required to and generally do not use these classifications for investments. However, not-for-profit hospitals, in order to be comparable to their investor-owned counterparts, generally do.

The classification of securities as trading and available for sale is driven by the intent and ability to hold them. Health care entities that use discretionary money managers are able to demonstrate the ability to hold the securities but not the intent, since the timing decisions on purchases and sales are made by the money manager. Trading securities are reported as current assets.

Since not-for-profit entities do not have comprehensive income, the unrealized gains and losses on available for sale securities are reported *after* the performance indicator. Dunhill classifies its investments as current because they are considered trading securities. (See the discussion of the performance indicator later in this chapter.)

Securities include various types of stocks and bonds and are discussed in more detail in Chapter Eight.

Properties and Equipment, Net

Depreciation

A measure of the extent to which a tangible asset (such as plant or equipment) has been used up or consumed.

Accumulated Depreciation

The total amount of depreciation taken on an asset since it was put into use.

This category of assets represents the major capital investments in the facility. Three types of assets are included in this category: land, plant, and equipment. *Plant* refers to buildings (fixed, immovable objects), *land* refers to property, and *equipment* includes a wide variety of durable items from beds to CAT scanners. Land, plant, and equipment are recorded on the entity's books at cost, and over time, plant and equipment are depreciated. Land is not depreciated. Land improvements are depreciated unless there is no way to estimate their useful lives. This may occur when land is being prepared for its intended purpose. *Depreciation* is an estimate of the extent to which the plant or equipment has been used up during the accounting period. Depreciation is a noncash item.

The word *net* in *properties and equipment, net*, means that the total amount of depreciation taken up to this point in time has been subtracted from the original cost. To derive properties and equipment, net, the total amount of depreciation taken since the asset was put into use (called *accumulated depreciation*) is subtracted from the original cost of the asset (called *plant and equipment*). Assuming the original cost is $4,126,149 and

---

EXHIBIT 2.7 CALCULATION OF PROPERTIES AND EQUIPMENT, NET

Account Title	Amount (in thousands)	Explanation
Properties and equipment	$4,126,149	The original cost of the land, plant, and equipment.
– Accumulated depreciation	–1,824,381	An estimate of the amount by which the assets have been used up, which is equal to the total amount of depreciation taken since the organization acquired the assets; by convention, plant and equipment depreciate, land does not.
Properties and equipment, net	$2,301,768	The original cost minus the amount by which the assets have been depreciated (used up).

---

accumulated depreciation is $1,824,381, then properties and equipment, net, would be calculated as $2,301,768 (in thousands) (Exhibit 2.7).

By convention, plant and equipment are always kept on the books in their own accounts at their original cost until the assets are modified or sold. Similarly, the total amount of depreciation is kept in a separate account, accumulated depreciation. In this way, those looking at the balance sheet are always able to know (1) the original cost of the assets, (2) how much they have been depreciated, and (3) their current book value (original cost less depreciation). More detail is available in the notes.

The FASB requires that whenever events or changes in circumstances indicate that the carrying value of a long-lived asset or asset group may not be recoverable, its value must be reduced by an impairment loss. This can occur when there is a downturn in the economy that affects the real estate market. It can also happen when a facility is no longer being used for its intended purpose and there is not a market for it that will cover its cost minus accumulated depreciation.

For example, inpatient volumes may decline and the board of a small community hospital may decide that the facility should be used for outpatient services only. In this instance the facility would be grouped with other assets and liabilities at the lowest level for which identifiable cash flows are measured, and compared to the fair value of the asset group. This type of evaluation takes specialized skills and use of a valuation specialist is recommended when the entity does not have the expertise in-house.

Other Assets

Other assets is a catchall account used for noncurrent assets not included in the other categories of noncurrent assets.

Goodwill

Goodwill is the term used for what an entity is buying in an acquisition when it pays cash and assumes liabilities in excess of the fair value of the assets acquired. Goodwill represents the future earnings power of the acquired entity. Goodwill is no longer amortized. However, it must be evaluated for impairment every year.

Liabilities

The preceding section focused on how assets are presented on the balance sheet. We now turn to a discussion of the liabilities of a health care entity. *Liabilities* are probable sacrifices of economic benefits. Although it is tempting to describe liabilities as what an entity owes to its creditors, some liabilities, such as a malpractice reserve, are simply an estimate. As with assets, liabilities are divided into two categories: current and noncurrent (see Exhibit 2.8).

Current Liabilities
Financial obligations due within one year.

Current Liabilities

Current liabilities are the financial obligations (or current portion of malpractice or other reserves) that, due to their contractual terms, are expected to be paid within one year. Common account categories include

- Current portion of long-term debt
- Accounts payable and accrued expenses (including payroll)
- Estimated third-party payor settlements
- Other current liabilities

Each of these accounts is discussed below.

Current Portion of Long-Term Debt

This account contains the amount of the entity's long-term debt that is expected to be paid off within one year. For example, if a home health agency has executed a five-year note payable, the principal amount due this year is reported in this account. The remainder is listed under noncurrent liabilities. This information is sometimes reported in the account *notes payable*, which reports the amount of short-term (less than one year) obligations for which a formal note has been signed.

EXHIBIT 2.8 LIABILITIES SECTION OF THE EXHIBIT 2.3 BALANCE SHEET (IN THOUSANDS)

Liabilities and net assets	2012
Current liabilities	
Commercial paper	$55,008
Short-term borrowings	511,301
Current portion of long-term debt	17,052
Accounts payable	182,390
Accrued expenses	145,688
Salaries, wages, and related liabilities	237,921
Estimated payables to third-party payors	146,092
Other current liabilities	72,377
Total current liabilities	1,367,829
Long-term debt, net of current portion	1,254,717
Self-insurance reserves	237,960
Accrued pension and retiree health costs	603,877
Other long-term liabilities	247,601
Total liabilities	$3,711,984

Accounts Payable and Accrued Expenses

Accounts payable are obligations to pay suppliers who have sold the health care entity goods or services on credit. *Accrued expenses* are expenses that arise in the normal course of business that have not yet been paid. Included in this category are salaries, wages, and interest. Sometimes accrued expenses are presented in separate accounts, such as

- Salaries and wages payable
- Interest payable

Key Point Accrued expenses are liabilities and are reflected in the balance sheet.

Estimated Third-Party Payor Settlements

This account represents an estimate of funds to be repaid to third-party payors. *Third-party payors* are entities such as insurance companies and governmental agencies that pay on behalf of patients. This account is necessary because much of the payment process is done using estimates. For example, Medicare (actually, a contractor or fiscal intermediary acting on Medicare's behalf) makes periodic payments to a hospital, based on the claims (i.e., bills) it has received and processed. The prospective payment system under which most health care entities are paid provides for retrospective adjustments for, for example, billing denials, coding changes, and settlements with third-party payors. With the advent of value-based reimbursement, 1 percent of Medicare payments will be held back to be paid out as bonuses to those that perform at or above targets on quality measures. As more fully discussed in Chapter Thirteen, this percentage will increase up to 2 percent over time. This process too will give rise to estimated third-party payor settlements.

The amount that appears on the balance sheet under *estimated third-party payor settlements* is an estimate of how much the hospital will need to return to the third parties due to overpayments by the third parties. Conversely, the same account can appear on the asset side representing the amounts due the hospital due to underpayments by a payor or settlements. Management will calculate this estimate based in large part on historical information. In addition to amounts based on claims submitted, estimated third-party payor settlements may also include advances from third parties to support the day-to-day needs of the entity, but this is not typical (see Chapter Five).

Other Current Liabilities

Other current liabilities includes all current liabilities not elsewhere presented in the current liabilities section. The accounts summarized in this category may be presented on their own lines or they may be detailed in the notes if they are material in amount. Increasingly, a major item in this account is deferred revenue.

Deferred revenue consists of fees that have been collected in advance. It represents cash that is received before the service is rendered by the entity. Accordingly, it is an obligation that will, upon performance, become revenue. For example, health care entities may receive capitation payments from health plans. Capitated payments are often in the form of a specific amount per member per month (PMPM) and require that the provider receiving the payments provide a prescribed set of services for the population covered by these payments. When the health care entity receives the capitated payment, it incurs an obligation to provide service. Thus, it records the amount received as an obligation (liability). After the obligation is satisfied (the time that the payment covers has passed), the deferred revenue is taken out of the deferred revenue account and recorded as revenue. Capitation payments are generally made by the beginning of the month in which the service is to be provided.

Noncurrent Liabilities

Noncurrent liabilities are obligations that will be paid back over a period longer than one year. Most long-term liabilities fall into two categories: mortgages and bonds payable, and estimates for malpractice or self-insured risks such as a self-funded health benefit or worker's compensation arrangement.

Net Assets

The final category of the balance sheet is *net assets* (Exhibit 2.9). The term *net assets* is used to reflect the community's interest in the assets of the not-for-profit entity. In an investor-owned entity, this category is the stockholders' interest in the entity's assets. In both instances, it is equal to the entity's assets minus its liabilities. Thus, in not-for-profit health care entities, the terms in the basic accounting equation are rearranged to derive net assets as follows:

$$\text{Net assets} = \text{Assets} - \text{Liabilities}$$

Third-Party Payors
Commonly referred to as *third parties*, these are entities that pay on behalf of patients.

Noncurrent Liabilities
The financial obligations not due within one year.

Noncontrolling Interest
The amount of a partially owned subsidiary entity that the parent does not own. In the not-for-profit parent's consolidated financial statement, this noncontrolling interest is reported as a separate component of the appropriate class of net assets. This distinguishes it from the other components of the net assets of the parent. The effects of donor-imposed restrictions on a partially owned subsidiary's net assets would also be reported in that net asset class. See Appendix A for an example.

EXHIBIT 2.9 NET ASSETS SECTION OF THE EXHIBIT 2.3 BALANCE SHEET (IN THOUSANDS)

	2012
Net assets	
Unrestricted net assets	2,761,115
Noncontrolling ownership interest in subsidiaries	11,413
Total unrestricted net assets	2,772,528
Temporarily restricted net assets	64,266
Total temporarily restricted net assets	64,266
Permanently restricted net assets	31,252
Total permanently restricted net assets	31,252
Total net assets	2,868,046

Key Point The net assets section of the not-for-profit health care provider's balance sheet is analogous to the owner's equity section of an investor-owned entity's balance sheet.

For example, going back to the full Dunhill consolidated balance sheet for 2012 (Exhibit 2.3), subtracting the amount of total liabilities ($3,711,984) from the value of the total assets ($6,580,030) equals net assets of $2,868,046.

In the presentation of net assets on the balance sheet, not-for-profit health care entities must categorize net assets into three categories of restrictions:

- Unrestricted net assets
- Temporarily restricted net assets
- Permanently restricted net assets

All net assets *not* restricted by donors are considered *unrestricted net assets*. Net assets that are restricted by donors, however, must be shown on the balance sheet as temporarily or permanently restricted (see Exhibit 2.10 and Perspective 2.3). An example of a temporary restriction is the donation of land by a county to a hospital with the provision that the hospital cannot sell it for five years, or a donation of cash that is restricted to the purchase of a piece of equipment. An example of a permanent restriction is a restriction on an endowment that allows the health care entity to spend the investment return according to its spending policy but not the corpus (or principal), which remains permanently restricted.

Stockholders' Equity

Investor-owned health care entities use a different form of presentation in the stockholders' equity section of the balance sheet (see Exhibit 2.11). The terms used in the stockholders' equity section (i.e., *par value of the stock, excess of par value,* and *retained earnings*) are technical and beyond the scope of this text.

Comprehensive Income and Its Relationship to the Performance Indicator

Although it will not be discussed in depth here, an investor-owned entity will have *other comprehensive income or loss*. This is the change in equity of a business enterprise during a given period from transactions and other events and circumstances stemming from nonowner sources. It includes

EXHIBIT 2.10 EXAMPLES OF TYPES OF RESTRICTIONS ON ASSETS

Temporarily Restricted

Amounts of funding that are restricted to the purchase of a new piece of equipment.

Permanently Restricted

Endowments. The amount that can be spent is now limited by state law under the Uniform Prudent Management of Institutional Funds Act. It states that all earnings on donor-restricted endowments must go into temporarily restricted net assets until appropriated by the board according to its adopted prudent spending policy. Note that the board can also appropriate assets for expenditure even when the return on investments for the period is not as large as the appropriation. This feature in the law was designed to give not-for-profit entities the ability to maintain constant spending. So in times when the market is doing well and return is higher the return will not all be spent, and when return is lower there is *excess return from other periods* that can be spent.

EXHIBIT 2.11 ILLUSTRATION OF THE STOCKHOLDERS' EQUITY SECTION OF THE BALANCE SHEET FOR AN INVESTOR-OWNED HEALTH CARE ORGANIZATION (IN THOUSANDS)

	20X2	20X1
Equity		
LifePoint Hospitals, Inc. stockholders' equity		
Preferred stock, $0.01 par value; 10,000,000 shares authorized; no shares issued	—	—
Common stock, $0.01 par value; 90,000,000 shares authorized; 63,233,088 and 61,450,098 shares issued at December 31, 2011 and 2010, respectively	0.6	0.6
Capital in excess of par value	1,354.8	1,289.4
Accumulated other comprehensive loss	—	(4.0)
Retained earnings	1,066.9	904.0
Common stock in treasury, at cost, 14,925,875 and 9,991,316 shares at December 31, 2011 and 2010, respectively	(477.1)	(302.5)
Total LifePoint Hospitals, Inc. stockholders' equity	1,945.2	1,887.5
Noncontrolling interests	14.4	3.8
Total equity	1,959.6	1,891.3

all changes in equity during the period except those resulting from investments by owners and distributions to owners. For example, other comprehensive income will include the income (loss) from operating activities (and discontinued operations) as well as the changes from such other circumstances as net pension obligations, the fair value of interest rate swaps or other hedging derivatives, foreign currency translation, and the fair value of investments available for sale. Not-for-profit entities do not use the concept of comprehensive income. The performance indicator serves that function. Accordingly, these activities are reported below the performance indicator.

Key Point Stockholders' equity in investor-owned entities consists of the stock and retained earnings.

Notes to Financial Statements (Footnotes)

Notes are an integral part of the financial statements. Because the information in the body of the statement is presented in summary form, additional key information must be presented in the notes. The quantity of footnote disclosures has increased significantly over the last several years as financial accounting has become more complex in response to the business environment. The content of the notes is generally prescribed by GAAP. However, an entity can disclose more than is required. For example, not-for-profit entities sometimes include more information in their footnotes than is required by GAAP in order to help a potential donor to understand the level of commitment the entity has to its mission.

Notes are required to contain a summary of significant accounting policies followed by the composition of significant balance sheet accounts; disclosure about which assets are restricted and for what purpose; the composition of property and equipment along with the depreciation method used and range of useful lives; the fair value of investments; the composition of both long-term and short-term debt, including the maturity and interest rates; the amount of professional liability insurance for malpractice; and whether there are suits filed against the entity that may adversely affect its financial position. This is not a comprehensive list but it suggests the extent of the disclosures required by GAAP. Exhibit A.9, in the appendix to this chapter, provides a detailed example of certain notes required to be included in a set of not-for-profit financial statements.

PERSPECTIVE 2.3 USING THE NOTES TO THE FINANCIAL STATEMENTS TO UNDERSTAND THE COMPOSITION OF DEBT

Policymakers, potential lenders, and bond credit rating agencies may want to know whether a health care entity's debt is tax exempt or taxable, when that debt comes due, and what interest rate the entity pays on that debt. The answers can be found in the notes to the financial statement. For example, Exhibit A.9, Note 5, indicates that Dunhill Health System has $1,199 million of tax-exempt revenue and refunding bonds due over the next thirty-six years at interest rates from 2.375 percent to 6.625 percent. Note 5 gives the balance, rate, and maturity information for $55 million of additional long-term debt and for $511 million of short-term borrowings, and discloses that an aggregate of $126 million in principal payments is due over the next three years.

EXHIBIT 2.12 COMPARISON OF THE TIME FRAMES COVERED BY THE BALANCE SHEET AND BY THE STATEMENT OF OPERATIONS

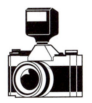

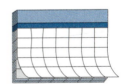

The *balance sheet* presents a snapshot of the organization as of a point in time.

The *statement of operations* presents a summary of revenues and expenses over a period of time.

The Statement of Operations

As opposed to the balance sheet, which summarizes the entity's total assets, liabilities, and net assets at a *particular point in time*, the *statement of operations* is a summary of the entity's revenues and expenses over a *period of time* (Exhibit 2.12). The period is usually the time between statements, such as a quarter, half-year, or fiscal year. The statement of operations is analogous to, but is different from, the income statement of an investor-owned entity (Exhibit 2.13). For investor-owned entities, the statement can be defined as either an income statement or a statement of operations.

EXHIBIT 2.13 COMPARISON OF THE HEADINGS AND MAJOR SECTIONS OF THE BODY OF THE INCOME STATEMENT FOR INVESTOR-OWNED AND NOT-FOR-PROFIT HEALTH CARE ORGANIZATIONS

Investor-Owned

Title

Body

Consolidated Statement of Income

Revenues (patient service revenue less contractual allowances, charity care, and bad debt expense followed by other types of revenue if disclosed separately)

− Operating expenses

Income from continuing operations before income taxes

− Provision for income taxes

Income from continuing operations

+ Income from discontinued operations, net of income taxes

Net income

− Net income attributable to noncontrolling interests

Net income attributable to entity

Title

Consolidated Statement of Comprehensive Income

Body

Net income

+ Other comprehensive income, net of income taxes

Comprehensive income

− Net income attributable to noncontrolling interests

Comprehensive income attributable to entity

Not-for-Profit

Title

Body

Consolidated Statement of Operations

Unrestricted revenues (patient service revenue less contractual allowances, charity care, and bad debt expense followed by other types of revenue if disclosed separately)

Net assets released from restrictions

Total unrestricted revenue

− Total expenses

Operating income

+/− Nonoperating items

Excess of revenue over expenses

− Excess of revenue over expenses attributable to noncontrolling income

Excess of revenue over expenses, net of noncontrolling interest

Unrestricted net assets

Excess of revenue over expenses

+/− Items shown below the performance indicator

Increase/decrease in unrestricted net assets before discontinued operations

Discontinued operations

Increase in unrestricted net assets

Temporarily restricted net assets

Increase in temporarily restricted net assets

Permanently restricted net assets

Increase in permanently restricted net assets

Increase in net assets

Net assets, beginning of year

Net assets, end of year

Exhibits A.5 to A.7 in the chapter appendix present an example of the financial statements for an investor-owned entity.

Not-for-profit health care entities present information related to their activities in two separate statements: a statement of operations and a statement of changes in net assets. The statement of operations reports all the changes in unrestricted net assets for the period. GAAP permits these two statements to be combined into one (see Exhibit 2.13).

Exhibits 2.14a and 2.14b display the statement of operations for one year and the statement of changes in net assets for Dunhill Health System, a not-for-profit health care entity. Dunhill, like most other health systems, combines the two statements. Because they are large, they are each shown on two pages. The first page shows the operating and nonoperating revenues and expenses culminating in the excess of revenues over expenses. The second page begins with the excess of revenues over expenses and then shows the items required to be excluded from the performance indicator (or below the line), the changes in temporarily restricted net assets, and the changes in permanently restricted net assets.

Key Point The statement of operations uses the accrual basis of accounting, which summarizes how much the entity earned and the resources it used to generate that income during a period of time. It does not use the cash basis of accounting, which focuses on the cash that actually came in and went out. This is discussed in detail in the next chapter.

Key Point The statement of operations does not represent the cash flow of the entity. Instead, it represents how much the entity earned, its gains and other sources of revenue, and the resources it used during the accounting period.

Unrestricted Revenue

This section of the statement of operations represents what most people think of as the revenues of the entity (Exhibit 2.15). The term *revenues* refers to the amounts either earned by the entity or donated to it. *Gains* can come from transactions such as selling assets for more than their carrying value (such as selling a building or other investment). *Other support* includes such items as appropriations from governmental entities and unrestricted donations. *Net patient service revenue* generally makes up the largest portion of unrestricted revenue, gains, and other support in not-for-profit business entities. Some entities have capitated contracts or a health plan. The revenue resulting from those arrangements is called *premium revenue*. As reform moves forward it is likely that the industry will see even more of these arrangements.

 Key Point As explained in detail in Chapter Three, revenues represent amounts earned by the entity, not the amount of cash it received during the period.

Net Patient Service Revenue

Gross patient service revenue is the amount the health care entity would have earned if all the payors paid full charges. However, as discussed under patient accounts receivable, many payors receive discounts, called *contractual allowances*. In addition, most health care entities also provide some free care to indigent patients, called *charity care*. In reporting net patient service revenue, a health care entity must subtract amounts both for contractual allowances and for charity care. Thus, the amount reported on the statement of operations is net patient service revenue, which equals gross patient service revenue minus contractual allowances and charity care. In addition, for years beginning after June 30, 2012, some entities will be deducting bad debt expense here as well.

Provision for Bad Debts

The *provision for bad debts*, also called *bad debt expense* or *uncollectibles expense*, is the estimate of patient accounts receivable that will not be collected. It does not include charity care or contractual allowances, for they have already been deducted to derive patient accounts receivable.

In June 2011, the FASB issued an amendment to the professional literature requiring those health care entities that do not assess the patient's ability to pay at the point of service to present bad debt expense as a reduction of revenue. This will mainly affect those hospitals that have emergency departments, because typically emergency patients are not evaluated for their ability to pay at the point of service. More and more hospitals are evaluating the patient's ability to pay in other patient delivery settings. And other health care entities, such as physician practices, home health entities, and the like, will do the same. Note that the Dunhill financial statements and the LifePoint financial statements reflect this presentation. (See Exhibits 2.14a and A.5.)

EXHIBIT 2.14a ANNOTATED COMBINED STATEMENT OF OPERATIONS AND CHANGES IN NET ASSETS FOR A SAMPLE NOT-FOR-PROFIT HOSPITAL

1 Title. The name of the organization, the name of the financial statement, and the period(s) of time for which information is being provided.

2 Unrestricted revenue, gains, and other support. The income of the organization derived from providing patient service, the sale of assets for more than their book value, contributions, appropriations, and assets released from restriction.

Net patient service revenue. Revenue earned from patient care minus the amounts the organization does not expect to collect because of contractual discounts.

Premium revenue. Revenue earned from capitated contracts.

Other revenue. Revenue derived from such sources as support services, investments, and certain contributions.

3 Provision for bad debts. An estimate of the amount of money owed the organization that will not be collected.

4 Net assets released from restriction. Funds formerly restricted by a donor, now available for general use to run the organization.

5 Expenses. Expenses are a measure of the resources used to generate revenue. (Those expenses listed that are self-evident have not been defined.)

Depreciation and amortization. Measures of the use of long-lived assets during the accounting period.

Other. A catch-all category for miscellaneous expenses and losses, including utilities, rent, telephone, travel, etc.

6 Operating income. Unrestricted revenue, gains, and other support minus expenses and losses. Traditionally, this is a measure of the income earned from health care–related endeavors.

7 Nonoperating items. Nonoperating items generally relate to investment gains and losses, goodwill, loss from early extinguishment of debt and other items that do not recur and would therefore distort operating income if they were not separated. Note that income taxes are a very real part of a hospital system. Although rarely material, they are amounts related to income that is unrelated to the hospital's exempt purpose. Such income is appearing more and more as hospitals try to find new sources of revenue.

8 Excess of revenue over expenses. This is the performance indicator. It is analogous to net income in an investor-owned entity. It is the measure of operations.

9 Excess of revenue over expenses, net of noncontrolling interest. The amount of excess of revenues over expenses that is related to the entity's percentage of ownership of subsidiaries.

Dunhill Health System
Consolidated Statement of Operations and Changes in Net Assets
Year Ended June 30, 2012
(in thousands)

2 Unrestricted revenue	
Net patient service revenue	$ 4,402,759
3 Provision for bad debts	(265,850)
Net patient service revenue less provision for bad debts	4,136,909
Capitation and premium revenue	234,822
4 Net assets released from restrictions	7,103
Other revenue	385,416
Total unrestricted revenue	4,764,250
5 Expenses	
Salaries and wages	1,971,053
Employee benefits	436,580
Contract labor	46,722
Total labor expenses	2,454,355
Supplies	820,513
Purchased services	491,716
Depreciation and amortization	269,880
Occupancy	184,312
Medical claims and capitation purchased services	97,526
Interest	55,388
Other	237,628
Total expenses	4,611,318
6 Operating income	152,932
7 Nonoperating Items	
Investment (loss) income	(11,655)
Change in market value and cash payments of interest rate swaps	(82,039)
Loss from early extinguishment of debt	(5,892)
Gain on bargain purchase and inherent contribution	137,658
Other, including income taxes	15,291
Total nonoperating items	53,363
8 Excess of revenue over expenses	206,295
Less excess of revenue over expenses attributable to noncontrolling interest	5,402
9 Excess of revenue over expenses, net of noncontrolling interest	$ 200,893

The accompanying notes are an integral part of the consolidated financial statements.

The statement of operations (also called the statement of activities) provides a summary of the organization's revenue and expenses over a period of time. This statement illustrates the operations of Dunhill for the year. Note that Dunhill, like most not-for-profit health systems, chooses to present a combined statement of operations and changes in net assets. It is shown on two pages.

EXHIBIT 2.14b ANNOTATED COMBINED STATEMENT OF OPERATIONS AND CHANGES IN NET ASSETS FOR A SAMPLE NOT-FOR-PROFIT HOSPITAL

1 Title. The name of the organization, the name of the financial statement, and the period(s) of time for which information is being provided.

2 Unrestricted net assets. This is the beginning of the section that bridges the statement of operations and the changes in net assets. The performance indicator reports the results of operations, and the remainder of unrestricted net assets are below that performance indicator.

3 Excess of revenue over expenses. This is the performance indicator. It is analogous to net income in an investor-owned entity.

4 Net assets released from restrictions for capital acquisitions. This account is required to be reported outside the performance indicator because it is related to assets released from donor restrictions on long-lived assets. Those related to operations go in the operating section.

5 Increase in unrestricted net assets before discontinued operations. Some entities find that they need to discontinue a service line or segment of the business. These amounts are excluded from the performance indicator.

6 Increase in unrestricted net assets. The total effects for the year on unrestricted net assets.

7 Temporarily restricted net assets. Those changes in net assets that are affected by a donor's timing or purpose restriction.

8 Net assets released from restrictions. The net assets released from restrictions are removed here and inserted as a positive number in unrestricted net assets. Only in this way can the amounts be used. The $9,222 in item 4 and the $7,103 (in item 4 on the statement of operations) = $16,325.

9 Permanently restricted net assets. Those changes in net assets that are affected by a donor's restriction on the net assets into perpetuity.

10 Increase in net assets. The sum of the changes in unrestricted, temporarily restricted, and permanently restricted net assets.

11 Net assets, beginning of year. The amount of net assets at the beginning of the year.

12 Net assets, end of year. The amount of net assets at the end of the year. This number agrees with the balance sheet.

1	**Dunhill Health System**	
	Consolidated Statement of Operations and Changes in Net Assets	
	Year Ended June 30, 2012	
	(in thousands)	
2	Unrestricted net assets	
3	Excess of revenue over expenses	$206,295
4	Net assets released from restrictions for capital acquisitions	9,222
	Net change in retirement plan related items	130,487
	Other	195
5	Increase in unrestricted net assets before discontinued operations	346,199
	Discontinued operations—Greater Suffolk Health System (GSHS)	
	Net change in retirement plan related items	58,731
	(Loss) from operations	(58,620)
6	Increase in unrestricted net assets	346,310
7	**Temporarily restricted net assets**	
	Contributions	32,120
8	Net assets released from restrictions	(16,325)
	Other	1,409
	Increase in temporarily restricted net assets	17,204
9	**Permanently restricted net assets**	
	Contributions for endowment funds	4,067
	Net investment (loss)	(261)
	Other	(387)
	Increase in permanently restricted net assets	3,419
10	Increase in net assets	366,933
11	Net assets, beginning of year	2,501,113
12	**Net assets, end of year**	$2,868,046

The statement of changes in net assets provides a summary of changes in the organization's unrestricted, temporarily restricted, and permanently restricted net assets over a period of time. Note that Dunhill, like most not-for-profit health systems, chooses to present a combined statement of operations and changes in net assets. It is shown on two pages.

EXHIBIT 2.15 ABBREVIATED STATEMENT OF OPERATIONS FROM EXHIBIT 2.14a, EMPHASIS ON UNRESTRICTED REVENUE (IN THOUSANDS)

	2012
Unrestricted revenue	
Net patient service revenue	$4,402,759
Provision for bad debts	(265,850)
Net patient service revenue less provision for bad debts	4,136,909
Capitation and premium revenue	234,822
Net assets released from restrictions	7,103
Other revenue	385,416
Total unrestricted revenue	4,764,250
Expenses	
Salaries and wages	1,971,053
Employee benefits	436,580
Contract labor	46,722
Total labor expenses	2,454,355
Supplies	820,513
Purchased services	491,716
Depreciation and amortization	269,880
Occupancy	184,312
Medical claims and capitation purchased services	97,526
Interest	55,388
Other	237,628
Total expenses	4,611,318
Operating Income	152,932
Nonoperating items	
Investment (loss) income	(11,655)
Change in market value and cash payments of interest rate swaps	(82,039)
Loss from early extinguishment of debt	(5,892)
Gain on bargain purchase and inherent contribution	137,658
Other, including income taxes	15,291
Total nonoperating items	53,363
Excess of revenue over expenses	206,295
Less excess of revenue over expenses attributable to noncontrolling interest	5,402
Excess of revenue over expenses, net of noncontrolling interest	$ 200,893

The accompanying notes are an integral part of the consolidated financial statements.

EXHIBIT 2.16 CALCULATION OF NET PATIENT SERVICE REVENUES

Account Title	Amount (in thousands)	Explanation
Gross patient service revenue	$4,444,582	The amount the health care organization earned at full retail price. This amount cannot be reported on financial statements because it does not recognize that all payors do not pay full charges.
— Provision for bad debts	−$265,850	Since Dunhill has an emergency department it does not assess the patient's ability to pay at the point of service. Bad debt expense goes up as a reduction of revenue.
— Contractual allowances	−31,068	Discounts given to third parties (large-scale purchasers of health care services).
— Charity care discounts	−10,755	The amount of full charges the organization will not attempt to collect because the patient has been certified as unable to pay; usually reported only in the footnotes.
Net patient service revenue less provision for bad debts	4,136,909	Full price charges less contractual allowances and charity care discounts. This is the amount reported on the financial statements, for it is felt to be a realistic estimate of how much revenue the health care organization has actually earned.

For example, assume that a health care entity's gross patient service revenues were $4,444,582 (in thousands). Its bad debt expense was $265,850, contractual allowances $31,068, and charity care $10,755. Then the net patient service revenue for 20X1 would be $4,136,909, as shown in Exhibit 2.16.

Premium Revenue

Premium revenue is revenue earned from capitated contracts, or it could be health plan revenue if the entity has a health plan. It is not earned solely through the delivery of service but rather through a combination of the passage of time (during which the entity is available to provide service when necessary) and actually delivering service as agreed during that contract period. This is more fully discussed in Chapter Thirteen.

Other Revenue

Other revenue (sometimes referred to as *other operating revenue*) is derived from several sources: appropriations and grants, support services, income from investments, and revenue from contributions. Appropriations are monies provided by governmental agencies on an ongoing basis, usually for operating purposes. Grants are funds awarded to a health care entity for special purposes. These are known as *exchange transactions* because the revenue earned is the result of work performed by the health care entity. These transactions are therefore classified as unrestricted. Governmental grants come with numerous compliance requirements, generally including a defined period of availability of funds.

Support services include such things as parking fees, cafeteria sales, and revenue from the gift shop. These services support the operations of patient care.

Although some health care entities report their investment income, (i.e., interest income, dividends, and gains) in this category, it is also possible to report it under Non-operating items, which is below operating income.

Net Assets Released from Restriction

Net assets released from restriction are funds reclassified to unrestricted accounts from temporarily restricted net assets. As discussed earlier, when donations are made with restrictions on them the entity is obliged to use those amounts for the purpose or with the timing specified by the donor. This use could take the form of purchasing equipment or transferring the income earned from restricted investments to unrestricted accounts. This is referred to as a *release from restriction*. The amount is deducted from the temporarily restricted net asset section of the statement of changes in net assets and added to the unrestricted revenue section of the statement of operations (see Exhibit 2.14).

Expenses

Although most of the expenses listed in Exhibit 2.17 are self-evident, several of them are discussed briefly here.

EXHIBIT 2.17 ABBREVIATED STATEMENT OF OPERATIONS FROM EXHIBIT 2.14b, EMPHASIS ON EXPENSES (IN THOUSANDS)

	2012
Unrestricted revenue	
Net patient service revenue	$4,402,759
Provision for bad debts	(265,850)
Net patient service revenue less provision for bad debts	4,136,909
Capitation and premium revenue	234,822
Net assets released from restrictions	7,103
Other revenue	385,416
Total unrestricted revenue	4,764,250
Expenses	
Salaries and wages	1,971,053
Employee benefits	436,580
Contract labor	46,722
Total labor expenses	2,454,355
Supplies	820,513
Purchased services	491,716
Depreciation and amortization	269,880
Occupancy	184,312
Medical claims and capitation purchased services	97,526
Interest	55,388
Other	237,628
Total expenses	4,611,318
Operating income	152,932
Nonoperating items	
Investment (loss) income	(11,655)
Change in market value and cash payments of interest rate swaps	(82,039)
Loss from early extinguishment of debt	(5,892)
Gain on bargain purchase and inherent contribution	137,658
Other, including income taxes	15,291
Total nonoperating items	53,363
Excess of revenue over expenses	206,295
Less excess of revenue over expenses attributable to noncontrolling interest	5,402
Excess of revenue over expenses, net of noncontrolling interest	$200,893

Key Point On the statement of operations, expenses are a measure of the amount of resources used or consumed in providing a service, not cash outflows.

Depreciation and Amortization

Depreciation and *amortization* reflect the amount of a noncurrent asset used up during the accounting period. Depreciation is a measure of how much of a tangible asset (such as a building or equipment) has been used up during the accounting period. For example, if a facility buys new examining room equipment for $10,000 and expects it to last ten years, the accountant might record $1,000 in depreciation each year, on the assumption that one-tenth of the equipment is used up each year.

Amortization is a measure of how much of an intangible asset (such as debt issuance cost and goodwill) has been used up during the accounting period. Both of these expenses are noncash expenses.

Amortization
The allocation of the acquisition cost of debt to the period that it benefits.

Key Point Depreciation and amortization are noncash expenses.

Interest

Interest is the cost to borrow money. If interest is 10 percent per year, then the cost to borrow $1,000 for one year is $100.

Other Expenses

Other expenses is a catchall category for miscellaneous operating expenses that are not considered significant enough to be listed separately. This category includes all general and administrative expenses, rent, utilities, and contracted services not included in the other categories. Although they are grouped in this example, they may be reported separately.

Operating and Nonoperating Items

The FASB requires that not-for-profit health care entities present an intermediate measure of operations. This can be expressed as *excess of revenue over expenses, revenues and gains over expenses and losses, earned income,* or *performance earnings*. However, within a class or classes of changes in net assets, a not-for-profit entity may classify items as operating and nonoperating, expendable and nonexpendable, earned and unearned, recurring and nonrecurring, or in various other ways. Exhibit 2.18 illustrates the

Operating Income
Operating income is a classification within *excess of revenues over expenses*, which separates revenues earned through health care-related activities (*operating income*) and those earned from other than health care-related activities (*nonoperating items*). Note that nonoperating items are most often a mixture of revenues, gains, *and* losses. Investment income (loss) is reported as nonoperating.

EXHIBIT 2.18 CONSOLIDATED STATEMENTS OF OPERATIONS AND CHANGES IN NET ASSETS FROM EXHIBIT 2.14a, EMPHASIS ON NONOPERATING ITEMS (IN THOUSANDS)

Dunhill Health System
Consolidated Statements of Operations and Changes in Net Assets
Year Ended June 30, 2012
(in thousands)

Unrestricted revenue	
Net patient service revenue	$ 4,402,759
Provision for bad debts	(265,850)
Net patient service revenue less provision for bad debts	4,136,909
Capitation and premium revenue	234,822
Net assets released from restrictions	7,103
Other revenue	385,416
Total unrestricted revenue	4,764,250
Expenses	
Salaries and wages	1,971,053
Employee benefits	436,580
Contract labor	46,722
Total labor expenses	2,454,355
Supplies	820,513
Purchased services	491,716
Depreciation and amortization	269,880
Occupancy	184,312
Medical claims and capitation purchased services	97,526
Interest	55,388
Other	237,628
Total expenses	4,611,318
Operating income	152,932
Nonoperating items	
Investment (loss) income	(11,655)
Change in market value and cash payments of interest rate swaps	(82,039)
Loss from early extinguishment of debt	(5,892)
Gain on bargain purchase and inherent contribution	137,658
Other, including income taxes	15,291
Total nonoperating items	53,363
Excess of revenue over expenses	206,295
Less excess of revenue over expenses attributable to noncontrolling interest	5,402
Excess of revenue over expenses, net of noncontrolling interest	$ 200,893

contrast between operating and nonoperating items in a statement of operations.

Excess of Revenues over Expenses

Excess of revenues over expenses is analogous to *income from continuing operations* (profit) in an investor-owned entity. However, not-for-profit business entities are prohibited from using the more common term *net income*. This item, traditionally referred to as the *bottom line* in investor-owned entities, is not actually the bottom line in the statement of operations because not-for-profit health care entities do not have other comprehensive income, the way that investor-owned entities do. Accounting literature created the term *performance indicator* to describe this intermediate measure.

Net Income
Equivalent to *excess of revenue over expenses* for a not-for-profit entity.

People in the industry refer to this point in the combined statement of operations and statement of changes in net assets as *the line*.

Items Reported outside the Performance Indicator (below the line)

Items that are reported outside the performance indicator (below the line) include the following:

- Transactions with owners or transfers to or from other entities that control the reporting entity, are controlled by it, or are under common control with it.
- Receipt of restricted contributions (these are included in the statement of changes in net assets in the temporarily or permanently restricted category).
- Contributions of long-lived assets such as property and equipment, and assets released from donor restrictions related to such long-lived assets.
- Items related to retirement benefits, effective portion of the gain or loss on derivative instruments related to hedging activities, and foreign currency translation adjustments.
- Extraordinary items and the effect of discontinued operations.
- Unrealized gains or losses on investments other than trading securities.
- Investment returns restricted by donors or law.

- Investment losses from endowment funds that reduce the corpus below its original value, and amounts restoring the endowment fund.
- An inherent contribution from an acquisition.

It is not necessary for health care managers to understand all of these items in great detail unless they are in the accounting or finance function. It is simply enough to understand that these items are not related to ongoing operations. Certain of the more common of these items are discussed below.

Change in Net Unrealized Gains and Losses on Investments Other Than Trading Securities

Although the guidelines pertaining to this item are complex, for most not-for-profit health care entities the amount reported here is the change in equity interest in stocks that do not trade in the public market, such as venture capital funds or limited partnerships in a physician practice. It is called *unrealized* because until the asset is disposed of (i.e., sold), the gain or loss occurs only on the books. Once the investment is disposed of, the gain or loss becomes a *realized* gain or loss.

For example, assume that on the last day of last year, an entity purchased $1,000,000 of stock in a public company. One year later, the stock is worth $1,300,000. The entity must report a $300,000 *unrealized* gain. Conversely, if the stock was sold for $1,300,000 during the year, the entity would report a $300,000 *realized* gain.

Increases in Long-Lived Unrestricted Net Assets

Increases in unrestricted long-term assets resulting from donations are not considered operating items but are reported below the performance indicator.

 Key Point Rather than being reported under *unrestricted revenue*, increases relating to the donation of unrestricted net assets for capital acquisitions are reported under *excess of revenue over expenses*.

Transfers to Parent

Another item that affects unrestricted net assets but is not an operating item is the transfer of assets to corporate headquarters (*transfer to parent*).

Extraordinary Items

Extraordinary items reflect unusual *and* infrequent gains or losses from such things as acts of nature (e.g., hurricanes or earthquakes). Paying off a loan early (generally through refinancing), which is referred to as *extinguishment of debt*, can also be an extraordinary item. Before classifying any of these items as extraordinary, it is important that both the *unusual* and the *infrequent* criteria be met. For example, if the entity is in the habit of refinancing or if hurricanes are a frequent occurrence due to the entity's geographical location, these items may just be gains or losses. Note that Dunhill considers the early extinguishment of debt to be a nonoperating loss, not an extraordinary item (Exhibit 2.18).

The Statement of Changes in Net Assets

A third financial statement is the statement of changes in net assets. Its purpose is to explain why there was a change from one year to the next in the entire net asset section of the balance sheet (Exhibit 2.4). There are two major reasons why the net asset section of the balance sheet changes from year to year: increases (decreases) in unrestricted net assets as discussed earlier and changes in temporarily and permanently restricted net assets, which are not included on the statement of operations. Note that as discussed above, many health care entities combine this statement with the statement of operations, producing a statement of operations and changes in net assets. Exhibit 2.19 illustrates the consolidated statement of changes in net assets apart from the consolidated statement of operations.

Key Point The statement of changes in net assets repeats some of the information found on the statement of operations to explain changes in unrestricted net assets but also adds information about changes in restricted net assets.

Like the other statements, the statement of changes in net assets has a descriptive heading, a body, and notes. The body of the statement of changes in net assets, as shown in Exhibit 2.19, is organized to represent the changes in each of the three categories of restrictions of net assets: unrestricted, temporarily restricted, and permanently restricted. The information in the first section, unrestricted net assets, summarizes

EXHIBIT 2.19 CONSOLIDATED STATEMENTS OF OPERATIONS AND CHANGES IN NET ASSETS FROM EXHIBIT 2.14, EMPHASIS ON NET ASSETS (IN THOUSANDS)

Dunhill Health System
Consolidated Statements of Operations and Changes in Net Assets
Years Ended June 30, 2012 and 2011
(in thousands)

	2012
Unrestricted net assets	
Excess of revenue over expenses	$206,295
Net assets released from restrictions for capital acquisitions	12,381
Net change in retirement plan related items	127,328
Other	195
Increase in unrestricted net assets before discontinued operations	346,199
Discontinued operations—Greater Suffolk Health System (GSHS)	
Net change in retirement plan related items	58,731
Loss from operations	(58,620)
Increase in unrestricted net assets	346,310
Temporarily restricted net assets	
Contributions	32,120
Net assets released from restrictions	(16,325)
Other	1,409
Increase in temporarily restricted net assets	17,204
Permanently restricted net assets	
Contributions for endowment funds	4,067
Net investment (loss)	(261)
Other	(387)
Increase in permanently restricted net assets	3,419
Increase in net assets	366,933
Net assets, beginning of year	2,501,113
Net assets, end of year	$2,868,046

the information from the statement of operations. The information in the remainder of the statement of changes in net assets reflects changes in restricted accounts.

Changes in Unrestricted Net Assets

The unrestricted net assets (see Exhibit 2.19) section begins with the excess of revenue over expenses (performance indicator), which comes directly from the statement of operations. During the year 2012, Dunhill Health System's excess of revenue over expenses was $206,295 (in thousands), and those items that are reported outside the performance indicator (or below the line), that is, adjustments for net assets released from restrictions for capital acquisitions, net change in retirement plan, and other related accounts, increased unrestricted net assets before discontinued operations by $346,199. Adjusting for items related to the discontinued operations of the Greater Suffolk Health System resulted in a net increase in unrestricted net assets of $346,310.

Key Point The unrestricted section of the statement of changes in net assets shows how the various items on the statement of operations contributed to the changes in unrestricted net assets.

Changes in Temporarily Restricted Net Assets

During 2012, Dunhill Health System received $32,120 in restricted contributions, released $16,325 from temporary restrictions, and had adjustments of other accounts of $1,409. A portion of the assets released from restriction (in the amount of $12,381) is shown below excess of revenue over expenses in the net assets released from restrictions for capital acquisitions account because it is to be used for the acquisition of long-lived capital assets.

Changes in Permanently Restricted Net Assets

For Dunhill Health System the changes in permanently restricted net assets in 2012 were an increase of $4,067 for a permanently restricted endowment contribution and an investment loss of $261 (net), as well as a decline of $387 in other permanent endowment accounts (Exhibit 2.19).

The Statement of Cash Flows

The *statement of cash flows* answers the question, Where did cash come from and where did it go? Although some may believe that the statement of operations answers this question, it does not. The cash flow statement takes the accrual basis financial statements that report activity as it was earned and expended or committed for expenditure, and converts it to the actual flow of cash. Like the other statements, the statement of cash flows has a descriptive heading, a body, and notes (see Exhibits 2.20 and A.4). The statement of cash flows covers the same time period as the statement of operations and the statement of changes in net assets do.

The body of the statement is organized into the following sections:

- Cash flows from operating activities
- Cash flows from investing activities
- Cash flows from financing activities
- Net increase (decrease) in cash and cash equivalents

The statement also discloses key noncash investing and financing transactions such as the issuance of stock for debt payment or for the acquisition of a company. These disclosures are at the bottom of the statement.

There are two forms of this statement; the most common, called the *indirect method*, has been presented here. The other form is called the *direct method*. The first section of the statement shown here is cash flows from operating activities.

EXHIBIT 2.20 ANNOTATED STATEMENT OF CASH FLOWS FOR SAMPLE NOT-FOR-PROFIT HOSPITAL

The statement of cash flows provides a summary of the cash inflows and outflows during the year.

1 **Title**. The name of the organization, the name of the financial statement, and the period(s) for which the information is being provided.

2 **Cash flows from operating activities**. This section explains the changes in cash resulting from the normal operating activities of the organization. It begins by presenting the change in net assets from the statement of changes in net assets. However, since the statement of changes in net assets is prepared on the accrual basis of accounting to show revenues when earned not when cash was received, and expenses when resources were used rather than when they were paid for, the remainder of this section makes adjustments to convert the changes in current assets and liabilities and other operating accounts to actual cash flows. This is explained in more detail in the next chapter.

3 **Cash flows from investing activities**. This section explains cash inflows and outflows resulting from investing activities such as purchasing and selling investments or from investing in the organization itself by, for example, purchasing or selling plant, property, or equipment.

4 **Cash flows from financing activities**. This section explains cash inflows and outflows resulting from financing activities such as obtaining grants and endowments, or from borrowing or paying back long-term debt. It also includes transfers to and from the parent corporation.

5 **Net increase (decrease) in cash and cash equivalents**. The total of cash flows from operating, investing, and financing activities.

6 **Cash and cash equivalents at beginning of year**. The amount of cash and cash equivalents that the organization had at the beginning of the year.

7 **Cash and cash equivalents at end of year**. The amount of cash and cash equivalents that the organization had at the end of the year.

8 **Supplemental information**. Additional information of use to the reader of the statement. This is limited to noncash investing and financing information, including cash paid for interest.

(Continued)

EXHIBIT 2.20 (CONTINUED)

1

Dunhill Health System
Consolidated Statement of Cash Flows
Year Ended June 30, 2012
(in thousands)

2 **Operating activities**

(Decrease) increase in net assets	$366,933
Adjustments to reconcile change in net assets to net cash provided by operating activities:	
Depreciation and amortization	269,880
Provision for bad debts	(265,850)
Deferred retirement loss (gain) arising during the year	175,414
Cumulative effect of a change in accounting principle	0
Change in net unrealized and realized gains on investments	73,007
Change in market values of interest rate swaps	77,981
Undistributed equity earnings from unconsolidated affiliates	(14,077)
Loss (gain) on disposals of property and equipment	(285)
Restricted contributions and investment income received	(8,844)
Restricted net assets acquired related to UMHS and NDHS	(16,882)
Gain: bargain purchase agreement & inherent contribution—UMHS and NDHS	(94,732)
Net change in retirement plan items due to transfer of shares of GSHS	(12,211)
Loss on transfer of shares of the GSHS	15,770
Decrease in noncontrolling interest due to transfer of the BCHS	51,713
Loss from extinguishment of debt	5,688
Gain on sales of unconsolidated affiliates	(2,107)
Other adjustments	1,681
Changes in, excluding assets acquired	
Patient accounts receivable	(303,988)
Other assets	(23,056)
Accounts payable and accrued expenses	28,750
Estimated receivables from and payables to third-party payors, net	5,129
Self-insurance reserves	21,799
Accrued pension and retiree health costs	(39,720)
Other liabilities	(8,871)
Total adjustments	(63,811)
Net cash provided by operating activities	303,122

3 **Investing activities**

Purchases of investment	(1,135,476)
Proceeds from sales of investments	1,155,328
Purchases of property and equipment	(267,650)
Acquisition of subsidiaries, net of $51.2 million and $5.4 million cash assumed in 2012 and 2011, respectively	(57,216)
Dividends received from unconsolidated affiliates and other changes	15,098
(Increase) decrease in assets limited as to use	512
Proceeds received from the transfer of shares of GSHS	10,284
Proceeds from sale of unconsolidated affiliates	2,370
Proceeds from disposal of property and equipment	2,281
Net cash used in investing activities	(274,469)

4 **Financing activities**

Proceeds from issuance of debt	611,092
Repayments of debt	(557,544)
Net increase (decrease) in commercial paper	16,980
Increase in financing costs and other	(5,634)
Restricted net assets acquired related to UMHS and NDHS	17,027
Proceeds from restricted contributions and restricted investment income	14,283
Net cash provided by financing activities	96,204

5	**Net increase (decrease) in cash and cash equivalents**	124,857
6	**Cash and cash equivalents, beginning of year**	302,511
7	**Cash and cash equivalents, end of year**	$427,368
8	**Supplemental disclosures and cash flow information**	
	Cash paid for interest (net of amounts capitalized)	$55,314
	New capital lease obligations for buildings and equipment	3,176
	Accruals for purchases of property and equipment and other long-term assets	21,327
	Unsettled investment trades, purchases	6,408
	Unsettled investment trades, sales	7,022

Cash Flows from Operating Activities

This section identifies the cash inflows and outflows resulting from the normal operations of an entity. Because most entities do not have this information readily available, they derive it by starting with the increase (decrease) in net assets from the statement of changes in net assets and then making adjustments to convert this accrual-based information into cash flows.

Assume for the purposes of illustration that the entity began with no assets or liabilities. During its first week in operation, only two transactions occurred: $150,000 worth of services were rendered, and patients paid $50,000 of this amount. Thus the balance sheet would show *cash* of $50,000, *patient accounts receivable* of $100,000, and *net assets* of $150,000. Hence, the increase in net assets since the last period would be $150,000 (Exhibit 2.21).

Key Point *Cash flows from operating activities* identifies cash flow from the operations of the entity.

To estimate cash flows from operations, however, net assets must be adjusted for changes in accounts that really do not result in cash inflows or outflows. In this case the $100,000 that is still owed from the $150,000 in changes in net assets is subtracted to determine how much cash actually came in ($150,000 − $100,000 = $50,000). This process occurs in order to convert the changes in net assets account, which was derived using the accrual basis of accounting, into an estimate of actual cash flows: net cash provided from operating activities.

Cash Flows from Investing Activities

The second section of the statement of cash flows is *cash flows from investing activities*. This section shows cash inflows and outflows from such accounts as

- Purchase of plant, property, and equipment
- Purchase of long-term investments
- Proceeds from sale of plant, property, and equipment
- Proceeds from sale of long-term investments

EXHIBIT 2.21 DERIVING NET CASH PROVIDED BY OPERATING ACTIVITIES BY ADJUSTING CHANGE IN NET ASSETS FOR ITEMS THAT DO NOT AFFECT CASH FLOWS

Sample Not-for-Profit Hospital

Balance Sheets

January 7, 20X1, and January 1, 20X1

	1/7/20X1	1/1/20X1		1/7/20X1	1/1/20X1
Cash	$50,000	$0	Liabilities	$0	$0
Patient accounts receivable	100,000	0	Net assets	150,000	0
Total assets	$150,000	$0	Liabilities and net assets	$150,000	$0

Sample Not-for-Profit Hospital

Statement of Cash Flows

for the Period Ended January 7, 20X1

	1/7/20X1	1/1/20X1
Cash flows from operating activities		
Changes in net assets	$150,000	$0
Increase in patient accounts receivable	100,000	0
Net cash provided by operating activities	**$50,000**	$0

 Key Point Investing by an entity includes investing in itself (such as when an entity buys new equipment).

Information found in this section is derived from changes in the non-current assets section of the balance sheet from one period to the next. It reports both the purchase or sale (or both) of outside investments and the purchase or sale (or both) of noncurrent assets, such as plant and equipment, which will be used to provide services. In the latter case, the entity is investing in itself.

Cash Flows from Financing Activities

In this section of the statement of cash flows, we identify the changes in cash flows resulting from financing activities. These include

- Transfers to parent
- Proceeds from selected contributions
- Proceeds from issuance of long-term debt
- Repayment of long-term debt
- Interest from restricted investments if interest income is also restricted

Key Point Repayment and issuance of long-term debt are identified in *cash flow from financing activities* in the statement of cash flows.

Cash and Cash Equivalents at the End of the Year

This is the "bottom line" of the statement of cash flows and is the same as the *cash and cash equivalents* amount that appears on the balance sheet. The latter is calculated by adding the net increase (decrease) in cash and cash equivalents for the year to the beginning balance of the cash and cash equivalents. The net increase (decrease) in cash and cash equivalents for the year on the statement of cash flows is computed by adding together the cash flows from the operating, investing, and financing activities, respectively. In Exhibit 2.20, the cash and cash equivalents at the end of 20X1 is $427,368 (in thousands).

Summary

This chapter examined the basic financial statements of not-for-profit, business-oriented health care entities: the balance sheet, the statement of operations, the statement of changes in net assets, and the statement of cash flows. Each of these statements is organized in the same way with a heading, a body, and notes. The notes are grouped together and presented after all four statements have been provided. They are considered an integral part of the financial statements.

The balance sheet presents a snapshot of the entity as of a point in time (usually the last day of the fiscal year). The body of the balance sheet has three major sections: assets, liabilities, and net assets. The balance sheet is so named because *Assets = Liabilities + Stockholders' Equity.* This fundamental accounting equation is expressed as Assets = Liabilities + Stockholders' Equity in investor-owned health care entities and Assets = Liabilities + Net Assets in not-for-profit, business-oriented health care entities.

Assets are the resources of the entity, liabilities are the obligations of the entity to pay its creditors, and net assets are the residual, or the difference between assets and liabilities. Assets are divided into two main sections: current and noncurrent. Current assets will be used or consumed within one year. Noncurrent assets will provide benefit to the entity for periods longer than one year. Liabilities are also classified into current and noncurrent categories. Current liabilities are those that must be paid within one year. Noncurrent liabilities will be due in more than one year. If part of a liability, such as a mortgage, is due within one year and the rest is due beyond one year, then the part due within one year is classified in the current section, and the remainder is presented under noncurrent liabilities. Revenues received in advance, such as capitated fees, are liabilities, classified as deferred revenue. They are considered liabilities because the entity has the obligation to deliver service. They are not recognized as revenues until they are earned.

Net assets are the stakeholders' interest in the entity's assets. The stakeholders of not-for-profit entities are generally assumed to be the community members. Net assets are presented in three categories: unrestricted, temporarily restricted, and permanently restricted. Unrestricted net assets are not constrained by donors. Restricted net assets are funds that have limitations imposed on them by outside donors.

The statement of operations is analogous to, but not the same as, the traditional income statement. The performance indicator, the excess of revenues over expenses, is the dividing line between those items that are considered to be related to the operations of the entity and those that are not. It is an earnings measure of the not-for-profit entity, in the same way that net income is for an investor-owned entity. The statement of change in net assets recaps the change in unrestricted net assets and adds the changes in temporarily and permanently restricted net assets.

The final financial statement of not-for-profit health care entities is the statement of cash flows. Its purpose is to summarize where the entity's cash came from and how it was spent during the year. It summarizes cash flows in three major categories: cash flows from operating activities, cash flows from investing activities, and cash flows from financing activities. This statement is necessary because the statement of operations is based on the accrual basis of accounting and reports the actual activity of the entity but not the cash flows.

KEY TERMS

a.	Accumulated depreciation	**o.**	Held to maturity security
b.	Amortization	**p.**	Liabilities
c.	Assets	**q.**	Liquidity
d.	Available for sale security	**r.**	Long-lived asset
e.	Basic accounting equation	**s.**	Net assets
f.	Charity care discounts	**t.**	Net income
g.	Classified balance sheet	**u.**	Noncurrent assets
h.	Comparative financial statements	**v.**	Noncurrent liabilities
		w.	Notes to the financial statements
i.	Current assets		
j.	Current liabilities	**x.**	Operating income
k.	Deferred revenue	**y.**	Performance indicator
l.	Depreciation	**z.**	Stockholders' equity
m.	Fair value	**aa.**	Third-party payors
n.	Goodwill	**bb.**	Trading security

Key Equations

- General accounting equation:

$$\text{Assets} = \text{Liabilities} + \text{Stockholders' Equity}$$

- Basic accounting equation (not-for-profit entities):

$$\text{Assets} = \text{Liabilities} + \text{Net Assets}$$

- Basic accounting equation (for-profit entities):

$$\text{Assets} = \text{Liabilities} + \text{Stockholders' Equity}$$

REVIEW QUESTIONS AND PROBLEMS

1. **Definitions**. Define the terms in the key terms list.

2. **Financial statement terminology**.

   a. What are each of the major financial statements commonly called in for-profit health care entities? In not-for-profit health care entities?

   b. Describe the three major sections common to all financial statements.

3. **Balance equation**. What is the primary accounting equation that describes the balance sheet of a not-for-profit, business-oriented health care entity?

4. **Balance sheet**. The following questions relate to the balance sheet:

   a. What is the name of this statement in not-for-profit health care entities?

   b. What are its main sections in investor-owned health care entities?

   c. What are its main sections in not-for-profit health care entities?

   d. What is deducted from gross patient accounts receivable to arrive at net patient accounts receivable?

   e. What are some examples of deferred revenue?

   f. What kinds of restrictions are put on net assets?

5. **Statement of operations**. The following questions relate to the statement of operations of not-for-profit health care entities:

   a. What are the major reductions of revenue taken to get from gross to net patient service revenue?

   b. What are major components of expenses?

   c. What is the performance indicator?

   d. How do net assets get released from restriction?

6. **Statement of changes in net assets**. The following questions relate to the statement of changes in net assets:

   a. What is the purpose of this statement?

   b. What are the main sections of this statement?

   c. What is the difference between permanently restricted and temporarily restricted net assets?

7. **Statement of cash flows**. The following questions relate to the statement of cash flows of a not-for-profit health care entity:

   a. What are the statement's main sections?

   b. What is the purpose of this statement?

8. **Financial statement element.** Where in the financial statements does importa[...] atory information appear?

9. **Financial statement element.** In which financial statement would an entity identify its purchase of long-term investments?

10. **Accounting methods.** How does the accrual basis of accounting differ from the cash basis of accounting?

11. **Balance sheet.** The following are account balances as of September 30, 20X1, for Ray Hospital. Prepare a balance sheet at September 30, 20X1. (*Hint:* net assets will also need to be calculated.)

what you have are take en the day

Givens

(a) asset

(l) liabilities

a	Gross plant, property, and equipment	– $70,000,000
	Accrued expenses	$6,000,000
a	Cash	– $8,000,000
a	Net accounts receivable	– $15,500,000
l	Accounts payable	$7,000,000
l	Long-term debt	$45,000,000
a	Supplies	– $3,000,000
a	Accumulated depreciation	– $5,000,000

ex) value of house ↓

12. **Balance sheet.** The following are account balances as of September 30, 20X1, for Stone Hospital. Prepare a balance sheet at September 30, 20X1. (*Hint:* net assets will also need to be calculated.)

Givens

a	Gross plant, property, and equipment	$65,000,000
a	Cash	$6,000,000
a	Net accounts receivable	$12,700,000
l	Accrued expenses	$5,200,000
a	Inventory	$5,300,000
l	Long-term debt	$22,500,000
l	Accounts payable	$8,300,000
a	Accumulated depreciation	– $28,500,000

13. **Statement of operations.** The following are annual account balances as of September 30, 20X1, for Snead Hospital. Prepare the portion of the statement of operations ending with operating income for the 12-month period ending September 30, 20X1.

Givens

Net patient revenue	$720,000
Interest expense	$18,000
Net assets released from restriction for operations	$220,000
Depreciation expense	$65,000
Labor expense	$444,000
Provision for bad debt	$7,000
Supply expense	$144,000

14. **Statement of operations.** The following are annual account balances as of September 30, 20X1, for Moore Hospital. Prepare a statement of operations for the 12-month period ending September 30, 20X1.

Givens

Patient service revenue (net of contractuals)	$950,000
Supply expense	$255,000
Net assets released from restriction for operations	$45,000
Depreciation expense	$35,000
Transfer to parent corporation	$9,500
Labor expense	$300,000
Provision for bad debts	$12,000
Unrealized gains from available for sale securities	$150,000

15. **Multiple statements.** The following are account balances as of September 30, 20X1, for Exton Outpatient Center. Prepare (a) a balance sheet, (b) a statement of operations, and (c) a statement of changes in net assets for September 30, 20X1.

Givens

Insurance expense	$55,000
Depreciation expense	$33,000
Cash	$61,000
General expense	$255,000
Patient revenue (net of contractuals)	$1,100,000
Transfer to parent corporation	$55,000
Net accounts receivable	$350,000
Beginning balance, unrestricted net assets	$275,000
Ending balance, temporarily restricted net assets	$48,000
Accounts payable	$23,000
Wages payable	$37,000
Beginning balance, temporarily restricted net assets	$70,000
Prepaid expenses	$8,000
Provision for bad debts	$8,000
Long-term debt	$270,000

Labor expense	$470,000
Supply expense	$65,000
Accumulated depreciation	$450,000
Gross plant, property, and equipment	$900,000
Ending / beginning balance, permanently restricted net assets	$35,000
Net assets released from temporary restriction	$22,000
Ending balance, unrestricted net assets	$456,000

16. **Multiple statements**. The following are account balances (in thousands) on September 30, 20X1, for Marview Medical Center. Prepare (a) a balance sheet, (b) a statement of operations, and (c) a statement of changes in net assets for September 30, 20X1.

Givens (in '000s)

Administrative expense	$35,000
Depreciation expense	$33,000
Cash	$42,000
General expense	$85,000
Patient revenue (net of contractuals)	$555,000
Transfer to parent corporation	$7,000
Gross accounts receivable	$53,000
Beginning balance, unrestricted net assets	$155,600
Ending balance, temporarily restricted net assets	$5,000
Accounts payable	$24,000
Wages payable	$14,000
Beginning balance, temporarily restricted net assets	$13,000
Prepaid expenses	$8,000
Provision for bad debt expense	$6,500
Long-term debt	$482,300
Labor expense	$144,000
Supply expense	$61,000
Accumulated depreciation	$100,000
Gross plant, property, and equipment	$660,000
Ending / beginning balance, permanently restricted net assets	$11,000
Net assets released from restriction for operations	$8,000
Ending balance, unrestricted net assets	$356,300
Uncollectibles in accounts receivable	$5,000
Accrued expenses	$4,100
Inventory	$9,000
Temporary investments	$9,200
Premium revenue	$6,200
Other revenue	$3,000
Long-term investments, unrestricted	$222,000
Current portion of long-term debt	$1,500

17. **Statement of cash flows.** The following are account balances (in thousands) at December 31, 20X1, for Sunview Hospital. Prepare a statement of cash flows for the year ended December 31, 20X1. (*Hint*: the amounts have been stated as positive or negative numbers as they affect cash flow.)

Givens (in '000s)

Decrease in prepaid expenses	$2,500
Payments on long-term debt	($7,000)
Cash and cash equivalents at beginning of the year	$24,000
Increase in inventory	($3,300)
Increases in long-term debt	$175,000
Decrease in accrued expenses	($2,400)
Change in net assets	$6,500
Sale of long-term investments	$31,000
Increase in other current liabilities	$2,600
Depreciation	$6,600
Payments on capital lease	($6,100)
Purchases of equipment	($177,000)
Increase in net account receivables	($50,000)
Increase in accounts payable	$40,000

18. **Statement of cash flows.** The following are account balances (in thousands) at December 31, 20X1, for Hilltop Hospital. Prepare a statement of cash flows for the year ended December 31, 20X1. (*Hint*: the amounts have been stated as positive or negative numbers as they affect cash flow.)

Givens (in '000s)

Increase in prepaid expenses	($8,000)
Increase in accrued expenses	$6,000
Cash and cash equivalents at beginning of the year	$62,000
Proceeds from restricted contribution	$119,000
Change in net assets	$12,000
Increase in net account receivables	($27,000)
Sale of equipment	$46,000
Decrease in other current liabilities	($6,100)
Depreciation	$43,000
Decrease in inventory	$8,000
Purchase of long-term investments	($111,000)
Payments on long-term debt	($72,000)
Decrease in accounts payable	($13,000)

19. **Multiple statements.** The following are account balances (in thousands) for Lima Health Plan. Prepare (a) a balance sheet and (b) an income statement for the year ended December 31, 20X0.

Givens (in '000s)

Income tax benefit of operating loss	$8,000
Net property and equipment	$2,000
Physician services expense	$164,000
Premium revenue	$125,000
Marketing expense	$11,000
Compensation expense	$13,000
Interest income and other revenue	$6,000
Outside referral expense	$4,000
Medicare revenue	$131,000
Occupancy and depreciation expense	$2,000
Medical claims payable	$37,000
Accounts receivable	$3,000
Emergency room expense	$14,000
Inpatient services expense	$101,000
Interest expense	$2,000
Medicaid revenue	$35,000
Owners' equity	$61,500
Cash and cash equivalents	$97,000
Long-term debt	$3,500
Other administrative expense	$2,000

20. **Multiple statements.** The following are account balances (in thousands) at September 30, 20X1, for Media Health Plan. Prepare (a) a balance sheet and (b) an income statement.

Givens (in '000s)

Income tax expense	$600
Prepaid expenses	$3,000
Physician services expense	$7,000
Premium revenue	$23,000
Cash and cash equivalents	$18,900
Marketing expense	$600
Compensation expense	$1,900
Other noncurrent assets	$3,100
Interest income and other revenue	$2,100
Accrued expenses	$3,700
Outside referral expense	$4,000

Claims payable—medical	$18,000
Medicare revenue	$9,000
Occupancy and depreciation expense	$400
Owners' equity	$5,300
Emergency room expense	$2,400
Net property and equipment	$5,000
Premium receivables	$2,800
Inpatient service expense	$8,400
Notes payable	$1,700
Interest expense	$900
Unearned premium revenue	$2,000
Medicaid revenue	$7,000
Long-term debt	$2,100
Other administrative expense	$600

21. **Multiple statements.** The following are account balances (in thousands) at September 30, 20X1, for Louis Medical Center. Prepare (a) a balance sheet, (b) a statement of operations, and (c) a statement of changes in net assets for September 30, 20X1.

Givens (in '000s)

Inventory	$7,000
Patient revenue (net of contractual allowance)	$220,000
Gross plant, property, and equipment	$161,900
Net accounts receivable	$65,000
Ending balance, temporarily restricted net assets	$9,300
Wages payable	$18,000
Long-term debt	$104,000
Supply expense	$18,000
Net assets released from temporary restriction	$3,500
Depreciation expense	$20,000
General expense	$40,000
Provision for bad debt expense	$12,000
Cash and cash equivalents	$7,500
Transfer to parent corporation	($3,300)
Beginning balance, unrestricted net assets	$70,000
Accounts payable	$12,000
Beginning balance, temporarily restricted net assets	$12,800
Interest expense	$6,500
Labor expense	$77,600
Accumulated depreciation	$90,000
Long-term investments	$108,000
Ending balance, unrestricted net assets	$116,100

22. **Multiple statements.** The following are account balances (in thousands) at September 30, 20X1, for Sharpe Medical Center. Prepare (a) a balance sheet, (b) a statement of operations, and (c) a statement of changes in net assets for September 30, 20X1.

Givens (in '000s)

Inventory	$4,000
Patient revenue (net of contractuals)	$302,000
Gross plant, property, and equipment	$375,000
Net accounts receivable	$85,000
Ending balance, temporarily restricted net assets	$6,000
Wages payable	$6,600
Long-term debt	$218,400
Supply expense	$34,000
Net assets released from temporary restriction	$7,000
Depreciation expense	$44,000
General expense	$95,000
Provision for bad debt expense	$4,500
Cash and cash equivalents	$18,000
Transfer to parent corporation	($3,900)
Beginning balance, unrestricted net assets	$239,400
Accounts payable	$11,000
Beginning balance, temporarily restricted net assets	$13,000
Interest expense	$6,000
Labor expense	$123,000
Accumulated depreciation	$22,000
Long-term investments	$20,000
Ending balance, unrestricted net assets	$238,000

23. **Multiple statements.** The following are account balances (in thousands) at September 30, 20X1, for Putman Outpatient Center. Prepare (a) a balance sheet, (b) a statement of operations, and (c) a statement of changes in net assets for September 30, 20X1.

Givens (in '000s)

Insurance expense	$70,000
Cash	$23,000
Patient revenue (net of contractuals)	$614,000
Net accounts receivable	$25,000
Ending balance, temporarily restricted net assets	$8,700
Wages payable	$9,100
Prepaid expenses	$1,100
Long-term debt	$191,700
Supply expense	$66,000

Gross plant, property, and equipment	$556,000
Net assets released from temporary restriction	$8,000
Depreciation expense	$10,000
General expense	$95,000
Transfer to parent corporation	($8,000)
Beginning balance, unrestricted net assets	$203,400
Accounts payable	$21,000
Beginning balance, temporarily restricted net assets	$16,700
Provision for bad debt expense	$5,400
Labor expense	$145,000
Accumulated depreciation	$99,000
Long-term investments	$150,400
Ending balance, unrestricted net assets	$426,000

24. **Multiple statements.** The following are account balances (in thousands) at September 30, 20X1, for Chester Hospital. Prepare (a) a balance sheet, (b) a statement of operations, and (c) a statement of changes in net assets for September 30, 20X1.

Givens (in '000s)

Provision for bad debt expense	$10,200
Cash	$12,600
Patient revenues (net of contractuals)	$188,000
Net accounts receivable	$15,300
Ending balance, temporarily restricted net assets	$13,700
Wages payable	$7,800
Inventory	$4,400
Long-term debt	$39,000
Supply expense	$21,000
Gross plant, property, and equipment	$175,000
Net assets released from temporary restriction	$3,300
Depreciation expense	$10,000
General expense	$36,000
Transfer to parent corporation	($3,300)
Beginning balance, unrestricted net assets	$160,600
Accounts payable	$12,000
Beginning balance, temporarily restricted net assets	$17,000
Interest expense	$1,800
Labor expense	$105,000
Accumulated depreciation	$35,000
Long-term investments, restricted	$64,800
Ending balance, unrestricted net assets	$164,600

25. **Multiple statements.** The following are account balances (in thousands) at September 30, 20X1, for Upper Merion Hospital. Prepare (a) a balance sheet, (b) a statement of operations, and (c) a statement of changes in net assets for September 30, 20X1.

Givens (in '000s)

Provision for bad debt	$23,800
Cash	$30,000
Patient revenue (net of contractuals)	$275,000
Net accounts receivable	$42,100
Ending balance, temporarily restricted net assets	$15,900
Wages payable	$6,500
Inventory	$2,800
Long-term debt	$143,000
Supply expense	$55,000
Gross plant, property, and equipment	$290,000
Net assets released from temporary restriction	$2,100
Depreciation expense	$13,000
General expense	$19,000
Transfer to parent corporation	($2,800)
Beginning balance, unrestricted net assets	$234,000
Accounts payable	$15,000
Beginning balance, temporarily restricted net assets	$18,000
Interest expense	$9,000
Labor expense	$119,000
Accumulated depreciation	$35,000
Long-term investments	$120,000
Ending balance, unrestricted net assets	$269,500

Appendix A: Financial Statements for Sample Not-for-Profit and For-Profit Hospitals, and Notes to Financial Statements

EXHIBIT A.1 CONSOLIDATED BALANCE SHEETS FOR DUNHILL HEALTH SYSTEM

Dunhill Health System
Consolidated Balance Sheets
June 30, 2012 and 2011
(in thousands)

Assets	2012	2011
Current assets		
Cash and cash equivalents	$427,368	$302,511
Investments	1,246,310	105,480
Assets limited or restricted as to use, current portion	15,780	5,721
Patient accounts receivable, net of allowance for doubtful accounts of $98.6 million and $105.4 million in 2012 and 2011, respectively	532,715	418,986
Estimated receivables from third-party payors	64,077	51,238
Other receivables	74,389	65,420
Inventories	75,450	66,082
Assets held for sale	0	81,375
Prepaid expenses and other current assets	81,233	61,389
Total current assets	2,517,322	1,158,202
Assets limited or restricted as to use, noncurrent portion		
Held by trustees under bond indenture agreements	28,403	4,308
Self-insurance, benefit plans and other	228,732	116,588
By Board	1,204,519	1,097,238
By donors	58,753	62,471
Total assets limited or restricted as to use, noncurrent portion	1,520,407	1,280,605
Property and equipment, net	2,301,768	2,348,617
Investments in unconsolidated affiliates	73,912	62,317
Goodwill	60,322	59,028
Intangible assets, net of accumulated amortization of $5.1 million and $4.4 million in 2012 and 2011, respectively	35,711	12,798
Other assets	70,588	63,522
Total assets	$6,580,030	$4,985,089

Liabilities and net assets	2012	2011
Current liabilities		
Commercial paper	$55,008	$53,722
Short-term borrowings	511,301	607,189
Current portion of long-term debt	17,052	16,237
Accounts payable	182,390	155,481
Accrued expenses	145,688	72,907
Salaries, wages, and related liabilities	237,921	188,058
Estimated payables to third-party payors	146,092	79,650
Other current liabilities	72,377	103,210
Total current liabilities	1,367,829	1,276,454
Long-term debt, net of current portion	1,254,717	734,775
Self-insurance reserves	237,960	151,517
Accrued pension and retiree health costs	603,877	168,911
Other long-term liabilities	247,601	152,319
Total liabilities	3,711,984	2,483,976
Net assets		
Unrestricted net assets	2,761,115	2,378,170
Noncontrolling ownership interest in subsidiaries	11,413	48,048
Total unrestricted net assets	2,772,528	2,426,218
Temporarily restricted net assets	64,266	46,145
Noncontrolling ownership interest in subsidiaries		917
Total temporarily restricted net assets	64,266	47,062
Permanently restricted net assets	31,252	27,660
Noncontrolling ownership interest in subsidiaries	0	173
Total permanently restricted net assets	31,252	27,833
Total net assets	2,868,046	2,501,113
Total liabilities and net assets	$6,580,030	$4,985,089

The accompanying notes are an integral part of the consolidated financial statements.

Dunhill Health System
Consolidated Statements of Operations and Changes in Net Assets
Years Ended June 30, 2012 and 2011
(in thousands)

	2012	2011
Unrestricted revenue		
Patient service revenue (net of contractual allowances and discounts)	$4,402,759	$4,075,321
Provision for bad debts	(265,850)	(223,478)
Net patient service revenue less provision for bad debts	4,136,909	3,851,843
Capitation and premium revenue	234,822	189,750
Net assets released from restrictions	7,103	6,728
Other revenue	385,416	299,532
Total unrestricted revenue	4,764,250	4,347,853
Expenses		
Salaries and wages	1,971,053	1,863,278
Employee benefits	436,580	442,088
Contract labor	46,722	25,794
Total labor expenses	2,454,355	2,331,160
Supplies	820,513	652,871
Purchased services	491,716	433,605
Depreciation and amortization	269,880	242,232
Occupancy	184,312	170,298
Medical claims and capitation purchased services	97,526	95,620
Interest	55,388	44,714
Other	237,628	211,688
Total expenses	4,611,318	4,182,188
Operating income	152,932	165,665
Nonoperating items		
Investment (loss) income	(11,655)	251,666
Change in market value and cash payments of interest rate swaps	(82,039)	15,780
Loss from early extinguishment of debt	(5,892)	(6,648)
Gain on bargain purchase and inherent contribution	137,658	—
Other, including income taxes	15,291	(18,752)
Total nonoperating items	53,363	242,046
Excess of revenue over expenses	206,295	407,711
Less excess of revenue over expenses attributable to noncontrolling interest	5,402	4,732
Excess of revenue over expenses, net of noncontrolling interest	$200,893	$402,979

The accompanying notes are an integral part of the consolidated financial statements.

EXHIBIT A.3 CONSOLIDATED STATEMENTS OF OPERATIONS AND CHANGES IN NET ASSETS FOR DUNHILL HEALTH SYSTEM

Dunhill Health System
Consolidated Statements of Operations and Changes in Net Assets (continued)
Years Ended June 30, 2012 and 2011
(in thousands)

	2012	2011
Unrestricted net assets		
Excess of revenue over expenses	$206,295	$407,711
Net assets released from restrictions for capital acquisitions	9,222	5,181
Net change in retirement plan related items	130,487	116,618
Cumulative effect of change in accounting principle		(4,159)
Other	195	(4,096)
Increase in unrestricted net assets before discontinued operations	346,199	521,255
Discontinued operations—Greater Suffolk Health System (GSHS)		
Net change in retirement plan related items	58,731	
Loss from operations	(58,620)	4,804
Costs associated with transfer of shares		(898)
Increase in unrestricted net assets	346,310	525,161
Temporarily restricted net assets		
Contributions	32,120	10,141
Net investment gain		4,217
Net assets released from restrictions	(16,325)	(11,239)
Other	1,409	1,095
Increase in temporarily restricted net assets	17,204	4,214
Permanently restricted net assets		
Contributions for endowment funds	4,067	257
Net investment (loss)	(261)	1,777
Other	(387)	42
Increase in permanently restricted net assets	3,419	2,076
Increase in net assets	366,933	531,451
Net assets, beginning of year	2,501,113	1,969,662
Net assets, end of year	$2,868,046	$2,501,113

EXHIBIT A.4 CONSOLIDATED STATEMENTS OF CASH FLOWS FOR DUNHILL HEALTH SYSTEM

Dunhill Health System
Consolidated Statements of Cash Flows
Years Ended June 30, 2012 and 2011
(in thousands)

	2012	2011
Operating activities		
Increase in net assets	$366,933	$531,451
Adjustments to reconcile change in net assets to net cash provided by operating activities		
Depreciation and amortization	269,880	242,232
Provision for bad debts	(265,850)	(223,478)
Deferred retirement loss (gain) arising during the year	175,414	(285,774)
Cumulative effect of a change in accounting principle	0	5,691
Change in net unrealized and realized gains on investments	73,007	(54,102)
Change in market values of interest rate swaps	77,981	8,367
Undistributed equity earnings from unconsolidated affiliates	(14,077)	(11,572)
Loss (gain) on disposals of property and equipment	(285)	715
Restricted contributions and investment income received	(8,844)	(2,351)
Restricted net assets acquired related to UMHS and NDHS	(16,882)	0
Gain: bargain purchase agreement and inherent contribution—UMHS and NDHS	(94,732)	0
Net change in retirement plan items due to transfer of shares of GSHS	(12,211)	0
Loss on transfer of shares of the GSHS	15,770	0
Decrease in noncontrolling interest due to transfer of the BCHS	51,713	0
Loss from extinguishment of debt	5,688	1,708
Gain on sales of unconsolidated affiliates	(2,107)	(2,791)
Other adjustments	1,681	5,528
Changes in, excluding assets acquired		
Patient accounts receivable	(303,988)	(247,805)
Other assets	(23,056)	(18,511)
Accounts payable and accrued expenses	28,750	18,588
Estimated receivables from and payables to third-party payors, net	5,129	(31,076)
Self-insurance reserves	21,799	(5,999)
Accrued pension and retiree health costs	(39,720)	(90,212)
Other liabilities	(8,871)	11,389
Total adjustments	(63,811)	(679,453)
Net cash provided by (used in) operating activities	303,122	(148,002)
Investing activities		
Purchases of investment	(1,135,476)	(954,083)
Proceeds from sales of investments	1,155,328	998,212
Purchases of property and equipment	(267,650)	(350,211)
Acquisition of subsidiaries, net of $51.2 million and $5.4 million cash assumed in 2012 and 2011, respectively	(57,216)	(49,772)
Dividends received from unconsolidated affiliates and other changes	15,098	12,453
(Increase) decrease in assets limited as to use	512	(1,127)
Proceeds received from the transfer of shares of GSHS	10,284	43,881
Proceeds from sale of unconsolidated affiliates	2,370	6,840
Proceeds from disposal of property and equipment	2,281	3,418
Net cash used in investing activities	(274,469)	(290,389)
Financing activities		
Proceeds from issuance of debt	611,092	217,546
Repayments of debt	(557,544)	(172,089)
Net increase (decrease) in commercial paper	16,980	(27,560)
Increase in financing costs and other	(5,634)	(2,150)
Restricted net assets acquired related to UMHS and NDHS	17,027	0
Proceeds from restricted contributions and restricted investment income	14,283	3,289
Net cash provided by financing activities	96,204	19,036
Net increase (decrease) in cash and cash equivalents	124,857	(419,355)
Cash and cash equivalents, beginning of year	302,511	721,866
Cash and cash equivalents, end of year	$427,368	$302,511
Supplemental disclosures and cash flow information		
Cash paid for interest (net of amounts capitalized)	$55,314	$58,971
New capital lease obligations for buildings and equipment	3,176	568
Accruals for purchases of property and equipment and other long-term assets	21,327	21,344
Unsettled investment trades, purchases	6,408	3,281
Unsettled investment trades, sales	7,022	8,591

The accompanying notes are an integral part of the consolidated financial statements.

EXHIBIT A.5 CONSOLIDATED STATEMENTS OF OPERATIONS FOR LIFEPOINT HOSPITALS, INC.

LifePoint Hospitals, Inc.
Consolidated Statements of Operations
for the Years Ended December 31, 2011, 2010, and 2009
(in millions)

	2011	2010	2009
Revenues before provision for doubtful accounts	$3,544.6	$3,262.4	$2,962.7
Provision for doubtful accounts	518.5	443.8	375.4
Revenues	3,026.1	2,818.6	2,587.3
Salaries and benefits	1,364.7	1,270.3	1,170.9
Supplies	469.5	443.0	409.1
Other operating expenses	682.4	605.2	538.0
Other income	(26.7)	—	—
Depreciation and amortization	165.8	148.5	143.0
Interest expense, net	107.1	108.1	103.2
Debt extinguishment costs	—	2.4	—
Impairment charges	—	—	1.1
Total operating expenses	2,762.8	2,577.5	2,365.3
Income from continuing operations before income taxes	263.3	241.1	222.0
Provision for income taxes	97.8	82.4	80.3
Income from continuing operations	165.5	158.7	141.7
Income (loss) from discontinued operations, net of income taxes	0.2	(0.1)	(5.1)
Net income	165.7	158.6	136.6
Less: Net income attributable to noncontrolling interests	(2.8)	(3.1)	(2.5)
Net income attributable to LifePoint Hospitals, Inc.	$162.9	$155.5	$134.1

This exhibit omits per share data contained in the consolidated statements of operations, and these statements are also called "consolidated income statements."

LifePoint Hospitals, Inc.
Consolidated Statements of Comprehensive Income
for the Years Ended December 31, 2011, 2010, and 2009
(in millions)

	2011	2010	2009
Net income	$165.7	$158.6	$136.6
Other comprehensive income, net of income taxes			
Unrealized gains on changes in fair value of interest rate swap, net of income tax provisions of $2.8, $7.1, and $5.9 for the years ended December 31, 2011, 2010, and 2009, respectively	4.0	13.4	10.9
Other comprehensive income	4.0	13.4	10.9
Comprehensive income	169.7	172.0	147.5
Less: Net income attributable to noncontrolling interests	(2.8)	(3.1)	(2.5)
Comprehensive income attributable to LifePoint Hospitals, Inc.	$166.9	$168.9	$145.0

EXHIBIT A.6 CONSOLIDATED BALANCE SHEETS FOR LIFEPOINT HOSPITALS, INC.

LifePoint Hospitals, Inc.
Consolidated Balance Sheets
December 31, 2011 and 2010
(in millions)

	2011	2010
ASSETS		
Current assets		
Cash and cash equivalents	$126.2	$207.4
Accounts receivable, less allowances for doubtful accounts of $537.4 and $459.8 at December 31, 2011 and 2010, respectively	430.6	387.3
Inventories	87.2	84.6
Prepaid expenses	26.4	13.9
Income taxes receivable	1.6	5.5
Deferred tax assets	125.7	99.7
Other current assets	42.3	24.7
Total current assets:	840.0	823.1
Property and equipment, at cost		
Land	93.5	85.9
Buildings and improvements	1,631.6	1,532.9
Equipment	1,084.0	950.2
Construction in progress (estimated cost to complete and equip after December 31, 2011, is $80.7)	105.7	39.4
	2,914.8	2,608.4
Accumulated depreciation	(1,084.4)	(939.8)
Net property and equipment	1,830.4	1,668.6
Deferred loan costs, net	21.7	27.2
Intangible assets, net	89.5	73.1
Other	19.8	20.2
Goodwill	1,568.7	1,550.7
Total assets	$4,370.1	$4,162.9
LIABILITIES AND EQUITY		
Current liabilities		
Accounts payable	$99.6	$89.0
Accrued salaries	103.1	101.4
Interest rate swap	—	7.9
Other current liabilities	168.2	124.6
Current maturities of long-term debt	1.9	1.4
Total current liabilities	372.8	324.3
Long-term debt	1,595.4	1,570.5
Deferred income tax liabilities	259.0	211.2
Reserves for self-insurance claims and other liabilities	139.1	131.8
Long-term income tax liability	18.0	18.5
Total liabilities	2,384.3	2,256.3
Redeemable noncontrolling interests	26.2	15.3
Equity		
LifePoint Hospitals, Inc. stockholders' equity		
Preferred stock, $0.01 par value; 10,000,000 shares authorized; no shares issued	—	—
Common stock, $0.01 par value; 90,000,000 shares authorized; 63,233,088 and 61,450,098 shares issued at December 31, 2011 and 2010, respectively	0.6	0.6
Capital in excess of par value	1,354.8	1,289.4
Accumulated other comprehensive loss	—	(4.0)
Retained earnings	1,066.9	904.0
Common stock in treasury, at cost, 14,925,875 and 9,991,316 shares at December 31, 2011 and 2010, respectively	(477.1)	(302.5)
Total LifePoint Hospitals, Inc. stockholders' equity	1,945.2	1,887.5
Noncontrolling interests	14.4	3.8
Total equity	1,959.6	1,891.3
Total liabilities & stockholders' equity	$4,370.1	$4,162.9

Source: LifePoint's Form 10-K of December 2011, filed with the Securities and Exchange Commission.

EXHIBIT A.7 CONSOLIDATED STATEMENTS OF CASH FLOWS FOR LIFEPOINT HOSPITALS, INC.

LifePoint Hospitals, Inc.
Consolidated Statements of Cash Flows
for the Years Ended December 31, 2011, 2010, and 2009
(in millions)

	2011	2010	2009
Cash flows from operating activities			
Net income	$165.7	$158.6	$136.6
Adjustments to reconcile net income to net cash provided by operating activities			
(Income) loss from discontinued operations	(0.2)	0.1	5.1
Stock-based compensation	24.0	22.4	22.3
Depreciation and amortization	165.8	148.5	143.0
Amortization of physician minimum revenue guarantees	19.8	17.1	13.6
Amortization of convertible debt discounts	24.3	22.6	21.1
Amortization of deferred loan costs	5.9	7.1	8.3
Debt extinguishment costs	—	2.4	—
Deferred income taxes (benefit)	23.1	(29.0)	(7.2)
Reserve for self-insurance claims, net of payments	18.0	10.3	16.8
Increase (decrease) in cash from operating assets and liabilities, net of effects from acquisitions and divestitures			
Accounts receivable	(29.5)	(39.1)	(3.5)
Inventories and other current assets	(20.1)	(5.4)	(6.9)
Accounts payable and accrued expenses	2.9	13.2	(10.7)
Income taxes payable/receivable	3.9	48.8	9.9
Other	(2.4)	(1.9)	1.9
Net cash provided by operating activities—continuing operations	401.2	375.7	350.3
Net cash provided by (used in) operating activities—discontinued operations	0.3	(1.6)	(0.4)
Net cash provided by operating activities	401.5	374.1	349.9
Cash flows from investing activities			
Purchases of property and equipment	(219.9)	(168.7)	(166.6)
Acquisitions, net of cash acquired	(121.0)	(184.9)	(81.4)
Other	(1.2)	-	3.9
Net cash used in investing activities—continuing operations	(342.1)	(353.6)	(244.1)
Net cash provided by investing activities—discontinued operations	—	—	19.6
Net cash used in investing activities	342.1)	(353.6)	(224.5)
Cash flows from financing activities			
Proceeds from borrowings	—	400.0	—
Payments of borrowings	(0.1)	(255.2)	(13.5)
Repurchases of common stock	174.6)	(152.1)	(3.1)
Payment of debt financing costs	(0.4)	(13.7)	—
Proceeds from exercise of stock options	39.0	20.4	10.8
Proceeds from employee stock purchase plans	1.2	1.0	1.0
Distributions to noncontrolling interests, net of proceeds	(1.8)	(2.4)	(4.2)
(Repurchases) sales of redeemable noncontrolling interests	(2.3)	3.1	(0.8)
Capital lease payments and other	(1.6)	(1.4)	(4.1)
Net cash used in financing activities	(140.6)	(0.3)	(13.9)
Change in cash and cash equivalents	(81.2)	20.2	111.5
Cash and cash equivalents at beginning of year	207.4	187.2	75.7
Cash and cash equivalents at end of year	$126.2	$207.4	$187.2
Supplemental disclosure of cash flow information			
Interest payments	$79.2	$71.0	$76.1
Capitalized interest	$2.0	$0.8	$1.1
Income taxes paid, net	$71.0	$62.5	$75.4

Source: LifePoint's Form 10-K of December 2011, filed with the Securities and Exchange Commission.

EXHIBIT A.8 CONSOLIDATED STATEMENTS OF STOCKHOLDERS' EQUITY FOR LIFEPOINT HOSPITALS, INC.

LifePoint Hospitals, Inc.
Consolidated Statements of Stockholders' Equity
for the Years Ended December 31, 2011, 2010, and 2009
(in millions)

	Common Stock		Capital in Excess of Par Value	Accumulated Other Comprehensive Income (Loss)	Retained Earnings	Treasury Stock	Noncontrolling Interests	Total
	Shares	Amount						
Balance at January 1, 2009	53.4	$0.6	$1,212.6	$(28.3)	$614.4	$(147.3)	$3.5	$1,655.5
Net income					134.1		2.5	136.6
Other comprehensive income				10.9				10.9
Exercise of stock options and tax benefits of stock-based awards	0.8		11.8					11.8
Stock activity in connection with employee stock purchase plan	-		1.0					1.0
Stock-based compensation	0.8		22.3					22.3
Repurchases of common stock, at cost	(0.2)					(3.1)		(3.1)
Cash distributions to noncontrolling interests, net of proceeds			(1.3)				(2.9)	(4.2)
Balance at December 31, 2009	54.8	0.6	1,246.4	(17.4)	748.5	(150.4)	3.1	1,830.8
Net income					155.5		3.1	158.6
Other comprehensive income				13.4				13.4
Exercise of stock options and tax benefits of stock-based awards	0.7		19.7					19.7
Stock activity in connection with employee stock purchase plan	0.1		1.0					1.0
Stock-based compensation	0.4		22.4					22.4
Repurchases of common stock, at cost	(4.5)					(152.1)		(152.1)
Cash distributions to noncontrolling interests, net of proceeds			(0.1)				(2.4)	(2.5)
Balance at December 31, 2010	51.5	0.6	1,289.4	(4.0)	904.0	(302.5)	3.8	1,891.3
Net income					162.9		2.8	165.7
Other comprehensive income				4.0				4.0
Exercise of stock options and tax benefits of stock-based awards	1.3		43.5					43.5
Stock activity in connection with employee stock purchase plan	-		1.2					1.2
Stock-based compensation	0.4		24.0					24.0
Repurchases of common stock, at cost	(4.9)					(174.6)		(174.6)
Noncash change in noncontrolling interests as a result of acquisition and other			(3.7)				10.0	6.3
Cash proceeds from (cash distributions to) noncontrolling interests			0.4				(2.2)	(1.8)
Balance at December 31, 2011	48.3	$0.6	$1,354.8	$-	$1,066.9	$(477.1)	$14.4	$1,959.6

EXHIBIT A.9 SELECTED ACCOUNTING POLICIES AND OTHER FOOTNOTES FOR DUNHILL HEALTH SYSTEM

1.   **Summary of Significant Accounting Policies (in part)**

   a.   *Principles of consolidation.* The consolidated financial statements include the accounts of Dunhill Health System (the "Health System") and all of its wholly owned, majority owned, and controlled entities. Investments where the Health System holds less than 20% of the ownership interest are accounted for using the cost method. All other investments not controlled by the Health System are accounted for using the equity method of accounting. The Health System has included its equity share of income or losses from investments in unconsolidated affiliates in other revenue in the consolidated statements of operations and changes in net assets. In accordance with accounting principles generally accepted in the United States (GAAP), noncontrolling interests and the changes in noncontrolling interests have been disclosed in the notes to the financial statements. All material intercompany transactions and account balances have been eliminated in consolidation.

   b.   *Use of estimates.* The preparation of financial statements in conformity with GAAP requires management of the Health System to make assumptions, estimates, and judgments that affect the amounts reported in the consolidated financial statements, including the notes thereto, and related disclosures of commitments and contingencies, if any. The Health System considers the following to be critical accounting policies because they require significant judgments and estimates: recognition of net patient service revenue, which is reduced by both contractual allowances and the provision for doubtful accounts; recorded values of investments; reserves for losses and expenses related to health care professional and general liability; and risks and assumptions for measurement of pension and retiree medical liabilities. Management relies on historical experience and other assumptions believed to be reasonable in making its judgment and estimates. Actual results could differ materially from those estimates.

   c.   *Cash and cash equivalents.* For purposes of the consolidated statements of cash flows, cash and cash equivalents include certain investments in highly liquid debt instruments with original maturities of three months or less.

   d.   *Investments.* Investments, inclusive of assets limited or restricted as to use, include marketable debt and equity securities. Investments in equity securities with readily determinable fair values and all investments in debt securities (except those intended to be held to maturity) are measured at fair value and are classified as trading securities. Investments also include investments in commingled funds and other investments structured as limited liability corporations or partnerships. Commingled funds and investment funds that hold securities directly are stated at the fair value of the underlying securities, as determined by the administrator, based on readily determinable market values. Limited liability corporations and partnerships are accounted for under the equity method.

e. *Investment earnings.* Investment earnings include interest and dividends, realized gains and losses on investments, unrealized gains and losses, and equity earnings. Investment earnings on assets held by trustees under bond indenture agreements, assets designated by the Board for debt redemption, and assets deposited in trust funds by a captive insurance company for self-insurance purposes in accordance with industry practices are included in other revenue in the consolidated statements of operations and changes in net assets. Investment earnings from all other unrestricted investments and board designated funds are included in nonoperating investment income unless the income or loss is restricted by donor or law.

f. *Assets limited or restricted as to use.* Assets limited as to use is composed of amounts set aside by the Board for future capital improvements, future funding of retirement programs and insurance claims, retirement of debt, and other purposes over which the Board retains control. The Board may, at its discretion, subsequently use these funds for other purposes. Assets held by trustees under the bond indenture and self-insurance trust and benefit plan arrangements are also included. This caption also includes assets that are specifically restricted as to use by donors.

g. *Donor restricted gifts.* Unconditional promises to give cash and other assets to the Health System's various subsidiaries are reported at fair value at the date the promise is received. Conditional promises to give and indications of intentions to give are reported at fair value at the date the gift is received. The gifts are reported as either temporarily or permanently restricted support if they are received with donor stipulations that limit the use of the donated assets. When a donor restriction expires, that is, when a stipulated time restriction ends or purpose restriction is accomplished, temporarily restricted net assets are reclassified to unrestricted net assets and reported in the consolidated statements of operations and changes in net assets as net assets released from restrictions. Donor restricted contributions whose restrictions are met within the same year as received are reported as unrestricted contributions in the consolidated statements of operations and changes in net assets.

h. *Property and equipment.* Property and equipment, including internal-use software, are recorded at cost, if purchased, or at fair value at the date of donation, if donated. Depreciation is provided over the estimated useful life of each class of depreciable asset and is computed using either the straight line or an accelerated method and includes capital lease and internal-use software amortization. The useful lives of these assets range from 2 to 50 years. Interest costs incurred during the period of

(Continued)

construction of capital assets are capitalized as a component of the cost of acquiring those assets.

Gifts of long-lived assets such as land, buildings, or equipment are reported as unrestricted support and are excluded from the excess of revenue over expenses, unless explicit donor stipulations specify how the donated assets must be used. Gifts of long-lived assets with explicit restrictions that specify how the assets are to be used and gifts of cash or other assets that must be used to acquire long-lived assets are reported as restricted support.

i. *Temporarily and permanently restricted net assets.* Temporarily restricted net assets are those whose use by the Health System has been limited by donors to a specific time period or purpose. Permanently restricted net assets have been restricted by donors to be maintained by the Health System in perpetuity.

j. *Patient accounts receivable, estimated receivables from and payables to third-party payors, and net patient service revenue.* The Health System has arrangements with third-party payors that provide for payments to the Health System's subsidiaries at amounts different from established rates. Patient accounts receivable and net patient service revenue are reported at the estimated net realizable amounts from patients, third-party payors, and others for services rendered. Estimated retroactive adjustments under reimbursement agreements with third-party payors are included in net patient service revenue and estimated receivables from and payables to third-party payors. Retroactive adjustments are accrued on an estimated basis in the period the related services are rendered and adjusted in future periods, as final settlements are determined.

The Health System recognizes significant amounts of patient service revenue at the time services are rendered even though it does not assess the patient's ability to pay. Accordingly, bad debt expense is shown as a reduction of revenue on the statement of operations. Estimated receivables from third-party payors include amounts receivable from Medicare and state Medicaid meaningful use programs.

k. *Allowance for doubtful accounts.* Substantially all of the Health System's receivables are related to providing health care services to patients. Accounts receivable are reduced by an allowance for amounts that could become uncollectible in the future. The Health System's estimate for its allowance for doubtful accounts is based upon management's assessment of historical and expected net collections from payors.

l. *Premium and capitation revenue.* The Health System has certain subsidiaries that arrange for the delivery of health care services to enrollees through various contracts with providers and common provider entities. Enrollee contracts are negotiated on a yearly basis. Premiums are due monthly and are recognized as revenue during the period in which the Health System is obligated to provide services to enrollees. Premiums received prior to the period of coverage are recorded as deferred revenue and included in accrued expenses in the consolidated balance sheets.

Certain of the Health System's subsidiaries have entered into capitation arrangements whereby they accept the risk for the provision of certain health care services to health plan members. Under these agreements, the Health System's subsidiaries are financially responsible for services provided to the health plan members by other institutional health care providers. Capitation revenue is recognized during the period for which the subsidiary is obligated to provide services to health plan enrollees under capitation contracts. Capitation receivables are included in other receivables in the consolidated balance sheets.

Reserves for incurred but not reported claims have been established to cover the unpaid costs of health care services covered under the premium and capitation arrangements. The premium and capitation arrangement reserves are classified with accrued expenses in the consolidated balance sheets. The liability is estimated based on actuarial studies, historical reporting, and payment trends. Subsequent actual claim experience will differ from the estimated liability due to variances in estimated and actual utilization of health care services, the amount of charges, and other factors. As settlements are made and estimates are revised, the differences are reflected in current operations. The Health System limits a portion of its liability through stop loss reinsurance.

m. *Excess of revenue over expenses*. The consolidated statement of operations and changes in net assets includes the excess of revenue over expenses. Changes in unrestricted net assets, which are excluded from excess of revenue over expenses, consistent with industry practice, include the effective portion of the change in market value of derivatives that meet hedge accounting requirements, permanent transfers of assets to and from affiliates for other than goods and services, contributions of long-lived assets received or gifted (including assets acquired using contributions, which by donor restriction were to be used for the purposes of acquiring such assets), net change in postretirement plan related items, discontinued operations, extraordinary items, and cumulative effects of changes in accounting principles.

Adopted Accounting Pronouncements

n. In July 2011, the Health System adopted new accounting principles related to the "Presentation of Insurance Claims and Related Insurance Recoveries," which provides clarification to companies in the health care industry on the accounting for professional liability and other similar insurance. This guidance states that receivables related to insurance recoveries should not be netted against the related claim liability and such claim liabilities should be determined without considering insurance recoveries. The adoption of this guidance resulted in an asset and liability being recorded in the consolidated financial statements at June 30, 2012, of $58.2 million in self-insurance, benefit plans and other, and in self-insurance reserves.

(Continued)

o. In July 2011, the Health System adopted new accounting principles related to the "Presentation and Disclosure of Patient Service Revenue, Provision for Bad Debts, and the Allowance for Doubtful Accounts for Certain Health Care Entities." This guidance requires certain health care entities to present the provision for bad debts related to patient service revenues as a deduction from revenue, net of contractual allowances and discounts, versus as an expense in the statement of operations. In addition, it requires enhanced disclosures regarding revenue recognition policies and the assessment of bad debt. Implementation resulted in a reduction of net patient service revenue, operating revenue, and operating expense, but had no impact on operating income in the statement of operations and changes in net assets.

2. Net Patient Service Revenue

A summary of the payment arrangements with major third-party payors follows:

Medicare. Acute inpatient and outpatient services rendered to Medicare program beneficiaries are paid primarily at prospectively determined rates. These rates vary according to a patient classification system that is based on clinical, diagnostic, and other factors. Although the majority of services are reimbursed using prospective payment mechanisms, certain items are reimbursed at a tentative rate with final settlement determined after submission of annual cost reports and audits thereof by the Medicare fiscal intermediaries.

Medicaid. Reimbursement for services rendered to Medicaid program beneficiaries includes prospectively determined rates per discharge, per diem payments, discounts from established charges, fee schedules, and cost reimbursement methodologies with certain limitations. Cost reimbursable items are reimbursed at a tentative rate with final settlement determined after submission of annual cost reports and audits thereof by the Medicaid fiscal intermediaries.

Other. Reimbursement for services to certain patients is received from commercial insurance carriers, health maintenance organizations, and preferred provider organizations. The basis for reimbursement includes prospectively determined rates per discharge, per diem payments, and discounts from established charges.

The Health System recognizes patient service revenue associated with services provided to patients who have third-party payor coverage on the basis of contractual rates for the services rendered. For uninsured patients that do not qualify for charity care the Health System recognizes revenue on the basis of its standard rates for services provided (or on the basis of discounted rates, if negotiated or provided by policy). On the basis of historical experience, a significant portion of the Health System's uninsured patients will be unable or unwilling to pay for the services provided. Therefore, the Health System records a significant provision for bad debts related to uninsured patients in the period in which the services are provided. Patient service revenue, net of contractual allowances and discounts but before the provision for bad debts, recognized in the period from these major payor sources, is as follows:

	Third-Party Payors	Self-Pay	Total All Payors
Patient service revenue (net of contractual allowances and discounts)	$3,701,400	$701,359	$4,402,759

3. Summary of Net Patient Service Revenue

During the years ended June 30, 2012 and 2011, 33% and 32% of net patient service revenue was recognized under the Medicare program and 53% and 55% was recognized from other payor contracts and patients, respectively. During the years ended June 30, 2012 and 2011, 9% of net patient service revenue was received under state Medicaid and indigent care programs. Laws and regulations governing the Medicare and Medicaid programs are complex and subject to interpretation. Compliance with such laws and regulations can be subject to future government review and interpretation as well as significant regulatory action including fines, penalties, and exclusion from the Medicare and Medicaid programs.

Charity care. The Health System provides care to patients who meet certain criteria under its charity care policy without charge or at amounts less than its established rates. Because the Health System does not pursue collection of amounts determined to qualify for charity care, they are not reported as net patient service revenue in the consolidated statements of operations and changes in net assets.

A summary of net patient service revenue for the years ended June 30 is as follows:

	2012	2011
	(in thousands)	
Gross charges		
Acute inpatient	$2,354,900	$2,233,393
Outpatient, nonacute inpatient, and other	2,731,277	2,458,608
Gross patient service revenue	5,086,177	4,692,001
Less		
Allowance for doubtful accounts	(265,850)	(223,478)
Contractual and other allowances	(297,030)	(267,703)
Charity care charges	(290,825)	(263,851)
Allowance for self-insured health benefits	(95,563)	(85,126)
Net patient service revenue less provision for bad debts	$4,136,909	$3,851,843

(Continued)

4. Property and Equipment

A summary of property and equipment at June 30 is as follows:

	2012	2011
	(in thousands)	
Land	$208,409	$247,442
Buildings and improvements	2,238,364	2,280,923
Equipment	1,492,327	1,398,451
Total	3,939,100	3,926,816
Less accumulated depreciation and amortization	(1,824,381)	(1,676,411)
Construction in progress	187,049	98,212
Property and equipment, net	$2,301,768	$2,348,617

5. Long-Term Debt and Other Financing Arrangements

A summary of short-term borrowings and long-term debt at June 30 is as follows:

	2012	2011
	(in thousands)	
Short-term borrowings		
Variable rate demand bonds with contractual maturities through 2052. Interest payable monthly at rates ranging from 0.01% to 0.78% during 2012 and from 0.03% to 0.91% during 2011.	$511,301	$607,189
Long-term debt		
Tax-exempt revenue bonds and refunding bonds, fixed rate term and serial bonds, payable at various dates through 2048. Interest rates range from 2.375% to 6.625% during 2012 and 2011.	$1,199,251	$692,923
Notes payable to banks. Interest payable at rates ranging from 2.1% to 9.3%, fixed and variable, payable in varying monthly installments through 2023.	2,371	5,670
Capital lease obligations (excluding imputed interest of $19.4 million and $17.2 million at June 30, 2012 and 2011, respectively.	28,598	32,404
Mortgage obligations. Interest payable at rates ranging from 4.3% to 6.1% during 2012 and 6.1% during 2011.	27,500	18,047
Long-term debt	1,257,720	749,044
Less current portion	(17,052)	(16,237)
Unamortized bond premiums	14,049	1,968
Long-term debt	$1,254,717	$734,775

Contractually obligated principal repayments on short-term borrowings and long-term debt are as follows:

Years ending June 30	Short-Term Borrowings	Long-Term Debt
	(in thousands)	
2013	15,806	17,052
2014	17,814	27,541
2015	16,388	31,258
2016	15,076	24,615
2017	13,869	23,511
Thereafter	$432,348	$1,133,743
Total	$511,301	$1,257,720

Note

1. The phrase *investor-owned* is used to distinguish a for-profit entity from a not-for-profit entity or governmental entity.

CHAPTER 3

PRINCIPLES AND PRACTICES OF HEALTH CARE ACCOUNTING

The financial viability of a health care organization results from numerous decisions made by various people, including caregivers, administrators, boards, lenders, community members, and politicians. These decisions eventually result in an organization's acquiring and using resources to provide services, to incur obligations, and to generate revenues. One of the major roles of accounting is to record these transactions and report the results in a standardized format to interested parties. This chapter shows how a series of typical transactions at a health center are recorded on the books and how these records are used to produce the four major financial statements for a not-for-profit, business-oriented health care organization. The recording and reporting process can be time consuming, but changes are continually being made to automate it (see Exhibit 3.1 and Perspective 3.1).

The Books

As the transactions of a health care organization occur (such as the purchase of supplies), they are recorded chronologically in a "book" called a *journal*. Today, this book is more likely to be a computer than a paper journal requiring manual entries. Periodically (simultaneously when using most computer programs), these transactions are summarized by account (i.e., *cash, equipment, revenues*, etc.) into another book called a *ledger*. With these two books, the organization has both a chronological listing of transactions and the current balance in each account (see Exhibit 3.2.). The totals for each account in the ledger are used to prepare the four financial statements. Although this procedure is simple to conceptualize,

LEARNING OBJECTIVES

- Record financial transactions.
- Understand the basics of accrual accounting.
- Summarize transactions into financial statements.

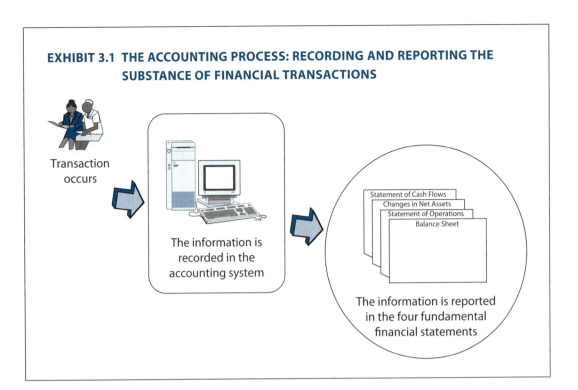

EXHIBIT 3.1 THE ACCOUNTING PROCESS: RECORDING AND REPORTING THE SUBSTANCE OF FINANCIAL TRANSACTIONS

Transaction occurs

The information is recorded in the accounting system

Statement of Cash Flows
Changes in Net Assets
Statement of Operations
Balance Sheet

The information is reported in the four fundamental financial statements

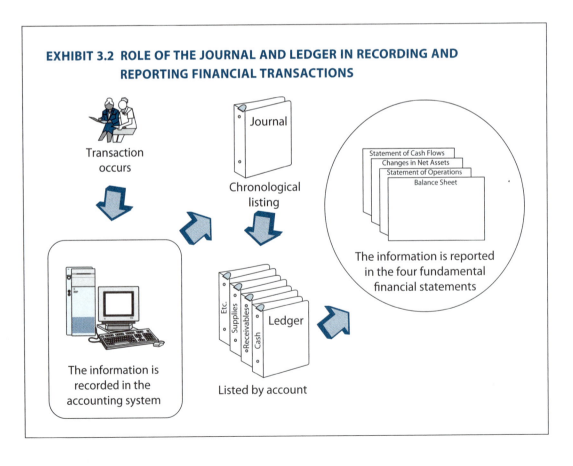

EXHIBIT 3.2 ROLE OF THE JOURNAL AND LEDGER IN RECORDING AND REPORTING FINANCIAL TRANSACTIONS

Transaction occurs

Journal

Chronological listing

The information is recorded in the accounting system

Etc.
Supplies
Receivables
Cash

Ledger

Listed by account

Statement of Cash Flows
Changes in Net Assets
Statement of Operations
Balance Sheet

The information is reported in the four fundamental financial statements

PERSPECTIVE 3.1 ELECTRONIC HEALTH RECORD HAS FINANCIAL REPORTING VALUE AS WELL

As more hospitals implement electronic health records, they are using these tools to integrate the clinical and financial aspects of these records. For example, one hospital in Georgia selected a particular system (Chart Access) because it gave the hospital the ability to use a clinical system that can be combined with its financial system. Using cloud-based technology, managers in the hospital can download reports that assist them in gaining perspectives on what is happening from both a clinical and financial perspective. For example, the financial reports include information on patient insurance and account information as well as hospital information related to accounts receivables and payables. More important, the system can provide one statement that lists patient account information from an array of care providers, including outpatient and postacute providers.

As a result patients will no longer have to receive multiple statements from each provider.

Source: Adapted from Information systems; healthcare providers choose integrated enterprise system from prognosis HIS to meet emerging industry challenges, *Investment Weekly News*, February 25, 2012.

ensuring the financial statements are prepared accurately and in a timely manner is quite involved, as Perspective 3.1 shows.

A fairly standard set of account categories is used by all health care organizations. The accounts used in the financial statements in Chapter Two constitute an important part of the standard set of account categories (and each of these accounts may contain subcategories).

Cash and Accrual Bases of Accounting

Before introducing examples of recording and reporting transactions, the difference between cash and accrual accounting needs to be discussed. The *cash basis of accounting* focuses on the flows of cash in and out of the organization, whereas the *accrual basis of accounting* focuses on the flows of resources and the revenues those resources help to generate. This discussion begins with a focus on the cash basis of accounting, for it is more intuitive. The focus then turns to the accrual basis of accounting, which is the system the accounting profession applies to health care organizations.

Cash Basis of Accounting

The way the cash basis of accounting records transactions is similar to the way most people keep their personal checkbooks: revenues are recorded

Cash Basis of Accounting
An accounting method that tracks when cash was received and when cash was expended, regardless of when services were provided or resources were used.

Accrual Basis of Accounting
An accounting method that aligns the flow of resources and the revenues those resources helped to generate. It records revenues when earned and resources when used, regardless of the flow of cash in or out of the organization. This is the standard method in use today.

EXHIBIT 3.3 COMPARISON OF THE CASH AND ACCRUAL BASES OF ACCOUNTING

	Cash Basis of Accounting	Accrual Basis of Accounting
Revenues are recognized	When cash is received	When revenues are earned
Expenses are recognized	When cash is paid out	When resources are used

---

when cash is received, and expenses are recorded when cash is paid out (see Exhibit 3.3). For example, if an organization delivers a service to a patient, the revenue from that patient is recorded when received. Expenses are recorded as they are paid (such as when the staff are paid). The advantages of this method of accounting are that cash flows can be tracked and it is simple. Its main disadvantages are that it does not match revenues with the resources used to generate those revenues, and the financial reports under the cash basis of accounting are susceptible to managerial manipulation. Incidentally, large health care systems have internal auditors to provide assurance that cash dollars are spent for their declared specific purposes (see Perspective 3.2).

Accrual Basis of Accounting

The accrual basis of accounting overcomes the disadvantages of the cash basis of accounting by recognizing revenues when they are earned and expenses when resources are used (Exhibit 3.3). The advantages of the accrual basis of accounting are that (1) it keeps track of revenues generated and resources used as well as cash flows, (2) it matches revenues with the resources used to generate those revenues, and (3) the financial statements provide a broader picture of the provider's operation. Its main disadvantages are that it is more difficult to implement and it, too, is open to manipulation, often by bending accounting rules. Keeping track of revenues and resource use can be a technologically intensive endeavor (see Perspective 3.3).

An Example of the Effects of Cash Flows on Profit Reporting under Cash and Accrual Accounting

Exhibit 3.4 illustrates how the cash basis of accounting is vulnerable to management's manipulation of revenues and expenses. Assume a health

PERSPECTIVE 3.2 FUNCTIONS OF INTERNAL AUDIT DEPARTMENT

Many hospitals have established internal audit teams. The primary function of the audit team is to ensure that hospitals comply with their financial record keeping, especially with respect to daily cash management and the reporting and recording of revenues and expenses. They are typically staffed with individuals with financial experience, but these teams may also include personnel with clinical backgrounds as well, such as nursing. One of the functions of the auditors is to ensure departments do not game the budget system. For example personnel within a department may purchase a piece of equipment in stages so it is treated as a supply expense rather than being reviewed as a capital expenditure. A second function of the internal auditors is to ensure compliance that the department utilized its capital funds for the requested equipment. Auditors sometime find that capital dollars allocated for an obsolete piece of critical equipment were used to purchase a totally unrelated newer piece of equipment. Additional duties also include reviewing repair and maintenance programs and complying with asset disposal regulations.

Source: Adapted from Steve Womack, Tap your internal audit department to support capital management, *Healthcare Financial Management*, 2011;65(3):134.

PERSPECTIVE 3.3 ACCURATELY CAPTURING PATIENT REVENUE IS ALSO A KEY COMPONENT FOR HEALTH IT

A critical access hospital (CAH) hired a vendor to implement a web-based charge master system that allows medical staff to access detailed information to record the code and charge for a specific service. One section of the federal government's stimulus package of 2009 was the "HITECH Act," which approved close to $20 billion to go toward health care information technology. The vast majority of this funding was related to financial incentives to encourage hospitals and physician practices to invest in IT infrastructure and training and in electronic health records. Hospitals that received this funding are required to implement certified electronic health information systems. One of the requirements hospitals must meet in implementing an electronic health record, if they are to qualify for federal funding under the HITECH Act, is to possess the information technology and software to transmit medical data via the EHR as well as to translate those data into accurate charge data. In contrast to larger hospitals, smaller facilities, like CAHs, have smaller IT budgets and fewer full-time IT staff to help them meet these requirements; however, there are vendors that tailor their systems to critical access hospitals.

Source: Adapted from Electronic medical records: Ellenville Regional Hospital selects Craneware solution to ensure accurate chargemaster data prior to EHR implementation, *Investment Weekly News*, October 8, 2011.

EXHIBIT 3.4 MANAGEMENT MANIPULATION UNDER THE CASH BASIS OF ACCOUNTING

Situation

During the accounting period, a health care organization has earned $12,000 in revenues and consumed $4,000 in resources.

Assume Three Scenarios

1. Management wants to show a high profit, so although it collects full payment of $12,000, it delays paying its bills until after the end of the accounting period.

2. Management wants to show low profit, perhaps to encourage more donations. It pays the bills, $4,000, but discourages patients and third parties from paying until after the end of the accounting period.

3. Accrual basis of accounting rules are followed, and the organization records revenues earned of $12,000 and resources used to generate those revenues of $4,000.

	Scenario 1	Scenario 2	Scenario 3
Revenues reported	$12,000	$0	$12,000
Expenses reported	$0	$4,000	$4,000
Profit reported	$12,000	($4,000)	$8,000

Points

- Management can manipulate reported profits through its payment and collection policies under the cash basis of accounting.

- Revenues are not necessarily matched with the resources used to generate those revenues under the cash basis of accounting.

---

care organization earned $12,000 in revenues and had $4,000 in expenses. In scenario 1, management wants to show a high profit, so although it collects full payment of $12,000, it delays paying its bills until after the end of the accounting period; therefore the reported profit is $12,000. In scenario 2, management wants to show low profit (perhaps so it can encourage more donations). In this case, management pays all its bills, $4,000, but sends out its own bills late so that payment is not received from patients and third parties until after the end of the accounting period; reported profit under this scenario is –$4,000. Scenario 3 follows the accrual basis of accounting rules, and management records revenues earned of $12,000 and resources used to generate those revenues of $4,000, which shows a profit of $8,000. Thus, under accrual accounting, the organization cannot influence reported profit by accelerating or slowing cash inflows and out-flows. Revenues *must* be recorded when they are earned and expenses recorded when resources are used. Perspective 3.4 shows the importance of accurate record keeping and how systems can go astray.

Generally accepted accounting principles recommend that health care organizations use the accrual basis of accounting. This does not mean, however, that having information about cash flows is any less important than is having information about revenues and the resources used to gener-ate those revenues.

PERSPECTIVE 3.4 HEALTHSOUTH: A CASE OF ACCOUNTING FRAUD

HealthSouth, a hospital management company with a chain of rehabilitation hospitals, reported a $440 million tax refund from the Internal Revenue Service. This accounting aberration stemmed from HealthSouth's tax payment on $2.7 billion of fraudulent income it reported to the IRS in 2003. In essence, HealthSouth paid taxes on income that was not real.

Federal investigators found substantial accounting fraud in the company in 2003. Several senior executives pleaded guilty for their involvement in this accounting fraud case. However, Health-South's chief executive, Richard M. Scrushy, was not found guilty of these accounting fraud charges at his trial in 2005, although he was later sentenced to prison on an unrelated federal bribery conviction.

Although the company was profitable, the former chief financial officer of the company indi-cated that one of the major underlying motives for committing this accounting fraud was the financial pressure to show more profits so that the company could meet Wall Street's earnings expectations. The irony of this accounting scheme is that the company's actual earnings were not high enough to pay the taxes on the fraudulent profits. As a result, the company issued debt to help pay off the tax liability. In addition, this financial leverage position contributed to more than $3.6 billion in debt. Under new management, HealthSouth has lowered its outstand-ing debt to $1 billion, and it intends to use the tax refund to reduce this debt position even further.

Source: Adapted from K. Whitmire, Profits aren't real, but the refund is, *New York Times*, October 21, 2007, www .nytimes.com/2007/10/21/business/21suits.html.

Recording Transactions

This section and the problems at the back of the chapter illustrate a step-by-step approach to posting transactions. To make this approach easier to follow, all amounts billed are equal to the contracted rate, and the provider does not assess the patient's ability to pay at the point of service. Therefore the only reduction of revenue that needs to be considered is for bad debt.

Assume Windmill Point Outpatient Center is a not-for-profit, business-oriented health care organization that had the transactions summarized in Exhibit 3.5 during 20X1, its first year of operation. Exhibit 3.6 presents the journal and ledger entries that record the transactions listed in Exhibit 3.5. Because the transactions are recorded chronologically by row, the rows serve as the journal. Because each account has its own column, summarized at the bottom, the columns serve as the ledger. These transactions are being recorded in part so that the four financial statements can be prepared. These statements allow interested parties to make informed judgments about the financial health of the organization.

Rules for Recording Transactions

Two rules must be followed to record transactions under the accrual basis of accounting:

1.   At least two accounts must be used to record a transaction.

    a.   Increase (decrease) an *asset* account whenever assets are acquired (used).

    b.   Increase (decrease) a *liability* account whenever obligations are incurred (paid for).

    c.   Increase a *revenues, gains, or other support* account when revenues are earned, a gain occurs, or other support is received.

    d.   Increase an *expense* account when an asset is used. Net assets increase when unrestricted revenues, gains, and other support increase, and net assets decrease when expenses occur.

There are additional rules that must be followed for donations; however, these rules can become complex and are beyond the scope of this text.

2.   After each transaction, the fundamental accounting equation must be in balance:

$$Assets = Liabilities + Net\ Assets$$

EXHIBIT 3.5 SAMPLE TRANSACTIONS FOR WINDMILL POINT OUTPATIENT CENTER, JANUARY 1, 20X1–DECEMBER 31, 20X1

During the year, the center had these transactions:

1. The center received $600,000 in unrestricted contributions.

2. The center obtained a $500,000 bank loan at 6 percent interest; $20,000 in principal is due this year.

3. The center purchased $450,000 of plant and equipment (P&E). It paid cash for the purchase.

4. The center purchased $100,000 of supplies on credit. The vendor expects payment within 30 days.

5. The center provided $500,000 of billable services. Payment has not yet been received.

6. On the first day of the year, the center received $250,000 in capitation payment from an HMO. In other words, the HMO paid the center $250,000 in advance on a per member per year (PMPY) basis to provide for the health care needs of its enrollees over the next year.

7. In the provision of services to all patients, the center incurred $300,000 in labor expenses, which it paid for in cash.

8. In the provision of services to all patients, the center used $80,000 of supplies.

9. The center paid $10,000 in advance for one year's insurance.

10. The center paid for $90,000 of the $100,000 of supplies purchased in transaction 4.

11. Patients or their third parties paid the center $400,000 of the $500,000 they owed (see transaction 5).

12. During the year, the center made a $50,000 cash payment toward its bank loan; $20,000 went toward the principal, and $30,000 went to pay the full amount of interest due.

13. The center transferred $25,000 to its parent corporation.

At the end of the year, the center recognized the following:

14. Since the last payday, employees have earned wages of $35,000.

15. Equipment has depreciated $45,000.

16. The $10,000 insurance premium was for one year. That time has now expired.

17. The health center has fulfilled the health care service obligation it took on, because the $250,000 in capitated payments were for one year (transaction 6), which has now expired. This revenue is now considered earned.

18. $20,000 of the note payable (transaction 2) is due within the next year.

19. Provision for bad debt is estimated to be $5,000.

20. $60,000 is set aside for the beginning of the next fiscal year, to be used toward purchase of new computer equipment.

EXHIBIT 3.6 LISTING OF FINANCIAL TRANSACTIONS FOR WINDMILL POINT OUTPATIENT CENTER

Windmill Point Outpatient Center
Journal and Ledger
For the Period January 1 - December 31, 20X1

Transaction	ASSETS									LIABILITIES			NET ASSETS				
	Cash	Assets Limited as to Use	Accounts Receivable	Allowance for Doubtful Accounts	Supplies	Prepaid Expenses	Long-term Investments	Plant & Equipment (P&E)	Accumulated Depreciation	Current Liabilities	Deferred Revenues	Non-Current Liabilities	Revenues, Gains and Other Support	Expenses	Transfer to Parent	Unrestricted Net Assets	Restricted Net Assets
Beginning balance	$0	$0	$0	$0	$0	$0	$0	$0	$0	$0	$0	$0	$0	$0	$0	$0	$0
1 Contribution	600,000												600,000				
2 Long-term bank loan	500,000									20,000		480,000					
3 Purchased P & E with cash	-450,000							450,000									
4 Purchased supplies on credit					100,000					100,000							
5 Patient services on credit			500,000										500,000				
6 Received HMO capitation	250,000										250,000						
7 Paid labor	-300,000													-300,000			
8 Used supplies					-80,000									-80,000			
9 Prepaid insurance	-10,000					10,000											
10 Paid cash for supplies	-90,000									-90,000							
11 Patients paid accounts	400,000		-400,000														
12 Paid bank loan & interest	-50,000									-20,000				-30,000			
13 Transferred funds to parent	-25,000														-25,000		
14 Wages earned but not paid										35,000				-35,000			
15 Depreciation									-45,000					-45,000			
16 Expired insurance						-10,000								-10,000			
17 Capitation earned											-250,000		250,000				
18 Current portion of debt										20,000		-20,000					
19 Provision bad debt				-5,000									-5,000				
20 IS funds set aside	-60,000	60,000															
Balances after adjustments	765,000	60,000	100,000	-5,000	20,000	0	0	450,000	-45,000	65,000	0	460,000	1,345,000	-500,000	-25,000	0	0
Operating income																845,000	
Closing income from operations to unrestricted net assets													-500,000 845,000			845,000 -25,000	
Transfer to parent																820,000	
Ending balances	765,000	60,000	100,000	-5,000	20,000	0	0	450,000	-45,000	65,000	0	460,000					
Balances with summarized net assets	$765,000	$60,000	$100,000	-$5,000	$20,000	$0	$0	$450,000	-$45,000	$65,000	$0	$460,000				$820,000	$0

The Recording Process

The following is an outline of the transactions listed in Exhibit 3.6.

1. The center received $600,000 in unrestricted contributions.

   a. Because cash was received, the cash account (an asset) is increased by $600,000.

   b. Because an unrestricted contribution for operating purposes was received, revenues, gains, and other support is increased by $600,000. If Exhibit 3.6 were not constrained for space, the transaction would be more accurately recorded in *other revenue*, a subcategory of revenues, gains, and other support.

Caution: Under accrual accounting, revenues are recognized when earned. Because the receipt of an unrestricted donation *that can be used for operating purposes* is not earned in the same sense that patient revenues are, such donations are recorded in the related account other revenue, under revenues, gains, and other support. It is also possible to report it under nonoperating items, which is below operating income.

2. The center obtained a $500,000 bank loan at 6 percent interest; $20,000 in principal is due this year.

   a. Because cash was received, cash (an asset) is increased by $500,000.

   b. Because the center borrowed $500,000, it must recognize this as a liability. The part due this year ($20,000) is a current liability. The part not due this year ($480,000) is a noncurrent liability. Thus, *notes payable* under *current liabilities* is increased by $20,000, and notes payable under *noncurrent liabilities* is increased by $480,000.

Caution: Notice that although cash was received, no revenues were recognized. Under accrual accounting, revenues are recognized when they are earned. In this case the cash received did not represent earnings, just the borrowing of funds. Also, this transaction involved three accounts, not just two: cash and notes payable under both current liabilities and noncurrent liabilities. However, the fundamental accounting equation still remains in balance.

A common error is to record interest expense at this time. Because interest is a *usage* fee, interest is recognized when the borrower keeps the funds, not when the borrowing takes place. (This is shown in transaction 12.)

3.   The center purchased $450,000 of properties and equipment. It paid cash for the purchase.

   a.   Because cash was paid, cash (an asset) is decreased by $450,000.

   b.   Because properties and equipment were purchased, *properties and equipment* (an asset) is increased by $450,000.

Caution: Notice that although cash was paid, no expense was recognized. Under accrual accounting, expenses are recognized as assets are used, and the center has not yet used the plant and equipment. (This is shown in transaction 15.)

---

4.   The center purchased $100,000 of supplies on credit. The vendor expects payment within thirty days.

   a.   Because supplies increased, *supplies* (an asset) is increased by $100,000.

   b.   Because the vendor is owed $100,000, and the payment is due within thirty days, the current liability, *accounts payable*, is increased by $100,000.

Caution: Notice that although supplies were purchased, no supplies expense was recognized. Under accrual accounting, expenses are recognized when resources are used or consumed, and the center has not yet used the supplies. (This is shown in transaction 8.)

---

5.   The center provided $500,000 of billable services to noncapitated patients. Payment has not yet been received.

   a.   Although the patients received services, they have not paid. Therefore, *accounts receivable* (an asset) is increased by $500,000 to show that the organization has a right to collect the money it is owed.

   b.   Because revenue was earned by providing services, *patient revenues*, a net asset subaccount, is increased by $500,000.

Caution: Under accrual accounting, revenues are recognized when earned. Therefore, although no cash was received, revenues are increased because the service was performed.

---

6.   On the first day of the year, the center received $250,000 in capitation prepayment from an HMO. This means the HMO paid the center

$250,000 in advance on a per member per year (PMPY) basis to take care of the medical needs of all its enrollees over the next year.

a. Because cash was received, cash (an asset) is increased by $250,000.

b. The center has an obligation to provide services to the capitated patients. Therefore, *deferred revenues* (a liability) is increased by $250,000.

Caution: Under accrual accounting, revenues are recognized when they are earned. Although cash was received, the revenues will be earned only when the coverage period expires. (This is shown in transaction 17.)

7. In the provision of services to all patients, the center incurred $300,000 in labor expenses, which it paid for in cash.

a. Because cash was paid out, cash (an asset) is decreased by $300,000.

b. Because labor, a resource, was used, *expenses*, a net asset, is increased. Because expenses decrease net assets, it is recorded as a negative number.

Caution: Because cash was paid in recognition of the use of resources, expenses would have been recognized under either the cash or accrual bases of accounting.

8. In the provision of services to all patients, the center used $80,000 of supplies.

a. The organization now has $80,000 less in supplies. Therefore, supplies (an asset) is decreased by $80,000.

b. Because $80,000 of supplies has been used, *supplies expense* is increased by $80,000. Because expenses decrease net assets, it is recorded as a negative number.

Caution: Although no cash was paid, the expense is recognized because resources have been used. Recall that no expense was recognized when the resource was purchased in transaction 4.

9. The center paid a $10,000 premium in advance for one year's insurance coverage.

a. Because cash was paid out, cash (an asset) is decreased by $10,000.

b. $10,000 purchased the right to be covered by insurance for the entire year. Therefore, *prepaid insurance* (an asset) is increased by $10,000.

Caution: Under accrual accounting, expenses are recognized when assets are used. Thus, although cash has been paid out, no expense was recognized. The expense will be recognized as the right to be covered by insurance is used up (with the passage of time). (This is shown in transaction 16.)

10. The center paid for $90,000 of the $100,000 of supplies purchased in transaction 4.

a. Because cash was paid, cash (an asset) is decreased by $90,000.

b. Because the center no longer owes $90,000 of the $100,000 liability, accounts payable (a liability) is decreased by $90,000.

Caution: Although cash has been paid out, no expense was recognized because no resources were used.

11. Patients or their third parties paid the center $400,000 of the $500,000 they owed (see transaction 5).

a. Because cash was received, cash (an asset) is increased by $400,000.

b. Because payment has been received, the organization no longer has the right to collect this $400,000 from patients. Therefore, accounts receivable (an asset) is decreased by $400,000.

Caution: Notice that although cash was received, no revenues were recognized. Under accrual accounting, revenues are recognized when they are earned. The revenue was recognized when it was earned in transaction 5.

12. During the year, the center made a $50,000 cash payment toward its bank loan; $20,000 was for principal, and $30,000 was to pay the full amount of interest due.

a. Because cash was paid out, cash (an asset) is decreased by $50,000.

b. Because $20,000 of the loan has been paid off, notes payable (a liability) is decreased by $20,000.

c. Because the center paid $30,000 for the use of the $500,000 loan (6 percent interest rate), *interest expense* (a net asset) is increased by $30,000. Because expenses decrease net assets, it is recorded as a negative.

Caution: Remember, interest expense was *not* recognized when the loan was taken in transaction 2. Interest, the right to use someone else's money, is recognized over time, as the loan is outstanding.

13. The center transferred $25,000 to its parent corporation.

a. Because cash was paid out, cash (an asset) is decreased by $25,000.

b. Because the organization now has $25,000 less in assets, *transfer to parent* (a net asset) is decreased by $25,000. This is recorded as a negative because it has the effect of decreasing unrestricted net assets (like expenses that are also recorded as negatives).

Caution: Although cash has been paid out, no expense is recognized because no resources were used.

14. Since the last payday, employees have earned wages of $35,000.

a. Because the center owes its employees $35,000, it must recognize this obligation by increasing *wages payable* (a liability) by $35,000.

b. Because the center used $35,000 of labor, it must increase *labor expense* (a liability) by $35,000. Because expenses decrease net assets, the increase in expenses is recorded as a negative number.

Caution: Although no cash was paid, the expense was recognized because labor resources have been used.

15. Equipment has depreciated $45,000.

a. To keep a cumulative record of the amount of depreciation taken on the assets, the center must increase *accumulated depreciation* (a *contra-asset account*) by $45,000. An increase in a contra-asset account results in a decrease in the value of the assets. Thus, the accumulated depreciation is subtracted from the amount in the equipment account to find the book value of the equipment.

b. Because the organization has used up $45,000 of the equipment, it must increase *depreciation expense* (a net asset account) by

Contra-asset
An asset that, when increased, decreases the value of a related asset on the books. Two primary examples are accumulated depreciation, which is the contra-asset to properties and equipment, and the allowance for uncollectibles, which is the contra-asset to accounts receivable. For example, by convention, the historical cost of a fixed asset is kept on the books in its own account under properties and equipment, and the amount of depreciation that has accumulated on that asset is kept in a related account called accumulated depreciation. To find the book value of the fixed asset, the accumulated depreciation is subtracted from the amount in properties and equipment. Patient service revenues (the asset) and allowance for uncollectibles (the contra-asset) work the same way.

$45,000. Because expenses decrease net assets, the increase in expenses is recorded as a negative number.

Caution: Although no cash was paid, the depreciation expense is recognized because resources have been used.

16. The $10,000 of insurance coverage was for one year. That time has now expired.

   a. Because the organization no longer has the $10,000 of insurance coverage it purchased, it must decrease *prepaid insurance* (an asset) by $10,000.

   b. Because the organization used up the right it purchased to be covered by insurance for one year, it must increase the *insurance expense* account by $10,000. The expense is recognized when the resource is used, not when the insurance is purchased (see transaction 9). Because expenses decrease net assets, the increase in expenses is recorded as a negative number.

Caution: Although no cash was paid, the insurance expense is recognized because the right to be covered by insurance has been "used up."

17. The center has fulfilled its health care service obligations under the $250,000 capitated arrangement in transaction 6. This revenue is now considered earned.

   a. The center no longer has the obligation to provide service to these HMO enrollees. Therefore, it must reduce *unearned HMO revenues* (a liability) by $250,000.

   b. By covering the health care needs of the HMO enrollees for one year, the center earned $250,000. Therefore, revenues, gains, and other support is increased by $250,000. The specific account that would be increased under revenues, gains, and other support is *premium revenue*. Incidentally, note that revenue was not recognized when the cash was received (see transaction 6).

Caution: Although no cash was received, revenues are recognized when earned.

18. $20,000 of the note payable is due within the next year.

   a. Because the organization must pay $20,000 next year, the center must increase notes payable (a current liability) by $20,000.

    b. Because it no longer owes $20,000 over the long term, the center decreases notes payable (a noncurrent liability) by $20,000.

19. Provision for bad debt is estimated to be $5,000.

    a. The estimate of how much of the accounts receivable will *not* be paid is placed in a contra-asset account called the *allowance for uncollectibles*. Therefore, the allowance for uncollectibles is increased by $5,000 and is recorded as a negative. By increasing the allowance for uncollectibles, *net patient accounts receivable* is decreased.

    b. By estimating uncollectibles, the organization is recognizing that there are certain patient accounts receivable it will not be able to collect. This is part of doing business. Essentially, the organization is using up the right to collect the funds without actually collecting anything. It recognizes this use of resources by increasing provision for *bad debt expense* by $5,000. Because expenses decrease net assets, the increase in expenses is recorded as a negative number. The $5,000 provision for bad debt will reduce net patient revenues by this amount, so it would be recorded in a *contra-revenue* account.

Key Point The terms *allowance for doubtful accounts, allowance for uncollectible accounts*, and *allowance for bad debt* are used interchangeably in practice. Similarly, the terms *provision for bad debt* and *bad debt expense* are used interchangeably in practice.

Caution: Although no cash was paid, the bad debt expense (provision for bad debt) is recognized in the same time period as the earning occurred. If the organization did not recognize this expense at this time, it would be matching one year's bad debt with the revenues earned in a future year.

Key Point If nothing else were done, the value of the allowance for uncollectibles would grow indefinitely. To avoid this, when deemed uncollectible, specific accounts are written off, and the allowance for uncollectibles and the accounts receivable are both reduced by an equal amount.

20. $60,000 is set aside by the board to be used next year to help purchase a new information system.

a.   Because cash was set aside, cash (an asset) is decreased by $60,000.

b.   Because the board designated these funds for a specific use next year, *assets limited as to use* (a current asset) is increased by $60,000.

Caution: Because no resource has been consumed, there is no expense.

Developing the Financial Statements

Once the transactions have been analyzed and recorded, the organization can develop the four financial statements: the balance sheet, the statement of operations, the statement of changes in net assets, and the statement of cash flows.

The Balance Sheet

The balance sheet presents the assets, liabilities, and net assets for a health care provider. To construct a balance sheet for Windmill Point Outpatient Center (Exhibit 3.7), the information from the transaction recording sheet (Exhibit 3.6) is used to develop a snapshot of the organization's financial position at year's end.

Assets

For Windmill Point Outpatient Center, total current assets ($940,000) equals the sum of all cash ($765,000), assets limited as to use ($60,000), net accounts receivable ($95,000: accounts receivable of $100,000 less the allowance for uncollectibles of $5,000), supplies ($20,000), and prepaid assets ($0). Properties and equipment, net is $405,000. This is computed by taking the original purchase of $450,000 and subtracting the $45,000 of accumulated depreciation. Thus total assets are $1,345,000, which is the sum of current and noncurrent assets.

Liabilities

Windmill Point Outpatient Center has a balance of $65,000 in current liabilities: $10,000 for supplies ($100,000 purchased less $90,000 paid for); $35,000 in wages payable; and $20,000, the current portion of the long-term debt. There are no deferred revenues, but there is $460,000 of the long-term portion of the loan remaining, which is a noncurrent liability. The sum of these accounts, $525,000, is the total liabilities.

EXHIBIT 3.7 BALANCE SHEET FOR WINDMILL POINT OUTPATIENT CENTER

Windmill Point Outpatient Center Balance Sheet
for the Periods Ending December 31, 20X1 and 20X0

		12/31/20X1	12/31/20X0
Current assets			
Cash		$765,000	$0
Gross accounts receivable	100,000		
(less allowance for uncollectibles)	(5,000)		
Net accounts receivable		95,000	0
Supplies		20,000	0
Assets limited as to use		60,000	0
Prepaid expenses		0	0
Total current assets		940,000	0
Noncurrent assets			
Long-term investments (net)		0	0
Plant, property, and equipment	450,000		
(less accumulated depreciation)	(45,000)		
Net plant, property, and equipment		405,000	0
Total noncurrent assets		405,000	0
Total assets		**$1,345,000**	**$0**

	12/31/20X1	12/31/20X0
Current liabilities		
Accounts payable	$10,000	$0
Wages payable	35,000	0
Notes payable	20,000	0
Total current liabilities	65,000	0
Noncurrent liabilities	460,000	0
Total liabilities	525,000	0
Net assets		
Unrestricted	820,000	0
Temporarily restricted	0	0
Permanently restricted	0	0
Total net assets	820,000	0
Total liabilities and net assets	**$1,345,000**	**$0**

Net Assets

Net assets equal $820,000. This net asset balance is computed by summing the beginning balance of $0, the increase in unrestricted net assets of $820,000, and $0 in temporarily restricted and permanently restricted net assets.

The Statement of Operations

As with the balance sheet, the information in Exhibit 3.6 is used to develop a statement of operations for Windmill Point Outpatient Center (Exhibit 3.8). However, because the transactions that make up this statement were

EXHIBIT 3.8 STATEMENT OF OPERATIONS FOR WINDMILL POINT OUTPATIENT CENTER

Windmill Point Outpatient Center
Statement of Operations
for the Periods Ending December 31, 20X1 and 20X0

	12/31/20X1	12/31/20X0
Revenues		
Unrestricted revenues, gains and other support		
Net patient service revenue	$500,000	$0
Less provision for bad debts	($5,000)	
Net patient service revenue after provision	$495,000	
Premium revenue	250,000	0
Other revenue	600,000	0
Total revenues	1,345,000	0
Expenses		
Labor expense	335,000	0
Supplies expense	80,000	0
Interest expense	30,000	0
Insurance expense	10,000	0
Depreciation and amortization	45,000	0
Total expenses	500,000	0
Operating income	845,000	0
Excess of revenues over expenses	845,000	0
Contribution of long-lived assets	0	0
Transfers to parent	(25,000)	0
Increase in unrestricted net assets	**$820,000**	**$0**

recorded in an abbreviated form, it is necessary to refer also to the first column of Exhibit 3.6 to identify the specific nature of the transactions classified under unrestricted revenues, gains, and other support and also under expenses.

Unrestricted Revenues, Gains, and Other Support

The revenues of Windmill Point Outpatient Center are classified into three categories: net patient revenue earned after the provision of bad debt, $495,000; premium revenue earned from capitated patients, $250,000; and unrestricted contributions, which are presented in the category other revenue, $600,000. These revenues total $1,345,000.

Operating Expenses

Operating expenses are costs that are incurred in the day-to-day operation of the business. Exhibit 3.8 shows that the operating expense of $500,000 is made up of $335,000 labor expense ($300,000 paid for and $35,000 not yet paid for), $80,000 supplies expense, $30,000 interest expense, $10,000 insurance expense, and $45,000 depreciation expense.

Operating Income and Excess of Revenues over Expenses

Operating income is the difference between unrestricted revenues, gains, and other support and expenses. For Windmill Point Outpatient Center, operating income is $845,000. Because there are no *nonoperating income* items, this is also equal to *excess of revenues over expenses*, the net income of the organization.

Increase in Unrestricted Net Assets

As shown in Exhibit 3.8, the increase in unrestricted net assets, $820,000, for Windmill Point Outpatient Center is calculated as the operating income, $845,000, minus the transfers to parent ($25,000).

The Statement of Changes in Net Assets

The third financial statement is the statement of changes in net assets (the statement of changes in owners' equity or stockholders' equity for a for-profit business). Its purpose is to explain the changes in net assets from one period to the next (Exhibit 3.9). This statement reflects increases and decreases in net assets for both restricted and unrestricted net asset accounts. For Windmill Point Outpatient Center, the ending balance of net assets, $820,000, is the sum of the beginning total net assets account for the year, $0; the changes in unrestricted net assets for the year, $820,000

EXHIBIT 3.9 STATEMENT OF CHANGES IN NET ASSETS FOR WINDMILL POINT OUTPATIENT CENTER

Windmill Point Outpatient Center
Statement of Changes in Net Assets
for the Periods Ending December 31, 20X1 and 20X0

	12/31/20X1	12/31/20X0
Unrestricted net assets		
Excess of revenues over expenses	$845,000	$0
Contribution of long-lived assets	0	0
Transfers to parent	(25,000)	0
Increase in unrestricted net assets	820,000	0
Temporarily restricted net assets		
Restricted contribution	0	0
Increase in temporarily restricted net assets	0	0
Permanently restricted net assets		
Increase in permanently restricted net assets	0	0
Increase in net assets	820,000	0
Net assets, beginning of year	0	0
Net assets, end of year	$820,000	$0

(from the statement of operations); and contributions made to the temporarily restricted net asset accounts, $0.

The Statement of Cash Flows

Because accrual accounting is used, the statement of operations provides information about how much revenue was generated and the amount of resources used to generate those revenues. However, the statement of operations does not tell how much cash came into the organization and how much went out. That is the purpose of the statement of cash flows (see Exhibit 3.10). The construction of the statement of cash flows is beyond this introductory text. Most standard introductory accounting texts can provide more detailed information.

This statement is organized into three major sections: cash flows from operating activities, cash flows from investing activities, and cash flows from financing activities. Whereas the sections on investing and financing

EXHIBIT 3.10 STATEMENT OF CASH FLOWS FOR WINDMILL POINT OUTPATIENT CENTER

Windmill Point Outpatient Center
Statement of Cash Flows
for the Periods Ending December 31, 20X1 and 20X0

	12/31/20X1	12/31/20X0
Cash flows from operating activities		
Change in net assets	$820,000	$0
Depreciation expense	45,000	0
– Increase in temporarily restricted net assets	0	0
+ Transfers to parent	25,000	0
– Increase in net accounts receivable	(95,000)	0
– Increase in inventory	(20,000)	0
+ Increase in accounts payable	10,000	0
+ Increase in wages payable	35,000	0
Net cash provided by operating activities	820,000	0
Cash flows from investing activities		
Purchase of assets limited as to use	(60,000)	0
Purchase of plant, property, and equipment	(450,000)	0
Net cash flow used in investing activities	(510,000)	0
Cash flows from financing activities		
Transfers to parent	(25,000)	0
Increase in long-term debt	480,000	0
Net cash provided by financing activities	455,000	0
Net increase in cash and cash equivalents	765,000	0
Cash and cash equivalents, beginning of year	0	0
Cash and cash equivalents, end of year	$765,000	$0

activities are relatively straightforward, the section on cash flows from operating activities is not. The latter begins with changes in net assets and then makes adjustments required by the accrual basis of accounting.

Cash flows from investing activities include cash transactions involving the purchase or sale of properties and equipment, and the purchase or sale of long-term investments. Cash flows from financing activities include changes in noncurrent liability accounts, such as an increase or decrease in long-term debt (including the current portion), any increase in temporarily or permanently restricted assets, and the recognition of the transfer of cash funds to the parent corporation.

That *transfers to parent* appears twice in this statement can be confusing. It appears in the cash flows from operating activities section to show that there was $25,000 more cash available from operations than is shown in changes in net assets, which is the beginning point for calculating cash flows from operating activities. Because the inflow is included in the cash flows from operating activities, the cash outflow is then shown as a cash flow from financing activities.

Summary

The financial viability of a health care organization is the result of numerous decisions made by a variety of people including caregivers, administrators, boards, lenders, community members, and politicians. These decisions eventually result in the organization's acquiring and using resources to provide services, incur obligations, and generate revenues. One of the major roles of accounting is to record these transactions in a standardized format and to report the results to interested parties. This chapter shows how a series of typical transactions of a health center are recorded on the books, and how these records are used to produce the four major financial statements of a not-for-profit, business-oriented health care organization.

Transactions are recorded using either the cash basis of accounting or the accrual basis of accounting. In the *cash basis* of accounting, revenues are recognized when cash is received, and expenses are recognized when cash is paid. In the *accrual basis* of accounting, revenues are recognized when earned, and expenses are recognized when resources are used. The accrual basis of accounting must be used by health care organizations.

Two rules must be followed to record transactions under the accrual basis of accounting:

1. At least two accounts must be used to record a transaction.
   a. Increase (decrease) an *asset* account whenever assets are acquired (used).
   b. Increase (decrease) a liability account whenever obligations are incurred (paid for).
   c. Increase a *revenues, gains, or other support* account when revenues are earned, a gain occurs, or other support is received.

d. Increase an *expense* account when an asset is used. Net assets increase when unrestricted revenues, gains, and other support increase, and net assets decrease when expenses occur.

There are additional rules that must be followed for donations; however, these rules can become complex and are beyond the scope of this text.

2. After *each* transaction, the fundamental accounting equation must be in balance:

$$\text{Assets} = \text{Liabilities} + \text{Net Assets}$$

KEY TERMS

a. Accrual basis of accounting
b. Cash basis of accounting
c. Contra-asset

REVIEW QUESTIONS AND PROBLEMS

1. **Definitions.** Define the key terms in the list above.

2. **Accrual versus cash basis of accounting.** Explain the difference between the accrual basis of accounting and the cash basis of accounting. What are the major reasons for using accrual accounting?

3. **Accrual accounting.** How are revenues and expenses defined under accrual accounting?

4. **Journal versus ledger.** What are the purposes of a journal and a ledger?

5. **Adjustment of three accounts.** Give two examples of transactions that involve the adjustment of three accounts, rather than the usual two accounts.

6. **Contra-asset.** Give an example of a contra-asset, and explain how it is recorded on the ledger as a transaction.

7. **Prepaid expense.** Explain what a prepaid expense is and how it is recorded on the ledger as a transaction.

8. **Timing of transactions.** How would transactions differ if supplies were (a) completely paid for and consumed in one period or (b) paid for in one period but not used until the next period?

9. **Timing of transactions**. Are transactions recorded on a fiscal-year basis or a calendar-year basis? Does it have to be one or the other; if so, why?

10. **For-profit versus not-for-profit transactions**. What are the major differences in recording transactions for a for-profit organization versus a not-for-profit one, or are there any?

11. **Transactions plus multiple statements**. List and record each transaction for the Claymont Outpatient Clinic, under the accrual basis of accounting, at December 31, 20X1. Then develop a balance sheet as of December 31, 20X1, and a statement of operations for the year ended December 31, 20X1.

   a. The clinic received a $10,000,000 unrestricted cash contribution from the community. (*Hint*: this transaction increases the unrestricted net assets account.)

   b. The clinic purchased $4,500,000 of equipment. The clinic paid cash for the equipment.

   c. The clinic borrowed $2,000,000 from the bank on a long-term basis.

   d. The clinic purchased $550,000 of supplies on credit.

   e. The clinic provided $8,400,000 of services on credit.

   f. In the provision of these services, the clinic used $420,000 of supplies.

   g. The clinic received $800,000 in advance to care for capitated patients.

   h. The clinic incurred $4,500,000 in labor expenses and paid cash for them.

   i. The clinic incurred $2,230,000 in general expenses and paid cash for them.

   j. The clinic received $6,000,000 from patients and their third parties in payment of outstanding accounts.

   k. The clinic met $440,000 of its obligation to capitated patients (transaction g).

   l. The clinic made a $400,000 cash payment on the long-term loan.

   m. The clinic also made a cash interest payment of $40,000.

   n. A donor made a temporarily restricted donation of $370,000, which is set aside in temporary investments.

   o. The clinic recognized $400,000 in depreciation for the year.

   p. The clinic estimated that $850,000 of patient accounts would not be received, and established a provision for bad debt.

12. **Transactions plus multiple statements**. The following are the financial transactions for the Family Home Health Care Center, a not-for-profit, business-oriented organization. Beginning balances at January 1, 20X1, for its assets, liabilities, and net assets accounts are shown in the following list.

Givens

Cash	$5,500
Accounts receivable	$60,000
Allowance for uncollectibles	$4,500
Supplies	$13,000
Long-term investments	$42,000
Properties and equipment	$880,000
Accumulated depreciation	$90,000
Short-term accounts payable	$42,000
Other current liabilities	$3,000
Long-term debt	$680,000
Unrestricted net assets	$169,000
Permanently restricted net assets	$12,000

List and record each transaction under the accrual basis of accounting. Then develop a balance sheet as of December 31, 20X1 and 20X0, and a statement of operations for the year ended December 31, 20X1.

a.   The center purchased $4,000 of supplies on credit.

b.   The center provided $430,000 of home health services on credit.

c.   The center consumed $9,000 of supplies in the provision of its home health services.

d.   The center provided $250,000 of home health services, and patients paid for services in cash.

e.   The center paid cash for $5,000 of supplies in the provision of its home health services.

f.   The center paid $24,000 in cash for supplies previously purchased on credit.

g.   A donor established a $87,000 permanent endowment fund (in the form of long-term investments) for the center. (*Hint*: this transaction increases the permanently restricted net assets account.)

h.   The center collected $250,000 from patients for outstanding receivables.

i.   The center paid $300,000 in cash toward labor expense.

j.   The center paid $90,000 in cash toward its long-term loan.

k.   The center purchased $35,000 in small equipment on credit. The amount is due within one year.

l.   The center incurred $40,000 in general expenses. The center used cash to pay for the general expenses.

m. The center incurred $8,000 in interest expense for the year. A cash payment of $8,000 was made to the bank.

n. The center made a $9,000 cash transfer to its parent corporation.

o. The center recognized labor expense of $4,500 but does not incur a cash payment.

p. The center recognized depreciation expenses of $20,000.

q. The center estimated it would not collect $85,000 of the patient accounts receivable, and established a provision for bad debt.

13. **Statement of operations.** The following is a list of account balances for Krakower Healthcare Services, Inc. on December 31, 20X1. Prepare a statement of operations as of December 31, 20X1. (*Hint*: when net assets are released from restriction, the restricted account is decreased, and the unrestricted account is increased. It is recognized under revenues, gains, and other support.)

Givens

Supply expense	$60,000
Transfer to parent corporation	$18,000
Provision for bad debt expense	$10,000
Depreciation expense	$35,000
Labor expense	$80,000
Interest expense	$7,000
Administrative expense	$50,000
Net patient service revenues	$220,000
Net assets released from restriction	$30,000

14. **Statement of operations.** The following is a list of account balances (in thousands) for the Kirkland County Hospital on September 30, 20X1. Prepare a statement of operations as of September 30, 20X1. (*Hint*: unrestricted donations are recognized under revenues, gains, and other support.)

Givens

Labor expense	$12,000
Provision for bad debt	$3,200
Supplies expense	$4,800
Unrestricted cash donation for operations	$2,300
Net patient service revenues	$34,000
Professional fees	$8,550
Transfer to parent corporation	$1,450
Other revenues from cafeteria and gift shop	$1,000
Depreciation expense	$1,600
Income from investments (unrestricted investments)	$3,000
Administrative expense	$3,900

15. **Statement of cash flows**. The following is a list of account balances for Hover Hospital on June 30, 20X1. Prepare a statement of cash flows as of June 30, 20X1.

Givens

Transfer to parent corporation	$40,000
Proceeds from sale of fixed equipment	$2,290,000
Principal payment on bonds payable	$780,000
Purchase of fixed equipment	$5,300,000
Beginning cash balance	$6,500,000
Cash from operating activities	$3,900,000
Principal payment on notes payable	$6,500

16. **Multiple statements**. The following is a list of accounts (in thousands) for St. Paul's Hospital on December 31, 20X1. Prepare a balance sheet and statement of operations as of December 31, 20X1. (*Hints*: (a) unrestricted contributions increase the unrestricted net assets account, and they are a part of revenues, gains, and other support; (b) Net Assets = Total Assets − Total Liabilities.)

Givens

Interest expense	$1,800
Net patient revenues, net of contractuals only	$113,000
Unrestricted contributions	$2,300
Cash	$5,500
Other noncurrent assets	$18,200
Temporary investments	$8,800
Gross accounts receivable	$42,400
Professional expense	$3,200
Other current liabilities	$2,100
Accrued expenses	$10,000
Accounts payable	$11,500
Other revenues	$19,000
Long-term debt	$11,600
Administrative and medical supplies expense	$29,000
Gross plant and equipment	$85,000
Labor expense	$78,000
Prepaid expenses	$2,100
Deferred revenue	$2,800
Inventory	$2,200
Depreciation expense	$7,500
Provision bad debt expense	$12,000
Accumulated depreciation	$38,000
Nonoperating gains	$1,800
Allowance for uncollectibles	$20,000

17. **Transactions plus multiple statements**. St. Catherine's Diagnostic Center had the following ending balances at December 31, 20X0, for its assets, liabilities, and net assets accounts.

Givens

Cash and temporary investments	$300,000
Accounts receivable	$2,500,000
Allowance for uncollectibles	$200,000
Inventory	$205,000
Plant and equipment	$5,800,000
Accumulated depreciation	$312,000
Accounts payable	$230,000
Other short-term notes payable	$30,000
Long-term bonds payable	$400,000
Unrestricted net assets	$7,632,800
Temporarily restricted net assets	$200

List and record each 20X1 transaction under the accrual basis of accounting. Then develop a balance sheet at end-of-years 20X0 and 20X1 and a statement of operations and a statement of changes in net assets for the year ended December 31, 20X1.

a. The center collected $2,000,000 in cash from outstanding accounts receivable.

b. The center purchased $2,000,000 of inventory on credit.

c. The center provided $9,100,000 of patient services on credit.

d. The center incurred $4,660,000 of labor expenses, which it paid in cash.

e. The center consumed $1,930,000 of supplies from its inventory in the provision of its diagnostic services.

f. The center paid $45,000 in cash for outstanding short-term notes payable.

g. The center collected $7,650,000 in cash from outstanding accounts receivable.

h. The center paid $1,800,000 in cash for outstanding accounts payable.

i. The center issued $3,800,000 in long-term bonds that it must pay back.

j. The center purchased $3,000,000 in new equipment using a short-term note payable.

k. The center incurred $51,000 in interest expense, which it paid in cash.

l. The center incurred $1,050,000 in general expenses, which it paid in cash.

m. The center made a cash payment of $780,000 toward principal payment of its outstanding bonds.

n. A local corporation gave an unrestricted $46,000 cash donation. (*Hint*: this transaction increases the unrestricted net assets account.)

o. The center received, in cash, $4,000 in interest income from unrestricted temporary investments.

p. The center transferred $518,000 in cash to its parent corporation.

q. The center incurred an annual depreciation expense of $95,000.

r. The center estimated that its provision for bad debt expense is $12,000.

18. **Transactions plus multiple statements.** Ambulatory Center, Inc., had the following ending balances for its assets, liabilities, and net assets accounts as of December 31, 20X0.

Givens

Cash	$33,000
Accounts receivable	$60,000
Allowance for uncollectibles	$20,000
Inventory or supplies	$8,200
Prepaid insurance	$1,800
Long-term investments	$20,000
Plant, property, and equipment	$3,800,000
Accumulated depreciation	$1,750,000
Short-term accounts payable	$79,000
Accrued expenses	$15,000
Long-term debt	$1,055,000
Unrestricted net assets	$903,300
Permanently restricted net assets	$100,700

List and record each 20X1 transaction under the accrual basis of accounting. Then develop a balance sheet for end-of-years 20X0 and 20X1 and a statement of operations and a statement of changes in net assets for the year ended December 31, 20X1.

a. The center made a cash payment of $65,000 to pay off outstanding accounts payable.

b. The center received $14,000 in cash from a donor who temporarily restricted its use. (*Hint*: this transaction increases the temporarily restricted net assets account.)

c. The center provided $3,100,000 of services on credit.

d. The center consumed $4,000 of supplies in the provision of its ambulatory services.

e. The center paid off accrued interest expense of $17,500 in cash.

f. The center collected $2,650,000 in cash from outstanding accounts receivable.

g. The center incurred $17,000 in general expenses that it paid for in cash.

h. The center made a $200,000 cash principal payment toward its long-term debt.

i. The center collected $380,000 in cash from outstanding accounts receivable.

j. The center received $19,000 in cash from an HMO for future capitated services.

k. The center purchased $4,000 of supplies on credit.

l.   The center earned, but did not receive, $3,900 in income from its restricted net assets. The income can be used for general operations. (*Hint*: this transaction increases interest receivable and is also recorded under revenues, gains, and other support.)

m.   The center's temporarily restricted asset account released $3,500 from its restricted account to its unrestricted account for operations. (*Hint*: the transfer gets recorded under revenues, gains, and other support.)

n.   The center incurred $5,000 in interest expense. The interest expense was recorded but not yet paid in cash.

o.   The center incurred $2,560,000 in labor expenses, which it paid for in cash.

p.   The center paid $4,000 in advance for insurance expense.

q.   The center transferred $4,000 in cash to its parent corporation.

r.   The center incurred $200,000 in depreciation expense.

s.   The center's prepaid insurance of $2,400 expired for the year.

t.   The center estimated $6,800 in bad debt and established a provision for bad debt expense for the year.

19.   **Transactions plus multiple statements.** Happy Valley Hospital, Inc., had the following ending balances (in thousands) for its assets, liabilities, and net assets as of December 31, 20X0.

Givens

Cash	$2,900
Accounts receivable	$44,000
Allowance for uncollectibles	$6,000
Inventory or supplies	$3,000
Prepaid insurance	$700
Long-term investments	$93,000
Plant, property, and equipment	$155,000
Accumulated depreciation	$80,000
Short-term accounts payable	$8,500
Accrued expenses	$19,000
Long-term debt	$49,000
Unrestricted net assets	$127, 200
Temporarily restricted net assets	$7,900
Permanently restricted net assets	$1,000

List and record each 20X1 transaction under the accrual basis of accounting. Then develop a balance sheet for end-of-years 20X0 and 20X1 and a statement of operations and a statement of changes in net assets for the year ended December 31, 20X1.

a.   The hospital made a cash payment of $3,100,000 toward outstanding accounts payable.

b. The hospital received $5,200,000 in cash from a donor who temporarily restricted its use. (*Hint*: this transaction increases the temporarily restricted net assets account.)

c. The hospital provided $123,000,000 of services on credit.

d. The hospital consumed $2,630,000 of supplies in the provision of its ambulatory services.

e. The hospital paid cash for incurred interest expense of $3,800,000.

f. The hospital collected $114,000,000 in cash from outstanding accounts receivable.

g. The hospital incurred $4,000,000 in general expenses that it paid for in cash.

h. The hospital made a $3,800,000 cash principal payment toward its long-term debt.

i. The hospital collected $25,000,000 in cash from outstanding accounts receivable.

j. The hospital purchased $30,000,000 of supplies on credit.

k. The hospital earned, but did not receive, $2,000,000 in income from its restricted net assets. The income can be used for general operations. (*Hint*: this transaction increases interest receivable and is also recorded under revenues, gains, and other support.)

l. The hospital incurred $1,300,000 in interest expense, but not yet paid for in cash.

m. The hospital incurred $60,000,000 in labor expenses, which it paid for in cash.

n. The hospital made a cash payment of $2,300,000 in advance for insurance expense.

o. The hospital transferred $1,200,000 in cash to its parent corporation.

p. The hospital incurred $8,000,000 in depreciation expense.

q. The hospital's prepaid insurance of $2,500,000 expired for the year.

r. The hospital estimated $700,000 in bad debt and established a provision for bad debt expense for the year.

20. **Transactions plus multiple statements**. Glenwood Hospital had the following ending balances (in thousands) for its assets, liabilities, and net assets accounts as of December 31, 20X0.

Givens

Cash	$8,000
Accounts receivable	$58,000
Allowance for uncollectibles	$8,000
Inventory or supplies	$4,900
Prepaid insurance	$1,500
Long-term investments	$230,000
Plant, property, and equipment	$250,000
Accumulated depreciation	$90,000
Short-term accounts payable	$20,000
Accrued expenses	$8,700
Long-term debt	$165,000
Unrestricted net assets	$251,400
Temporarily restricted net assets	$4,200
Permanently restricted net assets	$5,100

List and record each 20X1 transaction under the accrual basis of accounting. Then develop a balance sheet for end-of-years 20X0 and 20X1 and a statement of operations and a statement of changes in net assets for the year ended December 31, 20X1.

a. The hospital made a cash payment of $7,100,000 toward outstanding accounts payable.

b. The hospital collected $34,000,000 in cash from outstanding accounts receivable.

c. The hospital provided $236,000,000 of services on credit.

d. The hospital consumed $3,100,000 of supplies in the provision of its ambulatory services.

e. The hospital paid cash for incurred interest expense of $4,100,000.

f. The hospital purchased $36,000,000 in long-term investments and used cash for this purpose.

g. The hospital incurred $8,100,000 in general expenses that it paid for in cash.

h. The hospital made a $3,900,000 cash principal payment toward its long-term debt.

i. The hospital collected $141,000,000 in cash from outstanding accounts receivable.

j. The hospital purchased $6,100,000 of supplies on credit.

k. The hospital earned, but did not receive, $330,000 in income from its restricted net assets. The income can be used for general operations. (*Hint*: this transaction increases interest receivable and is also recorded under revenues, gains, and other support.)

l. The hospital incurred $720,000 in interest expense, which it paid for in cash.

m. The hospital incurred $93,000,000 in labor expenses, which it paid for in cash.

n. The hospital made a cash payment of $730,000 in advance for insurance expense.

o. The hospital transferred $1,050,000 in cash to its parent corporation.

p. The hospital incurred $5,300,000 in depreciation expense.

q. The hospital's prepaid insurance of $620,000 expired for the year.

r. The hospital recognized $1,000,000 in bad debt for the year and established a provision of bad debt for this amount.

s. The hospital made a cash payment of $14,100,000 for radiology equipment.

CHAPTER 4

FINANCIAL STATEMENT ANALYSIS

The financial performance of health care organizations is of interest to numerous individuals and groups, including administrators, board members, creditors, bondholders, community members, and governmental agencies (see Perspectives 4.1 and 4.2). Chapters Two and Three examined the four main financial statements of health care organizations and the accounting methods underlying the preparation of these statements. This chapter shows how to analyze the financial statements of health care organizations to help answer questions about the organization that produced them:

- Is the organization profitable? Why or why not?
- How effective is the organization in collecting its receivables?
- Is the organization in a good position to pay its bills?
- How efficiently is the organization using its assets?
- Are the organization's plant and equipment in need of replacement?
- Is the organization in a good position to take on additional debt?

Three approaches are commonly used to analyze financial statements: *horizontal analysis*, *vertical analysis*, and *ratio analysis*. Each of these approaches is examined using the financial statements shown in Exhibit 4.1, Newport Hospital's statement of operations and balance sheet. For simplicity, the statement of operations contains only operating items.

LEARNING OBJECTIVES

- Analyze the financial statements of health care organizations using horizontal analysis, vertical (common-size) analysis, and ratio analysis.

- Calculate and interpret liquidity ratios, profitability ratios, activity ratios, and capital structure ratios.

PERSPECTIVE 4.1 FITCH CREDIT RATING AGENCIES CONSIDER KEY FINANCIAL RATIOS IN REVIEWING A HEALTH CARE SYSTEM'S CREDIT RATING

Novant is a regional health care system with thirteen hospitals in North Carolina and Virginia that has a strong credit rating of AA– from Fitch Rating, which is one notch below the highest rating of AAA. Novant has been able to maintain this high credit rating of AA– because of its consistent operating performance over the last three years, adequate liquidity, strong market position, and extensive physician network. For example, in the first six months of 2012, Novant's cash flow margin was 10.2 percent, which matched the 10.2 percent median benchmark for an AA rating. However, Fitch's credit issues projecting into the future relate to Novant's loss of market share in selected markets and its increased leverage position. Novant's debt to total capital (which includes both long-term debt and equity) was 46.3 percent, compared to an AA median of 33.9 percent. Furthermore, its debt service coverage ratio is 3.8x, which indicates its operating cash flow is almost four times its debt service payments for the first six months of 2012, as compared to a median benchmark value of 4.8x. Novant needs to address these concerns in the near future in order to avoid a downgrading of its credit rating from AA–.

Source: Adapted from Fitch affirms Novant Health, Inc. System's (NC) revs at "AA–": outlook stable, *Business Wire*, September 26, 2012.

 Caution: The financial statements presented in this chapter have been simplified from those presented in Chapter Two to facilitate the application of the tools and techniques presented in this chapter.

 ## Horizontal Analysis

Horizontal Analysis

A method of analyzing financial statements that looks at the percentage change in a line item from one year to the next. It is computed by the formula (Subsequent Year − Previous Year) / Previous Year.

Horizontal and vertical analyses are two of the most commonly used techniques to analyze financial statements; each is based on percentages. *Horizontal analysis* looks at the percentage change in a line item from one year to the next. A horizontal analysis of Newport Hospital's statement of operations and balance sheet is presented in Exhibit 4.2 and serves as the basis for the discussion in this section. Horizontal analysis uses the formula:

$$\left(\frac{\text{Subsequent Year} - \text{Previous Year}}{\text{Previous Year}}\right)100 = \text{Percentage Change}$$

The goal is to answer the question, What is the percentage change in a line item from one year to the next year? For example, using Newport Hospital's statement of operations in Exhibit 4.2, the change in operating

PERSPECTIVE 4.2 IMPORTANT RATIOS USED BY HEALTH CARE ADVISORS TO ASSESS FINANCIAL PERFORMANCE OF HOSPITALS

A senior executive at a major health care financial advisory firm recommends that CEOs and CFOs follow the trends of five key financial ratios within the health care industry relative to their organization's operational and market conditions. These financial ratios are the (1) operating margin, (2) cash flow margin, (3) days cash on hand, (4) long-term debt to total capital, and (5) capital expenditures relative to depreciation expense. The financial advisor gave this example: a hospital had higher days cash on hand relative to the industry benchmark; however, the hospital also had an aging plant, declining utilization, and falling market share. Overall, the hospital was not leveraging its cash position to address the downward trend in these areas. To act strategically, the hospital needed to use its high liquidity position, or days cash on hand ratio, to help it borrow tax-exempt debt to achieve a higher credit rating. By issuing tax-exempt debt, the hospital could replace or renovate the hospital and/or purchase new medical equipment to help attract physicians and patients. This in turn would increase its patient volume as well as recapture its lost market share. As a result the hospital could generate higher revenues, which in turn would lead to an improvement in its operating margin ratio and cash flow, and build its days cash on hand ratio.

Source: Adapted from S. Rodak, 5 key financial ratios healthcare providers should track, *Becker's Hospital Review,* May 20, 2012, www.beckershospitalreview.com/racs-/-icd-9-/-icd-10/5-key-financial-ratios-healthcare-providers -should-track.html.

income from 20X0 (where 20X0 is the base year) to 20X1 using horizontal analysis would be

$$\left(\frac{\$330,909-\$1,054,186}{\$1,054,186}\right)100=-68.6 \text{ percent}$$

Key Point Three approaches to analyzing financial statements are horizontal analysis, vertical analysis, and ratio analysis.

A problem with horizontal analysis is that percentage changes can hide major dollar effects. For example, on the one hand, Newport had an 80.9 percent change in interest expense, which was the result of a $223,621 change from 20X0 to 20X1 ($500,000 − $276,379) (see the statement of operations in Exhibit 4.1); on the other hand, the 9.4 percent change in total operating expenses was a $915,605 change (Exhibit 4.2).

EXHIBIT 4.1 STATEMENT OF OPERATIONS AND BALANCE SHEET FOR NEWPORT HOSPITAL

Newport Hospital Statement of Operations for the Years Ended December 31, 20X1 and 20X0

	12/31/20X1	12/31/20X0
Operating revenues		
Net patient revenues	$10,778,272	$10,566,176
Other operating revenues	233,749	253,517
Total operating revenues	11,012,021	10,819,693
Operating expenses		
Salaries and benefits	5,644,880	5,345,498
Supplies	1,660,000	1,529,680
Insurance	1,536,357	1,551,579
Depreciation and amortization (1)	383,493	420,238
Interest	500,000	276,379
Other	956,382	642,133
Total operating expenses	10,681,112	9,765,507
Operating income	330,909	1,054,186
Nonoperating revenue	185,000	165,000
Excess of revenues over expenses	515,909	1,219,186
Increase (decrease) in unrestricted net assets	**$515,909**	**$1,219,186**

(1) The hospital did not incur any amortization expense for this time period; therefore, the entire account represents depreciation expense.

EXHIBIT 4.1 CONTINUED

Newport Hospital Balance Sheet December 31, 20X1 and 20X0

	12/31/20X1	12/31/20X0
Assets		
Current assets		
Cash and marketable securities	$363,181	$158,458
Patient accounts receivables net of uncollectible accounts	1,541,244	1,400,013
Inventories	346,176	316,875
Prepaid expenses	163,734	78,788
Other current assets	100,000	0
Total current assets	2,514,335	1,954,134
Noncurrent assets		
Gross plant, property, and equipment	7,088,495	6,893,370
(less accumulated depreciation)	(2,781,741)	(2,398,248)
Net plant, property, and equipment	4,306,754	4,495,122
Long-term investments	3,414,732	4,525,476
Other assets	640,915	340,853
Total noncurrent assets	8,362,401	9,361,451
Total assets	**$10,876,736**	**$11,315,585**
Liabilities and net assets		
Current liabilities		
Accounts payable	$387,646	$166,600
Salaries payable	135,512	529,298
Notes payable	500,000	2,359,524
Current portion of long-term debt	372,032	338,996
Total current liabilities	1,395,190	3,394,418
Long-term liabilities		
Bonds payable	6,938,891	6,009,484
Total long-term liabilities	6,938,891	6,009,484
Total liabilities	8,334,081	9,403,902
Net assets		
Unrestricted	1,901,739	1,570,830
Temporary restricted	328,000	40,853
Permanently restricted	312,916	300,000
Total net assets	2,542,655	1,911,683
Total liabilities and net assets	**$10,876,736**	**$11,315,585**

EXHIBIT 4.2   HORIZONTAL ANALYSIS OF THE STATEMENT OF OPERATIONS AND BALANCE SHEET FOR NEWPORT HOSPITAL

Newport Hospital Statement of Operations for the Years Ended December 31, 20X1 and 20X0

	20X1	20X0	Percentage Change 20X1–20X0
Operating revenues			
Net patient revenues	$10,778,272	$10,566,176	2.0%
Other operating revenues	233,749	253,517	−7.8%
Total operating revenues	11,012,021	10,819,693	1.8%
Operating expenses			
Total operating expenses	10,681,112	9,765,507	9.4%
Operating income	330,909	1,054,186	−68.6%
Nonoperating revenue	185,000	165,000	12.1%
Excess of revenues over expenses	515,909	1,219,186	−57.7%
Increase (decrease) in unrestricted net assets	**$515,909**	**$1,219,186**	−57.7%

Newport Hospital Balance Sheet December 31, 20X1 and 20X0

	20X1	20X0	Percentage Change 20X1–20X0
Assets			
Current assets	$2,514,335	$1,954,134	28.7%
Noncurrent assets	8,362,401	9,361,451	−10.7%
Total assets	**$10,876,736**	**$11,315,585**	−3.9%
Liabilities			
Current liabilities	$1,395,190	$3,394,418	−58.9%
Long-term liabilities	6,938,891	6,009,484	15.5%
Total liabilities	8,334,081	9,403,902	
Net assets			
Total net assets	2,542,655	1,911,683	33.0%
Total liabilities and net assets	**$10,876,736**	**$11,315,585**	−3.9%

Key Point When using horizontal analysis, (1) small percentage changes can mask large dollar changes from one year to the next, and (2) large percentage changes from year to year may be relatively inconsequential in terms of dollar amounts. The latter situation usually occurs when the base year shows a small dollar amount.

Horizontal analysis is also often used to compare changes from one year to the next over several years. The following example analyzes five consecutive years of Newport Hospital's operating income (not shown in the exhibits):

	20X0	20X1	20X2	20X3	20X4
Operating income	$1,054,186	$330,909	$500,098	$1,232,565	$1,453,567
Percentage change from previous year		−68.6%	51.1%	146.5%	17.9%

Note that the year 20X0 in the above table and ensuing discussion represents the first year of the next decade. The change from 20X1 to 20X2 is calculated as follows:

$$\left(\frac{\$500,098 - \$330,909}{\$330,909}\right)100 = 51.1 \text{ percent}$$

This analysis shows how successful the organization was in increasing operating income from one year to the next. A disadvantage of this approach is that it does not answer the question, How much overall change has there been since 20X0? Trend analysis supplies an answer to this question.

Trend Analysis

Instead of looking at single-year changes, *trend analysis* compares changes over a longer period of time by comparing each year with a base year. The formula for a trend analysis is

$$\left(\frac{\text{Any Subsequent Year} - \text{Base Year}}{\text{Base Year}}\right)100$$

Trend Analysis
A type of horizontal analysis that looks at changes in line items compared with a base year.

Applying this formula to operating income for the same five-year period used to illustrate horizontal analysis yields the following results:

	20X0	20X1	20X2	20X3	20X4
Operating income	$1,054,186	$330,909	$500,098	$1,232,565	$1,453,567
Percentage change from 20X0		−68.6%	−52.6%	16.9%	37.9%

For instance, the change from 20X0 to 20X4 is calculated as follows:

$$\left(\frac{\$1,453,567 - \$1,054,186}{\$1,054,186}\right)100 = 37.9 \text{ percent}$$

Thus from 20X0 (the base year) to 20X4, operating income rose 37.9 percent. Note that the average annual increase of 9.5 percent (37.9 percent / 4 years) is different from that obtained by simply averaging the increases or decreases each year.

Vertical (Common-Size) Analysis

Vertical Analysis
A method of analyzing financial statements that answers the general question: What percentage of one line item is another line item? Also called *common-size analysis* because it converts every line item to a percentage, thus allowing comparisons among the financial statements of different organizations. One can determine, for example, which organization has the highest percentage of its assets as current assets.

The purpose of *vertical analysis* is to answer the general question, What percentage of one line item is another line item? The formula to use in this case is

$$\frac{\text{Line Item of Interest}}{\text{Base Line Item}}100$$

For instance, Newport Hospital might want to know if net patient revenues have increased as a percentage of total operating revenues or, similarly, what percentage the operating expenses are of its operating revenues. The top section of Exhibit 4.3 computes all line items in Newport Hospital's statement of operations as a percentage of total operating revenues. In 20X0, total operating expenses were 90.3 percent of total operating revenues [($9,765,507 / $10,819,693) × 100], but by 20X1, they had increased to 97 percent of total operating revenues [($10,681,112 / $11,012,021) × 100]. This information provides some insight as to why Newport Hospital experienced the 68.6 percent decrease in operating income observed in the horizontal analysis.

Although the focus up until now has been on the statement of operations, vertical analysis is useful for analyzing the balance sheet as well, as shown in the bottom of Exhibit 4.3, which presents all line items as a percentage of total assets. By using total assets as a base, the reader can ask such questions as, Has the composition of the balance sheet changed appreciably from 20X0 to 20X1? In this example, total liabilities decreased from 83.1 percent of total assets in 20X0 to 76.6 percent in 20X1.

Two points can be noted from this information: in 20X1, debt was used to finance 76.6 percent of Newport Hospital's assets, whereas in 20X0 it

EXHIBIT 4.3 VERTICAL (COMMON-SIZE) ANALYSIS FOR THE STATEMENT OF OPERATIONS AND BALANCE SHEET FOR NEWPORT HOSPITAL

Newport Hospital Statement of Operations for Years Ended December 31, 20X1 and 20X0

	20X1	Percentage of Total Revenues	20X0	Percentage of Total Revenues
Operating revenues				
Net patient revenues	$10,778,272	97.9%	$10,566,176	97.7%
Other operating revenues	233,749	2.1%	253,517	2.3%
Total operating revenues	11,012,021	100.0%	10,819,693	100.0%
Operating expenses				
Total operating expenses	10,681,112	97.0%	9,765,507	90.3%
Operating income	330,909	3.0%	1,054,186	9.7%
Nonoperating revenue	185,000	1.7%	165,000	1.5%
Excess of revenues over expenses	515,909	4.7%	1,219,186	11.3%
Increase (decrease) in unrestricted net assets	**$515,909**	4.7%	**$1,219,186**	11.3%

Newport Hospital Balance Sheet December 31, 20X1 and 20X0

	20X1	Percentage of Total Assets	20X0	Percentage of Total Assets
Assets				
Current assets	$2,514,335	23.1%	$1,954,134	17.3%
Noncurrent assets	8,362,401	76.9%	9,361,451	82.7%
Total assets	**$10,876,736**	100.0%	**$11,315,585**	100.0%
Liabilities				
Current liabilities	$1,395,190	12.8%	$3,394,418	30.0%
Long-term liabilities	6,938,891	63.8%	6,009,484	53.1%
Total liabilities	8,334,081	76.6%	9,403,902	83.1%
Net assets				
Total net assets	2,542,655	23.4%	1,911,683	16.9%
Total liabilities and net assets	**$10,876,736**	100.0%	**$11,315,585**	100.0%

Leveraged

The degree to which an organization is financed by debt.

was used to finance over 83 percent; and the use of long-term debt to finance assets grew from 53.1 percent of total assets in 20X0 to 63.8 percent in 20X1. In other words, Newport is more highly leveraged in 20X1 than it was in 20X0.

Key Point Vertical analysis is also called common-size analysis because it converts every line item to a percentage, thus allowing comparisons between the financial accounts of organizations of different sizes.

Exhibit 4.4 presents common-size financial statements for a small community hospital and a large community hospital. The larger facility has a smaller percentage of its assets, 75 percent, in plant and equipment, compared with 88 percent for the smaller facility. However, the smaller facility has a lower proportion of its capital structure, 58 percent, in total debt, compared with 70 percent for the larger facility. The larger facility also has a higher percentage of its revenues from net patient revenues (97 percent) than does the smaller facility (83 percent). Although there are no benchmarks to compare these percentages with, they can elicit questions as to why the differences exist.

Ratio Analysis

Although horizontal and vertical analyses are easy to calculate and commonly used, *ratio analysis* is the preferred approach for gaining an in-depth understanding of financial statements. A *ratio* expresses the relationship between two numbers as a single number. For instance, the current ratio expresses the relationship between current assets and current liabilities. This provides an indication of the organization's ability to cover current obligations with current assets (the ability to pay short-term debt).

Ratio

An expression of the relationship between two numbers as a single number.

Categories of Ratios

Ratios are generally grouped into four categories: liquidity, profitability, activity, and capital structure.

Liquidity ratios answer the question, How well is the organization positioned to meet its short-term obligations? *Profitability ratios* answer the question, How profitable is the organization? *Activity ratios* answer the question, How efficiently is the organization using its assets to produce revenues? *Capital structure ratios* answer the questions, How are the organization's assets financed?, and, How able is the organization to take on new debt? Exhibit 4.5 shows what the ratios would be for Newport Hospital and compares them with industry norms. The remaining sections of this chapter will describe how these results were derived.

EXHIBIT 4.4 COMMON-SIZE FINANCIAL STATEMENTS FOR A SMALL AND A LARGE HOSPITAL

Small Community Hospital
Balance Sheet December 31, 20X0[a]

		Percentage of Total Assets
Current assets	$1,000	10%
Net plant and equipment	9,000	88%
Other assets	200	2%
Total assets	10,200	100%
Current liabilities	900	9%
Long-term debt	5,000	49%
Total liabilities	5,900	58%
Net assets	4,300	42%
Total liabilities and net assets	$10,200	100%

Small Community Hospital
Statement of Operations December 31, 20X0[a]

		Percentage of Total Revenues
Net patient revenues	$10,000	83%
Investment income	2,000	17%
Total operating revenues	12,000	100%
Operating expenses	10,000	83%
Income from operations	2,000	17%
Excess of revenues over expenses	2,000	17%
Increase in net assets	$2,000	17%

Large Community Hospital
Balance Sheet December 31, 20X0[a]

		Percentage of Total Assets
Current assets	$15,000	22%
Net plant and equipment	50,000	75%
Other assets	2,000	3%
Total assets	67,000	100%
Current liabilities	12,000	18%
Long-term debt	35,000	52%
Total liabilities	47,000	70%
Net assets	20,000	30%
Total liabilities and net assets	$67,000	100%

Large Community Hospital
Statement of Operations December 31, 20X0[a]

		Percentage of Total Revenues
Net patient revenues	$68,000	97%
Investment income	2,000	3%
Total operating revenues	70,000	100%
Operating expenses	65,000	93%
Income from operations	5,000	7%
Excess of revenues over expenses	5,000	7%
Increase in net assets	$5,000	7%

[a]Note: All figures other than percentages are expressed in thousands.

EXHIBIT 4.5 NEWPORT HOSPITAL RATIOS FOR 20X0 AND 20X1, AND OPTUM AND CMS MEDIAN RATIO VALUES

Ratios	Benchmark Small Hospitals' Optum & CMS Median Ratio[a]	Newport Ratios		Desired Position	Current Year Position[c]	Trend Position
		20X1	20X0			
Liquidity ratios						
Current ratio	2.11	1.80	0.58	Above	−15% Unfavorable	Increasing
Quick ratio[b]	1.52	1.36	0.46	Above	−10% Unfavorable	Increasing
Acid test ratio[b]	0.30	0.26	0.05	Above	−13% Unfavorable	Increasing
Days in accounts receivable	49	52	48	Below	7% Unfavorable	Increasing
Days cash on hand	86	134	183	Above	56% Favorable	Decreasing
Average payment period	50	49	133	Below	−1% Favorable	Decreasing
Revenue, expense and profitability ratios						
Operating revenue per adjusted discharge	$7,448	$5,647	$6,011	Above	−24% Unfavorable	Decreasing
Operating expense per adjusted discharge	$7,197	$5,477	$5,425	Below	−24% Favorable	Stable
Salary and benefit expense as percentage of operating expense[b]	40%	53%	55%	Below	32% Unfavorable	Decreasing
Operating margin	0.03	0.03	0.10	Above	0% Favorable	Decreasing
Nonoperating revenue	0.04	0.02	0.02	Varies	−58% Unfavorable	Increasing
Return on total assets	0.04	0.05	0.11	Above	36% Favorable	Decreasing
Return on net assets	0.08	0.20	0.64	Above	154% Favorable	Decreasing
Activity ratios						
Total asset turnover ratio	1.07	1.01	0.96	Above	−5% Unfavorable	Increasing
Net fixed assets turnover ratio	2.12	2.56	2.41	Above	21% Favorable	Increasing
Age of plant ratio	10.31	7.25	5.71	Below	−30% Favorable	Increasing
Capital structure ratios						
Long-term debt to net assets ratio	0.21	2.73	3.14	Below	1200% Unfavorable	Decreasing
Net assets to total assets ratio	0.54	0.23	0.17	Above	−57% Unfavorable	Increasing
Times interest earned ratio	3.78	2.03	5.41	Above	−46% Unfavorable	Decreasing
Debt service coverage ratio	3.18	2.00	4.02	Above	−37% Unfavorable	Decreasing

[a]Because Newport Hospital has fewer than 100 beds, the Optum benchmark ratio values for bed size less than 100 is used.

[b]All ratio values, except for quick, acid test, and salary and benefit expense as a percentage of operating expense ratios, were obtained from Optum Insight, *2013 Almanac of Hospital Financial and Operating Indicators*, 2011/2010 median value data. The quick, acid test, and salary and benefit expense as a percentage of operating expense ratios were obtained from 2010 CMS cost report data.

[c]These percentages may be slightly off because they are computed from nonrounded ratio values.

Liquidity analysis: Newport's liquidity is improving, though several ratios are still considered unfavorable relative to the desired benchmark positions. The current and quick ratios are 15% and 10% below standard, respectively, while the most stringent acid test is 13% below standard. This suggests potential difficulty in being able to pay off immediate debt obligations, such as monthly payments, without having to tap into a reserve fund. In order for the current ratio to be at the 2.11 benchmark with given current liabilities, Newport would need an additional $430,000 in liquidity. However, Newport is nearly at benchmark for days in accounts receivable, suggesting sufficient control in collecting funds; its days cash on hand is still comfortably high; and the recently favorable average payment period shows that so far, Newport has been able to pay all of its bills in a timely manner.

Revenue, expense, and profitability analysis: While Newport's operating revenue per adjusted discharge has been stable and remains well below the norm, the declining operating revenue per adjusted discharge is of concern. This could arise from lower payor payment rates, or possibly poor chart documentation leading to an inability to code discharges appropriately at higher levels to generate additional income. Lower expenditures could be due to better control over labor and supply costs, though overall operating expense devoted to salary and benefit costs remains too high. Newport's operating margin is currently at benchmark, but has dropped precipitously over the past year. Return on total assets and return on net assets have also dropped precipitously, yet both remain above benchmark. Newport's low nonoperating revenue suggests that it needs to do a better job investing its money and generating income from sources other than simply direct patient care revenues.

Activity analysis: The total asset turnover and net fixed assets turnover ratios for Newport have both increased over the past year, but the former still subsides below benchmark, which implies that the hospital is not using its total assets more effectively to generate revenue. The age of plant ratio remains comfortably below benchmark, which indicates that Newport does not have a pressing need to upgrade its facilities, only to make better use of its existing assets.

Capital structure analysis: As indicated above, Newport fortunately doesn't need to upgrade its facilities in the near future, because it is quite highly leveraged, as evidenced by the long-term debt to net assets ratio. The ratio of 2.73 means that for every $1.00 in net assets, Newport has $2.73 in long-term debt, while the desired position is $0.21. Though net assets have increased (from approximately $1.9M to over $2.5M in the past year, see Exhibit 4.1), this amount as a proportion of total assets remains too low. On a similar note, the hospital's times interest earned and debt service coverage ratios have both plummeted below benchmark for similarly sized institutions, which makes potential creditors nervous about Newport's ability to take on additional debt if need be. This risk in turn would raise the cost of capital for Newport should it need to look to other funds.

Overall analysis: While Newport is able to hold its own at this point, the trends generally are not favorable. Receivables are being collected and bills are being paid in a timely manner right now, but this may not persist, and Newport has over two months of cash and investments in reserve if margins and cash flow get tight. The facility is not collecting as much as it could be in patient care revenues, and it has not fared well trying to generate income from other sources. Fortunately, Newport does not have a pressing need to upgrade its facilities, but these assets are currently not being used as effectively as they could be to generate much-needed income. The hospital is also already highly leveraged at this point and not in a good position to borrow if need be. In summary, Newport needs to be operating more efficiently with the resources available, because other alternative options are limited at this point.

Key Point Industry norms vary by hospital size. For purposes of the example used throughout this chapter, Newport is assumed to be a small hospital of fewer than 100 beds. Ratios for facilities of various sizes can be found later in the chapter in Exhibit 4.16a.

Key Point The term *benchmark* is used to indicate the desired level of performance an organization wishes to compare itself with.

Key Point The latest data available from Optum and the Centers for Medicare and Medicaid Services (CMS) are used as benchmarks in the remainder of the chapter.

Key Points to Consider When Using and Interpreting Ratios

1. *No one ratio is necessarily better than any other ratio.* It is often useful to use more than one ratio to help answer a question.

2. *Each ratio's terms offer clues about how to fix a problem.* For example, if the current ratio (Current Assets / Current Liabilities) is too low, it can be improved by increasing the numerator (Current Assets), by decreasing the denominator (Current Liabilities), or by doing both. However, changing the conditions to improve one ratio may affect other ratios as well.

3. *Most ratios are interpreted as follows: there are* n *dollars in the numerator for every dollar in the denominator.* Thus, a current ratio of 2.00 indicates that there are $2 in current assets for every $1 in current liabilities.

4. *A ratio can best be interpreted relative to a benchmark.* The benchmark may be the organization's past performance, a goal set by the organization, the performance of a comparison group (such as similar organizations), or some combination thereof. For example, a current ratio of 2.00 would probably be interpreted favorably if the industry benchmark were 1.75; however, it would probably be interpreted unfavorably if the industry benchmark were 2.50.

5. *There are several problems with using benchmarks for comparison in the health care industry.* Two of the most prominent are the availability and the reliability of the data:

   • *Finding appropriate data.* Not all segments of the health care industry have data available that can be used as benchmarks. For example, on the one hand, there are no complete, national-level ratio data on health departments or mental health centers. On the other hand, certain segments of the industry have excellent data. Optum benchmark ratio values provide excellent ratio information on hospitals on both a national and a regional basis. Alternatively, individual providers may join together to develop their own benchmarks.

Even when data are available, it is important to *compare an organization with similar organizations*. It might be highly inappropriate for a small rural hospital in North Dakota to use the ratios of large academic medical centers in Boston for comparison. Services such as Optum can provide data by size and location. The data are presented by both median and percentile, which means that an organization can set its own benchmarks relative to what it considers an appropriate comparison group.

- *Ensuring reliability of the data.* The same ratio may be calculated differently by different organizations, different sources of industry benchmarks, or both. For example, in calculating the days in accounts receivable, one organization may use the ending balance in accounts receivable, whereas another organization may use the average daily balance. *Therefore, when comparing organizations with one another or with benchmarks, it is necessary to make sure the same formula is being used* (see Perspective 4.3). There may be differences in practices and procedures among organizations that may not be immediately apparent to those using the information. For example, hospitals may use different depreciation or inventory valuation methods. This could have a profound effect on certain ratios.

6. *In general, a ratio should be neither too high nor too low relative to the benchmark.* For example, the acid test ratio [(Cash + Marketable Securities) / Current Liabilities] looks at an organization's ability to meet its short-term debt. Although an organization would like to have this ratio above the benchmark, a value too high may indicate too much cash on hand, which likely could be better invested elsewhere.

7. *Not only should a ratio be compared with a benchmark but also the trend of the ratio can help to interpret how well an organization is doing.* For example, an organization would feel differently about a ratio that was at the benchmark and declining versus a ratio that was at the benchmark and rising over the past five years.

8. *Because ratios are usually relatively small, relatively small differences may indicate large percentage deviations from the benchmark.* For

PERSPECTIVE 4.3 FORMULAS HOSPITALS REPORT USING TO CALCULATE NET DAYS IN ACCOUNTS RECEIVABLE

Hospital	Formula
Hospital 1	Gross Accounts Receivable − Uncollectibles / [(Gross Charges − Deductions) / Number of Days in Period]
Hospital 2	Net Patient Accounts Receivable / (Net Patient Service Revenue / 365)
Hospital 3	Net Accounts Receivable / Net Charges per Day
Hospital 4	Net Accounts Receivable / [(Gross Patient Service Revenue − Charity − Contractual Allowances − Bad Debt) / 365]
Hospital 5	Accounts Receivable + Reserve for Bad Debt + Contractual Adjustments / (Net Patient Revenue / Number of Days in the Period)
Hospital 6	Accounts Receivable / (Revenue Available / Days in Current Year)
Hospital 7	Net Patient Revenue / Operating Margin
Hospital 8	Net Accounts Receivable / (Net Revenue Past 3 Months / Days in Period)

Source: Contributed by Denise R. Smith, data analyst, Columbia Cape Fear Memorial Hospital.

example, if the organization's current ratio were 1.5 and the industry benchmark was 2.0, although this is only a 0.5 difference, the organization would be 25 percent below benchmark.

Caution: When comparing organizations to one another or against benchmarks, it is necessary to make sure the same formula is being used.

The remainder of this chapter uses ratio analysis to analyze the statement of operations and balance sheet for Newport Hospital (see Exhibit 4.1), using industry benchmarks for small hospitals.

Liquidity Ratios

Liquidity ratios answer the question, How well is the organization positioned to meet its current obligations? Six key ratios fall into this category: the current ratio, quick ratio, acid test ratio, days in accounts receivable, days cash on hand, and average payment period (Exhibit 4.6). Incidentally, by convention, the current ratio, quick ratio, and acid test ratio all have the word *ratio* in their title, but the other three ratios do not.

EXHIBIT 4.6 SELECTED LIQUIDITY RATIOS

Ratio	Formula	Benchmark[a]	Desired Position
Current ratio	$\dfrac{\text{Current Assets}}{\text{Current Liabilities}}$	2.11	Above
Quick ratio	$\dfrac{\text{Cash} + \text{Marketable Securities} + \text{Net Receivables}}{\text{Current Liabilities}}$	1.52	Above
Acid test ratio	$\dfrac{\text{Cash} + \text{Marketable Securities}}{\text{Current Liabilities}}$	0.30	Above
Days in accounts receivable	$\dfrac{\text{Net Patient Accounts Receivable}}{\text{Net Patient Revenues} / 365}$	49	Below
Days cash on hand	$\dfrac{\text{Cash} + \text{Marketable Securities} + \text{Long-Term Investments}}{(\text{Operating Expenses} - \text{Depreciation and Amortization Expenses}) / 365}$	86	Above
Average payment period (days)	$\dfrac{\text{Current Liabilities}}{(\text{Operating Expenses} - \text{Depreciation and Amortization Expenses}) / 365}$	50	Organizationally dependent

[a]Based on Optum and CMS approximate hospital median values.

Each of these liquidity ratios provides a different insight into Newport Hospital's liquidity. Notice that the first three ratios focus only on the balance sheet, each giving a little more stringent picture of the organization's ability to pay off its current liabilities. The last three ratios use information from both the statement of operations and the balance sheet to look at different aspects of liquidity: the ability of the organization to turn its receivables into cash, the actual amount of cash it has on hand to meet its short-term obligations, and how long it takes the organization to pay its bills.

Key Point *Liquidity ratios* measure a facility's ability to meet short-term obligations, collect receivables, and maintain a cash position.

Current Ratio

The current ratio (Current Assets / Current Liabilities) is one of the most commonly used ratios. The *current ratio* is the proportion of all current assets to all current liabilities. Values above the benchmark indicate either too many current assets, too few current liabilities, or both. Values below the benchmark indicate either too few current assets, too many current liabilities, or both. To calculate the current ratio (Exhibit 4.6a):

"do we have enough assets to pay off our current debts"

Step 1. Identify the dollar amount of current assets on the balance sheet.

Step 2. Identify the dollar amount of current liabilities on the balance sheet.

Step 3. Divide the current assets by the current liabilities.

Newport Hospital's current ratio increased from 0.58 in 20X0 to 1.80 in 20X1. The benchmark used for comparison is 2.11. Although the 20X1

EXHIBIT 4.6a NEWPORT'S CURRENT RATIO FOR 20X0 AND 20X1

Year	Current Ratio[a]	=	Current Assets	/	Current Liabilities
20X1	1.80	=	$2,514,335	/	$1,395,190
20X0	0.58	=	$1,954,134	/	$3,394,418

[a]Benchmark = 2.11.

value is still below the industry median, this dramatic increase in Newport's current ratio reflects a major improvement in liquidity according to this measure.

Quick Ratio

The *quick ratio* [(Cash + Marketable Securities + Net Accounts Receivable) / Current Liabilities] is commonly used in industries in which net accounts receivable is relatively liquid. Traditionally, this has not been the case in health care organizations. To compute the quick ratio (Exhibit 4.6b):

Step 1. Identify the dollar amounts of cash, marketable securities, and net accounts receivable on the balance sheet.

Step 2. Identify the dollar amount of current liabilities on the balance sheet.

Step 3. Divide the sum of cash, marketable securities, and net accounts receivable by current liabilities.

As with the current ratio, Newport Hospital's quick ratio improved from 20X0 to 20X1, but it is still approximately 10 percent below the industry benchmark of 1.52. To improve this ratio, Newport Hospital must either increase its current assets or decrease its current liabilities or both.

Acid Test Ratio

The *acid test ratio* [(Cash + Marketable Securities) / Current Liabilities] provides the most stringent test of liquidity. It looks at how much cash is on hand or readily available from marketable securities to pay off all current liabilities. This ratio is particularly useful if current liabilities contain a high

---

EXHIBIT 4.6b NEWPORT'S QUICK RATIO FOR 20X0 AND 20X1

Year	Quick Ratio[a]	=	(Cash + Marketable Securities	+	Net Accounts Receivable)	/	Current Liabilities
20X1	1.36	=	($363,181	+	$1,541,244)	/	$1,395,190
20X0	0.46	=	($158,458	+	$1,400,013)	/	$3,394,418

[a]Benchmark = 1.52.

EXHIBIT 4.6c NEWPORT'S ACID TEST RATIO FOR 20X0 AND 20X1

Year	Acid Test Ratio[a]	=	(Cash + Marketable Securities)	/	Current Liabilities
20X1	0.26	=	$363,181	/	$1,395,190
20X0	0.05	=	$158,458	/	$3,394,418

[a]Benchmark = 0.30.

---

percentage of accounts that must be paid off soon (such as wages payable), if collections of accounts receivable are slow, or both. To compute the acid test ratio (Exhibit 4.6c):

Step 1. Identify the dollar amounts of cash and marketable securities on the balance sheet.

Step 2. Identify the dollar amount of current liabilities on the balance sheet.

Step 3. Divide the sum of cash and temporary investments by current liabilities.

 Key Point The *current ratio, quick ratio,* and *acid test ratio* all measure the relationship of various current assets to current liabilities. The acid test ratio provides the most stringent test of liquidity of the three.

Newport's acid test ratio increased from 0.05 to 0.26 from 20X0 to 20X1. In this case there is a favorable trend, but a concern might be raised because Newport is still below the industry benchmark of 0.30. This means that Newport needs to increase its cash and marketable securities or decrease its current liabilities to meet the target figure.

Days in Accounts Receivable

The *days in accounts receivable ratio* [Net Patient Accounts Receivable / (Net Patient Revenues / 365)] provides an indication of how quickly a hospital is converting its receivables into cash. By dividing net patient accounts receivable by an average day's revenue (Net Patient Revenues / 365), this ratio provides an estimate of how many days' revenues have not yet been collected. Values above the benchmark indicate prob-

EXHIBIT 4.6d NEWPORT'S DAYS IN ACCOUNTS RECEIVABLE RATIO FOR 20X0 AND 20X1

Steps 1, 2

Year	Average Net Patient Revenues per Day		Net Patient Revenues	/	365 days
20X1	$29,530	=	$10,778,272	/	365 days
20X0	$28,948	=	$10,566,176	/	365 days

Steps 3, 4

Year	Days in Accounts Receivable[a]		Net Patient Accounts Receivable	/	Average Net Patient Revenues per Day
20X1	52	=	$1,541,244	/	$29,530
20X0	48	=	$1,400,013	/	$28,948

[a]Benchmark = 49.

lems relating to credit collection policies; values below the benchmark indicate ability to collect receivables on time. To calculate the days in accounts receivable ratio (Exhibit 4.6d):

Step 1. Identify the dollar amount of net patient revenues on the statement of operations.

Step 2. Divide net patient revenues by 365 to compute average net patient revenues per day.

Step 3. Identify the dollar amount of net patient accounts receivable on the balance sheet.

Step 4. Divide net patient accounts receivable by average net patient revenues per day.

 Key Point The term *average collection period* can be used interchangeably with *days in accounts receivable*.

Although it only took 4 days longer on average to collect receivables in 20X1 than it did in 20X0 (48 days versus 52 days), Newport Hospital has now risen above the benchmark of 49 days in the current year. Still, this generally indicates good performance in this area.

Days Cash on Hand

The *days cash on hand ratio* {(Cash + Marketable Securities + Long-Term Investments) / [(Operating Expenses − Depreciation and Amortization Expenses) / 365]} provides an indication of the number of days' worth of expenses an organization can cover with its most liquid assets: cash and marketable securities. The denominator [(Operating Expenses − Depreciation and Amortization Expenses) / 365] measures an average day's cash outflow. Depreciation and amortization are subtracted from operating expenses in the denominator because these are operating expenses but require no cash outflow. To compute the days cash on hand ratio (Exhibit 4.6e):

Step 1. Identify the dollar amounts of operating expenses and depreciation and amortization expenses on the statement of operations.

Step 2. Divide operating expenses minus depreciation and amortization expenses by 365 days to compute average cash operating expense per day.

EXHIBIT 4.6e NEWPORT'S DAYS CASH ON HAND RATIO FOR 20X0 AND 20X1

Year	Operating Expense per Day	=	(Operating Expenses	−	Depreciation & Amortization Expenses)	/ 365 Days
20X1	$28,213 / day	=	($10,681,112	−	$383,493)	/ 365 days
20X0	$25,603 / day	=	($9,765,507	−	$420,238)	/ 365 days

Year	Days Cash on Hand[a]	=	(Cash + Marketable Securities + Long-Term Investments)	/ Operating Expense per Day
20X1	134 days	=	$3,777,913	/ $28,213
20X0	183 days	=	$4,683,934	/ $25,603

[a]Benchmark = 86.

Step 3. Identify the dollar amounts of cash, marketable securities, and long-term investments on the balance sheet. Any long-term investments that are under assets limited as to use or board-designated accounts should also be included.

Step 4. Divide cash and marketable securities and long-term investments by the average cash operating expense per day (from step 2).

Newport Hospital has lowered its day's cash on hand from 183 days (20X0) to 134 days (20X1). Although this is still 48 days above the benchmark, it is viewed as unfavorable because these days are declining. This decline may stem from Newport either decreasing its cash, marketable securities, and long-term investments or increasing its operating expenses. System-affiliated hospitals may keep a low balance of cash on hand because they may transfer a large portion of cash to their parent organization each day. If an unusual amount of cash is needed, the parent will transfer back the needed amount. By doing this, the parent organization has larger amounts of cash available for investment purposes and in many cases is in a better position to invest cash than are the subsidiaries. In such instances, a low days cash on hand ratio in the subsidiary organization is not indicative of a problem.

Average Payment Period

The _average payment period ratio_ {Current Liabilities / [(Total Operating Expenses − Depreciation and Amortization Expenses) / 365]} is the counterpart to the days in accounts receivable ratio. It is a measure of how long, on average, it takes an organization to pay its bills. Because the denominator is a measure of an average day's payments for bills, dividing current liabilities by an average day's payment provides a measure of how many days bills have not been paid. To develop a creditworthy relationship and goodwill with vendors and suppliers, health care organizations should attempt to pay their bills on time. To calculate the average payment period ratio (Exhibit 4.6f):

Step 1. Identify the dollar amounts of total operating expenses and depreciation and amortization expenses on the statement of operations.

Step 2. Divide total operating expenses minus depreciation and amortization expenses by 365 days to compute average cash expense per day.

Step 3. Identify the dollar amount of current liabilities on the balance sheet.

Step 4. Divide the current liabilities by average cash expense per day.

EXHIBIT 4.6f NEWPORT'S AVERAGE PAYMENT PERIOD RATIO FOR 20X0 AND 20X1

Steps 1, 2

Year	Average Cash Expense per Day	=	(Operating Expenses	−	Depreciation & Amortization Expenses)	/ 365 Days
20X1	$28,213 / day	=	($10,681,112	−	$383,493)	/ 365 days
20X0	$25,603 / day	=	($9,765,507	−	$420,238)	/ 365 days

Steps 3, 4

Year	Average Payment Period Days[a]		Current Liabilities	/	Average Cash Expense per Day
20X1	49 days	=	$1,395,190	/	$28,213 / day
20X0	133 days	=	$3,394,418	/	$25,603 / day

[a]Benchmark = 50.

In the period of one year, Newport Hospital has decreased its average payment period from 133 days to 49 days and is now below the industry benchmark of 50 days.

Key Point *Days in accounts receivable, cash on hand,* and *average payment period* are all liquidity ratios that give an insight into how quickly cash is flowing in and out of the organization.

Liquidity Summary

From 20X0 to 20X1, Newport Hospital improved its ability to meet current obligations with current assets as indicated by its current, quick, and acid test ratios and its average payment period, although the first three are still considerably below their benchmarks (Exhibit 4.7). In terms of the relative amount of cash actually available, a mixed picture emerges. On the one hand, the acid test ratio, which indicates the amount of cash and marketable securities available to meet current liabilities, is below its desired position of being at the benchmark. Newport has a favorable position on its days in accounts receivable, which (see Exhibit 4.8) indicates that the

EXHIBIT 4.7 NEWPORT HOSPITAL'S CURRENT, QUICK, AND ACID TEST RATIOS IN 20X0 AND 20X1 COMPARED WITH THE BENCHMARK

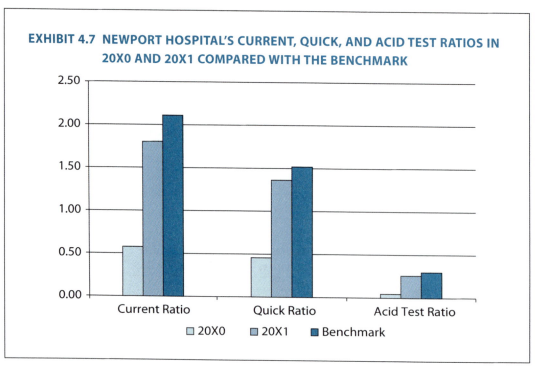

EXHIBIT 4.8 NEWPORT HOSPITAL'S DAYS IN ACCOUNTS RECEIVABLE, DAYS CASH ON HAND, AND AVERAGE PAYMENT PERIOD RATIOS FOR 20X0 AND 20X1 COMPARED WITH THE BENCHMARK

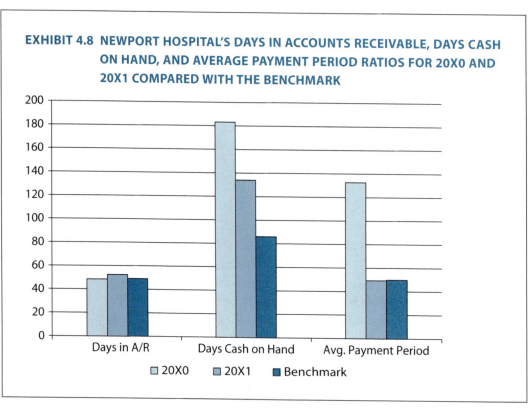

organization is performing well in turning its receivables into cash. This higher cash position may have kept its days cash on hand above its benchmark by 48 days, although the days cash on hand ratio did decline from 20X0 to 20X1.

In regard to collecting money owed and paying its bills, Newport's days in accounts receivable increased above the benchmark (which means that revenues will be converted to cash more slowly), while Newport has greatly decreased its average payment period (which will likely be well received by its suppliers). Fortunately, days cash on hand is still favorable, which should create some relief for the organization.

Revenue, Expense, and Profitability Ratios

There are several *revenue, expense, and profitability ratios*, each providing a different insight into the ability of a health care organization to produce a profit. The most commonly used ratios include operating revenue per adjusted discharge, operating expense per adjusted discharge, salary and benefit expense as a percentage of total operating expenses, operating margin, non-patient-service revenue, return on net assets, and return on total assets (Exhibit 4.9 and Perspective 4.4).

PERSPECTIVE 4.4 PROFITABILITY MARGIN INCREASED BY REDUCING OPERATING EXPENSES AND IMPROVING REVENUES

The upcoming annual budget for a hospital in Missouri required an improvement in the hospital's operating margin to 3.5 percent in order to help cover its interest expense. To improve its operating margin ratio, the hospital considered lowering the numerator of the ratio (its operating expenses) as well as improving the denominator of the ratio (its net patient revenues). To meet the budgeting goal of a 3.5 percent operating margin before interest expense, the hospital lowered its labor costs by reducing its staffing levels for the upcoming year and evaluating its vendor contracts to lower its medical supply costs. The hospital also projected higher patient revenue growth from hiring a new surgeon who was expected to "significantly affect projected volumes" in the operating room, laboratory, pharmacy, and other departments.

Source: S. Sterling, Hospital projects 2 percent profit, *Warrensburg* (MO) *Daily Star-Journal*, December 11, 2012, retrieved from McClatchy-Tribune Business News.

EXHIBIT 4.9 SELECTED REVENUE, EXPENSE, AND PROFITABILITY RATIOS

Ratio	Formula	Benchmark[a]	Desired Position
Operating revenue per adjusted discharge	$\dfrac{\text{Total Operating Revenues}}{\text{Adjusted Discharges}^{b}}$	$7,448	Above
Operating expense per adjusted discharge	$\dfrac{\text{Total Operating Expenses}}{\text{Adjusted Discharges}^{b}}$	$7,197	Below
Salary and benefit expense as percentage of operating expense	$\dfrac{\text{Salary and Benefit Expenses}}{\text{Total Operating Expenses}}$	40%	Below
Operating margin	$\dfrac{\text{Operating Income}}{\text{Total Operating Revenues}}$	0.03	Above
Nonoperating revenue ratio	$\dfrac{\text{Nonoperating Revenues}}{\text{Total Operating Revenues}}$	0.04	Organizationally dependent
Return on total assets[c]	$\dfrac{\text{Excess of Revenues over Expenses}}{\text{Total Assets}}$	0.04	Above
Return on net assets[d]	$\dfrac{\text{Excess of Revenues over Expenses}}{\text{Net Assets}}$	0.08	Above

[a]Based on Optum and CMS approximate hospital median values.
[b]Adjusted Discharges = Adjustment Factor × Total Discharges; Adjustment Factor = Total Gross Patient Revenues / Total Gross Inpatient Revenues. The adjustment factor expresses health care organizations' revenue activities in terms of inpatient acute-care services.
[c]Called *return on assets* in for-profit health care organizations and calculated as Net Income / Total Assets.
[d]Called *return on equity* in for-profit health care organizations and calculated as Net Income / Owners' Equity.

Operating Revenue per Adjusted Discharge

The *operating revenue per adjusted discharge* ratio (Total Operating Revenue / Adjusted Discharge) measures total operating revenues generated from the organization's patient care line of business based on its adjusted inpatient discharges. The adjusted discharge attempts to transform all of the health care provider's revenue, including outpatient revenue, into units representing inpatient care services. Discharges are adjusted by multiplying hospital total discharges by a factor defined as *gross patient revenue* divided by *gross inpatient revenue*. Other adjustments can be also made for case complexity (by dividing by case-mix index) and geographical wage differences (wage index); however, this textbook adjusts only for inpatient care services. The ratio measures the amount of operating revenue generated from its patient care services. To compute the operating revenue per adjusted discharge (Exhibit 4.9a):

Step 1. Identify operating revenue on the statement of operations.

Step 2. Identify adjusted discharges from utilization data.

Step 3. Divide operating revenue by adjusted discharges.

In 20X0, Newport Hospital was already well below the industry benchmark ($6,011 versus $7,448) but decreased even further to $5,647 in 20X1, reflecting the fact that total operating revenues related to patient care services decreased during this time.

Operating Expense per Adjusted Discharge

The *operating expense per adjusted discharge ratio* (Total Operating Expense / Adjusted Discharge) measures total operating expenses incurred

---

EXHIBIT 4.9a NEWPORT'S OPERATING REVENUE PER ADJUSTED DISCHARGE FOR 20X0 AND 20X1

Year	Operating Revenue per Adjusted Discharge[a]	=	Total Operating Revenue	/	Adjusted Discharges
20X1	$5,647	=	$11,012,021	/	1,950
20X0	$6,011	=	$10,819,693	/	1,800

[a]Benchmark = $7,448.

EXHIBIT 4.9b   NEWPORT'S OPERATING EXPENSE PER ADJUSTED DISCHARGE FOR 20X0 AND 20X1

Year	Operating Expense per Adjusted Discharge[a]	=	Total Operating Expense	/	Adjusted Discharges
20X1	$5,477	=	$10,681,112	/	1,950
20X0	$5,425	=	$9,765,507	/	1,800

[a]Benchmark = $7,197.

from providing its patient care services, and it is adjusted for inpatient discharges where adjusted discharges are calculated the same way as for the previous ratio. To compute the operating expense per adjusted discharge (Exhibit 4.9b):

Step 1. Identify total operating expenses on the statement of operations.

Step 2. Identify adjusted discharges from utilization data.

Step 3. Divide total operating expenses by adjusted discharges.

In 20X0, Newport Hospital's operating expense per adjusted discharge ratio was considerably below the industry benchmark ($5,425 versus $7,197) and remained virtually unchanged at $5,477 in 20X1, indicating that Newport has maintained control of its operating costs during this period.

Key Point The *operating revenue per adjusted discharge* measures the amount of operating revenues generated from the organization's patient care line of business patient, and the *operating expense per adjusted discharge* measures operating expenses incurred from providing patient care services.

Salary and Benefit Expense as a Percentage of Total Operating Expense

The salary and benefit expense as a percentage of total operating expense ratio (Total Salary and Benefit Expenses / Total Operating Expenses) measures the percentage of total operating expenses that are attributed to labor

EXHIBIT 4.9c NEWPORT'S SALARY AND BENEFIT EXPENSE AS A PERCENTAGE OF TOTAL OPERATING EXPENSE FOR 20X0 AND 20X1

Year	Salary and Benefit Expense as a Percentage of Total Operating Expense[a]	=	Salary and Benefit Expense	/	Total Operating Expense
20X1	53%	=	$5,644,880	/	$10,681,112
20X0	55%	=	$5,345,498	/	$9,765,507

[a]Benchmark = 40%.

costs. Labor costs are a major expense in the operation of a health care facility. To compute the salary and benefit expense as a percentage of total operating expenses (Exhibit 4.9c):

Step 1. Identify the total salary and benefit expenses on the statement of operations.

Step 2. Identify the total operating expenses on the statement of operations.

Step 3. Divide the total salary and benefit expenses by the total operating expenses.

In 20X0, Newport Hospital was well above the industry benchmark (55 percent versus 40 percent). However, the salary and benefit expense as a percentage of total operating expense has decreased to 53 percent in 20X1, reflecting the fact that Newport has lowered its labor costs during this period relative to its other costs.

Operating Margin

The *operating margin ratio* (Operating Income / Total Operating Revenues) measures profits earned from the organization's main line of business. The margin indicates the proportion of profit earned for each dollar of operating revenue—that is, the proportion of profit remaining after subtracting total operating expenses from operating revenues. To compute the operating margin (Exhibit 4.9d):

EXHIBIT 4.9d NEWPORT'S OPERATING MARGIN RATIO FOR 20X0 AND 20X1

Year	Operating Margin[a]	=	Operating Income	/	Total Operating Revenues
20X1	0.03	=	$330,909	/	$11,012,021
20X0	0.10	=	$1,054,186	/	$10,819,693

[a]Benchmark = 0.03.

Step 1. Identify the operating income on the statement of operations.

Step 2. Identify the total operating revenues on the statement of operations.

Step 3. Divide the operating income by total operating revenues.

In 20X0, Newport Hospital was considerably above the industry benchmark (10 percent versus 3 percent). Unfortunately, the operating-margin ratio has decreased to 3 percent in 20X1, reflecting the fact that total operating expenses have increased faster than have total operating revenues.

Nonoperating Revenue Ratio

The purpose of the *nonoperating revenue ratio* (Nonoperating Revenues / Total Operating Revenues) is to find out how dependent the organization is on patient-related net income. The higher the ratio, the less the organization is dependent on direct patient-related income and the more it is dependent on revenues from other, nonoperating sources. This ratio is becoming increasingly difficult to use to compare health care organizations because under recent accounting rules, there is considerable discretion as to what is classified as operating or nonoperating revenues. This results in two potential problems: to the extent that the ratio for any one organization is not calculated in exactly the same way as the benchmark, a comparison with the benchmark may be inappropriate; and when multiple organizations are being compared, to the extent they did not classify various items (such as interest expense) in exactly the same way, the comparisons may be invalid. Nonoperating revenue may include such accounts as interest income, dividends, gains from investment activities, and assets released from restricted investment accounts (Exhibit 4.9e):

EXHIBIT 4.9e NEWPORT'S NONOPERATING REVENUE RATIO FOR 20X0 AND 20X1

Year	Nonoperating Revenue Ratio[a]	=	Nonoperating Revenues	/	Total Operating Revenues
20X1	0.02	=	$185,000	/	$11,012,021
20X0	0.02	=	$165,000	/	$10,819,693

[a]Benchmark = 0.04.

Step 1. Identify the nonoperating revenues on the statement of operations.

Step 2. Identify the total operating revenues on the statement of operations.

Step 3. Divide the nonoperating revenues by the total operating revenues.

Newport's nonoperating revenue ratio is 2 percent for both 20X1 and 20X0, which is below the national benchmark of 4 percent. An increase in contributions and improved investment portfolio performance could raise the hospital's ratio value.

Return on Total Assets

In not-for-profit organizations, the *return on total assets ratio* is calculated as Excess of Revenues over Expenses / Total Assets. In for-profit organizations, it is called *return on assets* and is calculated as Net Income / Total Assets. It measures how much profit is earned for each dollar invested in assets. To compute the return on total assets ratio (Exhibit 4.9f):

Step 1. Identify the excess of revenues over expenses on the statement of operations.

Step 2. Identify total assets on the balance sheet.

Step 3. Divide the excess of revenues over expenses by total assets.

Newport Hospital's return on total assets ratio declined significantly over this time period (11 percent to 5 percent) and was only slightly above the benchmark of 4 percent in 20X1. One reason for this decrease could

EXHIBIT 4.9f NEWPORT'S RETURN ON TOTAL ASSETS RATIO FOR 20X0 AND 20X1

Year	Return on Total Assets[a]	=	Excess of Revenues over Expenses	/	Total Assets
20X1	0.05	=	$515,909	/	$10,876,736
20X0	0.11	=	$1,219,186	/	$11,315,585

[a]Benchmark = 0.04.

EXHIBIT 4.9g NEWPORT'S RETURN ON NET ASSETS RATIO FOR 20X0 AND 20X1

Year	Return on Net Assets[a]	=	Excess of Revenues over Expenses	/	Net Assets
20X1	0.20	=	$515,909	/	$2,542,655
20X0	0.64	=	$1,219,186	/	$1,911,683

[a]Benchmark = 0.08.

be that Newport's expenses have increased faster than have its revenues, thereby reducing the excess of revenues over expenses. To improve this ratio, Newport could increase operating revenues, decrease expenses, or decrease total assets (or all three).

Return on Net Assets

In not-for-profit organizations, this ratio is called *return on net assets* (Excess of Revenues over Expenses / Net Assets). In for-profit organizations, it is called *return on equity* and is calculated using the formula Net Income / Owners' Equity. In for-profit organizations, it measures the rate of return for each dollar in owners' equity. In not-for-profit health care organizations, it measures the rate of return for each dollar in net assets. To calculate the return on net assets ratio (Exhibit 4.9g):

Step 1. Identify the excess of revenues over expenses on the statement of operations.

Step 2. Identify the net assets on the balance sheet.

Step 3. Divide excess of revenues over expenses by net assets.

As was the case for the return on total assets ratio, the return on net assets ratio also decreased (from 64 percent in 20X0 to 20 percent in 20X1). Expenses growing faster than revenues contributed to this decrease. However, the return on net assets in 20X1 is still considerably above the industry benchmark of 8 percent.

It is important to note that the return on net assets ratio is magnified by the amount of debt financing. The higher the level of debt relative to net assets, the more the return on net assets is affected for a given level of profit or loss. Exhibit 4.10 provides an example of this phenomenon.

In case 1, the organization earns a profit (excess of revenues over expenses) of $100,000. Because there is no debt, the return on net assets is 10 percent ($100,000 / $1,000,000). However, in case 2, the assets are financed with 50 percent debt and 50 percent equity. Thus, the return to the owners is doubled (20 percent) because they have only half as much invested ($500,000 instead of $1,000,000), the remainder of the assets being financed by debt. Although debt results in higher returns when there is a profit (as in both cases 1 and 2), there is a greater loss in return on net assets when the organization is unprofitable (as illustrated in cases 3 and 4). As previously noted, financial leverage reflects the proportion of debt used in the organization's capital structure. Thus these cases show that debt increases the financial risk to the owners of a health care organization. It magnifies positive returns when there is a profit but negative returns when there is a loss. It also carries the added burden of fixed interest payments.

Key Point Higher debt increases financial risk by magnifying the returns on net asset or equity.

Revenue, Expense, and Profitability Summary

Newport Hospital has a favorable position with three of the five revenue and profitability ratios in 20X1 at or above the benchmark. For its two expense ratios, the operating expense per adjusted discharge ratio is the only one below the benchmark position, which reflects a desirable position. However, Newport has also shown a decline from 20X0 to 20X1 in six of the seven revenue, expense, and profitability ratios (see Exhibits 4.11a and 4.11b). This raises concerns about the control of revenues and expenses.

EXHIBIT 4.10 EXAMPLE OF HOW INCREASED DEBT MAGNIFIES GAINS AND LOSSES WHEN COMPUTING RETURN ON NET ASSETS

In Case 1, the organization has no debt. In Case 2, the organization has 50 percent of its assets financed by debt. In both cases, the organization makes a $100,000 profit, but the return on net assets is twice as high in Case 2.

Case 1: $100,000 Excess of revenues over expenses; no debt

Balance Sheet			Statement of Operations	
Assets	$1,000,000	Debt	$0	Excess of revenues over expenses	$100,000
		Net assets	$1,000,000		

Return on net assets = $100,000 / $1,000,000 = 0.10

Case 2: $100,000 Excess of revenues over expenses; 50 percent debt

Balance Sheet			Statement of Operations	
Assets	$1,000,000	Debt	$500,000	Excess of revenues over expenses	$100,000
		Net assets	$500,000		

Return on net assets = $100,000 / $500,000 = 0.20

In Case 3, the organization has no debt. In Case 4, the organization has 50 percent of its assets financed by debt. In both cases, the organization incurs a $100,000 loss, but the negative return on net assets is twice as much in Case 4.

Case 3: ($100,000) Excess of revenues over expenses; no debt

Balance Sheet			Statement of Operations	
Assets	$1,000,000	Debt	$0	Excess of revenues over expenses	($100,000)
		Net assets	$1,000,000		

Return on net assets = –$100,000 / $1,000,000 = –0.10

Case 4: ($100,000) Excess of revenues over expenses; 50 percent debt

Balance Sheet			Statement of Operations	
Assets	$1,000,000	Debt	$500,000	Excess of revenues over expenses	($100,000)
		Net assets	$500,000		

Return on net assets = –$100,000 / $500,000 = –0.20

Point: Increased debt magnifies both gains and losses when computing return on net assets.

EXHIBIT 4.11a NEWPORT HOSPITAL'S REVENUE AND EXPENSE PER ADJUSTED DISCHARGE FOR 20X0 AND 20X1 COMPARED WITH THE BENCHMARKS

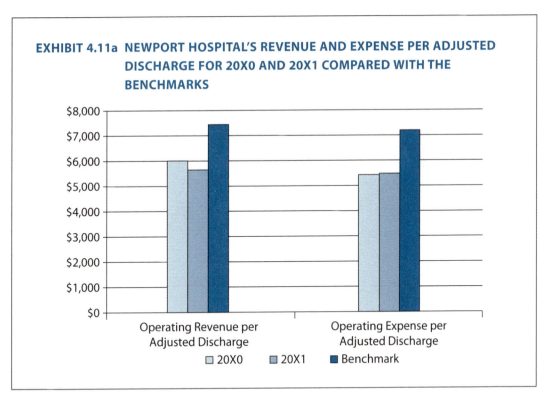

EXHIBIT 4.11b NEWPORT HOSPITAL'S EXPENSE AND PROFITABILITY RATIOS FOR 20X0 AND 20X1 COMPARED WITH THE BENCHMARKS

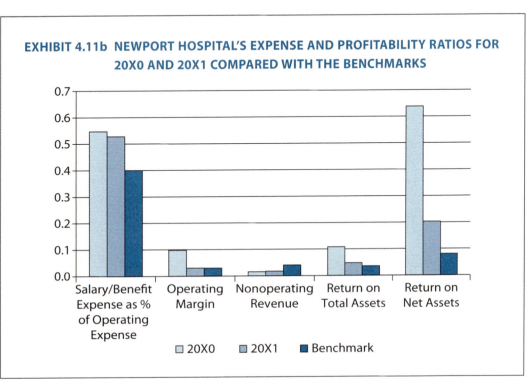

EXHIBIT 4.12 SELECTED ACTIVITY RATIOS

Ratio	Formula	Benchmark[a]	Desired Position
Total asset turnover ratio	$\dfrac{\text{Total Operating Revenues}}{\text{Total Assets}}$	1.07	Above
Fixed asset turnover ratio	$\dfrac{\text{Total Operating Revenues}}{\text{Net Plant And Equipment}}$	2.12	Above
Age of plant ratio	$\dfrac{\text{Accumulated Depreciation}}{\text{Depreciation Expense}}$	10.31	Below

[a]Based on Optum median values.

Activity Ratios

In general, *activity ratios* (Exhibit 4.12) ask the question, For every dollar invested in assets, how many dollars of revenue (not excess of revenues over expenses) are being generated? Most ratios in this category take the general form:

$$\frac{\text{Revenues}}{\text{Assets}}$$

Thus the more revenue generated, the higher the ratio.

Key Point Because many of the *activity ratios* ask the general question, How many dollars in revenue (the numerator) are being generated relative to [specific] assets (the denominator)?, activity ratios are also called *efficiency ratios.* The higher the ratio, the more efficiently the assets are being used.

Total Asset Turnover

The *total asset turnover ratio* (Total Operating Revenues / Total Assets) measures the overall efficiency of the organization's assets in producing revenue. It answers the question, For every dollar in assets, how many dollars of operating revenue are being generated? To calculate the total asset turnover ratio (Exhibit 4.12a):

EXHIBIT 4.12a NEWPORT'S TOTAL ASSET TURNOVER RATIO FOR 20X0 AND 20X1

Year	Total Asset Turnover[a]	=	Total Operating Revenues	/	Total Assets
20X1	1.01	=	$11,012,021	/	$10,876,736
20X0	0.96	=	$10,819,693	/	$11,315,585

[a]Benchmark = 1.07.

Step 1. Identify total operating revenues on the statement of operations.

Step 2. Identify total assets on the balance sheet.

Step 3. Divide total operating revenues by total assets.

For Newport Hospital, the ratio increased slightly from 20X0 to 20X1 and remained close to the benchmark. A value of 1.00 indicates that for every dollar of total assets, one dollar of total revenues is generated, which is approximately the benchmark.

Key Point Asset accounts reflect values at a specific point in time, which in turn can fail to account for seasonal changes in asset accounts. To deal with this problem, some analysts use an average of the beginning and ending year values for the fixed asset or current asset accounts. That convention, however, is not used in this text.

Fixed Asset Turnover

The *fixed asset turnover ratio* (Total Operating Revenues / Net Plant and Equipment) aids in the evaluation of the most productive assets, plant and equipment. To calculate the fixed asset turnover ratio (Exhibit 4.12b):

Step 1. Identify total operating revenues on the statement of operations.

Step 2. Identify net plant and equipment assets on the balance sheet.

Step 3. Divide total operating revenues by net plant and equipment (fixed) assets.

Key Point The *fixed asset turnover ratio* is a measure of how productive the fixed assets of the organization are in generating operating revenues.

EXHIBIT 4.12b　NEWPORT'S FIXED ASSET TURNOVER RATIO FOR 20X0 AND 20X1

Year	Fixed Asset Turnover[a]	=	Total Operating Revenues	/	Net Plant and Equipment
20X1	2.56	=	$11,012,021	/	$4,306,754
20X0	2.41	=	$10,819,693	/	$4,495,122

[a]Benchmark = 2.12.

Newport's fixed asset turnover ratio increased from 20X0 to 20X1 (2.41 to 2.56) and remains above the benchmark of 2.12. The fixed asset turnover value of 2.56 indicates that for every dollar of fixed assets, only $2.56 of operating revenues is being generated.

Key Point　Asset turnover ratios have an interesting property because of accrual accounting. When revenues (the numerator) stay the same, the ratio will continually increase from year to year because asset values (the denominator) decrease each year due to depreciation. This will occur until the assets are fully depreciated. To check how old the assets are, the *age of plant ratio* is used.

Caution:　Note that this text uses excess of revenues over expenses in the numerator for the profitability ratios *return on total assets* and *return on net assets*, and it uses total operating revenues in the numerator for the activity ratios *total asset turnover ratio* and *net asset turnover ratio*.

Age of Plant Ratio

The *age of plant ratio* (Accumulated Depreciation / Depreciation Expense) provides an indication of the average age of a hospital's plant and equipment. This ratio complements the fixed asset turnover ratio. High fixed asset turnover ratios may be an indication of lack of investment in fixed assets. If the average age of plant is high, it may indicate that the organization needs to replace its fixed assets shortly. If so, it would be important to look at other ratios to see how well positioned the organization is to finance the purchase of new assets. To compute the age of plant ratio (Exhibit 4.12c):

EXHIBIT 4.12c NEWPORT'S AGE OF PLANT RATIO FOR 20X0 AND 20X1

Year	Age of Plant[a]	=	Accumulated Depreciation	/	Depreciation Expense
20X1	7.25	=	$2,781,741	/	$383,493
20X0	5.71	=	$2,398,248	/	$420,238

[a]Benchmark = 10.31.

Step 1. Identify the accumulated depreciation on the balance sheet.

Step 2. Identify the depreciation expense on the statement of operations.

Step 3. Divide the accumulated depreciation by the depreciation expense.

Newport Hospital's average age of plant ratio has increased by over 1.5 years (5.71 to 7.25), but it is still more than 3 years below the industry benchmark of 10.31.

Activity Summary

Newport Hospital is below the benchmark on its total asset turnover ratio but above benchmark on its fixed asset turnover ratio, and it shows improvement from 20X0 to 20X1 for both (Exhibit 4.13). Its average age of plant is still well below the benchmark of 10.31 years, which indicates that the hospital has newer assets relative to the small hospital benchmark. Thus, because of the fixed asset ratio, a question should be raised regarding how efficiently the fixed assets are being used to generate revenue.

Capital Structure Ratios

Capital structure ratios answer two questions: How are an organization's assets financed?, and, How able is this organization to take on new debt? In many cases a greater understanding of these ratios (and answers to these questions) can be gained by examining the statement of cash flows to see if significant long-term debt has been acquired or paid off, or if there has been a sale or purchase of fixed assets. Capital structure ratios include *long-term debt to net assets, net assets to total assets, times interest earned,* and *debt service coverage* (Exhibit 4.14).

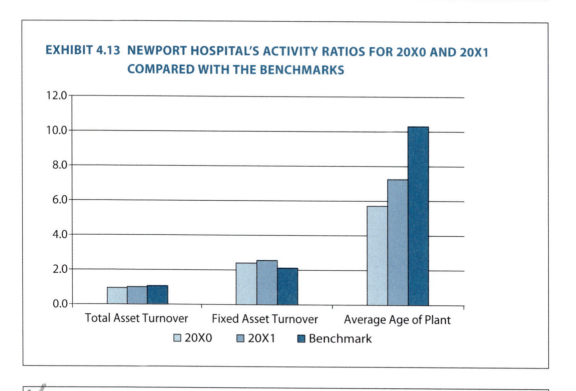

EXHIBIT 4.13 NEWPORT HOSPITAL'S ACTIVITY RATIOS FOR 20X0 AND 20X1 COMPARED WITH THE BENCHMARKS

EXHIBIT 4.14 SELECTED CAPITAL STRUCTURE RATIOS

Ratio	Formula	Benchmark[a]	Desired Position
Long-term debt to net assets ratio	$\dfrac{\text{Long-Term Debt}}{\text{Net Assets}}$	0.21	Below
Net assets to total assets ratio	$\dfrac{\text{Net Assets}}{\text{Total Assets}}$	0.54	Above
Times interest earned ratio	$\dfrac{\text{(Excess of Revenues over Expenses + Interest Expense)}}{\text{Interest Expense}}$	3.78	Above
Debt service coverage ratio	$\dfrac{\text{(Excess of Revenues over Expenses + Interest Expense + Depreciation and Amortization Expenses)}}{\text{(Interest Expense + Principal Payments)}}$	3.18	Above

[a]Based on Optum median values.

Key Point *Capital structure ratios* measure how an organization's assets are financed and how able the organization is to pay for the new debt.

Key Point One might also want to measure capital structure ratios by using the unrestricted net assets account rather than the combined restricted and unrestricted net assets values. The unrestricted net assets account represents the claim on assets that the provider could sell to meet debt payments.

Long-Term Debt to Net Assets

The *long-term debt to net assets ratio* (Long-Term Debt / Net Assets) measures the proportion of debt to net assets. In for-profit organizations, this ratio is called the *long-term debt to equity ratio* and is calculated by the formula Long-Term Debt / Owners' Equity. Although most organizations certainly want to finance a portion of their assets with debt, at a certain level an organization takes on too much debt and may find itself in a precarious position where it has difficulty both paying back its existing debt and borrowing additional funds. To calculate the long-term debt to net assets ratio (Exhibit 4.14a):

Step 1. Identify noncurrent debt on the balance sheet.

Step 2. Identify net assets on the balance sheet.

Step 3. Divide noncurrent debt by net assets.

Key Point The *long-term debt to net assets ratio* measures the proportion of assets financed by debt relative to the proportion not financed by debt.

EXHIBIT 4.14a NEWPORT'S LONG-TERM DEBT TO NET ASSETS RATIO FOR 20X0 AND 20X1

Year	Long-Term Debt to Net Assets[a]	=	Long-Term Debt	/	Net Assets
20X1	2.73	=	$6,938,891	/	$2,542,655
20X0	3.14	=	$6,009,484	/	$1,911,683

[a]Benchmark = 0.21.

Despite an increase in noncurrent debt, Newport Hospital's long-term debt to net assets ratio actually decreased from 20X0 to 20X1, due to the increase in net assets. Still, the 20X1 ending value (2.73) is over ten times the industry benchmark (0.21).

Net Assets to Total Assets

The *net assets to total assets ratio* (Net Assets / Total Assets) reflects the proportion of total assets financed by equity. In for-profit organizations, this ratio is called the *equity to total asset ratio* and is calculated by the formula Owners' Equity / Total Assets. Creditors desire a strong equity position with sufficient funds to pay off debt obligations. A high net asset or equity position is enhanced either through the retention of earnings or through private contributions from the community. In investor-owned facilities, retention of earnings and issuance of stock increase the equity. To calculate the net assets to total assets ratio (Exhibit 4.14b):

Step 1. Identify net assets on the balance sheet.

Step 2. Identify total assets on the balance sheet.

Step 3. Divide net assets by total assets.

In 20X1, Newport's ratio was less than half the industry benchmark (0.54), though it did increase from 0.17 (20X0) to 0.23 (20X1). Given this thin equity state, creditors probably would be cautious about lending funds to this facility in the future.

Times Interest Earned

The *times interest earned ratio* [(Excess of Revenues over Expenses + Interest Expense) / Interest Expense] enables creditors and lenders to evaluate

---

EXHIBIT 4.14b NEWPORT'S NET ASSETS TO TOTAL ASSETS RATIO FOR 20X0 AND 20X1

Year	Net Assets to Total Assets[a]	=	Net Assets	/	Total Assets
20X1	0.23	=	$2,542,655	/	$10,876,736
20X0	0.17	=	$1,911,683	/	$11,315,585

[a]Benchmark = 0.54.

EXHIBIT 4.14c NEWPORT'S TIMES INTEREST EARNED RATIO FOR 20X0 AND 20X1

Year	Times Interest Earned[a]	=	(Excess of Revenues over Expenses	+	Interest Expense)	/	Interest Expense
20X1	2.03	=	($515,909	+	$500,000)	/	$500,000
20X0	5.41	=	($1,219,186	+	$276,379)	/	$276,379

[a]Benchmark = 3.78.

a hospital's ability to generate the earnings necessary to meet interest expense requirements. In for-profit organizations, the ratio is calculated by the formula (Net Income + Interest Expense) / Interest Expense. The ratio answers the question, For every dollar in interest expense, how many dollars are there in profit? Interest expense is added back into the numerator so that the numerator reflects profit *before* taking interest into account. To calculate the times interest earned ratio (Exhibit 4.14c):

Step 1. Identify excess of revenues over expenses on the statement of operations.

Step 2. Identify interest expense on the statement of operations.

Step 3. Add together excess of revenues over expenses and interest expense and divide the total by interest expense.

Unfortunately, Newport's times interest earned ratio decreased precipitously from 20X0 (5.41) to 20X1 (2.03), falling well below the benchmark of 3.78. A continued decline in the times interest earned ratio may affect Newport's ability to borrow in the future.

Debt Service Coverage

A more robust measure of ability to repay a loan is the *debt service coverage ratio* [(Excess of Revenues over Expenses + Interest Expense + Depreciation and Amortization Expenses) / (Interest Expense + Principal Payments)]. In for-profit organizations, it is calculated as (Net Income + Interest Expense + Depreciation and Amortization Expenses) / (Interest Expense + Principal Payments). It answers the question, For every dollar the organization has to pay on debt service (Principal + Interest), what is

EXHIBIT 4.14d NEWPORT'S DEBT SERVICE COVERAGE RATIO FOR 20X0 AND 20X1

Steps 1–4

Year	Cash Flow before Interest	=	(Excess of Revenues over Expenses	+	Interest Expense	+	Depreciation Expense)
20X1	$1,399,402	=	($515,909	+	$500,000	+	$383,493)
20X0	$1,915,803	=	($1,219,186	+	$276,379	+	$420,238)

Steps 5

Year	Debit Service Coverage[a]	=	Cash Flow before Interest	/	(Interest Expense	+	Principal Payments)
20X1	2.00	=	$1,399,402	/	($500,000	+	$200,000)
20X0	4.02	=	$1,915,803	/	($276,379	+	$200,000)

[a]Benchmark = 3.18.

its approximate cash inflow during the year? This ratio is used extensively by investment bankers and bond rating agencies to evaluate a facility's ability to meet its total loan requirements, principal payments plus interest. Principal payments are usually presented in the statement of cash flows. Because it is not provided elsewhere in this chapter, assume that Newport's principal payments are $200,000 per year. Interest expense and depreciation expense are added to the excess of revenues over expenses account to develop an indication of cash flow before interest expense. To compute the debt service coverage ratio (Exhibit 4.14d):

Step 1. Identify excess of revenues over expenses on the statement of operations.

Step 2. Identify interest expense on the statement of operations.

Step 3. Identify principal payments on the statement of cash flows.

Step 4. Add the excess of revenues over expenses, interest expense, and depreciation and amortization expense from the statement of operations.

Step 5. Divide the sum from step 4 by the sum of the interest expense and principal payments.

Key Point *Debt service coverage ratio* is a critical ratio used by investment bankers because it reflects the proportion of the cash flow payments being used to pay off debt service payments.

Reconfirming the outcome of the times interest earned ratio, Newport also has placed itself in a precarious position in terms of meeting its interest and principal payments. It has fallen considerably below the benchmark of 3.18 and has dropped by half from 20X0 (4.02) to 20X1 (2.00). It currently has a cash flow before principal and interest payments of only 2.00 times its debt service payments. If this condition persists, Newport likely would find itself in technical default on its long-term obligations.

Capital Structure Summary

Newport Hospital decreased its debt position from 20X0 to 20X1; however, the remaining amount of debt is still too high and well above the industry benchmark. This is reflected in the capital structure ratios, which show that Newport's proportion of debt to net assets is still too high, albeit decreasing. More troublesome for Newport is its ability to pay its debt: both the times interest earned and debt service coverage ratios fell considerably below their benchmarks in 20X1 (Exhibit 4.15).

Summary of Newport Hospital's Ratios

Newport Hospital's ratios cause some concern. Most problematic are the capital structure ratios, which indicate that Newport Hospital is above the benchmark in debt and considerably below the benchmark in ability to pay

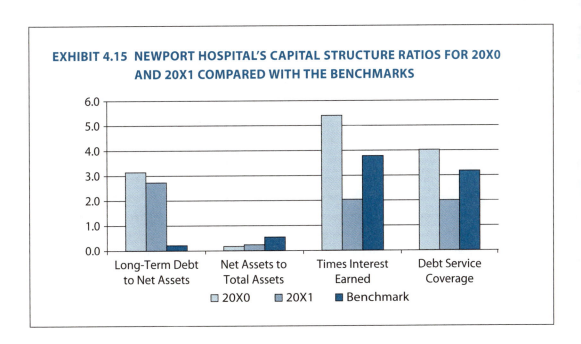

EXHIBIT 4.15 NEWPORT HOSPITAL'S CAPITAL STRUCTURE RATIOS FOR 20X0 AND 20X1 COMPARED WITH THE BENCHMARKS

it off. Though improving in liquidity from 20X0 to 20X1, it is still below the benchmark in its ability to meet current obligations with current assets, and is only at benchmark in its ability to collect on its receivables. Most of Newport's profitability ratios are above benchmark, but they are falling precipitously, indicating potential problems in its ability to pay off its short-term obligations. Although Newport Hospital seems to be using its assets more efficiently, as indicated by most of the activity ratios, this is likely due to the increasing age of its plant. Newport's capital structure ratios raise serious concerns about its ability to pay off current debt or to increase debt financing if it needed to replace properties and equipment in the near future.

Although this chapter has introduced the commonly used financial ratios, there are many others. Perspective 4.5 presents some used by HMOs.

PERSPECTIVE 4.5 KEY FINANCIAL RATIOS FOR HEALTH PLANS

Key financial ratios employed to assess and evaluate the financial performance of health plans include the medical loss ratio, administrative cost ratio, and total profit margin ratio. The *medical loss ratio* is defined as medical expenses divided by insurance premium revenues, and it measures the amount of the insurance revenues paid out as medical expenses and quality of care expenses. The *administrative cost ratio* measures the percentage of insurance premium revenues allocated for administrative costs, such as salary, marketing, and office expenses, and is defined as administrative costs divided by premium revenues. The *operating profit margin ratio* measures operating income earned by premium revenues. *Operating income* is defined as premium revenues less medical and quality of care expenses and administrative expenses.

Under health reform, risk-based insurance plans offering commercial, individual, and small group health insurance must pay out at least 80 percent of premium revenues in medical and quality of care expenses, while insurers offering large group insurance plans are required to pay out at least 85 percent of their premiums in medical and quality of care expenses. Except for small membership plans, health plans with a medical loss ratio (MLR) below their 80 or 85 percent regulation threshold must rebate their members the difference, which is measured as the percentage below the regulated value times the total premium revenues. For example, in California in 2011, Blue Cross of California paid out only 77 percent of its premium revenues from its small group plans in medical and quality of care expenses, which resulted in a $211 rebate per member; conversely, Kaiser paid out 91% of its premium revenues in medical and quality of care expenses and therefore did not have to pay a rebate, since its MLR was well above the regulated value of 80 percent. Aetna's MLR was at the 80 percent regulated value, and it did not have to pay a rebate to its small group members either.

In terms of operating profit margin ratio, Blue Cross generated 10 percent of its premium revenues as operating earnings, whereas Aetna and Kaiser earned 5.5 percent and 2 percent, respectively. (This 2011 information is summarized in the following table.) The CMS Center for Consumer Information & Insurance Oversight (CCIIO) lists all U.S. health insurers' medical loss ratio information, which provides the financial information to determine whether each health plan offering health insurance complies with the MRL regulation. This information is listed for each state by each market segment (individual, small group, and large group markets), and discloses any rebate that is paid. The website is listed in the table source note below.

Key Ratios 2011	Aetna Health Plan	Blue Cross	Kaiser
Medical loss	80.5%	77%	91%
Administrative cost	14%	13%	7%
Operating profit margin	5.5%	10%	2%
Rebate amount	$0	$38.5 million	$0
Rebate per policyholder	$0	$211	$0

Source: CMS Center for Consumer Information & Insurance Oversight (CCIIO), Medical Loss Ratio web page, retrieved December 2012 from www.cms.gov/CCIIO/Resources/Data-Resources/mlr.html.

Summary

The financial performance of health care organizations is of interest to numerous individuals and groups, including administrators, board members, creditors, bondholders, community members, and governmental agencies. This chapter presented three ways to analyze the financial statements of health care organizations: horizontal analysis, vertical analysis, and ratio analysis.

Horizontal analysis examines year-to-year changes in the line items of the financial statements. It answers the question, What is the percentage change from one year to the next in a particular line item (such as cash, long-term debt, or patient accounts receivable)? The formula for horizontal analysis is [(Subsequent Year − Base Year) / Base Year] × 100 = Percentage Increase (Decrease) between years.

A variant of horizontal analysis is trend analysis. Instead of comparing one line item with that of the previous year, trend analysis compares a line item from any subsequent year with that of the base year. Trend analysis answers the question, What is the percentage change from a base year? For example: How much have net patient service revenues increased between 20X4 and 20X0? The formula for trend analysis is (Any Subsequent Year − Base Year) / Base Year. As the name suggests, trend analysis is most useful when data for multiple periods are available. Generally, there are no recognized national benchmarks for either horizontal or trend analysis.

Vertical analysis compares one line item with another line item for the same period. It answers the question, What percentage of one line item is another line item? For example: What percentage of current assets is cash?, or, What percentage of operating revenues are operating expenses? Vertical analysis is also called common-size analysis because it allows comparison of organizations of different sizes by converting all items to percentages. As with horizontal analysis, there are no nationally recognized benchmarks.

Ratio analysis is the preferred approach for a detailed analysis of the financial statements of health care organizations. Ratio analysis asks the question, What is the ratio of one line item to another? For example: How many dollars are there in current assets compared with current liabilities? Because ratios are not limited to just one financial statement at a time, they may combine and compare items from several different financial statements. The four categories of ratios are liquidity, profitability, activity, and capital structure.

Liquidity ratios answer the question, How well is an organization positioned to meet its short-term obligations?

Revenue, expense, and profitability ratios answer two questions, How profitable is an organization?, and, How effective is it in controlling its operating costs and increasing its operating revenues?

Activity ratios answer the question, How efficiently is an organization using its assets to produce revenues?

Capital structure ratios answer two questions: How are an organization's assets financed?, and, How able is this organization to take on new debt?

Once calculated, these ratios are generally compared to some meaningful benchmark (historical, industry, etc.). Such comparisons yield clues as to how well an entity is functioning and how it might improve its operational performance, and financial position. Exhibit 4.16a presents financial ratios for U.S. hospitals overall and by bed-size categories. Exhibit 4.16b presents a summary of key financial ratios and their formulas.

EXHIBIT 4.16a FINANCIAL RATIOS FOR ALL U.S. HOSPITALS BY BED SIZE

Ratio	Optum & CMS Median Ratio[a] Hospital Industry	1–99 Beds	100–199 Beds	200–299 Beds	300–399 Beds	400+ Beds	Desired Position[b]
Liquidity ratios							
Current ratio	2.11	2.18	2.04	1.88	1.71	1.84	Above
Quick ratio	1.52	1.65	1.39	1.27	1.42	1.50	Above
Acid test ratio	0.30	0.35	0.18	0.20	0.20	0.38	Above
Days in accounts receivable	49	47	45	44	48	44	Below
Days cash on hand	86	85	81	102	76	119	Above
Average payment period, days	50	45	51	56	53	52	Below
Revenue, expense, and profitability ratios							
Operating revenue per adjusted discharge	$7,448	$7,086	$6,407	$6,766	$7,121	$7,517	Above
Operating expense per adjusted discharge	$7,197	$6,494	$6,112	$6,260	$6,819	$7,399	Below
Salary and benefit expense as a percentage of operating expense	40%	40%	38%	38%	38%	38%	Below
Operating margin	0.03	0.02	0.03	0.04	0.04	0.04	Above
Nonoperating revenue	0.04	0.05	0.03	0.05	0.07	0.17	Varies
Return on total assets	0.04	0.04	0.04	0.04	0.05	0.05	Above
Return on net assets	0.08	0.08	0.08	0.09	0.10	0.09	Above
Activity ratios							
Total asset turnover ratio	1.07	1.19	1.03	0.99	1.03	1.06	Above
Net fixed assets turnover ratio	2.12	2.17	2.03	2.11	2.04	2.21	Above
Age of plant ratio	10.31	10.41	10.12	11.97	10.93	11.19	Below
Capital structure ratios							
Long-term debt to net assets ratio	0.21	0.18	0.31	0.42	0.38	0.59	Below
Net assets to total assets ratio	0.54	0.58	0.51	0.47	0.52	0.48	Above
Times interest earned ratio	3.78	3.47	3.43	3.64	4.43	5.13	Above
Debt service coverage ratio	3.18	3.51	3.63	3.50	6.36	4.24	Above

[a]All ratio values, except for quick, acid test, and salary and benefit expense as a percentage of operating expenses, were obtained from Optum Insight, *2013 Almanac of Hospital Financial and Operating Indicators*, 2011/2010 median value data. The quick, acid test, and salary and benefit expense as a percentage of operating expense ratios were obtained from 2010 CMS cost report data.
[b]These are true up to a certain point. For example, in general the higher the better for the current ratio, but after a certain point, the organization might be better off investing some of the excess cash.

Key Equations

EXHIBIT 4.16b FORMULAS FOR KEY FINANCIAL RATIOS

Liquidity ratios	Formula
Current ratio	Current Assets / Current Liabilities
Quick ratio	(Cash + Marketable Securities + Net Receivables) / Current Liabilities
Acid test ratio	(Cash + Marketable Securities) / Current Liabilities
Days in accounts receivable	Net Patient Accounts Receivables / (Net Patient Revenues / 365)
Days cash on hand	(Cash + Marketable Securities + Long-Term Investments) / [(Operating Expenses − Depreciation and Amortization Expenses) / 365]
Average payment period, days	Current Liabilities / [(Operating Expenses − Depreciation and Amortization Expenses) / 365]

Revenue, expense, and profitability ratios	Formula
Operating revenues per adjusted discharge[a]	Total Operating Revenues / Adjusted Discharges
Operating expense per adjusted discharge[a]	Total Operating Expenses / Adjusted Discharges
Salary and benefit expense as percentage of operating expense	Total Salary and Benefit Expense / Total Operating Expenses
Operating margin	Operating Income / Total Operating Revenues
Nonoperating revenue ratio	Nonoperating Revenues and Other Income / Total Operating Revenues
Return on total assets[b]	Excess of Revenues over Expenses / Total Assets
Return on net assets[c]	Excess of Revenues over Expenses / Net Assets

Activity ratios	Formula
Total asset turnover ratio	Total Operating Revenues / Total Assets
Net fixed assets turnover ratio	Total Operating Revenues / Net Plant and Equipment
Age of plant ratio	Accumulated Depreciation / Depreciation Expense

Capital structure ratios	Formula
Long-term debt to net assets ratio[d]	Long-Term Debt / Net Assets
Net assets to total assets ratio[e]	Net Assets / Total Assets
Times interest earned ratio[f]	(Excess of Revenues over Expenses + Interest Expense) / Interest Expense
Debt service coverage ratio[g]	(Excess of Revenues over Expenses + Interest Expense + Depreciation and Amortization Expenses) / (Interest Expense + Principal Payments)

[a]Adjusted Discharges = (Total Gross Patient Revenue / Total Gross Inpatient Revenues) × Total Discharges.
[b]In for-profit health care organizations, calculated as Net Income / Total Assets.
[c]Called *return on equity* in for-profit health care organizations, and calculated as Net Income / Owners' Equity.
[d]Called *long-term debt to equity* in for-profit health care organizations, and calculated as Long-Term Debt / Owners' Equity.
[e]Called *equity to total assets* in for-profit health care organizations, and calculated as Owners' Equity / Total Assets.
[f]In for-profit health care organizations, calculated as (Net Income + Interest Expense) / Interest Expense.
[g]In for-profit health care organizations, calculated as (Net Income + Interest Expense + Depreciation and Amortization Expenses) / (Interest Expense + Principal Payments).

KEY TERMS

a. Financial leverage

b. Horizontal analysis

c. Ratio

d. Trend analysis

e. Vertical analysis

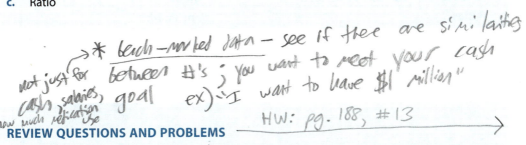

** bench-marked data - see if there are similarities
not just for between #'s; you want to meet your cash
(cash, salaries, goal ex) "I want to have $1 million"
how much reduction use*

REVIEW QUESTIONS AND PROBLEMS

HW: pg. 188, #13

1. **Definitions**. Define the key terms in the list above.

2. **Horizontal and vertical analyses**. Compare horizontal and vertical analyses, including trend analysis. How are they used? *pg. 138 + 142 + pg. 144*

3. **Vertical analysis**. Explain common-sized analysis. *pg. 144*

4. **Ratio analysis**. What is the purpose of ratio analysis? What are the four benchmark categories of ratios? *pg. 152-158 aka pg. 186*

5. **Medians**. Why is it that an industry median may not be an appropriate benchmark with which a particular organization wants to compare itself? *-b/c they don't include extreme outliers*

6. **Ratio interpretation**. How do the current, quick, and acid test ratios differ from the average payment period ratio? To what categories do these ratios belong? *liquidity ratios — includes expenses (read)*

7. **Ratio interpretation**. How do capital structure ratios and liquidity ratios differ in providing insight into an organization's ability to pay debt obligations? Identify two situations where an organization might have increasing activity ratios but declining profitability. *① hospital happened to not make a lot of profit + still needed to replace that MRI machine (total asset turnover) pg. 186*

8. **Ratio interpretation**. What is the difference between the operating margin ratio and a return on total assets ratio? What is the difference between operating revenue per adjusted discharge ratio and operating expense per adjusted discharge ratio? To what categories of ratios do these ratios belong? *revenue, expense, + profitability ratios*

9. **Ratio interpretation**. What capital structure ratio measures the ability to pay debt service payments? *debt service coverage ratio*

10. **Ratio interpretation**. How would you describe the plant and equipment status of a health care provider with an increasing age of plant ratio?

11. **Profitability analysis**. Compare the profitability ratios for Hightower Hospital with its industry benchmarks (Exhibit 4.17). Hightower has increased its patient volume,

② had to add a new wing

EXHIBIT 4.17 SELECTED RATIOS FOR HIGHTOWER HOSPITAL AND THE INDUSTRY BENCHMARKS

Revenue, Expense, and Profitability Ratios	Industry Benchmark	Hightower Hospital
Operating revenue per adjusted discharge	$5,900	$6,250
Operating expense per adjusted discharge	$5,700	$5,600
Salary and benefit expense as a percentage of total operating expense	52%	48%
Operating margin	0.02	0.04
Return on total assets	0.05	0.08
Nonoperating revenue ratio	0.08	0.12

negotiated higher rates for its managed care contracts, and lowered its labor expenses by outsourcing several support services.

12. **Ratio analysis.** Compare the capital structure ratios for Avon Hospital against industry benchmarks (Exhibit 4.18). Note that during this time period, Avon has refinanced its fixed rate debt with lower variable rate debt.

13. **Ratio analysis.** The statement of operations and balance sheet for Longwood Community Hospital for the years ended 20X0 and 20X1 are shown in Exhibits 4.19a and 4.19b. Compute the following ratios for both years: current, acid test, days in accounts receivable, average payment period, long-term debt to net assets, net assets to total assets, total asset turnover, fixed asset turnover, operating revenue per adjusted discharge, operating expense per adjusted discharge, salary and benefit expense as a percentage of total operating expense, return on total assets, and operating margin. After calculating the ratios, comment on Longwood's liquidity; efficient use of assets or activity ratios; revenue, expense, and profitability; and capital structure relative to its industry benchmarks for its respective bed size (listed in Exhibit 4.16a). Cite at least two meaningful ratios per

EXHIBIT 4.18 SELECTED RATIOS FOR AVON HOSPITAL AND THE INDUSTRY BENCHMARKS

Capital Ratios	Industry Benchmark	Avon Hospital (20X1)	Avon Hospital (20X0)
Debt service coverage	3.00	3.20	2.40
Times interest earned	4.00	4.90	3.00
Net assets to total assets	0.50	0.45	0.40
Long-term debt to net assets	0.50	0.55	0.60

EXHIBIT 4.19a STATEMENT OF OPERATIONS FOR LONGWOOD COMMUNITY HOSPITAL

Longwood Community Hospital
Statement of Operations for the Years Ended
December 31, 20X1 and 20X0 (in thousands)

	20X1	20X0
Revenues		
Net patient service revenue	$54,000	$53,000
Other revenue	1,000	500
Total operating revenues	55,000	53,500
Expenses		
Salaries and benefits	23,000	22,000
Supplies and other expenses	20,000	23,000
Depreciation	10,000	9,000
Total operating expenses	53,000	54,000
Operating income	2,000	(500)
Excess of revenues over expenses	2,000	(500)
Increase (decrease) in net assets	**$2,000**	**($500)**

EXHIBIT 4.19b BALANCE SHEET FOR LONGWOOD COMMUNITY HOSPITAL

Longwood Community Hospital

Balance Sheet December 31, 20X1 and 20X0 (in thousands)

	20X1	20X0
Current assets		
Cash and cash equivalents	$6,000	$4,000
Net patient receivables	10,000	8,500
Prepaid expenses	1,400	1,300
Total current assets	17,400	13,800
Noncurrent assets		
Plant, property, and equipment		
Gross plant, property, and equipment	27,000	24,000
(less accumulated depreciation)	(1,500)	(1,300)
Net plant, property, and equipment	25,500	22,700
Construction in progress	1,000	4,000
Total assets	**$43,900**	**$40,500**
Current liabilities		
Accounts payable	$500	$750
Salaries payable	7,800	9,000
Total current liabilities	8,300	9,750
Long-term liabilities		
Bonds payable	9,000	8,000
Total long-term liabilities	9,000	8,000
Net assets	26,600	22,750
Total liabilities and net assets	**$43,900**	**$40,500**

EXHIBIT 4.20a STATEMENT OF OPERATIONS FOR LOUISVILLE COMMUNITY HOSPITAL

Louisville Community Hospital
Statement of Operations for the Years Ended December 31,
20X1 and 20X0 (in thousands)

	20X1	20X0
Revenues		
Net patient service revenue	$23,000	$19,000
Net assets released from restriction	1,000	800
Total operating revenues	24,000	19,800
Expenses		
Salaries and benefits	13,000	9,000
Supplies and other expenses	7,000	6,000
Depreciation	2,500	2,000
General services	200	100
Total operating expenses	22,700	17,100
Operating income	1,300	2,700
Nonoperating income	4,000	2,500
Excess of revenue over expenses	5,300	5,200
Increase (decrease) in net assets	**$5,300**	**$5,200**

pick 1 for each group on pg. 186
+explain how that makes the company look good

category. Assume for this analysis that Longwood is a 350-bed facility and its adjusted discharges were 5,500 for 20X0 and 5,400 for 20X1.

14. **Ratio analysis**. Exhibits 4.20a and 4.20b show the statement of operations and balance sheet for Louisville Community Hospital for the years ended 20X0 and 20X1. Compute the following ratios for both years: current, quick, acid test, days in accounts receivable, days cash on hand, average payment period, operating revenue per adjusted discharge, operating expense per adjusted discharge, salary and benefit expense as a percentage of total operating expense, operating margin, nonoperating revenue, return on total assets and net assets, total asset turnover, fixed asset turnover, age of plant, long-term debt to net assets, and net assets to total assets. Comment on Louisville's liquidity; efficient use of assets; revenue, expense, and profitability; and capital structure, citing at least

EXHIBIT 4.20b BALANCE SHEET FOR LOUISVILLE COMMUNITY HOSPITAL

Louisville Community Hospital
Balance Sheet December 31, 20X1 and 20X0 (in thousands)

	20X1	20X0
Current assets		
Cash and cash equivalents	$700	$500
Net patient receivables	4,000	3,500
Inventory	950	750
Total current assets	5,650	5,250
Noncurrent assets		
Plant, property, and equipment		
Gross plant, property, and equipment	26,500	24,000
(less accumulated depreciation)	(18,000)	(17,000)
Net plant, property, and equipment	8,500	7,000
Board-designated funds	18,000	9,000
Total assets	**32,150**	**21,250**
Current liabilities		
Accounts payable	2,500	2,000
Accrued expenses	900	750
Total current liabilities	3,400	2,750
Long-term liabilities		
Bonds payable	6,500	8,000
Total long-term liabilities	6,500	8,000
Net assets	22,250	10,500
Total liabilities and net assets	**$32,150**	**$21,250**

one ratio per category. Use the national hospital industry benchmarks listed in Exhibit 4.16a for 125 beds, and assume that Louisville's adjusted discharges were 3,100 for 20X0 and 3,300 for 20X1.

15. **Ratio analysis**. Exhibit 4.21 lists the financial ratios for 189-bed Collingswood Community Hospital. Assess the revenue, expense, and profitability; liquidity; activity; and capital structure of Collingswood for 20X1. Explain why these financial measures changed between 20X0 and 20X1, and compare them to national industry benchmarks for Collingswood's bed size, using the data from Exhibit 4.16a.

EXHIBIT 4.21   SELECTED FINANCIAL RATIOS FOR COLLINGSWOOD COMMUNITY HOSPITAL

Ratio	20X1	20X0
Liquidity ratios		
Current ratio	3.05	2.01
Acid test ratio	0.65	0.35
Days in accounts receivable	48	60
Days cash on hand	215	120
Average payment period (days)	62	48
Revenue, expense, and profitability ratios		
Operating revenue per adjusted discharge	$7,200	$8,000
Operating expense per adjusted discharge	$6,934	$7,300
Salary and benefit expense as a percentage of total operating expense	43%	50%
Operating margin	0.04	0.08
Nonoperating revenue	0.15	0.04
Return on net assets	0.13	0.04
Activity ratios		
Total asset turnover ratio	0.90	1.20
Fixed asset turnover ratio	2.20	2.75
Age of plant	8.45	11.15
Capital structure ratios		
Debt service coverage ratio	2.75	4.00
Long-term debt to net assets (equity)	1.40	0.55
Net assets to total assets	0.42	0.65

16. **Ratio analysis.** Radnor Healthcare System, an 800-bed institution, is located in a highly competitive, urban market area. Using the financial ratios from Exhibit 4.22 for the current and previous years, evaluate Radnor's financial condition, focusing on revenue, expense, and profitability; liquidity; activity; and capital structure ratios, and compare them to national industry benchmarks for Radnor's bed size, using the data from Exhibit 4.16a.

17. **Ratio analysis,** unknown bed size. Compare Spring Hill Community Hospital's liquidity; revenue, expense, and profitability; activity; and capital structure ratios with its national industry benchmarks, using the data from Exhibits 4.16a and 4.23.

EXHIBIT 4.22 SELECTED FINANCIAL RATIOS FOR RADNOR HEALTHCARE SYSTEM

Ratio	20X1	20X0
Liquidity ratios		
Current ratio	1.85	2.10
Quick ratio	1.50	1.55
Acid test ratio	0.43	0.45
Days in accounts receivable	70	55
Days cash on hand	155	145
Average payment period (days)	60	55
Revenue, expense, and profitability ratios		
Operating revenue per adjusted discharge	$12,500	$11,000
Operating expense per adjusted discharge	$12,800	$10,500
Salary and benefit expense as a percentage of total operating expense	55%	50%
Operating margin	(0.05)	0.02
Nonoperating revenue	0.06	0.07
Return on assets	0.02	0.06
Activity ratios		
Total asset turnover ratio	1.12	0.99
Fixed asset turnover ratio	2.55	2.35
Age of plant	11.75	11.03
Capital structure ratios		
Long-term debt to equity	0.45	0.56
Equity to total assets	0.55	0.71
Debt service coverage ratio	2.85	3.05

18. **Ratio analysis**, unknown bed size. Exhibit 4.24 displays the financial ratios for St. Joe Hospital. Compare its liquidity; revenue, expense, and profitability; activity; and capital structure ratios to national industry benchmarks for all hospitals, using the data from Exhibit 4.16a.

19. **Ratio analysis**. Swift Community Hospital, a 310-bed facility, is a sole provider hospital in a rural New England area serving a large market. Recently, a wealthy philanthropist made a major contribution to the hospital's long-term investment fund. Assess Swift's profitability, liquidity, activity, and capital structure ratios. Using the financial ratios from Exhibit 4.25 for the current and previous years, evaluate Swift's financial condition, and also compare its ratios to national industry benchmarks for its bed size, using the data from Exhibits 4.16a.

20. **Ratio analysis**. Allen Community Hospital is a small, 95-bed hospital. The hospital just completed a major renovation of its facility, which has helped to attract new physicians and patients to the hospital. Assess Allen's revenue, expense, and profitability; liquidity; activity; and capital structure ratios. Using the financial ratios from Exhibit 4.26 for the current and previous years, evaluate Allen's financial condition and also compare its ratios to national industry benchmarks for its bed size, using the data from Exhibits 4.16a.

21. **Horizontal, vertical, and ratio analyses**. Exhibits 4.27a and 4.27b show the statement of operations and balance sheet for the 310-bed Wakeland Community Hospital for 20X0 and 20X1. Adjusted discharges for 20X0 and 20X1 are 25,000 and 26,000, respectively.

    a. Perform a horizontal analysis on both statements.

    b. Perform a vertical analysis on both statements relative to 20X0.

    c. Compute all the selected ratios listed in Exhibit 4.16a, and compare them with the industry benchmarks.

    Using these financial performance measures, evaluate the financial state of Wakeland Community. The debt principal payments each year are $5.5 million, whereas adjusted discharges, as mentioned, are 25,000 in 20X0 and 26,000 in 20X1.

22. **Horizontal, vertical, and ratio analyses**. Exhibits 4.28a and 4.28b show the statement of operations and balance sheet for the 375-bed Island Regional Medical Center for 20X0 and 20X1.

    a. Perform a horizontal analysis on both statements.

    b. Perform a vertical analysis on both statements relative to 20X0.

    c. Compute all the selected ratios listed in Exhibit 4.16a, and compare them with the benchmarks.

    Using these financial performance measures, evaluate the financial state of Island. The debt principal payments each year are $4,500,000, and adjusted discharges are 13,500 for 20X0 and 14,000 for 20X1.

EXHIBIT 4.23 SELECTED FINANCIAL RATIOS FOR SPRING HILL COMMUNITY HOSPITAL

Ratio	20X1	20X0
Liquidity ratios		
Current ratio	1.78	2.15
Quick ratio	1.29	1.55
Acid test ratio	0.18	0.35
Days in accounts receivable	82	60
Days cash on hand	60	100
Average payment period (days)	40	50
Revenue, expense, and profitability ratios		
Operating revenue per adjusted discharge	$7,900	$7,800
Operating expense per adjusted discharge	$8,200	$7,400
Salary and benefit expense as a percentage of total operating expense	55%	45%
Operating margin	(0.04)	0.05
Nonoperating revenue	0.06	0.01
Return on total assets	0.02	0.03
Return on net assets	0.08	0.05
Activity ratios		
Total asset turnover ratio	1.07	0.84
Fixed asset turnover ratio	2.70	1.46
Age of plant	9.26	11.08
Capital structure ratios		
Long-term debt to net assets	0.65	0.25
Net assets to total assets	0.35	0.52
Times interest earned	2.00	3.20
Debt service coverage ratio	2.50	3.70

EXHIBIT 4.24 SELECTED FINANCIAL RATIOS FOR ST. JOE HOSPITAL

Ratio	20X1	20X0
Liquidity ratios		
Current ratio	1.70	1.85
Acid test ratio	0.15	0.19
Days in accounts receivable	65	53
Days cash on hand	60	75
Average payment period (days)	65	50
Revenue, expense, and profitability ratios		
Operating revenue per adjusted discharge	$6,800	$6,800
Operating expense per adjusted discharge	$6,500	$6,700
Salary and benefit expense as a percentage of total operating expense	44%	47%
Operating margin	0.04	0.03
Return on total assets	0.06	0.05
Activity ratios		
Total asset turnover ratio	1.00	0.99
Fixed asset turnover ratio	1.90	1.80
Age of plant	8.34	10.89
Capital structure ratios		
Long-term debt to equity	0.20	0.35
Equity to total assets	0.60	0.50
Debt service coverage ratio	3.80	3.40

EXHIBIT 4.25 SELECTED FINANCIAL RATIOS FOR SWIFT COMMUNITY HOSPITAL

Ratio	20X1	20X0
Liquidity ratios		
Current ratio	3.12	1.95
Quick ratio	2.12	1.45
Acid test ratio	0.89	0.25
Days in accounts receivable	46	58
Days cash on hand	148	48
Average payment period (days)	50	56
Profitability ratios		
Operating margin	0.02	0.01
Nonoperating revenue	0.35	0.05
Return on assets	0.15	0.04
Activity ratios		
Total asset turnover ratio	0.80	0.90
Fixed asset turnover ratio	1.90	2.10
Age of plant	12.92	11.04
Capital structure ratios		
Long-term debt to net assets	0.25	0.60
Net assets to total assets	0.65	0.35
Debt service coverage ratio	3.50	2.25

EXHIBIT 4.26 SELECTED FINANCIAL RATIOS FOR ALLEN COMMUNITY HOSPITAL

Ratio	20X1	20X0
Liquidity ratios		
Current ratio	1.90	2.18
Acid test ratio	0.20	0.35
Days in accounts receivable	53	63
Days cash on hand	70	90
Average payment period (days)	75	50
Revenue, expense, and profitability ratios		
Operating revenue per adjusted discharge	$6,900	$6,500
Operating expense per adjusted discharge	$6,800	$6,600
Salary and benefit expense as a percentage of total operating expense	50%	45%
Operating margin	0.01	(0.01)
Return on assets	0.03	0.02
Activity ratios		
Total asset turnover	1.20	0.95
Fixed asset turnover	2.95	2.20
Age of plant	7.85	11.52
Capital structure ratios		
Long-term debt to equity	1.47	1.40
Equity to total assets	0.25	0.23
Debt service coverage ratio	2.00	3.02

EXHIBIT 4.27a STATEMENT OF OPERATIONS FOR WAKELAND COMMUNITY HOSPITAL

Wakeland Community Hospital
Statement of Operations for the Years Ended December 31,
20X1 and 20X0 (in thousands)

	20X1	20X0
Revenues		
Net patient service revenue	$225,000	$210,000
Other operating revenue	6,400	5,700
Total operating revenues	231,400	215,700
Operating expenses		
Salaries and benefits	124,173	110,167
Supplies and other expenses	85,000	61,000
Depreciation	12,000	11,300
Interest	4,500	2,500
Total operating expenses	225,673	184,967
Income from operations	5,727	30,733
Nonoperating income		
Investment income/contributions	7,500	8,500
Excess of revenue over expenses	13,227	39,233
Net income	**$13,227**	**$39,233**

EXHIBIT 4.27b BALANCE SHEET FOR WAKELAND COMMUNITY HOSPITAL

Wakeland Community Hospital
Balance Sheet December 31, 20X1 and 20X0 (in thousands)

	20X1	20X0
Current assets		
Cash and cash equivalents	$40,500	$35,500
Net patient accounts receivables	39,500	36,400
Inventories	3,800	4,000
Other current assets	6,500	5,200
Total current assets	90,300	81,100
Plant, property, and equipment		
Gross plant, property, and equipment	215,000	175,500
(Less accumulated depreciation)	(65,000)	(107,000)
Net property, plant, and equipment	150,000	68,500
Funded depreciation/board-designated funds		
Cash and short-term investments	185,000	110,000
Total assets	**$425,300**	**$259,600**
Current liabilities		
Accounts payable	$14,500	$8,500
Salaries payable	4,500	3,500
Notes payable	4,300	4,500
Total current liabilities	23,300	16,500
Long-term liabilities		
Bonds payable	60,000	27,500
Total long-term liabilities	60,000	27,500
Net assets	342,000	215,600
Total liabilities and net assets	**$425,300**	**$259,600**

EXHIBIT 4.28a STATEMENT OF OPERATIONS FOR ISLAND REGIONAL MEDICAL CENTER

Island Regional Medical Center
Statement of Operations for the Years Ended December 31,
20X1 and 20X0 (in thousands)

	20X1	20X0
Revenues		
Net patient service revenue	$116,500	$105,600
Other operating revenue	2,100	2,300
Total operating revenues	118,600	107,900
Expenses		
Salaries and benefits	74,800	65,300
Supplies and other expenses	34,500	32,300
Depreciation	5,500	4,500
Interest	1,200	1,300
Total operating expenses	116,000	103,400
Operating income	2,600	4,500
Nonoperating revenue	1,500	2,500
Excess of revenues over expenses	4,100	7,000
Increase (decrease) in net assets	**$4,100**	**$7,000**

23. **Horizontal, vertical, and ratio analyses**. Exhibits 4.29a and 4.29b show the statement of operations and balance sheet for Resort Hospital for 20X1 and 20X0. The debt principal payment each year for Resort is $1,300,000, and its adjusted discharges are 6,500 for 20X0 and 5,500 for 20X1.

   a. Perform horizontal and vertical analyses using the statement of operations.

   b. Perform horizontal and vertical analyses using the balance sheet.

   c. Compute all the selected ratios listed in Exhibit 4.16a.

   Evaluate the financial state of Resort Hospital, a 60-bed facility, using all of the above measures. Make the basis for the vertical analysis the year 20X0.

EXHIBIT 4.28b BALANCE SHEET FOR ISLAND REGIONAL MEDICAL CENTER

Island Regional Medical Center
Balance Sheet December 31, 20X1 and 20X0 (in thousands)

	20X1	20X0
Current assets		
Cash and cash equivalents	$9,800	$14,300
Net patient receivables	18,919	17,032
Inventory	1,840	1,800
Prepaid expenses	750	800
Total current assets	31,309	33,932
Plant, property, and equipment		
Gross plant, property, and equipment	72,000	65,000
(Less accumulated depreciation)	(37,000)	(32,000)
Net property, plant, and equipment	35,000	33,000
Long-term investments	48,000	42,000
Total assets	**$114,309**	**$108,932**
Current liabilities		
Accounts payable	$6,200	$6,800
Salaries payable	5,400	4,300
Total current liabilities	11,600	11,100
Long-term liabilities		
Bonds payable	55,000	65,000
Total long-term liabilities	55,000	65,000
Net assets	47,709	32,832
Total liabilities and net assets	**$114,309**	**$108,932**

EXHIBIT 4.29a STATEMENT OF OPERATIONS FOR RESORT HOSPITAL

Resort Hospital
Statement of Operations for the Years Ended December 31,
20X1 and 20X0 (in thousands)

	20X1	20X0
Revenues		
Net patient service revenue	$33,500	$30,500
Other operating revenue	2,600	2,500
Total operating revenues	36,100	33,000
Expenses		
Salaries and benefits	23,500	19,600
Supplies and other expenses	11,400	10,500
Depreciation	700	700
Interest	710	710
Total operating expenses	36,310	31,510
Operating income	(210)	1,490
Nonoperating revenue	6,500	1,200
Excess of revenue over expenses	**$6,290**	**$2,690**

24. **Horizontal, vertical, and ratio analyses**. Exhibits 4.30a and 4.30b show the balance sheet and income statement for the 660-bed Williams Academic Medical Center for the years 20X0 and 20X1. Assume that principal payments each year come to $5,500,000 and that adjusted discharges are 120,000 for 20X0 and 125,000 for 20X1.

    a. Perform full horizontal and vertical analyses on the balance sheet.

    b. Perform full horizontal and vertical analyses on the income statement.

    c. Calculate every ratio described in the chapter for both years, and compare these ratios with the benchmarks (Exhibit 4.16a).

    Discuss Williams's current financial position and future outlook based on these results. Make the basis for the vertical analysis the year 20X0.

EXHIBIT 4.29b BALANCE SHEET FOR RESORT HOSPITAL

Resort Hospital
Balance Sheet December 31, 20X1 and 20X0 (in thousands)

	20X1	20X0
Current assets		
Cash and cash equivalents	$1,500	$2,500
Net patient receivables	6,500	4,800
Inventory	400	350
Prepaid expenses	350	250
Total current assets	8,750	7,900
Plant, property, and equipment		
Gross plant, property, and equipment	22,000	19,500
(Less accumulated depreciation)	(12,700)	(12,000)
Net property, plant, and equipment	9,300	7,500
Long-term investments	16,500	10,500
Total assets	**$34,550**	**$25,900**
Current liabilities		
Accounts payable	$5,300	$3,800
Salaries payable	1,000	900
Total current liabilities	6,300	4,700
Long-term liabilities		
Bonds payable	1,200	2,500
Total long-term liabilities	1,200	2,500
Net assets	27,050	18,700
Total liabilities and net assets	**$34,550**	**$25,900**

EXHIBIT 4.30a BALANCE SHEET FOR WILLIAMS ACADEMIC MEDICAL CENTER

Williams Academic Medical Center
Balance Sheet December 31, 20X0 and 20X1 (in thousands)

	20X1	20X0
Current assets		
Cash and cash equivalents	$66,300	$63,500
Patient accounts receivables, net	105,000	125,000
Inventories	69,500	62,000
Other current assets	3,000	2,400
Total current assets	243,800	252,900
Plant, property, and equipment		
Gross plant, property, and equipment	1,040,000	976,000
(Less accumulated depreciation)	(254,000)	(326,000)
Net property, plant, and equipment	786,000	650,000
Long-term investments	195,000	175,000
Total assets	**$1,224,800**	**$1,077,900**
Current liabilities		
Accounts payable	$87,200	$89,000
Salaries payable	23,000	20,000
Notes payable	3,200	3,000
Other current liabilities	2,100	1,200
Total current liabilities	115,500	113,200
Noncurrent liabilities		
Bonds payable	466,500	461,000
Total noncurrent liabilities	466,500	461,000
Owners' equity	642,800	503,700
Total liabilities and equity	**$1,224,800**	**$1,077,900**

EXHIBIT 4.30b INCOME STATEMENT FOR WILLIAMS ACADEMIC MEDICAL CENTER

Williams Academic Medical Center
Income Statement for the Years Ended December 31, 20X0 and 20X1 (in thousands)

	20X1	20X0
Revenues		
Net patient revenues	$935,300	$735,200
Other operating revenues	47,000	35,600
Total operating revenues	982,300	770,800
Expenses		
Salaries and benefits	305,000	325,000
Supply expenses	102,500	105,000
Depreciation	55,000	32,800
Purchased services	85,000	84,000
Other expenses	314,500	172,000
Interest	28,700	12,500
Total operating expenses	890,700	731,300
Income from operations	91,600	39,500
Nonoperating income:		
Investment income and contributions	21,000	19,000
Total income before taxes	112,600	58,500
(Less income taxes)	(45,040)	(23,400)
Net income (loss)	**$67,560**	**$35,100**

CHAPTER 5

WORKING CAPITAL MANAGEMENT

Although noncurrent assets provide the capability to provide services, it is the combination of current assets and current liabilities that turns that capability into service. For example, an X-ray machine is useless without an adequate supply of film on hand or cash to pay the radiation technologists. This chapter begins with a discussion of working capital and then focuses on the management of working capital in the health care industry: cash and accounts receivable, which are key components of revenue cycle management.

The term *working capital* refers to both current assets and current liabilities. A related term, *net working capital*, refers to the *difference* between current assets and current liabilities. That is

Net Working Capital = Current Assets − Current Liabilities

Working Capital Cycle

In the day-to-day operations of an organization, an ongoing series of cash inflows and outflows pays for day-to-day expenses (such as supplies and salaries). The organization must have sufficient funds available to pay for these items on a timely basis. This is particularly problematic in health care, where it is not unusual for payments to be received more than two months after the patient or third party has been billed for the provided services.

Ideally, a health care organization will earn and receive sufficient funds from providing services to enable it to meet its current obligations with available cash. To do this requires managing the four phases of the working capital cycle (Exhibit 5.1):

LEARNING OBJECTIVES

- Define working capital and the revenue cycle.

- Understand working capital and revenue cycle management strategies.

- Construct a cash budget.

- Understand receivables and payables management.

Working Capital
Measures current asset and current liability accounts of the health care entity.

Net Working Capital
The difference between current assets and current liabilities.

EXHIBIT 5.1 THE WORKING CAPITAL CYCLE: THE IMPORTANCE OF TIMING IN MANAGING WORKING CAPITAL

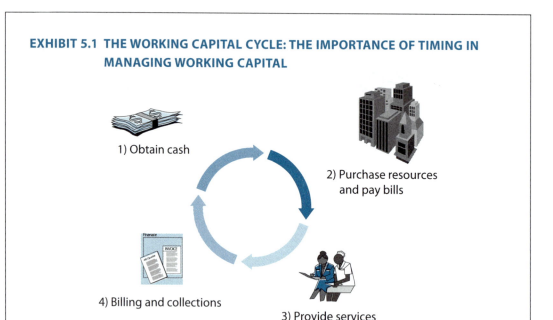

1) Obtain cash

2) Purchase resources and pay bills

4) Billing and collections

3) Provide services

- Obtaining cash
- Turning cash into resources, such as supplies and labor, and paying bills
- Using these resources to provide services
- Billing patients for the services, and collecting revenues so that the cycle can be continued

In regard to cash, managing the working capital cycle involves not only ensuring that total cash inflows cover cash outflows but also managing the timing of these flows. To the extent that payments come due before cash is available, the organization has to obtain cash from sources other than existing revenues, such as from investments or through short-term borrowing. To illustrate, suppose an organization starts the month of September with no working capital (see Exhibit 5.2). During the month, it delivers $20,000 worth of services but must pay $9,000 in staff salaries every fifteen days and $2,000 for supplies every thirty days. Situation 1 assumes that the full amount owed is collected during the month but is not received until the end of the month. Situation 2 assumes that the organization also collects the full amount owed but in two equal payments of $10,000 each, the first payment arriving after fifteen days and the second payment after thirty days.

EXHIBIT 5.2 THE EFFECTS OF TIMING ON WORKING CAPITAL NEEDS

		Situation 1				Situation 2		
	Account	Cash Inflows	Cash Outflows	Balance	Account	Cash Inflows	Cash Outflows	Balance
Day 1				$0				$0
Day 15	Revenues				Revenues	$10,000		
	Salaries		$9,000	($9,000)	Salaries		$9,000	$1,000
Day 30	Revenues	$20,000			Revenues	$10,000		
	Salaries		$9,000		Salaries		$9,000	
	Supplies		$2,000	$0	Supplies		$2,000	$0

In both cases, cash inflows ($20,000) equal cash outflows ($20,000). However, whereas in situation 2 there is always sufficient cash on hand to meet the payments when due, in situation 1 the organization will not be able to meet its first $9,000 payroll on day 15. To meet this obligation, it either must take cash out of existing reserves or borrow. However, even in situation 2, there is little margin for error. How much extra working capital an organization determines it must keep as a cushion is called its *working capital strategy*.

Working Capital Management Strategies

Working capital management strategy has two components: asset mix and financing mix. *Asset mix* is the amount of working capital an organization keeps on hand relative to its potential working capital obligations. *Financing mix* refers to how an organization chooses to finance its working capital needs.

Asset Mix Strategy

A health care provider's asset mix strategy falls on a continuum between aggressive and conservative (Exhibit 5.3). Under an *aggressive approach*, the health care organization attempts to maximize returns by investing excess funds in nonliquid assets expected to have relatively high earnings, such

Working Capital Strategy
The amount of working capital an organization determines it must keep as a cushion.

Asset Mix
The amount of working capital an organization keeps on hand relative to its potential working capital obligations.

Financing Mix
How an organization chooses to finance its working capital needs.

EXHIBIT 5.3 WORKING CAPITAL MANAGEMENT STRATEGIES

	Aggressive Strategy	**Conservative Strategy**
Goal	Maximize returns	Minimize risk
Liquidity	Low	High
Risk	High	Low
Return	High	Low

Liquidity

A measure of how quickly an asset can be converted into cash.

as buildings and equipment; yet it does so at the risk of lower *liquidity*, with increased chances of inventory stock-outs, lost customers from stringent credit policies, and lack of cash to pay employees and suppliers.

 Key Point A health care organization that utilizes an aggressive asset mix strategy seeks to maximize its returns by investing in nonliquid assets but faces the risk of lower liquidity.

Conversely, under a *conservative approach*, a health care organization seeks to minimize its risk of having insufficient short-term funds by maintaining higher liquidity. However, it does so at the cost of receiving lower returns because short-term investments typically earn a lower return than do long-term investments.

Financing Mix Strategy

Financing mix refers to how the organization chooses to finance its working capital needs. Temporary working capital needs result from short-term fluctuations, whereas permanent working capital needs arise from more ongoing factors, such as a permanent increase in patient volume. Borrowing for the short term at lower interest costs for short-term needs under normal conditions leads to a higher profit, because working capital is otherwise being invested optimally (everything else being equal), but this places the facility at risk because of possible higher debt payments if the need for additional borrowing arises. If the organization has long-term working capital financing needs, it is better off financing those needs with long-term financing under normal conditions. Facilities borrowing long

EXHIBIT 5.4 COMPARISON OF KEY CHARACTERISTICS OF SHORT- AND LONG-TERM BORROWING UNDER NORMAL CONDITIONS

	Short-Term	Long-Term
Interest rate[a]	Lower	Higher
Interest cost	Lower	Higher
Profit	Higher	Lower
Volatility risks	Variable	Fixed

[a]Short-term rates are typically lower than long-term rates.

term at higher interest costs to support ongoing working capital needs face lower earnings because they are paying higher interest than they would with low-cost short-term borrowing. Exhibit 5.4 compares the key characteristics of short-term and long-term borrowing. Overall, an aggressive working capital strategy involves maintaining a relatively low amount of working capital on hand and financing working capital shortfalls with short-term debt. For example, a hospital could follow an aggressive strategy by maintaining less cash and inventory on hand and increasing access to low-interest, short-term debt to cover shortfalls. This aggressive strategy would be expected to generate higher returns for the hospital because it would then be investing a smaller proportion of its total assets in low-return current assets and a higher proportion of its debt in low-interest, short-term debt. However, the risk to this greater return is lower liquidity because there would be an increased chance of not having the working capital available to meet short-term financing needs. For instance, hospitals may not have enough cash and inventory on hand to pay any unexpected current obligations that may come due, nor sufficient supplies to support a sudden increase in demand for hospital services. Another risk is that in a tight credit market, the cost to borrow short term may suddenly rise higher than would be expected, as occurred during the 2008 to 2009 recession.

In reality, the health care market and the risk tolerance of the health care provider may influence the provider's working capital strategy. On the one hand, a health care provider located in a market with little competition and a high degree of stability for services might consider a more aggressive

PERSPECTIVE 5.1 HEALTH CARE SYSTEMS FORMING ACOs TO ESTABLISH LINES OF CREDIT TO PAY OFF POTENTIAL LOSSES

As hospitals form accountable care organizations (ACOs), they must conform to the regulation of the Centers for Medicare and Medicaid Services (CMS) that an ACO must have the ability to pay back any financial losses. Under an ACO arrangement, a health care system's ACO faces potential losses if the cost of care for a specific condition is greater than the payment from CMS. One way to repay a potential shortfall is to obtain approval for a line of credit from a bank. For example, both Banner Health, a Phoenix-based health system, and OSF Healthcare System have arranged lines of credit with banks for their ACO requirement. These health care systems consider the line of credit the least expensive option to comply with the CMS regulation. Besides a line of credit, other options to cover any financial losses from an ACO are cuts to future payments, reinsurance, escrow accounts, and surety bonds.

Source: Adapted from M. Evans, Buffering risk: market aims to help ACOs navigate potential losses, *Modern Healthcare*, May 21, 2012;42:22.

approach, since it would be better able to forecast its working capital needs, especially in regard to cash and inventory. On the other hand, a provider in a competitive, unsettled market with fluctuating demand for services should choose a more conservative approach to working capital management. Unpredictable patient volume makes it difficult to estimate future needs for cash on hand and inventory, and to estimate how much revenue will be tied up in patient accounts receivable. Therefore, a provider may resign itself to having all these current asset accounts at a higher level than it would like, leaving a smaller proportion of long-term assets to generate the higher rates of return. Perspectives 5.1 and 5.2 illustrate the need to have adequate cash on hand to cover short-term losses.

Key Point There are three rules to follow, under normal conditions, to decide between short-term and long-term borrowing to finance working capital needs: (1) finance short-term working capital needs with short-term debt; (2) finance long-term working capital needs with long-term financing; and (3) finance fluctuating needs for working capital by employing a mixed strategy: finance a certain base amount with long-term financing, and as short-term situations arise, finance these with short-term debt.

PERSPECTIVE 5.2 MEDICAL PRACTICE PITFALLS WHEN BORROWING FROM BANKS

Physician practices have increased bank borrowing as they continue to finance their needs for new medical technology, especially for loans secured by the federal Small Business Administration (SBA). These secured loans among physician practices have more than doubled, from 625 loans in 2001 to over 1,500 loans in 2011. Pitfalls for physicians in such borrowing include (1) considering only the nearest bank and not conducting comparative shopping for lenders (when shopping for banks, physician practices should assess the experience of the bank in working with the bureaucratic intricacies of SBA-backed loans); (2) not matching the expected life of the new equipment with the term of the loan (one consultant noticed that practices were borrowing funds from a short-term line of credit to fund a piece of equipment that had a useful asset life of five years, whereas a loan term of five years would be a better match with the useful life of the equipment); (3) borrowing consistently from a line of credit to meet payroll (advisors do not recommend using a line of credit as a source of funds to meet payroll: the cash collections from billed insurance claims should be used to meet payroll, whereas lines of credit should be accessed for less routine situations, such as when starting a practice or hiring a new physician partner); and (4) not assessing and projecting the added cash flow needed to pay for the new technology project. Given the thin margins of some physician practices, especially those in primary care, the practice should try to estimate how it will generate extra cash flow from the new piece of equipment to pay off the loan. Some equipment, such as imaging, may increase volume and generate enough additional cash flow to meet the loan payments. However, an electronic medical record system, which supports the operations of the practice, may bring in revenues only from meaningful use incentives and not by directly increasing revenues. Therefore the practice must consider other sources of potential income or cost savings within the practice (e.g., reducing staff) to help pay for the loan.

Source: Adapted from E. Berry, 5 mistakes doctors make when borrowing money, *American Medical News*, posted April 9, 2012, www.amednews.com/article/20120409/business/304099975/4.

Cash Management

In general, the term *cash* refers not only to coin and currency but also to *cash equivalents*, such as interest-bearing savings and checking accounts. There are three major reasons for a health care provider to hold cash:

- Daily operations purposes
- Precautionary purposes
- Speculative purposes

Meeting daily operations purposes requires holding cash to pay day-to-day bills. Meeting precautionary purposes requires holding cash to meet unexpected demands, such as unforeseen maintenance. Meeting speculative purposes requires holding cash to take advantage of unexpected opportunities, such as buying a competing group practice that has decided to sell.

Key Point　There are three major reasons to hold cash: for daily operations purposes, precautionary purposes, and speculative purposes.

Sources of Temporary Cash

Normal Line of Credit

An agreement established by a bank and a borrower that establishes the maximum amount of funds that may be borrowed, and the bank may loan the funds at its own discretion.

Although it would be favorable to always have excess short-term funds available to invest, health care organizations often find that they need to borrow funds for short periods to meet their maturing obligations. The two primary sources of short-term funds are

- Bank loans
- Extension of credit from suppliers (i.e., trade payables)

Bank Loans

Revolving Line of Credit

An agreement established by a bank and a borrower that legally requires the bank to loan money to the borrower at any time requested, up to a prenegotiated limit.

There are two major types of *unsecured* (not backed by an asset) short-term loans offered by banks: lines of credit and transaction notes. The interest expense associated with these alternatives is a function of economic conditions and the credit background of the borrower.

Lines of Credit

There are two types of lines of credit: a normal line of credit and a revolving line of credit. A *normal line of credit* is an agreement established by the bank and the borrower that establishes the maximum amount of funds that may be borrowed, but the bank is not legally obligated to fulfill the borrower's credit request. In contrast, a *revolving line of credit* legally requires the bank to fulfill the borrower's credit request up to a prenegotiated limit.

Key Point　A revolving line of credit differs from a normal line of credit in that the revolving line of credit legally requires a bank to fulfill the borrower's credit request up to a prenegotiated limit.

Commitment Fees

In addition to the interest rate on a line of credit, financial institutions are also compensated through either commitment fees or compensating balances, or both. A *commitment fee* is a percentage of the *unused* portion of the credit line that is charged to the potential borrower. The annual fee, often between 0.25 percent and 0.50 percent, is a function of the credit risk of the borrower and the reason for the line of credit. For example, assume a health care organization has a line of credit of $4 million and borrows on average $2.5 million during the year. If the commitment fee rate were 0.25 percent, then the borrower would pay an annual fee of $3,750 [($4 million − $2.5 million) × 0.0025] to have the right to borrow the full $4 million essentially on demand. Sometimes an organization can negotiate with a bank to reduce or eliminate a commitment fee for a line of credit, especially if it has a favorable, long-standing history with the lending institution.

Compensating Balances

Under a *compensating balance* arrangement, the borrower is required to maintain a designated dollar amount on deposit with the bank. The balance requirement is generally a percentage (perhaps 10 to 20 percent) of the total credit line or a percentage of the unused portion of the credit line. The effect of the compensating balance is to increase the *true* or *effective* interest rate that the borrower must pay. The effective interest rate is calculated using the following formula:

$$\text{Effective Interest Rate} = \frac{(\text{Interest Expense on Amount Borrowed} + \text{Total Fees})}{(\text{Amount Borrowed} - \text{Compensating Balance})}$$

Assume Community Healthcare Provider borrowed $600,000 during the year on a credit line of $1 million with an interest rate of 9 percent with no fees. Using this formula, the interest expense in the numerator is $54,000 (9 percent × $600,000). The amount borrowed in the denominator is $600,000, and the compensating balance is 10 percent of the unused portion of the line of credit (0.10 × $400,000), or $40,000. Thus, the effective interest rate, using the equation given above, is 9.64 percent [($54,000 + $0) / ($600,000 − $40,000)].

$$9.64\% = \frac{(\$54,000 + \$0)}{(\$600,000 - \$40,000)}$$

Transaction Notes

The second type of bank loan commonly used for short-term borrowing by health care providers is a transaction note. A *transaction note* is a

Commitment Fee
A percentage of the unused portion of a credit line that is charged to the potential borrower.

Compensating Balance
A designated dollar amount on deposit with a bank that a borrower is required to maintain.

Effective Interest Rate
The true interest rate that a borrower pays.

Transaction Note

A short-term, unsecured loan made for some specific purpose.

short-term, unsecured loan made for some specific purpose, such as financing inventory purchases. Transaction notes have compensating balance requirements. The borrower obtains the loan by signing a promissory note, or IOU. The terms of the transaction note (maturity and cost) are similar to those for the line of credit.

Trade Credit or Payables

Trade Credit

Short-term credit offered by the supplier of a good or service to the purchaser.

Trade Payables

Short-term debt that results from supplies purchased on credit for a given length of time. This allows an organization to use the supplier's money to pay for the purchase up until the time it pays the supplier the amount owed.

Instead of relying solely on an external lending source to obtain cash, an organization can generate cash by controlling its outflow, but the health care organization must have strict cash disbursement policies and procedures in effect. When a health care organization buys on credit, it is in fact using the supplier's money to pay for the purchase up until the time it pays the supplier the amount owed. These credit obligations are called *trade payables* (often referred to as *accounts payable*). Thus, one of the most important areas to address in cash management is that of either accepting or rejecting discounts offered by suppliers for early payment. These discounts are often stated as

2/10 net 30

This means that full payment is due within thirty days (*net 30*), but a 2 percent discount is offered if the payment is made within ten days after the sale (*2/10*) (Exhibit 5.5). Although at first glance it may seem optimal to delay payment for thirty days to retain cash on hand, in fact, depending on the credit terms, it is usually in the best interest of an organization to pay early and take the discount.

To compare the financial implications of taking a discount with the implications of not doing so, assume an organization receives an invoice

---

EXHIBIT 5.5 EXPLANATION OF COMMONLY USED DISCOUNT TERMS

A 2% discount is available if payment is made within 10 days.

↑

2/10 net 30

↓

If the payment isn't made within 10 days, the full payment is due within 30 days.

for $1,000 with terms of 2/10 net 30. If the organization pays within ten days, it receives a 2 percent discount worth $20 (0.02 × $1,000) and therefore has to pay only $980 ($1,000 − $20). If the payment isn't made until thirty days, the health care organization has to pay the full $1,000. Although it is clear that if the organization takes the discount it is paying less than it would by holding onto its cash longer, the true cost of paying later may not be so apparent. Understanding this cost involves switching perspectives.

Key Point Depending on a health care organization's credit terms for its trade payables, it is usually in the best interest of an organization to pay early and take the discount.

A common way to approach this situation is to think that paying $1,000 by thirty days would be the "normal" management action, and paying $980 early would be the alternative action. From this perspective, the savings from taking the discount is $20 (see Exhibit 5.6). However, a better way to

---

EXHIBIT 5.6 TWO APPROACHES TO CONCEPTUALIZING THE COST ASSOCIATED WITH NOT TAKING A DISCOUNT

Situation: Community Healthcare Provider receives a bill for $1,000 for supplies purchased. The terms of the bill are *2/10 net 30.*

A common way to think about this situation....

The bill:	$1,000
Discounted price	$ 980
Discount	$ 20

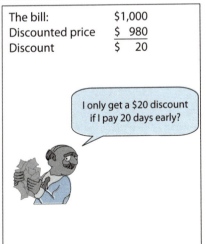

I only get a $20 discount if I pay 20 days early?

A better way to approach this situation....

The bill:	$ 980
Bill + interest	$1,000
Interest to borrow $980 for 20 days	$ 20

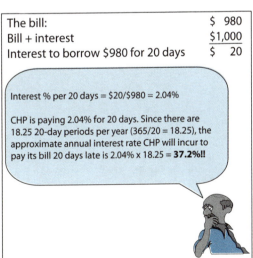

Interest % per 20 days = $20/$980 = 2.04%

CHP is paying 2.04% for 20 days. Since there are 18.25 20-day periods per year (365/20 = 18.25), the approximate annual interest rate CHP will incur to pay its bill 20 days late is 2.04% x 18.25 = **37.2%!!**

approach this decision is to consider the discounted price ($980) within ten days as the "real" price, and the full price paid by thirty days ($1,000) as the "penalty" price, because of the supplemental interest charge for not paying within the discount period. In other words, the organization would be paying $20 in interest ($1,000 − $980) to keep the $980 for an extra twenty days (the time between day 10 and day 30).

To determine the *approximate interest rate* the health care organization would pay to keep the $980 for an extra 20 days, use the formula given in Exhibit 5.7.

The calculation shows that the approximate annual interest rate is 37.2 percent. That is, by not taking the discount within ten days and instead waiting to pay until day 30, the health care organization is paying the annual equivalent of 37.2 percent interest to borrow $980. Thus, if the organization has the $980, it should take the discount unless it can earn this much interest by investing the $980 elsewhere, or it should borrow the $980 on a short-term basis if it can do so at a rate less than 37.2 percent.

Approximate Interest Rate

The interest rate incurred by not taking advantage of a supplier's discount offer on bills paid early. The formula in this chapter gives an approximate annual interest rate. A more precise method of calculation can be found in more advanced texts.

EXHIBIT 5.7 CALCULATING THE APPROXIMATE INTEREST RATE ASSOCIATED WITH NOT TAKING TRADE DISCOUNTS

1. Assume: $1,000 invoice is received for the purchase of medical supplies with terms **2/10 net 30**.

2. To calculate the **approximate interest rate,** the following formula is used:

$$\text{Approximate Interest Rate} = \frac{\text{Discount \%}}{1 - \text{Discount \%}} \times \frac{365}{\text{\# days until full payment is due} - \text{last day for discount}}$$

$$\frac{0.02}{1 - 0.02} = 0.0204 = 2.04\%$$

This is the interest rate for one 20-day period. The rate is somewhat higher than 2%, because $20 is being paid to borrow $980, not $1,000.

$$\frac{365}{30 - 10} = 18.25$$

This calculation is used to annualize the rate. In this case, there are 18.25 periods during a year. That is, if the facility kept paying 2.04% to borrow for 20 days at a time all year long, the process would be done 18.25 times.

Thus, to determine the approximate interest rate for one year, the interest rate for one period is multiplied by the number of periods in a year.

3. Approximate Interest Rate = 0.0204 × 18.25 = 0.372 = 37.2%

EXHIBIT 5.8 ILLUSTRATION OF HOW NOT TAKING A DISCOUNT AT VARIOUS DISCOUNT RATES AND EXTENDING PAYMENTS AFFECTS THE APPROXIMATE INTEREST RATE PAID

Approximate Annual Interest Rates Associated with Selected Discounts for Payment within 10 Days

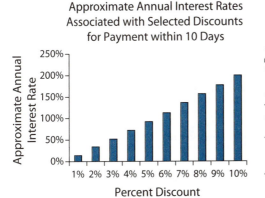

Percent Discount

Note: The approximate interest rate increases dramatically as the discount percent increases, holding the number of days in the discount period constant.

Interest Rates Associated with Selected Number of Days between the End of the Discount Period and Payment

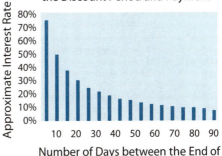

Number of Days between the End of the Discount Period and Payment

Note: The approximate interest rate decreases dramatically as the number of days between the last day for discount and the day the bill is paid increases.

Incidentally, the higher the discount being offered, the higher the approximate interest rate for not taking (or losing) the discount.

Exhibit 5.8 shows that the approximate interest rate decreases as the period of time after the discount date increases, until the bill is paid. Therefore, a prudent approach is to pay as late as possible within the discount period or, if the discount is not taken, to pay at the end of the net period. Although it is true that the approximate interest costs seem to decrease as the number of days the bill is not paid increases, at a certain point after the net period, new costs are encountered. These costs include late fees, loss of discounts in the future, loss of priority status with the supplier, and so forth.

Incidentally, in regard to the example used here, organizations that do weekly processing may find it virtually impossible to take advantage of a contract with terms such as *2/10 net 30*. In such cases, an organization may try to negotiate terms such as *2/15 net 35*, to give itself enough time to process the invoice and still meet the early payment deadline.

Revenue Cycle Management

The success of cash management is driven by the billing process. Ideally, a hospital bill is composed of a list of delivered services; therefore, at discharge, or even at any point during the service delivery process, the patient's bill reflects all services received. However, assembling the final bill can be a problem for many health care organizations, and for some this process may take weeks. Several hindrances can delay the billing process and collection of cash. For instance:

+ Patients who use more than one name or who have had name changes

+ Address changes or no address or phone number on file

+ Lack of clarity about who is responsible for paying the bill, or outdated insurance information

+ Specific requirements demanded by various insurers, such as retrospective reviews

A typical example might be an incoherent patient who is accepted into the emergency department for treatment. In its effort to turn around beds quickly to make room for the next patient, the hospital might discharge this patient when he or she is medically cleared but before complete billing information has been gathered. Or an uninsured patient may intentionally provide an expired insurance card or go under the name of an insured relative or friend to avoid payment. By the time the hospital realizes the problem, the claim has been denied and the patient is unreachable.

As a result of such problems, in recent years health care providers have implemented revenue cycle management techniques developed to help overcome billing-related problems. An essential component of an effective billing process is to have systematic, up-to-date, well-utilized billing policies and procedures in place, with the clear objective of ensuring fair, timely, and accurate invoicing. These management techniques define the goals, roles and responsibilities, and procedures to be used at various stages in the billing process. The revenue cycle includes several key processes, which are presented in Exhibit 5.9 and detailed below.

Scheduling or Preregistration

The normal revenue cycle begins with the patient's phone call to schedule an appointment. This starts the preregistration screening process, which gathers and verifies demographic and billing-related information before the patient enters the providing organization. Preregistration and admission screenings are important because they help the health care organization

EXHIBIT 5.9 THE REVENUE CYCLE MANAGEMENT PROCESS

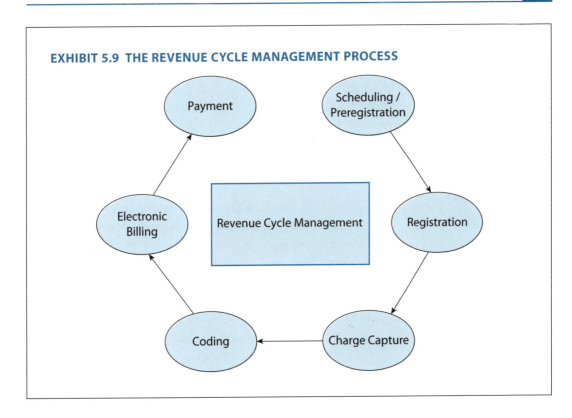

determine a patient's ability to pay by verifying name, address, employment status, and insurance coverage. Also in this process, the health care organization can make financial arrangements for patients who are unable to pay and can inform patients at the time of registration what they are responsible for paying under their insurance plans.

Registration

For patients who do not preregister (for example, an emergency room patient), hospitals need to try to follow the same processes used in preregistration in terms of insurance verification and ability to pay. Once they arrive at the facility, preregistered patients will encounter either a shortened registration process or, at some facilities, bypass the registration process altogether and report directly to the clinical area.

Charge Capture

The integration of a patient's financial and clinical information is critical to the revenue cycle. Correctly identifying the diagnostic and procedural codes when providing patient services is a critical step toward capturing charges and identifying billing items. The health care provider's management information system should allow easy interfacing among admissions or visits information, patient accounts, and medical records in a process that gathers and submits charge data in an accurate and timely manner. The primary objective for this system is the accurate, timely, and seamless transfer of data and information.

Coding

The primary objective of internal claims processing is to avoid claims denials. This involves the proper conduct of utilization review: preadmission certification and second opinions to verify medical necessity, verification of patient insurance, appropriate record keeping and patient classification, and the like. An important area to address is improper or incomplete medical record documentation and coding, which can result in delays and lost charges. For instance, failure of the medical staff to assign final diagnoses to the patient's medical record or to sign it can delay the timeliness of the billing submission process and hence the receipt of payment. Similarly, miscoding a diagnosis can also affect the funds the organization receives. Perspective 5.3 lists key reasons behind denied claims. The health care provider organization's bylaws should state the responsibility of physicians to fulfill these obligations.

Electronic Billing

Claims Scrubbing
The process of ensuring that billing claims contain all information required by an insurer before it will submit payment. Requirements include accurate patient demographics, consistency between coding and diagnoses, and preauthorization verification for the services provided. Good information systems can complete most of this work automatically and electronically.

Electronic billing is a process whereby bills are sent electronically to third parties through electronic data interfacing (EDI). This not only accelerates the transmission of bills but also provides an editing function (often called *claims scrubbing*) that reduces the number of processing errors and subsequent audits, ultimately decreasing turnaround time. Other related forms of technology can be used to enhance revenue performance (see Perspective 5.4).

Payment

Timely payment of a claim, especially if it is paid electronically, can speed up the cash flow payments. Electronic fund transfers going directly into designated bank accounts also provide a more secure and reliable process for hospitals to receive their cash. The major obstacle health care providers face is reconciling payments with the electronic remittance advice (ERA), which provides details on how the claims were paid by the third-party payor (i.e., insurer) or why they were denied, or both.

PERSPECTIVE 5.3 REASONS FOR DENIAL OF MEDICAL CLAIMS

Relative to the cost to process a clean electronic claim, it costs more to process a paper claim, and even more to process delayed claims on the back end after they have been previously denied. Claims denials also slow reimbursement, which can place stress on an organization's cash flow. (As a way to delay payment, insurers may provide only one denial reason at a time, rather than give all denial reasons at once.) Claims can be denied for a variety of reasons, including these:

- Policy number is incorrect (name and policy number do not match insurer files).

- Beneficiary is not covered by the insurer (for example, the insurance coverage has lapsed, or the patient is a dependent who is not a covered member on the policy).

- Provided service is deemed not reasonable nor medically necessary.

- Service provided is not a covered service under the patient's insurance policy.

- There has been duplicate billing.

- A procedure covered by a global payment is billed separately (unbundled services).

- Procedure code modifier is not provided.

- Diagnosis code does not match service provided.

- Procedure code does not match patient's gender, is inconsistent with the modifier used, or is inconsistent with the place of service.

- Diagnosis code is inconsistent with age, gender, procedure, and so forth.

Source: Adapted from M. Gamble, Top 21 reason codes for denied claims, *Becker Hospital Review*, July 31, 2012, www.beckershospitalreview.com/racs-/-icd-9-/-icd-10/top-21-reason-codes-for-denied-claims.html.

Key Point To achieve timely collection of billing, health care providers need to assess their management revenue cycle process, which includes the areas of scheduling, preregistration, charge capture, coding, electronic billing, and payment.

Collecting Cash Payments

Because health care providers depend primarily on third-party health plans to pay for patient bills, they constantly try to upgrade and improve their revenue cycle management processes to ensure timely and accurate cash collections. However, because more of the payment responsibility is now being shifted to patients through higher deductible health plans,

PERSPECTIVE 5.4 UPDATING EXISTING TECHNOLOGY TO IMPROVE THE PAYMENT PROCESS

Most health care systems continue to look for approaches to improve their collection of payments from third-party and individual payors. Sentara Healthcare in Norfolk, Virginia, an integrated delivery network with ten hospitals, records and evaluates how customer representatives respond to patient calls. Revenue cycle management personnel found that representatives were not responding completely to the customers' concerns, specifically with issues ranging from clinical effects of self-administered drugs to administrative questions related to authorizations, payment of bills, and financial assistance programs. Management decided to open the customer service center half an hour earlier and to use that time to train representatives on these issues. As a result, customer representatives began to emphasize a patient option to use the hospital's monthly automated payment system to pay bills, as opposed to sending in payments by mail. The representatives also negotiated payment terms with patients and helped them to apply for financial assistance. Management believes that addressing these issues during the training program contributed to a 37 percent increase in electronic payments from 2010 to 2011, which in turn resulted in a $2 million increase in revenues received through electronic payments.

Source: Adapted from K. Wagner, Leveraging existing technology to boost revenue cycle performance, *Healthcare Financial Management*, 2012;66(9):86–88.

health care providers also need to more proactively implement policies to obtain timely receipts for services from the patients. Cash payment should occur at the first encounter with a patient, especially for elective procedures and in cases where insurance coverage cannot be validated. For nonelective procedures and services for non-charity care cases, health care providers should be encouraged to develop programs to receive cash payment at the time of discharge. Accordingly, proper internal controls must be implemented to ensure accurate recording and depositing of cash payments. Finally, providers should use banking services to accept online credit card payments over the Internet and debit or credit card accounts for high-deductible health plans. By electronically accepting cash payments, health care providers can avoid the costs of billing and carrying accounts receivable. Health care providers can also employ other techniques to assist in collecting their payments, such as

• Decentralized collection centers and concentration banking

• Lockboxes

• Wire transfers

Decentralized Collection Centers and Concentration Banking

Decentralized collection centers and *concentration banking* allow health care providers to have payors send their payments to a nearby location (thus reducing *mail float*, the time spent in the mail before the payment reaches its destination). These collection centers deposit the payments they have received in the provider's local bank. Finally, the funds are transferred to a concentration bank, where the health care provider can draw on the cash for payments. This procedure is designed to help a health care provider reduce its mail and processing time, but there is a trade-off between the number of collection centers and the savings they provide versus the costs incurred to maintain accounts at a number of different financial institutions.

Lockboxes

Under the *lockbox* form of collection, a payor sends payments to a post office box located near a Federal Reserve bank or branch. The bank picks up the payments from the box and at various times during the day deposits these funds into the health care provider's account, processes the checks, and sends the facility a list of the payors and payments. Having the bank perform these duties enables the facility to reduce its mail and processing time. The decision to invest in the lockbox approach depends on whether the interest earned from the acceleration of funds exceeds the cost of having a lockbox. Lockboxes usually have a fixed fee and a variable rate calculated on a per check basis. An organization may be able to offset the costs of establishing a lockbox by freeing up internal staff who perform some of the functions that the bank will be taking over.

Lockbox
A post office box located near a Federal Reserve bank or branch that, for a fee, will pick up checks from the box and process them quickly.

Wire Transfers

Wire transfers eliminate mail and transit float. They are generally used in two ways: third parties electronically deposit payments into the health care organization's bank, and local banks serving parts of a multiprovider system electronically transfer cash from provider accounts at their local branches to the bank holding the system's corporate headquarters' account, from which all payments are disbursed. This minimizes the "excess cash" kept at subsidiaries and maximizes the amount at headquarters, which is responsible for investing all cash. However, this approach can be expensive because banks often charge two to four dollars per transfer. Nevertheless, one large central bank account may draw a better overall return than would several smaller accounts, and there is an increased likelihood that working capital funds would be available as needed, with less need to borrow. Related techniques are zero-balance accounts and sweep accounts, through which the bank automatically removes any excess cash from subsidiaries and places it in the account of the parent corporation.

Key Point Decentralized collection centers, concentration banking, lockboxes, and wire transfers are methods to reduce collection and transit float.

Investing Cash on a Short-Term Basis

After an organization has gone through the effort to collect its cash, it wants to ensure that the money is invested appropriately to generate a favorable return. Myriad short-term investment instruments exist, including treasury bills, certificates of deposit, commercial paper, and money market mutual funds. Some of the key attributes of these short-term investments are summarized in Exhibit 5.10.

Treasury Bills

Treasury bills (T-bills) are financial instruments purchased for a short term. Normally, they have maturities of thirteen, twenty-six, or fifty-two weeks and are sold in units of $100, with a minimum purchase of $100. Thus an investor can purchase $100, $1,000, $10,000, $15,000, $50,000, $100,000, $500,000, and up to $5 million of T-bills. Because they are issued by the government and are part of an active secondary market for buying and selling these securities, they are considered default-free and the most liquid short-term investment available. Instead of earning interest directly, T-bills are purchased at a discount and redeemed at face value when they mature. The discount represents the difference between the purchase price and the face value at time of maturity. Typically, the face value is presented on a $100 maturity value basis. If the discount price is $3, the purchase price is $97. Being virtually risk free and short term, T-bills offer low rates of return.

Negotiable Certificates of Deposit

Certificates of deposit (CDs) are issued by commercial banks as negotiable, interest-bearing, short-term certificates. In other words, when the deposit matures, the investor receives the interest earned plus the amount deposited. The maturities of CDs usually range from fourteen days to eighteen months. Small-value CDs are normally issued in $500 to $10,000 denomi-

EXHIBIT 5.10 KEY CHARACTERISTICS OF SELECTED SHORT-TERM INVESTMENTS

Investment	Denominations	Term	Where Purchased	Comments
Treasury bills	$100, $1,000, $10,000, $15,000, $50,000, $100,000, $500,000, and up to $5,000,000	Usually 13, 26, or 52 weeks	Banks, government	Most liquid and default free; purchased at a discount and redeemed at face value
Certificates of deposit (CDs)	Large: $100,000 to $1,000,000+ Small: $500 to $10,000	Usually 2 weeks to 18 months	Banks	Higher risk and higher yield than treasury bills; smaller amounts have lower returns than larger amounts
Commercial paper	$100,000+	1 to 270 days	Broker, dealer, or corporation	Higher risk and higher yield than CDs
Money market mutual funds	Varies; typically >$1,000	Varies (can be bought and sold on the market)	Mutual fund, broker, or bank	Highly liquid; higher risk and higher yield than commercial paper

nations. Large-value CDs are normally issued in $100,000 to $1 million denominations. Because of their size, large-value CDs earn a higher return than do small-value CDs. A *negotiable CD* is one that the investor may sell to someone else before maturity. *Nonnegotiable CDs* are offered in smaller denominations. CDs are not as liquid as T-bills and have a higher risk because they are issued by banks rather than the federal government. Because of this risk and illiquidity, investors demand a higher yield or return on CDs than they do on T-bills.

Commercial Paper

Commercial paper consists of negotiable promissory notes issued at a discount by large corporations (usually publicly traded) that need to raise internal capital. These instruments are issued for maturities of 1 to 270 days through a bank or a dealer that specializes in selling short-term securities. Commercial paper is sold in denominations of $100,000 or more. Because of the possibility of default from a major corporation, this security carries a higher credit risk than do T-bills or CDs and therefore requires a higher yield.

Money Market Mutual Funds

These funds, which require a minimum investment of $1,000, represent a pooling of investors' funds for the purchase of a diversified portfolio of short-term financial instruments, such as CDs, T-bills, and commercial paper. This pooling of funds allows small investors, such as rural health care facilities, to earn short-term money market rates on their investments. Furthermore, most money market funds offer an investor a high degree of liquidity by allowing withdrawals by check, telephone, and wire transfer.

 Key Point Some of the primary instruments for health care organizations to invest in on a short-term basis include treasury bills, certificates of deposit, commercial paper, and money market funds.

Forecasting Cash Surpluses and Deficits: The Cash Budget

To minimize costs and plan ahead to finance deficits and invest excess cash, a health care organization needs to clearly identify the timing of its cash inflows and outflows. The main vehicle for projecting cash inflows and outflows is a cash budget. Depending on the decision at hand, it may show inflows on a daily, weekly, monthly, quarterly, semiannual, annual, or multiyear basis. For instance, forecasts about weekly inflows and outflows are not needed for long-range planning, but monthly planning may require forecasting on a weekly or even daily basis. Much of the information for preparing the cash budget comes from the operating and capital budgets (discussed in Chapter Ten).

To illustrate cash inflows and outflows, a monthly cash budget for January through March 20X7 for Community Health Organization (CHO) is displayed in Exhibit 5.11.

Cash Inflows

Cash inflow estimates are generally derived from patient revenues; other operating revenues; proceeds from borrowing or stock issuances, or both

EXHIBIT 5.11 CASH BUDGET FOR COMMUNITY HEALTH ORGANIZATION FOR THREE MONTHS, BEGINNING JANUARY 20X7

Givens

1 Revenues:

Actual Patient Revenues, 20X6		Estimated Patient Revenues, 20X7	
October	$400,000	January	$500,000
November	$500,000	February	$600,000
December	$300,000	March	$700,000

2 Funds are received as follows: 50 percent within the month of service, 40 percent one month after service, and 10 percent two months after service.

3 "Other revenues" includes interest earned and are forecasted to be $44,000 in January, $55,000 in February, and $52,000 in March.

4 Cash outflows are forecasted to be $350,000, $450,000, $600,000, and $500,000 in January, February, March, and April, respectively.

5 "Cash outflows" are for the current month.

6 The ending cash balance for December was $50,000.

7 CHO desires a required cash balance of 40 percent of the following month's forecasted cash outflows.

CHO Cash Budget for the Quarter Ending March 31, 20X7

	Item	Formula	January	February	March	Total
	Cash inflows					
A	From October	Givens 1,2	$0	$0	$0	$0
B	From November	Givens 1,2	50,000	0	0	50,000
C	From December	Givens 1,2	120,000	30,000	0	150,000
D	From January	Givens 1,2	250,000	200,000	50,000	500,000
E	From February	Givens 1,2	0	300,000	240,000	540,000
F	From March	Givens 1,2	0	0	350,000	350,000
G	Other revenues	Given 3	44,000	55,000	52,000	151,000
H	Net cash inflows	Sum A:G	464,000	585,000	692,000	1,741,000
I	Forecasted cash outflows	Givens 4,5	350,000	450,000	600,000	1,400,000
J	**Monthly or quarterly net cash flow**	H − I	114,000	135,000	92,000	341,000
K	Beginning balance	a	50,000	180,000	240,000	50,000
L	**Cash before borrowing or investing**	J + K	164,000	315,000	332,000	391,000
M	Required cash balance	b	180,000	240,000	200,000	200,000
N	Surplus (deficit)	L − M	(16,000)	75,000	132,000	191,000
O	Investment of surplus in short-term investments	c	0	(75,000)	(132,000)	(207,000)
P	Short-term borrowing	d	16,000	0	0	16,000
Q	Ending cash balance	M + N + O + P	$180,000	$240,000	$200,000	$200,000

[a]January: Given 6: February/March: Row Q, previous month.
[b](Givens 4, 7) x (Row I), next month.
[c](− Row N), but only if there is a surplus.
[d](− Row N), but only if there is a deficit.

(for investor-owned organizations); and nonoperating contributions. To estimate cash receipts from patient revenues for the month, CHO needs to estimate the amounts of these revenues and when they will be received in cash. Assume that CHO forecasts the following revenues for 20X7, based on 20X6 data:

Actual Patient Revenues, 20X6		**Estimated Patient Revenues, 20X7**	
October	$400,000	January	$500,000
November	$500,000	February	$600,000
December	$300,000	March	$700,000

From its historical records, CHO estimates that it will collect 50 percent of revenues earned in the month of service, 40 percent the following month, and 10 percent two months after service has been delivered. All other revenues, such as contributions, appropriations, cash from sale of investments and used equipment, and interest income are expected to total $44,000, $55,000, and $52,000 in January, February, and March, respectively.

Based on this information, CHO can calculate cash inflows. For instance, February's cash inflows of $585,000 are composed of 50 percent of February's revenue ($600,000 × 0.50 = $300,000), 40 percent of January's revenue ($500,000 × 0.40 = $200,000), 10 percent of December's revenue ($300,000 × 0.10 = $30,000), plus the other revenues for February ($55,000), as given in Exhibit 5.11.

 Key Point The cash budget is the major budgetary tool for forecasting an organization's cash surplus and deficits over a given period of time.

Cash Outflows

CHO's cash outflows are estimated at $350,000, $450,000, $600,000, and $500,000 for January through April, respectively (Exhibit 5.11, Given 4). These outflows include such operating items as salaries and benefits, supplies, interest, capital expenditure outflows for equipment and land, and debt payments.

Ending Cash Balance

By subtracting cash outflows from net cash inflows, CHO can derive its monthly net cash flow. To this amount, it adds the beginning cash balance to calculate the cash available before borrowing or investing. For instance, in January there were net cash inflows of $464,000 and cash outflows of $350,000 that resulted in a $114,000 net cash inflow for the month (Exhibit 5.11, row J). When this is added to the $50,000 available at the beginning of the month (row K), CHO had $164,000 in cash before borrowing or investing (row L).

Although this number represents how much cash is available at the end of the month as a result of the normal cash flows during the month plus the beginning balance, many health care organizations are required to end a month (actually, begin the next month) with a certain minimum balance, called a *required cash balance*. When they are below this amount, they must borrow money, and when they are above, they invest the excess. In the case of CHO, the required cash balance is 40 percent of the next month's forecast cash outflows (row M, January, and row I, February: $180,000 / $450,000 = 0.40).

Here is an illustration of this process. CHO had $164,000 in January's cash balance before borrowing or investing (row L), but the required cash balance is $180,000 (0.40 × $450,000, February's cash outflows). Therefore, it must borrow $16,000 to make up the difference (row P). This results in an ending cash balance of $180,000 (row Q). If there had been a surplus, as in February (row N), CHO would have invested the excess funds (row O). Last, note that February's ending cash balance is higher than January's (row Q), $240,000 versus $180,000. This comes about because March's projected cash outflows are $600,000, whereas February's projected cash outflows are only $450,000 (row I), and 40 percent of the next month's projected cash outflows must be available at the end of each current month.

Required Cash Balance

The amount of cash an organization must have on hand at the end of the current period to ensure that it has enough cash to cover expected outflows during the next forecasting period.

Accounts Receivable Management

Accounts receivable, most of which is to be paid through third-party payors, constitutes approximately 75 percent of a health care provider's current assets. Unfortunately, having a large dollar amount tied up in accounts receivable means lost returns in other investment opportunities. Because third-party payors are volume purchasers of health care services, health care providers continuously face the problem of trying to control a largely external process in order to ensure the timely payment of accounts. Health care provider management does hold some degree of internal control with respect to processing payments. The earlier discussion introduced several ways to reduce float, including preadmission and admission screenings, computerized information systems, electronic billing, and billing and collection policies and procedures. These methods also reduce receivables because bringing cash in more quickly reduces the amount outstanding.

Methods to Monitor Accounts Receivable

Because most payments for services come well after the services have been provided, it is imperative that an organization closely monitor its outstanding balances. The tracking of outstanding accounts is often carried out through an analysis similar to that presented in Exhibit 5.12.

Net accounts receivable (row B) presents the total amount of receivables outstanding, both in total and by month. Thus, at the end of the first quarter, there are $6.4 million in receivables outstanding, of which $3.6 million are aged 1 to 30 days (row B), $2.0 million are aged 31 to 60 days, and $0.8 million are aged 61 to 90 days. For simplicity, assume that each month has thirty days and that all accounts are written off as bad debt after ninety days.

This information leads to an *aging schedule*, as shown in row C. Thus, at the end of the first quarter, of the $6.4 million in receivables outstanding, 56.3 percent was generated in the third and most recent month ($3.6M / $6.4M), 31.3 percent in the second month ($2.0M / $6.4M), and 12.5 percent in the first month ($0.8M / $6.4M). Row D in each quarter shows the revenues recorded during each of the three months of the quarter and for the quarter as a whole. Row E is the average daily patient revenue (Monthly Revenue / 30 Days, and Total Quarterly Revenue / 90 Days).

The information combined from rows A, B, and D yields two new measures: days in accounts receivable (row F) and receivables as a percentage of revenue (row G). Days in accounts receivable is calculated by dividing the net accounts receivable (row B) by the average daily patient revenue for the quarter (row E). For the first quarter, the average daily net revenue was $166,667 ($15.0M / 90 Days = $166,667 per Day), whereas the net accounts receivable is $6.4 million; therefore, the days in accounts receivable (row F) at the end of the quarter is 38.4 days ($6,400,000 / $166,667 = 38.4 Days). This same procedure can be applied to each month to show the number of days of outstanding receivables attributable to each month (using the quarter's average daily net revenue as the denominator).

The final item, receivables as a percentage of revenue (row G), is computed by dividing net accounts receivable (row B) for each thirty-day period by that month's net patient revenue (row D). For example, at the end of the first quarter, 60 percent of the third month's revenues ($3.6 / $6.0), 40 percent of the second month's revenues ($2.0 / $5.0), and 20 percent of the first month's revenues ($0.8 / $4.0) are all receivables out-

EXHIBIT 5.12 KEY MEASURES TO MONITOR ACCOUNTS RECEIVABLE

		Formula	Quarter 1 ($ in thousands)			
			Mar	Feb	Jan	Total
A	Days old at the end of the quarter[a]	Given	1–30	31–60	61–90	1–90
B	Net accounts receivable	Given	$3,600	$2,000	$800	$6,400
C	Aging schedule	(Row B) (month) / (row B) (total)	56.3%	31.3%	12.5%	
D	Net patient revenues	Given	$6,000	$5,000	$4,000	$15,000
E	Average daily patient revenue	(Row D) / No. of days in period (row A)	$200	$167	$133	$167
F	Days in accounts receivable	B / E				38.4
G	Receivables as a percentage of revenue	B / D	60%	40%	20%	

		Formula	Quarter 2 ($ in thousands)			
			Jun	May	Apr	Total
H	Days old at the end of the quarter[a]	Given	1–30	31–60	61–90	1–90
I	Net accounts receivable	Given	$6,900	$1,000	$200	$8,100
J	Aging schedule	(Row I) (month) / (row I) (total)	85.2%	12.3%	2.5%	
K	Net patient revenues	Given	$11,500	$2,500	$1,000	$15,000
L	Average daily patient revenue	(Row K) / No. of days in period (row H)	$383	$83	$33	$167
M	Days in accounts receivable	I / L				48.6
N	Receivables as a percentage of revenue	I / K	60%	40%	20%	

[a]For simplicity, each month is assumed to be 30 days.

Aging Schedule

A table that shows the percentage of receivables outstanding by the month they were incurred. This is often also called an *age trial balance*, or ATB.

standing (dollar figures expressed in millions). A similar analysis follows throughout for quarter 2 (rows H through N).

Receivables as a percentage of revenue is a better measure than days in accounts receivable to judge management's success in collecting revenues. In the example, it may appear as if collections are worsening because days in accounts receivable rose from 38.4 days for the first quarter to 48.6 days for the second quarter. However, receivables as a percentage of revenue shows that collections as a percentage of revenue for each thirty-day period remain the same for both quarters: 60 percent, 40 percent, and 20 percent. The reason for the discrepancy is that during the first quarter the highest percentage of revenues came in the early months, whereas in the second quarter most of the patient revenues occurred in the last month. Thus, the reason that the days in accounts receivable went up is not because collection efforts have changed but rather because the timing of the revenues varied (total revenues are $15 million in each quarter). Because patient revenues are higher in the earlier months of the first quarter, fewer receivables are outstanding later in the quarter. In turn, this outcome reduces the days in accounts receivable to 38.4 days, as well as reducing the percentage of older receivables outstanding.

 Key Point A common mistake is to infer that because days in accounts receivable is decreasing, collections are improving. This is not necessarily the case.

Methods to Finance Accounts Receivable

In addition to trying to improve its cash and receivables collections, an organization has two other options to bring funds in to meet cash needs: selling its accounts receivable, called *factoring*, and using receivables as collateral.

 Key Point Factoring and using receivables as collateral are two ways to receive cash advances from outstanding accounts receivable.

Factoring

Factoring is the selling of accounts receivable, usually to a bank, at a discount. There are two main reasons why a health care organization would decide to factor its accounts: it needs the cash currently tied up in receivables and cannot afford to wait to collect that money from patients and third parties, or it predicts that the benefits of selling the receivables at a discount will outweigh the possible returns it would receive by holding onto the accounts and trying to manage the collections process.

Typical discounts involved in factoring transactions range from 5 to 10 percent. In addition, the financing institution may impose a factoring fee equal to 15 to 20 percent of the value of the receivables. Under this arrangement, the financing institution purchasing the receivables takes on both control over the collection of the receivables and the associated risk. The more risky the collection of the accounts receivable, the higher the discount demanded by the bank and the higher the fees.

It is important to recognize that when a health care organization sells its receivables, another institution takes over the collections process. The potential ill will that may be generated as this other institution tries to collect these funds should receive serious consideration before factoring is undertaken. By law, Medicaid accounts receivable cannot be factored.

Pledging Receivables as Collateral

As noted earlier, health care organizations can negotiate a line of credit with a financial institution to cover temporary cash shortfalls. In such instances, the amount of receivables outstanding can be used as *collateral*. The cost of a line of credit is typically one to two percentage points above the prime rate, unless an organization has an excellent credit history, in which case it can negotiate for the prime rate or even slightly below it.

Methods to Monitor Revenue Cycle Performance

The previously mentioned accounts receivable measurements are tailored to senior management, who are interested in highly aggregated numbers. However, personnel involved in the day-to-day operation and evaluation of revenue cycle management, such as the director of patient financial services and service-line managing directors, may have an interest in more detailed measures related to the revenue cycle. *Cost to collect* is viewed by these managers as a key revenue cycle performance indicator because it measures the costs of all the departments involved in managing the revenue cycle processes. The majority of these costs relate to staff (salary, training, and benefits), information technology (hardware, software, and support), and telecommunications (a call center and long distance service). These operating costs are measured as a percentage of the actual cash collected during a given period (monthly, quarterly, or annually).

Exhibit 5.13 lists the key components of the cost to collect in two parts: unadjusted and adjusted. Net patient revenues (row A) presents the total amount of net revenues for the year, while revenue collected as cash during

Factoring
Selling accounts receivable at a discount, usually to a financial institution. The latter then assumes the responsibility of trying to collect on the outstanding payment obligations.

EXHIBIT 5.13 COST-TO-COLLECT METHOD TO MONITOR REVENUE CYCLE MANAGEMENT

	Cost to Collect Accounts Receivable: Unadjusted	Formula	($ in millions)
A	Net patient revenues	Given	$100
B	Cash collections	Given	$90
C	Cash as percentage of net patient revenues	B / A	90.0%
D	Costs incurred in collection	Given	$3
E	Cost-to-collect ratio	D / B	3.3%
	Cost to Collect Accounts Receivable: Adjusted for Human Intervention		
F	Cash collections incurring just EDI costs	Given	$45
G	Cash collections incurring human intervention	Given	$45
H	Costs incurred in collection	Given	$3
I	Less EDI costs	Given	($0.3)
J	Manual costs incurred in collection	H − I	$2.7
K	Cost to collect for high-cost claims	J / G	6.0%
L	Health care industry cost-to-collect standard	Given	2.0%

Source: Adapted and modified from Understanding your true cost to collect, *Healthcare Financial Management*, 2006;60(1, suppl 1–7).

Collateral

A tangible asset that is pledged as a promise to repay a loan. If the loan is not paid, the lending institution may, as a legal recourse, seize the pledged asset.

the year is presented in row B. Thus, 90 percent (row C, $90M / $100M) of the net patient revenues is collected as cash during the year. This health care provider incurred $3 million (row D) in operating costs to manage the revenue cycle processes; hence, the provider had a cost-to-collect ratio of 3.3 percent (row E, $3M / $90M). A reference statistic, the hospital industry's cost-to-collect benchmark, provided in row L, is 2 percent. Part of the reason this provider has a cost-to-collect ratio higher than the industry standard may be longer duration of claims. For example, this provider may have a large proportion of claims outstanding for more than 120 days; these require a heavier investment of resources to track and collect than do claims outstanding for 60 days. In addition, this provider may have fewer of the cleaner and highly accurate claims that consume less resource time to collect. Finally, this provider may need to invest in more up-front resources, both people and technology, to improve its efficiency in the revenue cycle process and to submit claims more cleanly, which in turn would lead to more efficient cash collections.

Health care providers should also conduct a detailed analysis of the cost-to-collect ratio by separating out clean claims or claims collected using only electronic services without human intervention. For example, in the lower half of Exhibit 5.13, row F shows the cash collected from claims needing only EDI as $45 million; whereas row G presents the balance of cash collections from row B that involved human intervention as also $45 million. The total cost to collect is $3 million (row H), but after excluding the EDI costs of $300,000 (row I), the revised cost to collect involving human intervention is $2.7 million (row J). The adjusted cost to collect then becomes 6 percent (row K), which is the $2.7 million in row J divided by $45 million from row G. This presents a much different picture, that of the high cost to collect claims needing human intervention.

The cost to collect should be trended over time as well as compared with an industry benchmark, which is typically around 2 percent to 3 percent. If the cost to collect is rising, potential reasons may be higher staff turnover; higher information technology costs in hardware, software, and personnel or higher outsourcing costs for billing or collections, or both; or other inefficiencies in the revenue cycle processes. Other key revenue cycle metrics are presented in Perspective 5.5.

Fraud and Abuse

Hospitals and other health care organizations must comply with numerous laws and restrictions established by regulation that address areas such as patient billing, cost reporting, physician transactions, and occupational health and safety. Given the rise in health care fraud and abuse, federal and state governments have a strong incentive to reduce any abusive practices in patient billing.

Efforts to eradicate fraud and abuse have significantly changed since the inception of the Medicare and Medicaid programs in 1965.[1] The first real federal effort was the Medicare-Medicaid Anti-Fraud and Abuse Amendments of 1977, which established Medicaid fraud control units. The next important initiative came when the False Claims Act was amended in the mid-1980s to strengthen the government's ability to identify and recover improper Medicare payments, providing for penalties up to $10,000 for false claims, along with treble damages. So even when the claims are not large individually, the penalties are. In 1996, health care fraud became a criminal activity above just making false claims, and the Health Care Fraud and Abuse Control Program was enacted as part of the antifraud

PERSPECTIVE 5.5   KEY REVENUE CYCLE AND ACCOUNTS RECEIVABLE METRICS

Key Revenue Cycle Performance Area	Relevant Metrics
Scheduling/preregistration	Physician referral compliance Percentage of preregistered accounts (inpatient and outpatient)
Registration	Percentage of insurance cards copied and on file Turnaround time until receipt of precertification from insurance company Inpatient admissions error rate Outpatient registration error rate Percentage of copays collected Cash receipts as a percentage of net revenues
Charge capture	Accuracy of recording billable supplies

Coding	Percentage of correct procedure codes
	Percentage of correct diagnostic codes
	Discharged not final billed (DNFB)
	    Accounts awaiting coding
	    Accounts awaiting dictation
	Proper coding of *present on admission* (POA) complications
	Case mix index based on submitted MS-DRGs

Electronic billing	Percentage of clean claims submitted Lag days from date of service until posting date
Payment	Average days in accounts receivable Percentage accounts receivable over 90 days Percentage accounts receivable over 120 days Percentage accounts receivable over 6 months (probably uncollectible accounts) Percentage of unpaid accounts Bad debt expense as a percentage of total gross revenues

Source: Adapted from J. Clark, Strengthening the revenue cycle: a 4-step method for optimizing payment, *Healthcare Financial Management*, 2008;62(10):44–46.

provisions of the Health Insurance Portability and Accountability Act (HIPAA). Now fraud carries a possible ten-year prison sentence along with the fines and penalties.

As discussed in Chapter One, recovery audit contractors (RACs) have been operating since 2003 to review, audit, and recover improper Medicare payments. Since they are paid on a contingency fee basis related to the overpayments they collect, this is a cost-effective program for CMS.

The Deficit Reduction Act of 2005 established the Medicaid Integrity Program, which is a federal effort to further address fraud and abuse in Medicaid. The government has made the issue of fraud and abuse a component of health care reform, and in May 2009 the Health Care Fraud Prevention and Enforcement Action Team was created. This group is an interagency task force, with members drawn from the Departments of Justice and Health and Human Services (HHS).

The Affordable Care Act provides CMS with more authority to screen providers and to refuse to do business with questionable ones. In addition, CMS has formed the Center for Program Integrity, which has helped to unify the various programs.

In fiscal year 2011, the combined efforts of CMS, the Department of Justice, and the HHS Office of Inspector General resulted in criminal charges for health care fraud against 1,430 defendants, resulting in 743 criminal convictions; initiated 977 new investigations of civil health care fraud; and recovered $4.1 billion. CMS also revoked the Medicare billing privileges of 4,850 providers and suppliers and deactivated an additional 56,733 billing numbers.

CMS is using what it refers to as the *twin pillar* approach, designed to make it easier for honest providers to get payment but more difficult for fraudulent ones. The twin pillars focus on provider payment and provider enrollment, using a claims-based predictive model and a provider screening system. These advanced analytical techniques include using algorithms and historical data to flag suspicious claims. This automatic screening process develops an individual risk score for each provider, which is not unlike an individual's credit score.

In addition, in late July 2012 the federal government formed the National Fraud Prevention Partnership, a voluntary public-private partnership involving federal and state governments, private insurance companies, and health care antifraud groups. Its goal is to prevent fraud before it occurs by sharing information on fraud schemes, utilized billing codes, and geographical fraud hotspots.[2]

To ensure compliance with laws and regulations, health care providers need to implement and maintain an effective corporate compliance plan. The plan should ensure that the corporate policies, practices, and culture promote the understanding of and adherence to appropriate legal requirements. The HHS Office of Inspector General (OIG) publishes model compliance guidance for all types of providers, from hospitals to physicians to medical billing companies. This guidance includes a list of the major types of fraud that can occur in that provider's setting. In addition, the OIG publishes a workplan each year (it can be accessed at oig.hhs.gov/reports-and-publications/archives/workplan).[3]

Although corporate compliance activities are expensive, they are nevertheless important to protect providers from actions against them that could prove to be even more costly.

Improving Revenue Cycle Processes

As health care reform has led to the imperative to do more with less, with an even greater emphasis on improved quality, the efficiency and effectiveness of the revenue cycle management process have become increasingly important. A more collaborative, patient-focused revenue cycle process will be necessary to address changes that continue to occur in the areas of patient access, insurance, and payment. This will become particularly

PERSPECTIVE 5.6 LEAN SIGMA IMPLEMENTATION LEADS TO REVENUE CYCLE IMPROVEMENTS

Bethesda Memorial Hospital in Boynton Beach, Florida, believes that its Lean Sigma efforts are paying off. In the two years that it has been using the techniques it has demonstrated

- Morale changes in the revenue cycle culture: staff work together to identify the root causes of issues and feel empowered to make changes

- A reduction, as a result of process standardization, in the *discharged but not final billed* rate, so that it is now below the benchmark standard

- Improved efficiency in coding, from using a worksheet to help coders organize notes when reviewing charts

- Streamlined processes for scheduling and registration, which have also shortened wait times and thus improved patient satisfaction

- Improved cash flow, as a result of standardization, transparency in metrics, and quicker billing

- A significant improvement in the clean claim rate

- Productivity increases, as a result of removing workflow bottlenecks and redundancies

Source: Adapted from J. DeGaspari, HFMA live: using lean concepts to improve revenue cycle, *Healthcare Informatics*, June 26, 2012. www.healthcare-informatics.com/blogs/john-degaspari/hfma-live-using-lean-concepts-improve-revenue-cycle.

important as hospitals continue to merge with or acquire other providers, and as accountable care organizations expand their role in the industry.

Revenue cycle improvement consumes significant effort and resources and is not merely a matter of improving upon the structure already in place. Providers must address issues being brought forth by increased regulatory oversight, including new rules and mandates; be able to collect complete and accurate information to meet elevated reporting standards; meet the challenges of preparing for ICD-10; and prepare for the inevitable RAC audits. And they must do all this while facing downward pressures in third-party reimbursements.

Many hospitals have turned to using Lean Six Sigma (also called Lean Sigma) disciplines to foster continuous improvement in their revenue cycle processes (see Perspective 5.6). Lean Sigma uses the concepts found in Six Sigma; however, it has the advantage of being a quicker process with less need for extensive training, implementation, and maintenance. But, like Six Sigma, it requires a culture change to ensure sustainable change and business outcomes. It also requires dedicated data collection efforts, decision support, and monitoring.

Summary

Working capital refers to the current assets and current liabilities of a health care organization. Working capital is important because it turns the capacity of an organization (its long-term assets) into services and revenues. All health care organizations must have sufficient working capital available at appropriate times to meet day-to-day needs.

The management of working capital involves managing the working capital cycle: (1) obtaining cash, (2) purchasing resources and paying bills, (3) delivering services, and (4) billing and collecting for services rendered. There are two components of a working capital management strategy: asset mix and financing mix. Asset mix is the amount of working capital the organization keeps on hand relative to its potential working capital obligations, whereas financing mix refers to how the organization chooses to finance its working capital needs. To determine its desired level of working capital, a health care facility must evaluate the risk versus return trade-off between overinvestment and underinvestment in working capital. A conservative approach with a higher investment in working capital increases an organization's liquidity but does so at the expense of lower returns. An aggressive approach with less investment in working capital decreases liquidity but frees funds to invest in the fixed assets that have higher returns. The decision to select either option or some comfortable medium depends on the health care provider's environment, financial condition, and risk tolerance.

A major component of current assets is cash and cash equivalents. There are three reasons to hold cash: for daily operations purposes, precautionary purposes, and speculative purposes. The sources of temporary cash are bank loans, trade credit and billing, collections, and disbursement policies and procedures. Types of bank loans include normal and revolving lines of credit and transaction notes. Lines of credit are usually preestablished and allow a health care organization to borrow money in a reasonably expeditious manner. Transaction notes are short-term, unsecured loans made for specific purposes, such as the purchase of supplies. Both of these borrowing methods may involve either a commitment fee or compensating balance.

A second important source of temporary cash is trade credit, which does not actually bring in cash but instead slows its outflow. Although not commonly thought of in this way, it is a loan by a vendor to the health care organization, and vendors often provide discounts for early payment. It is normally beneficial for a health care organization to take the discount. To determine the approximate interest rate, see formula 1 below. For the formula for the effective interest rate, see formula 2 below.

$$\text{Approximate Interest Rate} = \text{Discount \%} / (1 - \text{Discount \%}) \times (365 / \text{Net Period}) \qquad (1)$$

$$\text{Effective Interest Rate} = \frac{(\text{Interest Expense on Amount Borrowed} + \text{Total Fees})}{(\text{Amount Borrowed} - \text{Compensating Balance})} \qquad (2)$$

Because the approximate interest rate declines the longer the payment is delayed, a prudent policy is to make the payment as close to the last day of the discount period as is operationally feasible or, if the discount is not taken, on the last day of the net period. Although interest costs decrease as the number of days for which the bill is not paid increases, at a certain point new costs are encountered. These costs include late fees, loss of discounts in the future, loss of priority status with this supplier, and so forth.

To enhance the timely and accurate collection of receivables, health care organizations implement sophisticated revenue cycle management techniques. The six key elements of this process are scheduling or preregistration to gather as much information as possible in preparation for the patient's upcoming visit; registration of the patient on arrival to validate insurance information and review payment policies; systematic charge capture to ensure all services provided and supplies consumed have been recorded; coding audits to reconcile and maximize individual charges with services; electronic billing to submit invoice information in automated, standardized formats; and payment follow-up to track down and recover lost charges. The final step in the process underlines the need to use various methods to monitor revenue cycle management performance, including measurement of days in accounts receivable and calculating cost-to-collect ratios, among others.

There are several well-used techniques to reduce *collection float* (the time between the issuance of a bill and the monies being available for use) and *transit float* (the time it takes a check to clear the banking system). These techniques include using decentralized collection centers, lock-boxes, and electronic deposit of funds. The tools to reduce disbursement float include taking suppliers' discounts and using remote disbursement accounts.

A major function of cash management is to ensure that any excess cash is earning a reasonable return at an acceptable level of risk. There are four primary vehicles for short-term investment of cash: treasury bills, certificates of deposit, commercial paper, and money market mutual funds. These financial vehicles typically differ in degrees of risk, return, and initial outlay.

A well-managed cash strategy is based on accurate forecasting of cash flow. The principal tool for this is the cash budget. A cash budget should forecast not only cash inflows and outflows but also when excess cash will become available or when cash deficiencies that necessitate borrowing will occur.

In addition to managing cash, good working capital management involves managing accounts receivable. Most of the methods used to decrease accounts receivable are the same methods discussed under ways to speed up the inflows of cash. Managing receivables is based on good record keeping and periodic review. There are three main tools used to monitor receivables: creating an aging schedule, monitoring days in accounts receivable, and monitoring receivables as a percentage of revenues. Although days in accounts receivable is probably the most used ratio for monitoring receivables, it may be overly sensitive to the timing of revenues. Therefore receivables as a percentage of revenues is used to overcome this problem. Organizations can also improve their bottom line simply by keeping a well-trained staff, implementing good information systems, and maintaining good relations with payors. Finally, health care organizations need to develop a compliance program to ensure that their payroll, billing, and other financial transactions comply with governmental regulations.

Key Terms

a.	Aging schedule	l.	Liquidity
b.	Approximate interest rate	m.	Lockbox
c.	Asset mix	n.	Net working capital
d.	Claims scrubbing	o.	Normal line of credit
e.	Collateral	p.	Required cash balance
f.	Commitment fee	q.	Revenue cycle management
g.	Compensating balance	r.	Revolving line of credit
h.	Effective interest rate	s.	Trade credit
i.	Factoring	t.	Trade payables
j.	Financing mix	u.	Transaction note
k.	Health Insurance Portability and Accountability Act (HIPAA)	v.	Working capital
		w.	Working capital strategy

Key Equations

- Approximate interest rate:

$$\text{Approximate Interest Rate} = \text{Discount \%}/(1-\text{Discount \%}) \times (365/\text{Net Period})$$

- Effective interest rate:

$$2\%/(1-2\%) \times (365/20)$$

$$\text{Effective Interest Rate} = \frac{(\text{Interest Expense on Amount Borrowed} + \text{Total Fees})}{(\text{Amount Borrowed} - \text{Compensating Balance})}$$

REVIEW QUESTIONS AND PROBLEMS

1. **Definitions**. Define the key terms listed previously.
2. **Working capital**. What is the function of working capital?
3. **Working capital cycle**. In terms of cash flow, what are the stages of the working capital cycle?

4. **Working capital management strategy**. Describe the two components of a working capital management strategy.

5. **Asset mix strategies**. Compare aggressive and conservative asset mix strategies. The comparison should address goals, liquidity, and risk.

6. **Borrowing**. What is the difference between temporary and permanent working capital needs? What is the general rule about when to borrow long term or short term?

7. **Borrowing**. In terms of risk and return (profit), compare the advantages and disadvantages of both short- and long-term borrowing to meet working capital needs.

8. **Cash**. State the three reasons why a health care facility holds cash.

9. **Cash**. What are the main sources of temporary cash?

10. **Loans**. What is an unsecured loan?

11. **Loans**. What are the two types of unsecured bank loans? Describe each one.

12. **Compensating balance**. How do compensating balances affect the "true" interest rate the borrower pays?

13. **Discounts**. What does "1.5/15 net 25" mean?

14. **Discounts**. What is the formula to determine the approximate annual interest cost for not taking a discount? When should discounts be taken?

15. **Revenue cycle management**. What are the objectives of billing, credit, and collections policies?

16. **Revenue cycle management**. Why is preregistration important in the revenue cycle management process?

17. **Revenue cycle management**. What is the major obstacle that health care providers face in receiving their payments electronically?

18. **Revenue cycle management**. Identify two problems that can delay the billing process.

19. **Billing**. In the hospital's billing process, why is medical records a critical department?

20. **Revenue cycle management**. As more health care costs are shifted to the patient through high-deductible health plans, what policy can a health care provider implement to ensure timely payment for elective surgery procedures?

21. **Lockboxes**. Describe the lockbox technique for managing collection float.

22. **Revenue cycle management**. What is the critical step in capturing charges and identifying billing items?

23. **Investments**. Identify the alternatives for investing cash on a short-term basis, and discuss the general characteristics of each alternative.

24. **Accounts receivable**. List three ways to measure accounts receivable performance.

25. **Accounts receivable.** Two methods to monitor accounts receivable are as a percentage of net patient revenues and as days in accounts receivable. What factor can cause the former to be a better measure than the latter with regard to collections activities?

26. **Accounts receivable.** Identify and define two methods to finance accounts receivable.

27. **Trade credit discount.** Compute the approximate annual interest cost of not taking a discount, using each of the following scenarios. What conclusion can be drawn from the calculations?

 if pay in 10 days → 2% discount, if not one in 20 days full "

 a. 2/10 net 20.

 b. 2/10 net 30.

 c. 2/10 net 40.

 d. 2/10 net 50.

 e. 2/10 net 60.

28. **Trade credit discount.** Compute the approximate annual interest cost of not taking a discount using the following scenarios. What conclusion can be drawn from the calculations?

 a. 1/15 net 20.

 b. 1/15 net 30.

 c. 1/15 net 40.

 d. 1/15 net 50.

 e. 1/15 net 60.

29. **Trade credit discount.** Compute the approximate annual interest cost of not taking a discount using the following scenarios. What conclusion can be drawn from the calculations?

 a. 2/5 net 30.

 b. 2/10 net 30.

 c. 2/15 net 30.

 d. 2/20 net 30.

30. **Trade credit discount.** Compute the approximate annual interest cost of not taking a discount using the following scenarios. What conclusion can be drawn from the calculations?

 a. 1/5 net 30.

 b. 1/10 net 30.

 c. 1/15 net 30.

 d. 1/20 net 30.

31. **Trade credit discount.** Compute the approximate annual interest cost of not taking a discount using the following scenarios. What conclusion can be drawn from the calculations?

   a. 1/15 net 30.

   b. 2/15 net 30.

   c. 3/15 net 30.

   d. 4/15 net 30

32. **Trade credit discount.** Compute the approximate annual interest cost of not taking a discount using the following scenarios. What conclusion can be drawn from the calculations?

   a. 1/10 net 30.

   b. 2/10 net 30.

   c. 3/10 net 30.

   d. 4/10 net 30.

33. **Accounts receivable management.** Assume there are two physician groups, Lower Merion Physician Group and Penncrest Medical Practice, and both groups have contracts with two major health plans.

   a. Use the information that follows to compute Lower Merion's days in accounts receivable, aging schedule, and accounts receivable as a percentage of net patient revenues for Health Plan A and for Health Plan B for quarter 1, 20X2. Compare the two health plans to determine which plan is a faster payor. (*Hint*: For simplicity, assume that each month is thirty days. Dollar figures are expressed in thousands.)

Health Plan A, Quarter 1 20X2	Mar	Feb	Jan	Quarter
Days outstanding	1–30	31–60	61–90	1–90
Net accounts receivable	$2,520	$600	$280	$3,400
Net patient revenues	$6,300	$3,000	$700	$10,000
Health Plan B, Quarter 1 20X2	Mar	Feb	Jan	Quarter
Days outstanding	1–30	31–60	61–90	1–90
Net accounts receivable	$1,680	$600	$1,120	$3,400
Net patient revenues	$4,200	$3,000	$2,800	$10,000

   b. Use the information below to compute Penncrest's days in accounts receivable, aging schedule, and accounts receivable as a percentage of net patient revenues for Health Plan A and for Health Plan B for quarter 1, 20X2. Compare the two health plans to determine which plan is a faster payor. (*Hint*: For simplicity, assume that each month is thirty days. Dollar figures are expressed in thousands.)

Health Plan A, Quarter 1 20X2	Mar	Feb	Jan	Quarter
Days outstanding	1–30	31–60	61–90	1–90
Net accounts receivable	$4,500	$3,000	$1,500	$9,000
Net patient revenues	$8,000	$5,000	$2,000	$15,000
Health Plan B, Quarter 1 20X2	Mar	Feb	Jan	Quarter
Days outstanding	1–30	31–60	61–90	1–90
Net accounts receivable	$7,500	$1,000	$500	$9,000
Net patient revenues	$10,000	$3,000	$2,000	$15,000

34. **Accounts receivable management.** Given the information below, compute the days in accounts receivable, aging schedule, and accounts receivable as a percentage of net patient revenues for quarter 1 and quarter 2, 20X1. Compare the two quarters to determine if the organization's collection procedure is improving. (*Hint*: For simplicity, assume that each month is thirty days. Dollar figures are expressed in thousands.)

Quarter 1, 20X1	Sep	Aug	Jul	Quarter
Days outstanding	1–30	31–60	61–90	1–90
Net accounts receivable	$5,000	$3,000	$12,000	$20,000
Net patient revenues	$12,000	$6,000	$20,000	$38,000
Quarter 2, 20X1	Dec	Nov	Oct	Quarter
Days outstanding	1–30	31–60	61–90	1–90
Net accounts receivable	$13,000	$1,000	$6,000	$20,000
Net patient revenues	$20,000	$6,000	$12,000	$38,000

35. **Accounts receivable management.** Given the information below, compute the days in accounts receivable, aging schedule, and accounts receivable as a percentage of net patient revenues for quarter 1 and quarter 2, 20X1. Compare the two quarters to determine if the organization's collection procedure is improving. (*Hint*: For simplicity, assume that each month is thirty days. Dollar figures are expressed in thousands.)

Quarter 1, 20X1	Sep	Aug	Jul	Quarter
Days outstanding	1–30	31–60	61–90	1–90
Net accounts receivable	$500	$800	$3,700	$5,000
Net patient revenues	$1,000	$5,000	$9,000	$15,000
Quarter 2, 20X1	Dec	Nov	Oct	Quarter
Days outstanding	1–30	31–60	61–90	1–90
Net accounts receivable	$3,800	$800	$400	$5,000
Net patient revenues	$4,000	$5,000	$6,000	$15,000

36. **Accounts receivable management**. Given the information below, compute the days in accounts receivable, aging schedule, and accounts receivable as a percentage of net patient revenues for quarter 1 and quarter 2 of fiscal year 20X2, which runs from October 20X1 through September 20X2. Compare the two quarters to determine if the organization's collection procedure is improving. (*Hint*: For simplicity, assume that each month is thirty days. Dollar figures are expressed in thousands.)

Quarter 1, 20X1	Dec	Nov	Oct	Quarter
Days outstanding	1–30	31–60	61–90	1–90
Net accounts receivable	$1,000	$4,600	$14,000	$19,600
Net patient revenues	$4,000	$20,000	$36,000	$60,000
Quarter 2, 20X2	Mar	Feb	Jan	Quarter
Days outstanding	1–30	31–60	61–90	1–90
Net accounts receivable	$14,000	$4,600	$1,000	$19,600
Net patient revenues	$36,000	$20,000	$4,000	$60,000

37. **Compensating balance**. On January 2, 20X1, Uptown Hospital established a line of credit with First Union National Bank. The terms of the line of credit called for a $400,000 maximum loan with an interest rate of 3 percent. The compensating balance requirement is 5 percent of the total line of credit (with no additional fees charged).

   a. What would be the effective interest rate for Uptown Hospital if 50 percent of the total amount were used during the year?

   b. What would be the effective interest rate if only 25 percent of the total loan were used during the year?

   c. How would the answer to question a change if the additional fees were $500?

   d. How would the answer to question b change if the additional fees were $1,000?

38. **Compensating balance**. Tuckhoe Hospital wishes to establish a line of credit with a bank. The first bank's terms call for a $600,000 maximum loan with an interest rate of 3 percent and a $2,000 fee. The second bank, for the same line of credit, charges an interest rate of 4 percent but no fee. The compensating balance requirement is 5 percent of the total line of credit for either bank.

   a. What would be the effective interest rate for Tuckhoe Hospital from the first bank if 50 percent of the total amount were used during the year?

   b. What would be the effective interest rate for Tuckhoe Hospital from the first bank if 25 percent of the total amount were used during the year?

   c. What would be the effective interest rate for Tuckhoe Hospital from the second bank if 50 percent of the total amount were used during the year?

    d. What would be the effective interest rate for Tuckhoe Hospital from the second bank if 25 percent of the total amount were used during the year?

    e. Which bank would be the better choice for Tuckhoe Hospital?

39. **Cash budget.** Jim Zeeman Clinic provided the financial information in Exhibit 5.14. Prepare a cash budget for the clinic for the quarter ending March 20X1.

EXHIBIT 5.14　JIM ZEEMAN CLINIC

Givens

Revenues and Expenses

	Patient Revenues, 20X0			Estimated Patient Revenues, 20X1	
Given 1	October	$4,000,000	**Given 2**	January	$4,400,000
	November	$4,200,000		February	$4,600,000
	December	$4,400,000		March	$4,800,000

	Other Revenues, 20X1			Estimated Cash Outflows, 20X1[a]	
Given 3	January	$78,000	**Given 4**	January	$3,000,000
	February	$120,000		February	$3,200,000
	March	$200,000		March	$3,400,000
				April	$3,000,000

	Receipt of Payment for Patient Revenues and Services			Ending Cash Balances	
Given 5	Current month of service	60%	**Given 6**	December 20X0	$800,000
	1st month of prior service	30%		[b]	40%
	2nd month of prior service	10%			
	3rd+ months of prior service	0%			

[a]Cash outflows for the current month.
[b]The ending balance for each month as a percentage of the estimated cash outflows for the next month.

EXHIBIT 5.15 IOWA IMAGING CENTER

Givens

Revenues and Expenses

	Patient Revenues, 20X0			Estimated Patient Revenues, 20X1	
Given 1	October	$4,000,000	**Given 2**	January	$4,300,000
	November	$4,200,000		February	$4,350,000
	December	$4,300,000		March	$4,400,000

	Other Revenues, 20X1			Estimated Cash Outflows, 20X1[a]	
Given 3	January	$90,000	**Given 4**	January	$4,250,000
	February	$120,000		February	$4,300,000
	March	$140,000		March	$4,350,000
				April	$4,400,000

	Receipt of Payment for Patient Revenues and Services			Ending Cash Balances	
Given 5	Current month of service	60%	**Given 6**	December 20X0	$700,000
	1st month of prior service	30%		[b]	40%
	2nd month of prior service	10%			
	3rd+ month of prior service	0%			

[a]Cash outflows for the current month.
[b]The ending balance for each month as a percentage of the estimated cash outflows for the next month.

40. **Cash budget**. Iowa Imaging Center provided the financial information in Exhibit 5.15. Prepare a cash budget for the center for the quarter ending March 20X1.

41. **Cash budget**. Martha Zeeman Clinic provided the financial information in Exhibit 5.16. Prepare a cash budget for the clinic for the quarter ending March 20X1.

42. **Cash budget**. Rose Valley Rehab Facility provided the financial information in Exhibit 5.17. Prepare a cash budget for the facility for the quarter ending March 20X1.

EXHIBIT 5.16 MARTHA ZEEMAN CLINIC

Givens

Revenues

Patient Revenues, 20X0		Patient Revenues, 20X0		Estimated Patient Revenues, 20X1	
July	$4,500,000	October	$4,420,000	January	$4,600,000
August	$4,350,000	November	$4,210,000	February	$4,350,000
September	$4,530,000	December	$4,800,000	March	$4,220,000

Other Revenues, 20X1		Receipt of Payment for Patient Services / Revenues	
January	$98,000	Current month of service	45%
February	$130,000	1st month of prior service	25%
March	$125,000	2nd month of prior service	10%
		3–6 months of prior service	5%

Expenses[a]

Supplies Purchases, 20X0		Estimated Supplies Purchases, 20X1		Other Estimated Expenses, 20X1[a]			
					Nursing	Admin.	Other
October	$800,000	January	$1,000,000	January	$2,700,000	$80,000	$245,000
November	$1,000,000	February	$1,200,000	February	$2,750,000	$80,000	$335,000
December	$1,600,000	March	$1,400,000	March	$2,700,000	$80,000	$275,000
		April	$1,000,000	April	$2,450,000	$80,000	$205,000

Timing of Cash Payment for Supplies Purchases		Ending Cash Balances	
0%	Month purchased	December, 20X0	$1,800,000
60%	+1 month	[b]	50%
35%	+2 months		
5%	+3 months		

[a]All estimated expenses are cash outflows for the given month.
[b]The ending balance for each month as a percentage of the estimated cash outflows for the next month.

EXHIBIT 5.17 ROSE VALLEY REHAB FACILITY

Givens

Revenues					
Patient Revenues, 20X0		**Patient Revenues, 20X0**		**Estimated Patient Revenues, 20X1**	
July	$5,200,000	October	$5,500,000	January	$5,600,000
August	$5,400,000	November	$5,550,000	February	$5,500,000
September	$5,500,000	December	$5,600,000	March	$5,500,000

Other Revenues, 20X1		Receipt of Payment for Patient Services / Revenues	
January	$900,000	Current month of service	45%
February	$910,000	1st month of prior service	25%
March	$950,000	2nd month of prior service	10%
		3–6 months of prior service	5%

Expenses[a]							
Supplies Purchases, 20X0		**Estimated Supplies Purchases, 20X1**		**Other Estimated Expenses, 20X1[a]**			
					Nursing	**Admin.**	**Other**
October	$900,000	January	$1,000,000	January	$3,000,000	$200,000	$700,000
November	$950,000	February	$1,025,000	February	$3,100,000	$200,000	$675,000
December	$1,000,000	March	$1,050,000	March	$3,200,000	$200,000	$650,000
		April	$1,075,000	April	$3,300,000	$200,000	$525,000

Timing of Cash Payment for Supplies Purchases		Ending Cash Balances	
0%	Month purchased	December, 20X0	$700,000
60%	+1 month	[b]	50%
30%	+2 months		
10%	+3 months		

[a]All estimated expenses are cash outflows for the given month.
[b]The ending balance for each month as a percentage of the estimated cash outflows for the next month.

43. **Cash budget**. How would the cash budget in problem 41 change if new credit and collection policies were implemented such that collections resulted as follows:

    a. 30%: current month of patient revenues?

    b. 20% each: past months 1 and 2 of patient revenues?

    c. 10% each: past months 3 and 4 of patient revenues?

    d. 5% each: past months 5 and 6 of patient revenues?

44. **Cash budget**. How would the cash budget in problem 42 change if new credit and collection policies were implemented such that collections resulted as follows:

    a. 40%: current month of patient revenues?

    b. 15% each: past months 1 and 2 of patient revenues?

    c. 10% each: past months 3 and 4 of patient revenues?

    d. 5% each: past months 5 and 6 of patient revenues?

45. **Discounts**. Martha Zeeman Clinic (Exhibit 5.16) is going to take better advantage of credit terms offered by suppliers. The clinic has negotiated a 3 percent discount for all supplies purchased beginning in 20X1, if paid in full during the month of service with the credit terms listed below. How does this change the answer to problem 43?

    Timing of payment for 20X0 supply purchases

    55 percent: month purchased

    30 percent: first prior month

    10 percent: second prior month

    5 percent: third prior month

46. **Discounts**. Rose Valley Clinic (Exhibit 5.17) is going to take better advantage of credit terms offered by suppliers. The clinic has negotiated a 3 percent discount for all supplies purchased beginning in 20X1, if paid in full during the month of service, with the credit terms listed below. How does this change the answer to problem 44?

    Timing of payment for 20X0 supply purchases

    50 percent: month purchased

    30 percent: first prior month

    15 percent: second prior month

    5 percent: third prior month

47. **Revenue cycle management**. Malvern Hospital generated net patient revenues of $150 million for 20X1, and its cash collections were $125 million. The revenue cycle management costs to collect these revenues were $9 million.

    a. Compute Malvern's cost to collect for the year, and provide an assessment of how this cost compares with the hospital industry benchmark of 3 percent.

    b. Compute Malvern's cost to collect for the year if 55 percent of the cash collections during the year required human intervention and its EDI costs were $500,000. Provide an assessment of how this cost compares with the hospital industry benchmark of 3 percent.

48. **Revenue cycle management**. Penn Hospital generated net patient revenues of $225 million for 20X1, and its cash collections were $210 million. The revenue cycle management costs to collect these revenues were $8 million.

    a. Compute Penn's cost to collect for the year, and provide an assessment of how this cost compares with the hospital industry benchmark of 3 percent.

    b. Compute Penn's cost to collect for the year if 35 percent of the cash collections during the year required human intervention and its EDI costs were $600,000. Provide an assessment of how this cost compares with the hospital industry benchmark of 3 percent.

Notes

1. D. M. Berwick and A. D. Hackbarth, Eliminating waste in US health care, *JAMA*, 2012;307(14):1513–1516, doi: 10.1001/jama.2012.362.

2. T. R. Goldman, *Eliminating Fraud and Abuse*, Health Policy Brief, July 31, 2012, Health Affairs/Robert Wood Johnson Foundation.

3. U.S. Department of Health and Human Services, Office of Inspector General, *Work Plan: Fiscal Year 2013*, retrieved January 15, 2013, from oig.hhs.gov/reports-and-publications/archives/workplan/2013/Work-Plan-2013.pdf

CHAPTER 6

THE TIME VALUE OF MONEY

I s it better to receive $10,000 today or at the end of the year? The clear answer is today, for a variety of reasons:

- Certainty. A dollar in hand today is certain, whereas a dollar to be received sometime in the future is not.

- Inflation. During inflationary periods, a dollar will purchase less in the future than it will today. Thus, because of inflation, the value of the dollar in the future is less than it is today.

- Opportunity cost. A dollar today can be used or invested elsewhere. The interest forgone by not having the dollar to invest now is an opportunity cost.

The concept of *interest* determines how much an amount of money invested today will be worth in the future (its *future value*). It can also be used to determine how much a dollar received at some point in the future would be worth today (its *present value*) (see Exhibit 6.1). This chapter focuses on both future and present value, the basics of the *time value of money*, and that time value is essential to making long-term decisions (the focus of Chapter Seven). Perspective 6.1 provides an example of how the time value of money influences investment decisions.

Future Value of a Dollar Invested Today

What a dollar invested today will be worth in the future depends on the length of the investment period, the method used to calculate interest, and the interest rate. There are two types of methods to calculate interest: the simple method and compounding. Under the *simple*

LEARNING OBJECTIVES

- Explain why a dollar today is worth more than a dollar in the future.

- Define the terms future value and present value.

- Calculate the future value of an amount and an annuity.

EXHIBIT 6.1 COMPARISON OF FUTURE VALUE AND PRESENT VALUE CONCEPTS

Future Value (FV)—The worth in the future of an amount invested today,
or the worth in the future of a series of payments made over time.

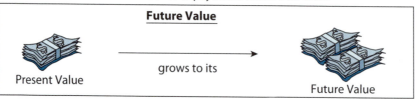

Future Value

Present Value   grows to its   Future Value

Present Value (PV)—The worth today of a future payment,
or the worth today of a series of payments made over time.

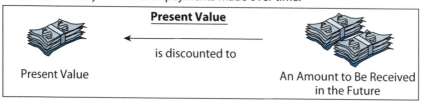

Present Value

Present Value   is discounted to   An Amount to Be Received
in the Future

PERSPECTIVE 6.1 THE TIME VALUE OF MONEY

A hospital CEO's decision to accept information technology (IT) incentive payments from the
Centers for Medicare and Medicaid Services (CMS) to install an electronic health record (EHR)
system is influenced by the time value of money and the risk that the organization may not
receive these payments in the future. Hospitals with health information technology systems
can accept incentive payments now or delay for one more year. Several factors, or underlying
forces, affect hospitals' decision making on whether to take the payments now. One factor is
the time value of money, which argues for payments received now rather than a year from now;
a second factor is the risk that government cutbacks will take funds away from the program;
and a third factor is the promotional advantage of being the first to introduce health IT into
the local market.

Source: Adapted from J. Conn, "To wait or not to wait . . . : decision to go for EHR incentive payments not a simple
one for providers," *Modern Healthcare*, 2011;41(39):10–11.

Opportunity Cost

Proceeds lost by forgoing
other opportunities.

interest method, interest is calculated only on the original principal each
year. When the *compound interest method* is used, interest is calculated on
both the original principal and on any accumulated interest earned up to
that point. Perspective 6.2 presents an example of what health care systems
are earning on their investments and how they allocate their investments.

PERSPECTIVE 6.2 WHAT ARE HOSPITALS AND HEALTH CARE SYSTEMS EARNING ON THEIR INVESTMENTS?

As health care systems grow by acquiring other hospitals and smaller health care systems, they are experiencing increased net worth in their investment portfolios. A survey of 90 health care organizations underscores the size of these portfolios. For example, Trinity Health in Michigan manages over $8.5 billion in investments, while Ascension Health possesses a $20 billion investment portfolio. The Mayo Clinic manages $9 billion, and UPMC in Pittsburgh has over $4.6 billion in investable assets. The typical allocation of investments across four major types of investments is as follows: 37 percent fixed income, 39 percent domestic and international equities, 17 percent alternative strategies, and 7 percent short-term securities and cash. Alternative strategies are to invest in high-risk and high-return investments such as hedge funds, private equity companies, and commodities and futures contracts. In 2010, the average returns on these asset classes were around 17 percent for domestic equities, 12 percent for international equities, 9 percent for alternative strategies, and 7 percent for fixed income. Dividends, realized and unrealized capital gains, and interest income earned on these funds typically accounted for more than one-third of a health care system's net income. As a result of cutbacks in Medicare, health care systems and hospitals face lower hospital reimbursement, which reduces their operating margins, thereby increasing their dependence on these investment returns to boost their overall earnings.

Source: Adapted from H. Bradford, Non-profits put investible assets under microscope, *Pensions & Investments*, March 19, 2012;40:3.

Exhibit 6.2, part A, uses the simple interest method to calculate how much $10,000 invested today at 10 percent interest would be worth in five years. Because the simple interest method calculates interest on the principal only, each year of investment would earn $1,000 interest (0.10 × $10,000). After five years, the net worth of the investment would be $15,000 ($10,000 plus $5,000 in interest).

Exhibit 6.2, part B, uses the same scenario to illustrate the difference of compounded interest. In the first year there is no difference between using the simple and compound interest methods because no interest has yet been earned. However, in the second and all subsequent years, more interest is earned using the compound interest method because 10 percent is earned on the original $10,000, plus 10 percent on the total amount of interest previously accumulated. Thus the future value of $10,000 invested at 10 percent interest after five years is $16,105 using compound interest, as compared with $15,000 using simple interest.

EXHIBIT 6.2 INVESTING $10,000 OVER FIVE YEARS AT 10 PERCENT, USING SIMPLE AND COMPOUND INTEREST

A. The future value of investing $10,000 over five years at 10 percent *simple* interest

A	B	C	D
	Total at	Interest	
	Beginning of	Earned	
Year	Year (D,	($10,000 ×	Amount at End
(Given)	Previous Year)	10%)	of Year[a] (B + C)
1	$10,000	$1,000	$11,000
2	$11,000	$1,000	$12,000
3	$12,000	$1,000	$13,000
4	$13,000	$1,000	$14,000
5	$14,000	$1,000	$15,000
Summary			
Beginning balance	$10,000		
Interest earned		$5,000	
Ending balance			$15,000

B. The future value of investing $10,000 over five years at 10 percent *compound* interest

E	F	G	H
	Total at		
	Beginning	Interest	Amount at
Year	of Year (H,	Earned	End of Year[a]
(Given)	Previous Year)	(F × 10%)	(F + G)
1	$10,000	$1,000	$11,000
2	$11,000	$1,100	$12,100
3	$12,100	$1,210	$13,310
4	$13,310	$1,331	$14,641
5	$14,641	$1,464	$16,105
Summary			
Beginning balance	$10,000		
Interest earned		$6,105	
Ending balance			$16,105

[a] Also called *future value.*

Key Point Simple interest calculates interest only on the original principal, whereas compound interest calculates interest on both the principal and on any accumulated interest. Thus the value in the future will always be higher when using compound interest than when using simple interest, except in the first period.

Key Point As commonly used, the term *future value* implies using the compound interest method. It is used in this way throughout this text unless noted otherwise.

The difference between the two methods is considerable and increases with time. After ten years, $10,000 invested at 10 percent simple interest would grow to $20,000; after twenty years it would be worth $30,000; and after fifty years it would grow to $60,000. The comparable numbers for compound interest are $25,937, $67,275, and $1,173,909, respectively. These differences are illustrated in Exhibit 6.3, which compares the constant rate of growth when using simple interest with the increasing growth rate when using compound interest.

Using a Formula to Calculate Future Value

One approach to calculating future value is to use the formula

$$FV = PV \times (1+i)^n$$

where PV is the present value (initial investment amount), i is the interest rate, and n is the number of time periods of the investment. This formula says that an investment's worth in the future, FV, equals the investment's present worth today, PV, multiplied by a factor, $(1 + i)^n$, that takes into account the compounded growth in interest over the lifetime of the investment.

For example, to calculate the future value of $10,000 in four years at 10 percent interest, the formula would be set up as follows:

$$FV = PV \times (1+i)^n$$
$$FV = \$10,000 \times (1+0.10)^4$$
$$FV = \$10,000 \times (1.4641)$$
$$FV = \$14,641$$

Future Value (FV)
What an amount invested today (or a series of payments made over time) will be worth at a given time in the future using the compound interest method, which accounts for the time value of money. Also see the definition of *present value*.

Time Value of Money
The concept that a dollar received today is worth more than a dollar received in the future.

Simple Interest Method
A method in which interest is calculated only on the original principal. The principal is the amount invested.

Compound Interest Method
A method in which interest is calculated on both the original principal and on all interest accumulated since the beginning of the investment time period.

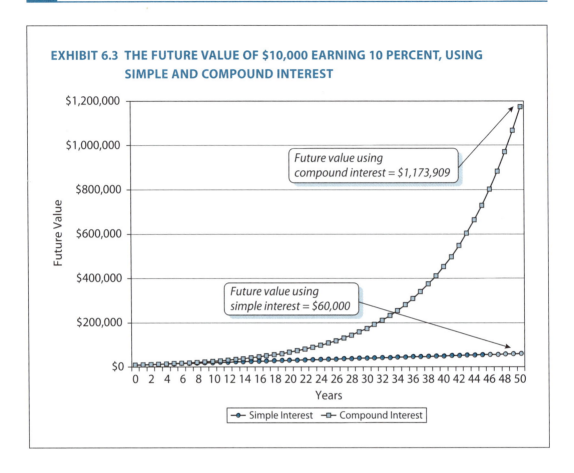

EXHIBIT 6.3 THE FUTURE VALUE OF $10,000 EARNING 10 PERCENT, USING SIMPLE AND COMPOUND INTEREST

Similarly, to calculate the future value of $10,000 earning 10 percent interest over five years, the formula would be set up as follows:

$$FV = PV \times (1+i)^n$$
$$FV = \$10,000 \times (1+0.10)^5$$
$$FV = \$10,000 \times (1.6105)$$
$$FV = \$16,105$$

Notice that these are the same numbers derived in Exhibit 6.2, part B, for four and five years, respectively.

Future Value Table

Table of factors that shows the future value of a single investment at a given interest rate.

Using Tables to Compute Future Value

An alternative to calculating the future value using the formula is to use a *future value table*. Table B.1, in Appendix B at the end of this chapter, contains a precalculated range of future value factors (FVF) using the

EXHIBIT 6.4 EXAMPLE OF HOW TO FIND THE FUTURE VALUE FACTOR AT 10 PERCENT INTEREST FOR 5 YEARS, USING TABLE B.1

			Interest Rate			
Period	2%	4%	6%	8%	10%	12%
1						
2						
3						
4						
5					→ 1.6105	

future value formula: $(1 + i)^n$. Across the top of the table, the column headings list various interest rates. The leftmost column in the table, containing the row headings, provides the number of compounding periods (annual, semiannual, quarterly, etc.). The cell where a row and a column intersect contains the corresponding future value factor (FVF). For example, as shown in Exhibit 6.4, the FVF to invest $10,000 at 10 percent for five years (abbreviated as $FVF_{10,5}$), is found by following the 10 percent column down to the fifth row (five years), to the number 1.6105. This number is then inserted into the following formula to derive the future value:

$$FV = PV \times FVF_{i,n}$$

in a manner similar to the last two steps in the formula approach:

$$FV = \$10,000 \times (1.6105)$$
$$FV = \$16,105$$

Key Point The *future value factor* (FVF) is $(1 + i)^n$, where i is the interest rate and n is the number of periods.

Key Point The formula to find the future value: Future Value = Present Value × Future Value Factor. It is abbreviated as $FV = PV \times FVF_{i,n}$ *or* $FV = PV(1 + i)^n$.

This is the same result calculated earlier by using the formula: $FV = PV \times (1 + i)^n$. Table B.1 can be used to find the FVF for interest rates up to 50 percent and as many as fifty periods.

EXHIBIT 6.5 USING EXCEL TO CALCULATE THE FUTURE VALUE FOR A SINGLE PAYMENT

EXHIBIT 6.5 USING EXCEL TO CALCULATE THE FUTURE VALUE FOR A SINGLE PAYMENT

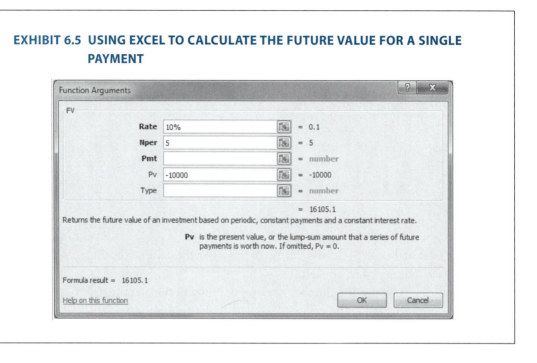

Using a Spreadsheet to Calculate Future Value

Most spreadsheets have easy-to-use financial functions that can calculate future value. For example, to calculate the future value of $10,000 at 10 percent interest over five years in Excel, use the FV function in the Financial category. Enter the rate (10%), the number of periods (5), and the present value as a negative number (−10,000) to represent the cash outflow of the investment. The future value, $16,105, is automatically calculated at the bottom (see Exhibit 6.5). Note that the future value is a positive number because it represents a cash inflow of the principal and interest at a later point in time.

Present Value (PV)

The value today of a payment (or series of payments) to be received in the future, taking into account the cost of capital (sometimes called *discount rate*). It is calculated using the formula: $PV = FV \times PVF$ or $PV = FV \times 1/(1+i)^n$.

Present Value of an Amount to Be Received in the Future

The focus until now has been on the future value of money invested today. The example showed that $10,000 invested by a clinic today will be worth $16,105 in five years at 10 percent compound interest each year. In this section, the question is turned around to become: How much is $16,105 to be received five years from now worth today? The value today of a payment (or series of payments) to be received in the future, taking into account the cost of capital, is the *present value*. Taking future values back to the present is also called *discounting*.

$$\text{Present Value} = \text{Future Value} \times \text{Present Value Factor}$$

Using a Formula to Calculate Present Value

Just as the present value is multiplied by a future value factor (FVF) to determine the future value, the future value is multiplied by a *present value factor* to calculate present value. The present value factor, $1 / (1 + i)^n$, is the inverse of the future value factor: $(1 + i)^n$.

Key Point The *present value factor* is the reciprocal of the future value factor and is calculated using the formula $1 / (1 + i)^n$.

Key Point The formula to find the present value is: Present Value = Future Value × Present Value Factor. It is abbreviated as: $PV = FV \times PVF_{i,n}$ *or* $PV = FV \times 1 / (1 + i)^n$.

Thus, using the formula, the present value of $16,105 at 10 percent interest for five years can be calculated as follows:

$$PV = FV \times 1/(1+i)^n$$
$$PV = \$16,105 \times 1/(1+0.10)^5$$
$$PV = \$16,105 \times 1/(1.6105)$$
$$PV = \$16,105 \times (0.6209)$$
$$PV = \$10,000$$

The $1 / (1.6105)$, which equals 0.6209, is the present value factor. It can be interpreted to mean that at 10 percent interest, a dollar received five years from now is worth only about 62 percent of its value in today's dollars. In the example, $16,105 received five years from now is worth only $10,000 in today's dollars.

Exhibit 6.6 illustrates the relationship between present value and future value. Just as $10,000 today grows to $16,105 over five years at 10 percent compound interest, $16,105 received five years from now is worth $10,000 today, assuming a 10 percent (discount) rate.

Key Point To find future value, *compound*. To find present value, *discount*. Discounting is the opposite of compounding. *Compound* toward the future; *discount* to the present.

Compounding
Converting a present value into its future value, taking into account the time value of money (see the previous definition of *compound interest method*). It is the opposite of discounting.

Discounting
Converting future cash flows into their present value, taking into account the time value of money. It is the opposite of compounding.

EXHIBIT 6.6 THE RELATIONSHIP BETWEEN PRESENT VALUE AND FUTURE VALUE AT 10 PERCENT AND 5 PERIODS

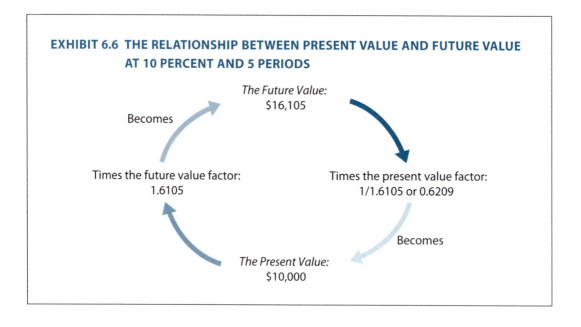

EXHIBIT 6.7 EXAMPLE OF HOW TO FIND THE PRESENT VALUE FACTOR AT 10 PERCENT INTEREST FOR 5 YEARS, USING TABLE B.3ª

Period	2%	4%	6%	8%	10%	12%
			Interest Rate			
1						
2						
3						
4						
5					0.6209	

ªThe present value factor for 10 percent interest over 5 periods is abbreviated as: $PVF_{10,5}$.

Using Tables to Compute Present Value

Just as Table B.1 contains a list of precalculated future value factors (FVFs) based on the formula $(1 + i)^n$, Table B.3 contains a list of present value factors (PVFs), based on the formula $1 / (1 + i)^n$. (Tables B.2 and B.4 will be discussed shortly.) Finding a present value factor in Table B.3 is analogous to finding a future value factor in Table B.1. The process of locating the present value factor for five years at 10 percent interest is illustrated in Exhibit 6.7.

This present value factor (PVF) can be used in the formula PV = FV × $PVF_{i,n}$ to derive the present value of $16,105 at 10 percent interest for five years:

$$PV = FV \times PVF_{10,5}$$
$$PV = \$16,105 \times 0.6209$$
$$PV = \$10,000$$

This is the same result derived by using the formula. Table B.3 can also be used to find the PVF for interest rates up to 50 percent and as many as fifty periods.

Using a Spreadsheet to Calculate Present Value

As with future value, most spreadsheets have basic financial functions that can calculate present value. For example, to calculate the present value of $16,105 at 10 percent interest for five years in Excel, select the PV function in the Financial category. Enter the rate (10%), the number of periods (5), and the future value as a negative number (−16,105). The present value, 9999.937908 ($10,000), is automatically calculated at the bottom (Exhibit 6.8).

EXHIBIT 6.8 USING EXCEL TO CALCULATE THE PRESENT VALUE FOR A SINGLE PAYMENT

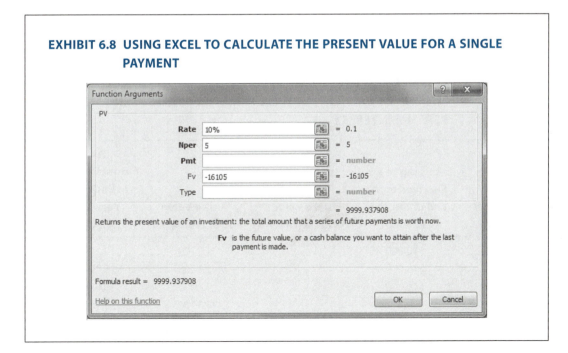

Future and Present Values of Annuities

The earlier discussion of present and future values shows how a single amount invested today grows over time and how a single amount to be received in the future is discounted to today's dollars. But sometimes, instead of a single amount, there is a series of payments. This section deals with a particular kind of series of payments called an annuity. An *annuity* is a series of equal payments made or received at equally spaced (regular) time intervals.

Annuity
A series of equal payments made or received at regular time intervals.

Future Value of an Annuity
What an equal series of payments will be worth at some future date, using compound interest. Also see the definitions of *future value factor of an annuity* and *present value of an annuity.*

Future Value of an Ordinary Annuity

This section shows how to determine what an annuity to be received or invested will be worth at some future date. Suppose a donor were going to give $10,000 per year at the end of each year for the next three years. What would the donation be worth at the end of three years if it earned 10 percent interest each period? Based on the information previously discussed, at the end of three years there would be $33,100, computed as shown in Exhibit 6.9.

Using Tables to Calculate the Future Value of an Ordinary Annuity

Rather than making three separate calculations (one for each year, as shown), a shortcut is to add the future value factors, which total 3.3100 $(1.2100 + 1.1000 + 1.000)$, then multiply the sum by $10,000. In this case,

---

EXHIBIT 6.9 CALCULATING THE FUTURE VALUE OF $10,000 TO BE RECEIVED AT THE END OF EACH OF THE NEXT THREE YEARS, ASSUMING 10 PERCENT INTEREST

Year (Given)	A Amount to Be Received at the End of the Year (Given)	B Future Value Formula (Given)	C Future Value Factor (Table B.1)	D Future Value at End of Year 3 (A × C)
1	$10,000	$(1 + i)^2$	1.2100	$12,100
2	$10,000	$(1 + i)^1$	1.1000	$11,000
3	$10,000	$(1 + i)^0$	1.0000	$10,000
Total			3.3100	$33,100

3.3100 × $10,000 = $33,100, the same value as seen in Exhibit 6.9. Rather than adding the factors for each of the three years, an alternative approach is to use a *future value factor of an annuity* (FVFA) table, such as Table B.2. Such tables contain the same figures as achieved by adding together the separate future value factors for each year. For example, in Table B.2, the future value factor of an annuity at 10 percent interest for three years, $FVFA_{10,3}$, is 3.3100, the same number derived by adding the future value factors for each of the three years in Exhibit 6.9. Thus, *whenever* a series of equal payments is to be made or received at the end of each period, the *future value of an annuity table* can be used, rather than computing the future value of each year's cash flow and adding the results.

Future Value Factor of an Annuity (FVFA)
A factor that when multiplied by a stream of equal payments equals the future value of that stream. Also see the definition of *present value factor of an annuity*.

Future Value of an Annuity Table
Table of factors that shows the future value of equal flows at the end of each period, given a particular interest rate.

$$FV = Annuity \times FVFA_{10,3}$$
$$FV = \$10,000 \times 3.3100$$
$$FV = \$33,100$$

Also note that a series of payments made or received at the end of each period is called an *ordinary annuity*, whereas a series of payments made or received at the beginning of each period is called an *annuity due* (discussed shortly).

Ordinary Annuity
A series of equal annuity payments made or received at the end of each period.

Key Point Whenever a series of payments is to be invested or received at the end of the year, an ordinary annuity table can be used to determine future value, rather than computing the future value of each year's cash flow.

Using a Spreadsheet to Calculate the Future Value of an Ordinary Annuity

Most spreadsheets can easily calculate the future value of an ordinary annuity. For example, in Excel, to calculate the future value of a series of $10,000 payments to be received at the end of each of three years, assuming a 10 percent interest rate, the financial FV function is again used. Enter the rate (10%), the number of periods (3), and the annuity, or Pmt, input value as a negative number (−10,000). The future value automatically appears at the bottom (Exhibit 6.10).

Future Value of an Annuity Due

The future value of an annuity table, such as Table B.2, is developed for ordinary annuities: cash flows that occur at the end of each period.

EXHIBIT 6.10 USING EXCEL TO CALCULATE THE FUTURE VALUE FOR AN ORDINARY ANNUITY PAYMENT

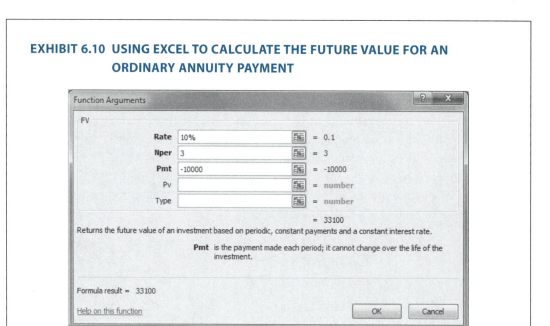

Sometimes however, a series of cash flows occurs at the beginning of each period, instead of at the end. Such an annuity is called an *annuity due*. The future value factor (FVF) for an annuity due is equal to the factor found on the future value of an ordinary annuity table for n + 1 years, less 1.

Suppose a lessee has agreed to pay an organization $10,000 today and at the beginning of each of the next four years, for a total of five $10,000 payments over five years. The organization thinks it can invest this money at 10 percent. To determine the future value of the investment after five years, the organization (1) takes the future value factor for an ordinary annuity in Table B.2 at 10 percent interest for $5 + 1 = 6$ years (7.7156); (2) subtracts 1 from this future value factor (7.7156 − 1 = 6.7156); and (3) multiplies this value by $10,000.

Annuity Due

A series of equal annuity payments made or received at the beginning of each period.

$$\text{FV annuity due} = (\text{FVFA}_{i,n+1} - 1) \times \text{annuity}$$
$$\text{FV annuity due} = (\text{FVFA}_{10,5+1} - 1) \times \$10,000$$
$$\text{FV annuity due} = (7.7156 - 1) \times \$10,000$$
$$\text{FV annuity due} = 6.7156 \times \$10,000$$
$$\text{FV annuity due} = \$67,156$$

This procedure can also be performed on a spreadsheet using the future value function. In Excel, the same function used to find an ordinary annuity is used (Exhibit 6.10), but a 1 is entered in the space for Type, to indicate that this is an annuity due.

Present Value of an Ordinary Annuity

As with future value, it is possible to calculate the *present value of an ordinary annuity* or an annuity due. Suppose a donor wants to give $10,000 per year at the end of each of the next three years. What is it worth today if the donations can earn 10 percent interest each period? One way to approach this problem would be to calculate the present value of each year's cash flow and then add them, which equals $24,869 (Exhibit 6.11).

Using Tables to Calculate the Present Value of an Ordinary Annuity
The same result can be derived by first adding the three present value factors (PVFs) $(0.9091 + 0.8264 + 0.7513 = 2.4869)$ and then multiplying the result by $10,000 (2.4869 \times \$10,000 = \$24,869)$, as shown in Exhibit 6.11. A shortcut is to use a *present value of an annuity table*, such as Table B.4. Such tables contain the same numbers as would be derived by adding the separate PVFs for each year (differences are due to rounding). For example, in Table B.4, the present value factor of an annuity (PVFA) at 10 percent interest for three years, $PVFA_{10,3}$, is 2.4869.

Present Value of an Annuity
What a series of equal payments in the future is worth today, taking into account the time value of money.

Present Value Factor of an Annuity (PVFA)
A factor that when multiplied by a stream of equal payments equals the present value of that stream.

Present Value of an Annuity Table
Table of factors that shows the value today of equal flows at the end of each future period, given a particular interest rate.

$$PV = Annuity \times PVFA_{10,3}$$
$$PV = \$10,000 \times 2.4869$$
$$PV = \$24,869$$

EXHIBIT 6.11 CALCULATING THE PRESENT VALUE OF $10,000 TO BE RECEIVED AT THE END OF EACH YEAR FOR THE NEXT THREE YEARS, ASSUMING 10 PERCENT INTEREST

	A	B	C	D
Year (Given)	Amount to Be Received at the End of the Year (Given)	Present Value Formula (Given)	Present Value Factor (Table B.3)	Present Value at End of Year 3 (A × C)
1	$10,000	$1/(1+i)^1$	0.9091	$9,091
2	$10,000	$1/(1+i)^2$	0.8264	$8,264
3	$10,000	$1/(1+i)^3$	0.7513	$7,513
Total			2.4869	$24,869

Key Point Whenever a series of payments is to be received at the end of the year, an ordinary annuity table can be used to determine its present value, rather than computing the present value of each year's cash flow.

Each factor in the present value of an annuity table is the sum of each of the present value factors for each year of the annuity. Present value annuity tables are set up to calculate values for ordinary annuities.

Using a Spreadsheet to Calculate the Present Value of an Ordinary Annuity

Most spreadsheets easily calculate the present value of an ordinary annuity (in Excel, this function is called PV). Exhibit 6.12 shows the result of entering the numbers in the appropriate categories to calculate the present value of a $10,000 annuity to be received at the end of each of the next three years, assuming 10 percent interest.

Present Value of an Annuity Due

Table B.4, which shows the present value factors (PVFs) for an ordinary annuity (PVFA), can be used to calculate the present value factor for an

EXHIBIT 6.12 USING EXCEL TO CALCULATE THE PRESENT VALUE FOR AN ORDINARY ANNUITY PAYMENT

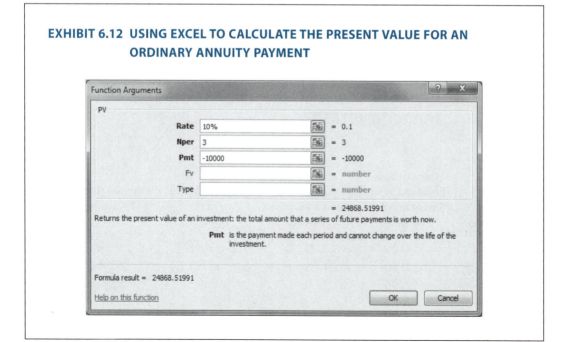

annuity due (PVFA). This is done by finding the PVF for n − 1 years and then adding 1 to this factor.

Suppose a lessee has agreed to pay an organization $10,000 today and at the beginning of each of the next four years, for a total of five $10,000 payments over five years. To find the present value of this series of payments, assuming an interest rate of 10 percent, the organization (1) determines the present value factor for an ordinary annuity from Table B.4 at 10 percent interest and 5 − 1 = 4 years (3.1699); (2) adds 1 to this factor to get the factor for an annuity due (3.1699 + 1 = 4.1699); and (3) multiplies this new factor by $10,000.

$$PV \text{ annuity due} = (PVFA_{i,n-1} + 1) \times \text{annuity}$$
$$PV \text{ annuity due} = (PVFA_{10,5-1} + 1) \times \$10,000$$
$$PV \text{ annuity due} = (3.1699 + 1) \times \$10,000$$
$$PV \text{ annuity due} = 4.1699 \times \$10,000$$
$$PV \text{ annuity due} = \$41,699$$

This procedure can also be performed on a spreadsheet using the present value function. In Excel, the function used to find an ordinary annuity is used (Exhibit 6.12), but a 1 is entered in the space for Type, to indicate that this is an annuity due.

Future and Present Value Calculations and Excel Functions for Special Situations

How to Compute Value When the Interest Rate Is Not Expressed as an Annual Rate

In the examples presented thus far, the interest rate has been expressed as an annual interest rate, and periods have been expressed in years. However, periods can also refer to other periods of time, such as months or days. If periods of time other than a year are being used, then the interest rate must be expressed for an equivalent period of time. For example, 12 percent annually is 1 percent a month.

Suppose an investment of $10,000 is invested at an interest rate of 12 percent and compounded semiannually for ten years. Because interest rates are always assumed to be annual unless stated otherwise, the formula must be adjusted to account for periods other than annual. The future value formula to compound at intervals more frequent than annual is

$$FV = PV \times (1+i/m)^{n \times m}$$

where i = annual interest rate, m = number of times per year that com-pounding occurs (e.g., $m = 4$ for quarterly, $m = 12$ for monthly), and n = number of years.

Using the figures in the example:

$$FV = PV \times (1+i/m)^{n \times m}$$
$$FV = \$10,000 \times (1+0.12/2)^{10 \times 2}$$
$$FV = \$10,000 \times (1+0.06)^{20}$$
$$FV = \$10,000 \times 3.2071$$
$$FV = \$32,071$$

Note that the final value, $32,071, is higher than it would have been had the same amount been invested and compounded annually rather than semiannually. For example, had it been compounded annually (using the standard formula $FV = PV \times FVF_{12,10}$), the future value factor (FVF) would have been 3.1058, yielding a future value of $31,058 ($10,000 × 3.1058). This discrepancy is not a mistake (see Exhibit 6.13). It happens because

EXHIBIT 6.13 EFFECT OF COMPOUNDING USING VARIOUS COMPOUNDING PERIODS

Givens

Initial amount	$10,000
Annualized interest rate	12%
Time horizon, years	10

Compounding Period	Future Value
Annually	$31,058
Semiannually	$32,071
Quarterly	$32,620
Monthly	$33,004
Daily	$33,195
Continuously	$33,201

compounding in the first instance is occurring twice per year rather than once per year, so interest is growing upon interest more frequently. With quarterly compounding over the same ten-year period (i.e., 3 percent per quarter for forty quarters), the future value would be still higher, and with monthly compounding (i.e., 1 percent per month for 120 months), still higher yet. Although the equation to calculate future value with continuous compounding is beyond the scope of this text, the key point here is that the more frequent the compounding for any given interest level and time period, the higher the future value.

Key Point The more frequent the compounding for any given interest level and time period, the higher the future value.

How to Compute Periodic Loan Payments Using Excel

Excel can also calculate periodic loan payments, using the PMT (payment) function. This function can only be used for loans that involve equal periodic payments over the length of the loan. Exhibit 6.14 provides an example of how to compute annual loan payments for a ten-year, $1 million loan that has an interest rate of 10 percent. Note that the present value is entered as a negative number (−$1,000,000) to make the final result

EXHIBIT 6.14 USING THE EXCEL PAYMENT FUNCTION TO COMPUTE LOAN PAYMENTS

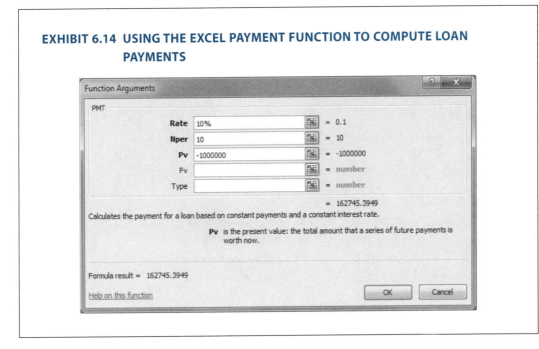

positive. This final result, $162,745, is interpreted to mean that by paying this annual amount under these conditions, the loan will be completely paid off at the end. This type of analysis is also called a *loan amortization*, which will be discussed in more detail in Chapter Eight.

How to Calculate the Compounded Growth Rate

When examining data, researchers often like to present the compounded growth rate for numerical data, such as revenues, expenses, and earnings, and an example is presented in Perspective 6.3. Suppose Memorial Hospital would like to determine the compounded growth rate for patient revenues between 20X0 and 20X7, as shown in Exhibit 6.15.

Solving this problem requires finding the compound growth rate (which is similar to compound interest) that causes 20X0 revenues to have a future value equal to 20X7 revenues (seven time periods into the future). To do this analysis:

- Step 1. Solve for FVF in the equation $FV = PV \times FVF_{i,n}$, where $FV = 20X7$ amount ($3,650,000) and $PV = 20X0$ amount ($2,123,000).

$$FV = PV \times FVF_{i,n}$$
$$\$3,650,000 = \$2,123,000 \times FVF_{i,7}$$
$$\$3,650,000 / \$2,123,000 = FVF_{i,7}$$
$$1.7192 = FVF_{i,7}$$

EXHIBIT 6.15 PATIENT REVENUES FOR MEMORIAL HOSPITAL

Year	Patient Revenues
20X0	$2,123,000
20X1	$2,245,000
20X2	$2,555,000
20X3	$2,700,000
20X4	$2,889,000
20X5	$3,145,000
20X6	$3,496,000
20X7	$3,650,000

PERSPECTIVE 6.3 AN ILLUSTRATION OF COMPOUND ANNUAL RATE OF GROWTH (CARG) IN HEALTH CARE

The pressure to reduce health care costs is creating growth opportunities in telehealth markets. Within the telemedicine market, revenues from the use of technology (hardware, software, and telecom) are expected to grow from $4.6 billion in 2011 to $11.3 billion in 2016, which represents a 19.8 percent compounded annual rate of growth during this time frame.

The compounded annual rate of growth in revenues for remote wireless patient monitoring devices is expected to rise annually by 4%, from $6.1 billion in 2010 to $8 billion in 2017, driven by an aging population and the movement toward monitoring a patient's medical progress at home. And even higher growth in profits is expected for some: one company that provides electronic health record and management service products to large and small group practices is expected to experience a compounded annual rate of growth in profits of 100 percent per year over the next five years.

Source: Statistics are from B. Dolan, Patient monitoring device market to hit $8B in 2017, MobiHealthNews, March 26, 2012; B. Monegain, Global telemedicine market pegged to more than double by 2016, *Healthcare IT News*, March 14, 2012; and eClinicalWorks announces eClinicalWorks care coordination portal, *Business Wire*, February 27, 2012.

- Step 2. Using Table B.1, compare the calculated FVF, 1.7192, against all FVF factors in the row for seven time periods to find the factor closest to 1.7192. The appropriate interest rate is the rate given at the top of that column. In this case, 1.7138 comes closest to 1.7192. Therefore, the appropriate interest rate is approximately 8 percent, which also represents the average compound growth rate per year in revenues from 20X0 to 20X7; however, year-to-year changes may be more or less than 8 percent.[1]

How to Calculate the Present Value of Perpetual Annuities

All the annuities in the earlier sections of this chapter were calculated using a finite number of time periods, such as ten years. In some instances, however, an organization needs to make an investment to generate an annuity (cash flow) for an infinite period. Such an annuity is called a *perpetual annuity*, or a *perpetuity*. For example, a donor may bequeath a large sum of money to a hospital under the condition that it generates a specified income every year for Alzheimer's research, and the donor may make no stipulation as to when the funds should be depleted and this research funding should cease. In this situation the hospital would treat the donation as a perpetuity.

The concept of perpetuities and the calculations involved are actually simple. If $1,000,000 were reinvested each year forever at an annual 10 percent interest rate, $100,000 in interest income could be extracted every year ($1,000,000 × 10%) without ever depleting the principal. Every year after withdrawal of the interest income, the investment would still be worth $1,000,000 in real terms. Looked at another way, how much principal would need to be invested at 10 percent to earn $100,000 per year forever? The answer is obviously $1,000,000. This leads to the formula for a perpetuity:

> Amount of Perpetuity = Initial Investment × Interest Rate

Thus, using this formula, to generate a $100,000 perpetuity at a 10 percent interest rate, $100,000 / 0.10, or $1,000,000, would be needed.

Suppose that in her will a wealthy donor has left a $2,500,000 donation to her alma mater's university hospital. The funds are to be used solely to buy gifts for pediatric cancer patients and to subsidize hotel costs for visiting parents. The donor's only son died at age eight from leukemia, and she wished to give other children hope and happiness. She stipulates in her will that no less than $150,000 in gift monies be available every year from the donation. It is at the hospital's discretion to decide how to invest the money prudently. What rate of return must the investment generate after the donor's death to ensure that her wishes be granted?

Perpetuity
An annuity for an infinite period of time. Also called a *perpetual annuity.*

The formula for a perpetuity can be rearranged to solve for rate of return, given the other two factors:

> Interest Rate = Amount of Perpetuity / Initial Investment
> Interest Rate = $150,000 / $2,500,000
> Interest Rate = 0.06 = 6%

Therefore, as long as the hospital can invest the $2,500,000 at a minimum 6 percent rate of return, the donor's wishes will be granted indefinitely.

How to Solve for the Interest Rate of a Loan with Fixed Payments

Assuming equal loan payments over the life of a loan, it is also possible to solve for the interest rate. If the present value of the loan, the loan payments over time, and the length of the loan are given, the unknown interest rate of the loan, i, can be determined.

For example, suppose Mt. Moriah Hospital needs to borrow $10,000 for a new computer system. The annual loan payments are $3,019 per year at the end of each year for the next four years. What is the interest rate of this loan? Using the present value formula for an ordinary annuity, solve for the interest rate, i:

$$PV = Annuity \times PVFA_{i,4}$$
$$\$10,000 = \$3,019 \times PVFA_{i,4}$$
$$\$10,000/\$3,019 = PVFA_{i,4}$$
$$3.3124 = PVFA_{i,4}$$
$$3.3124 = PVFA_{8,4}$$
$$i = 8\%^a$$

[a]In Table B.4, the PVFA equal or closest to 3.3124 is found in the row for four time periods. At this PVFA, the interest rate of this column heading is 8 percent.

This could also be done in a spreadsheet: for example, by using the RATE function in Excel, as shown in Exhibit 6.16. This is a four-year, $10,000 loan with equal annual payments of $3,019. This RATE function can be used only for loan payments that are equal over the life of the loan.

EXHIBIT 6.16 USING THE EXCEL RATE FUNCTION TO COMPUTE A LOAN RATE

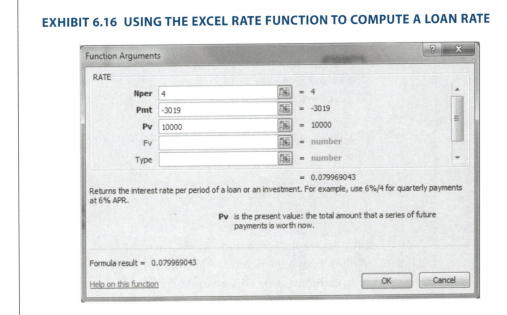

The loan payment value must be a negative value (cash outflow); the RATE function will give an incorrect value if both Pmt and Pv values are positive.

The prior example could also be used to solve for the time period (n), given an interest rate (i) of 8 percent instead, by going down the 8 percent column in the present value annuity table to the $PVFA_{8\%, n}$ of 3.3124 and going across to the period row of n to identify four periods or four years. The time period could also be derived in a spreadsheet, such as by using the NPER function in Excel. This is a four-year, $10,000 loan with equal annual payments of $3,019. This NPER function can be used only for loan payments that are equal over the life of the loan, and as before, the loan payment value must be entered as a negative value (cash outflow).

How to Solve for the Effective Interest Rate

Generally, if an interest rate for less than one year needs to be converted to an annualized rate, the effects of compounding may be ignored. For example, a monthly interest rate of 1 percent would convert into an annualized interest rate of 12 percent ($1\% \times 12$ months). However, if the annual stated, or *nominal*, rate of interest is compounded during the year, then a greater *effective* rate is earned or charged. For example, if a bank is willing to offer a hospital a bank loan that charges an annual 8 percent nominal rate but is compounded quarterly (four periods), then the hospital's effective rate is computed as in the following formula:

Effective Interest Rate $= [(1+$ Nominal Annual Rate $/$

$\qquad$ Compounding Periods$)^{\text{compounding periods}} - 1]$

$\qquad$ Effective Rate $= (1+.08/4)^4 - 1$

$\qquad$ Effective Rate $= (1+.02)^4 - 1$

In Table B.1, the future value factor for 2 percent and four periods is 1.0824.

$\qquad$ Effective Rate $= 1.0824 - 1$

$\qquad$ Effective Rate $= 8.24\%$

As a result, the hospital is charged more when the bank compounds the rate more often than once per year (the concept is similar to that presented earlier in Exhibit 6.13). This formula could also be computed in Excel by using the EFFECT function, as presented in Exhibit 6.17. Entering 8% in the Nominal rate box and 4 in the Npery box (number of annual

EXHIBIT 6.17 USING EXCEL TO CALCULATE THE EFFECTIVE INTEREST RATE

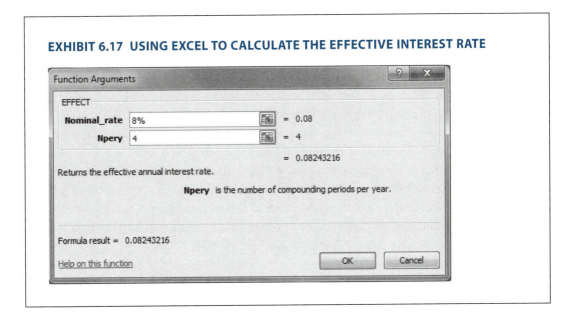

Function Arguments

EFFECT

Nominal_rate 8% = 0.08

Npery 4 = 4

= 0.08243216

Returns the effective annual interest rate.

Npery is the number of compounding periods per year.

Formula result = 0.08243216

Help on this function   OK   Cancel

compounding periods) results in an effective rate of 8.24 percent. (The nominal rate may also be lower than the effective rate due to up-front borrowing costs, as discussed in Chapter Five.)

Key Point In the Excel RATE and NPER functions, the Pmt box or loan payment box must be a negative value to represent cash outflows.

Summary

Future value is used to determine the value of dollar payments in the future, whereas present value indicates the current value of future dollars. Either simple interest, where interest is calculated only on the principal, or compound interest, where the interest is calculated on the principal *and* the interest, can be used to determine the future value of money. The compound interest method produces a larger sum of money in the future and is the standard method used.

The FVF, or $(1 + i)^n$, where i is the interest rate and n is the number of periods of the investment, is part of the formula to determine how much an investment will be worth in the future. The entire formula to find future value is: Future Value = Present Value × Future Value Factor, abbreviated as FV = PV × FVF$_{i,n}$ *or* FV = PV$(1 + i)^n$. The opposite formula calculates the present value: Present Value = Future Value × Present Value Factor, abbreviated as PV = FV × PVF$_{i,n}$ *or* PV = FV / $(1 + i)^n$. Similar formulas

Nominal Interest Rate
The stated annual interest rate of a loan, which does not account for compounding within the year.

Effective Interest Rate
The actual interest rate earned or charged, which is affected by the number of compounding periods during the year. The effective interest rate is higher than the nominal interest rate with compounding of interest.

Present Value Table

Table of factors that shows what a single amount to be received in the future is worth today, at a given interest rate.

are used to calculate the present value or future value of an annuity; all that changes is the factor. All these factors can be found in precalculated tables, which are known as *future value tables* and *present value tables*.

A series of payments to be paid or received at the end of each period is called an *ordinary annuity*. A series of payments to be paid or received at the beginning of each period is called an *annuity due*. The steps used to calculate each of these two types of annuities are somewhat different. An understanding of present and future values and annuities can be used to answer a number of key questions, such as, How much will an investment today be worth in the future?, and, What is the rate of return for a loan? This chapter also described special situations and applications. All calculations can be made either through the use of the accompanying tables in Appendix B or with the aid of a spreadsheet.

KEY TERMS

a. Annuity

b. Annuity due

c. Compound interest method

d. Compounding

e. Discounting

f. Effective interest rate

g. Future value

h. Future value factor

i. Future value factor of an annuity

j. Future value of an annuity

k. Future value of an annuity table

l. Future value table

m. Nominal interest rate

n. Opportunity cost

o. Ordinary annuity

p. Perpetuity

q. Present value

r. Present value factor

s. Present value factor of an annuity

t. Present value of an annuity

u. Present value of an annuity table

v. Present value table

w. Simple interest method

x. Time value of money

Key Equations

• Future value equation:

$$FV = PV \times (1+i)^n$$

- Future value formula:

$$FV = PV \times FVF_{i,n}$$

- Future value formula, annuity due:

$$FV = Annuity \times (FVFA_{i,n+1} - 1)$$

- Future value formula, ordinary annuity:

$$FV = Annuity \times FVFA_{i,n}$$

- Future value formula, period < 1 year:

$$FV = PV \times (1 + i/m)^{n \times m}$$

- Perpetuity formula:

$$Amount\ of\ Perpetuity = Initial\ Investment \times Interest\ Rate$$

- Present value equation:

$$PV = FV \times 1/(1+i)^n$$

- Present value formula:

$$PV = FV \times PVF_{i,n}$$

- Present value formula, annuity *(beginning)* due:

$$PV = Annuity \times (PVFA_{i,n-1} + 1)$$

- Present value formula, *(end)* ordinary annuity:

$$PV = Annuity \times PVFA_{i,n}$$

- Effective interest rate:

$$Effective\ Interest\ Rate = [(1 + Nominal\ Annual\ Rate\ /\ Compounding\ Periods)^{Compounding\ Periods} - 1]$$

REVIEW QUESTIONS AND PROBLEMS

1. **Definitions.** Define the key terms listed previously.

2. **Simple and compound interest.** What is the difference between simple interest and compound interest?

3. **Defining future value equation terms.** Write out the equation to find the future value of a single amount, and define each of the terms in it.

4. **Defining the exponent.** Does the n in the formula $(1 + i)^n$ always mean compounding on an annual basis?

5. **Multiple compounding periods in a year.** How should the future value equation be modified when compounding occurs more frequently than annually?

6. **Multiple compounding periods in a year.** What is the future value of $10,000 with an interest rate of 16 percent and one annual period of compounding? With an annual interest rate of 16 percent and two semiannual periods of compounding? With an annual interest rate of 16 percent and four quarterly periods of compounding?

7. **Multiple compounding periods in a year.** Referring to the answer to Question 6, explain why the investment increases in value when the number of compounding periods increases.

8. **Present and future value factors.** What is the relationship between the present value factor and the future value factor?

9. **Present value factor and discount rate.** What happens to the present value factor as the discount rate or the interest rate increases for a given time period? As the discount rate or the interest rate decreases?

10. **Relationship between an ordinary annuity and an annuity due.** Compare the present value of a $6,000 ordinary annuity at 10 percent interest for ten years with the present value of a $6,000 annuity due at 10 percent interest for eleven years. Explain the difference.

11. **Perpetuities.** How many years are there in a typical perpetuity?

12. **Factors.** What is the relationship between the future value factor for five years at 5 percent and the present value factor for five years at 5 percent?

13. **Future value of an annuity table.** In the future value annuity table, why is the future value factor for a one-year annuity equal to 1.00 at any interest rate?

14. **Present value of an amount and present value of an annuity.** What is the relationship between the present value of a single dollar payment formula and the present value of an ordinary annuity formula for the same number of years and the same discount rate? Assume a discount rate of 10 percent and an n value of five periods. Explain with an example.

15. If a nurse deposits $12,000 today in a real estate investment trust (REIT) and the interest is compounded annually at 7 percent, what will be the value of this investment:

= increase

   a. Five years from now?

   b. Ten years from now?

   c. Fifteen years from now?

   d. Twenty years from now?

16. If a nurse deposits $24,000 today in a mutual fund that is expected to grow at an annual rate of 8 percent, what will be the value of this investment:

   a. Three years from now?

   b. Six years from now?

   c. Nine years from now?

   d. Twelve years from now?

17. If a business manager deposits $60,000 in a bond fund at the end of each year for twenty years, what will be the value of her investment:

   a. At a compounded rate of 6 percent?

   b. At a compounded rate of 4 percent?

   What would the outcome be in each case if the deposits were made at the beginning of each year?

18. If a business manager deposits $60,000 in a bond fund at the end of each year for twenty years, what will be the value of his investment:

   a. At a compounded rate of 7 percent?

   b. At a compounded rate of 3 percent?

   What would the outcome be in each case if the deposits were made at the beginning of each year?

19. The chief financial officer of a home health agency needs to determine the present value of a $120,000 investment received at the end of year 5. What is the present value if the discount rate is

   a. 3 percent?

   b. 6 percent?

   c. 9 percent?

   d. 12 percent?

20. The chief financial officer of a home health agency needs to determine the present value of a $120,000 investment received at the end of year 20. What is the present value if the discount rate is

    a. 4 percent?

    b. 6 percent?

    c. 8 percent?

    d. 10 percent?

21. If a hospital received $7,500 in payments per year at the end of each year for the next twelve years from an uninsured patient who underwent an expensive operation, what would be the current value of these collection payments:

    a. At a 4 percent rate of return?

    b. At an 8 percent rate of return?

    If the funds were received at the beginning of the year, what would be the current value of these collection payments for each of the two rates of return?

22. If a hospital received $15,000 in payments per year at the end of each year for the next six years from an uninsured patient who underwent an expensive operation, what would be the current value of these collection payments:

    a. At a 3 percent rate of return?

    b. At a 6 percent rate of return?

    If the funds were received at the beginning of the year, what would be the current value of these collection payments for each of the two rates of return?

23. After completing her residency, an obstetrician plans to invest $25,000 per year at the end of each year into a low-risk retirement account. She expects to earn 5 percent for thirty-five years. What will her retirement account be worth at the end of those thirty-five years?

24. After completing his residency, an oncologist plans to invest $30,000 per year at the end of each year into a high-risk retirement account. He expects to earn 7 percent for thirty-five years. What will his retirement account be worth at the end of those thirty-five years?

25. Washington Memorial Hospital has just been informed that a private donor is willing to contribute $15 million per year at the beginning of each year for fifteen years. What is the current dollar value of this contribution if the discount rate is 6 percent?

26. Carson City Hospital has just been informed that a private donor is willing to contribute $20 million per year at the beginning of each year for fifteen years. What is the current dollar value of this contribution if the discount rate is 7 percent?

27. If Uptown clinic invested $3,000 in excess cash today, what would be the value of its investment at the end of three years:

    a. At a 16 percent annual rate compounded semiannually?

    b. At a 16 percent annual rate compounded quarterly?

28. If Summit Hospital invested $10,000 in excess cash today, what would be the value of its investment at the end of three years:

    a. At an 8 percent annual rate compounded semiannually?

    b. At an 8 percent annual rate compounded quarterly?

29. Erie General Hospital wants to purchase a new blood analyzing device today. Its local bank is willing to lend it the money to buy the analyzer at a 2 percent monthly rate. The loan payments will start at the end of the month and will be $2,600 per month for the next eighteen months. What is the purchase price of the device?

30. Memorial Hospital wants to purchase a new MRI machine today. Its local bank is willing to lend it the money to buy the MRI machine at a 1 percent monthly rate. The loan payments will start at the end of the month and will be $100,000 per month for the next thirty months. What is the purchase price of the MRI machine?

31. Regal Medical Center is starting an endowment fund to pay for the expenses of a medical research program. The expenses are $5 million per year, and the program is expected to last ten years. Assuming payments are made at the end of each year and the interest rate is 9 percent per year, what should be the initial size of the endowment?

32. Downtown Medical Center is starting an endowment fund to pay for the expenses of a community outreach pediatric program. The expenses are $800,000 per year, and the program is expected to last five years. Assuming payments are made at the end of each year and the interest rate is 7 percent per year, what should be the size of the initial endowment?

33. In 2010, James County Hospital's total patient revenues were $30 million. In 2019, patient revenues are expected to be $60 million. What is the compound growth rate in patient revenues over this time period?

34. In 2011, King County Hospital's total patient revenues were $15 million. In 2020, patient revenues are expected to be $38.37 million. What is the compound growth rate in patient revenues over this time period?

35. Upland Family Practice Center plans to invest $60,000 in a money market account at the beginning of each year for the next five years. The investment pays 3 percent annual interest. How much would this investment be worth after five years of investing?

36. Starting today and every six months thereafter for the next ten years, St. Joan's Hospital plans to invest $1,750,000 at 5 percent semiannual interest in an account. How much would this investment be worth after ten years of investing?

37. Dr. Rivas plans to retire today and would like an income of $500,000 per year for the next fifteen years, with the income payments starting one year from today. He will be able to earn interest of 6 percent per year compounded annually from his investment account. What must he deposit today in his investment account to achieve this income of $500,000 per year?

38. Today Hopewell Hospital lends its Home Health Care Center $938,510. The center expects to repay the loan in quarterly installments of $100,000 for three years, with the first payment starting one quarter from now. What annual interest rate is the hospital charging for this loan?

39. Big Sky Cancer Research Institute just received a $4 million gift to cover the salary for a permanent research scientist to study Hodgkin's disease, in perpetuity. What would be the required rate of return on the investment if the position paid an annual salary of

   a. $175,000 per year?

   b. $200,000 per year?

   c. $225,000 per year?

40. Upon the untimely and tragic death of their wealthy uncle, his heirs wanted to memorialize him with a named donation to the local hospital. They offered the hospital a choice of $60,000 annual payments forever or a lump sum payment of $700,000 today:

   a. What should be the decision if the hospital thinks it could earn an average of 5 percent annually on this donation?

   b. What should be the decision if the hospital thinks it could earn an average of 9 percent annually on this donation?

   c. What should be the decision if the hospital thinks it could earn an average of 13 percent annually on this donation?

41. Darby Hospital is borrowing $81 million for its medical office building. The annual interest rate is 4 percent. What will be the equal annual payments on the loan if the length of the loan is four years and payments occur at the end of each year?

42. Lima Nursing Home is investing in a restricted fund for a new assisted living home that will cost $16 million. How much does it need to invest each year to have $16 million in fifteen years:

   a. If the expected rate of return on the investment is 7 percent, and the hospital invests at the end of each year?

   b. If the expected rate of return on the investment is 7 percent, and the hospital invests at the beginning of each year?

43. Bishop Sheen Hospital is evaluating a lease arrangement for its ambulance fleet. The total value of the lease is $620,000. The hospital will be making equal monthly payments starting today.

   a. What is the monthly interest rate if the lease payments are $50,000 per month for twenty-four months?

   b. What is the monthly interest rate if the lease payments are $50,000 per month for thirty-six months?

c. What is the monthly interest rate if the lease payments are $60,000 per month for thirty-six months?

44. A wealthy philanthropist has established the following endowment for a hospital. The details of the endowment include the following:

a. A cash deposit of $19 million one year from now.

b. An annual cash deposit of $14 million per year for the next fifteen years. The first $14 million deposit will be made today.

c. At the end of year 15, the hospital will also receive a lump sum payment of $26 million.

Assuming the cost of money is 4 percent, what is the value of this endowment in today's dollars?

45. Devon Hospital is reviewing the details of several bank loans. Bank A offers a nominal rate of 8 percent compounded semiannually. Bank B offers a nominal rate of 8 percent compounded quarterly. Bank C offers a nominal rate of 8 percent compounded monthly. What is the effective rate of each loan, and which loan should the hospital accept?

46. Holy Spirit Hospital is reviewing the details of several bank loans. Bank A offers a nominal rate of 6 percent compounded semiannually. Bank B offers a nominal rate of 6 percent compounded quarterly. Bank C offers a nominal rate of 6 percent compounded monthly. What is the effective rate of each loan, and which loan should the hospital accept?

Appendix B: Future and Present Value Tables

Appendix B presents precalculated tables to assist in determining future and present values (FV and PV). Future value is used to determine the future value of dollar payments made earlier; present value indicates the current value of future dollars. Although the formulas to compute these values appear in Chapter Six, precalculated tables provide a quick and flexible reference for this information.

Appendix B presents this information in four ways. Table B.1 presents the future value factor (FVF) of $1: what the future value of a single investment today will be worth at a future time at a given interest rate. Table B.2 reflects the future value factor of an annuity (FVFA): what the future value of an annuity received or invested over equal time periods will be worth at a future time, given a specified interest rate and number of periods involved. Table B.3 provides the present value factor (PVF) of $1: how much a single, one time amount to be received in the future at a specified interest rate is worth today. Table B.4 reflects the present value factor of an annuity (PVFA): the amount an annuity is worth today at a specified rate from equal flows received at the end of a specified number of periods.

Table B.1 Future value factor of $1: $FVF_{i,n} = PV(1 + i)^n$; $FV = PV \times (FVF_{i,n})$

Period	1%	2%	3%	4%	5%	6%	7%	8%	9%	10%	11%	12%	13%	14%	15%
1	1.0100	1.0200	1.0300	1.0400	1.0500	1.0600	1.0700	1.0800	1.0900	1.1000	1.1100	1.1200	1.1300	1.1400	1.1500
2	1.0201	1.0404	1.0609	1.0816	1.1025	1.1236	1.1449	1.1664	1.1881	1.2100	1.2321	1.2544	1.2769	1.2996	1.3225
3	1.0303	1.0612	1.0927	1.1249	1.1576	1.1910	1.2250	1.2597	1.2950	1.3310	1.3676	1.4049	1.4429	1.4815	1.5209
4	1.0406	1.0824	1.1249	1.1699	1.2155	1.2625	1.3108	1.3605	1.4116	1.4641	1.5181	1.5735	1.6305	1.6890	1.7490
5	1.0510	1.1041	1.1593	1.2167	1.2763	1.3382	1.4026	1.4693	1.5386	1.6105	1.6851	1.7623	1.8424	1.9254	2.0114
6	1.0615	1.1262	1.1941	1.2653	1.3401	1.4185	1.5007	1.5869	1.6771	1.7716	1.8704	1.9738	2.0820	2.1950	2.3131
7	1.0721	1.1487	1.2299	1.3159	1.4071	1.5036	1.6058	1.7138	1.8280	1.9487	2.0762	2.2107	2.3526	2.5023	2.6600
8	1.0829	1.1717	1.2668	1.3686	1.4775	1.5938	1.7182	1.8509	1.9926	2.1436	2.3045	2.4760	2.6584	2.8526	3.0590
9	1.0937	1.1951	1.3048	1.4233	1.5513	1.6895	1.8385	1.9990	2.1719	2.3579	2.5580	2.7731	3.0040	3.2519	3.5179
10	1.1046	1.2190	1.3439	1.4802	1.6289	1.7908	1.9672	2.1589	2.3674	2.5937	2.8394	3.1058	3.3946	3.7072	4.0456
11	1.1157	1.2434	1.3842	1.5395	1.7103	1.8983	2.1049	2.3316	2.5804	2.8531	3.1518	3.4785	3.8359	4.2262	4.6524
12	1.1268	1.2682	1.4258	1.6010	1.7959	2.0122	2.2522	2.5182	2.8127	3.1384	3.4985	3.8960	4.3345	4.8179	5.3503
13	1.1381	1.2936	1.4685	1.6651	1.8856	2.1329	2.4098	2.7196	3.0658	3.4523	3.8833	4.3635	4.8980	5.4924	6.1528
14	1.1495	1.3195	1.5126	1.7317	1.9799	2.2609	2.5785	2.9372	3.3417	3.7975	4.3104	4.8871	5.5348	6.2613	7.0757
15	1.1610	1.3459	1.5580	1.8009	2.0789	2.3966	2.7590	3.1722	3.6425	4.1772	4.7846	5.4736	6.2543	7.1379	8.1371
16	1.1726	1.3728	1.6047	1.8730	2.1829	2.5404	2.9522	3.4259	3.9703	4.5950	5.3109	6.1304	7.0673	8.1372	9.3576
17	1.1843	1.4002	1.6528	1.9479	2.2920	2.6928	3.1588	3.7000	4.3276	5.0545	5.8951	6.8660	7.9861	9.2765	10.761
18	1.1961	1.4282	1.7024	2.0258	2.4066	2.8543	3.3799	3.9960	4.7171	5.5599	6.5436	7.6900	9.0243	10.575	12.375
19	1.2081	1.4568	1.7535	2.1068	2.5270	3.0256	3.6165	4.3157	5.1417	6.1159	7.2633	8.6128	10.197	12.056	14.232
20	1.2202	1.4859	1.8061	2.1911	2.6533	3.2071	3.8697	4.6610	5.6044	6.7275	8.0623	9.6463	11.523	13.743	16.367
21	1.2324	1.5157	1.8603	2.2788	2.7860	3.3996	4.1406	5.0338	6.1088	7.4002	8.9492	10.804	13.021	15.668	18.822
22	1.2447	1.5460	1.9161	2.3699	2.9253	3.6035	4.4304	5.4365	6.6586	8.1403	9.9336	12.100	14.714	17.861	21.645
23	1.2572	1.5769	1.9736	2.4647	3.0715	3.8197	4.7405	5.8715	7.2579	8.9543	11.026	13.552	16.627	20.362	24.891
24	1.2697	1.6084	2.0328	2.5633	3.2251	4.0489	5.0724	6.3412	7.9111	9.8497	12.239	15.179	18.788	23.212	28.625
25	1.2824	1.6406	2.0938	2.6658	3.3864	4.2919	5.4274	6.8485	8.6231	10.835	13.585	17.000	21.231	26.462	32.919
26	1.2953	1.6734	2.1566	2.7725	3.5557	4.5494	5.8074	7.3964	9.3992	11.918	15.080	19.040	23.991	30.167	37.857
27	1.3082	1.7069	2.2213	2.8834	3.7335	4.8223	6.2139	7.9881	10.245	13.110	16.739	21.325	27.109	34.390	43.535
28	1.3213	1.7410	2.2879	2.9987	3.9201	5.1117	6.6488	8.6271	11.167	14.421	18.580	23.884	30.633	39.204	50.066
29	1.3345	1.7758	2.3566	3.1187	4.1161	5.4184	7.1143	9.3173	12.172	15.863	20.624	26.750	34.616	44.693	57.575
30	1.3478	1.8114	2.4273	3.2434	4.3219	5.7435	7.6123	10.063	13.268	17.449	22.892	29.960	39.116	50.950	66.212
35	1.4166	1.9999	2.8139	3.9461	5.5160	7.6861	10.677	14.785	20.414	28.102	38.575	52.800	72.069	98.100	133.18
40	1.4889	2.2080	3.2620	4.8010	7.0400	10.286	14.974	21.725	31.409	45.259	65.001	93.051	132.78	188.88	267.86
45	1.5648	2.4379	3.7816	5.8412	8.9850	13.765	21.002	31.920	48.327	72.890	109.53	163.99	244.64	363.68	538.77
50	1.6446	2.6916	4.3839	7.1067	11.467	18.420	29.457	46.902	74.358	117.39	184.56	289.00	450.74	700.23	1,083.7

Period	16%	17%	18%	19%	20%	21%	22%	23%	24%	25%	30%	35%	40%	45%	50%
1	1.1600	1.1700	1.1800	1.1900	1.2000	1.2100	1.2200	1.2300	1.2400	1.2500	1.3000	1.3500	1.4000	1.4500	1.5000
2	1.3456	1.3689	1.3924	1.4161	1.4400	1.4641	1.4884	1.5129	1.5376	1.5625	1.6900	1.8225	1.9600	2.1025	2.2500
3	1.5609	1.6016	1.6430	1.6852	1.7280	1.7716	1.8158	1.8609	1.9066	1.9531	2.1970	2.4604	2.7440	3.0486	3.3750
4	1.8106	1.8739	1.9388	2.0053	2.0736	2.1436	2.2153	2.2889	2.3642	2.4414	2.8561	3.3215	3.8416	4.4205	5.0625
5	2.1003	2.1924	2.2878	2.3864	2.4883	2.5937	2.7027	2.8153	2.9316	3.0518	3.7129	4.4840	5.3782	6.4097	7.5938
6	2.4364	2.5652	2.6996	2.8398	2.9860	3.1384	3.2973	3.4628	3.6352	3.8147	4.8268	6.0534	7.5295	9.2941	11.391
7	2.8262	3.0012	3.1855	3.3793	3.5832	3.7975	4.0227	4.2593	4.5077	4.7684	6.2749	8.1722	10.541	13.476	17.086
8	3.2784	3.5115	3.7589	4.0214	4.2998	4.5950	4.9077	5.2389	5.5895	5.9605	8.1573	11.032	14.758	19.541	25.629
9	3.8030	4.1084	4.4355	4.7854	5.1598	5.5599	5.9874	6.4439	6.9310	7.4506	10.604	14.894	20.661	28.334	38.443
10	4.4114	4.8068	5.2338	5.6947	6.1917	6.7275	7.3046	7.9259	8.5944	9.3132	13.786	20.107	28.925	41.085	57.665
11	5.1173	5.6240	6.1759	6.7767	7.4301	8.1403	8.9117	9.7489	10.657	11.642	17.922	27.144	40.496	59.573	86.498
12	5.9360	6.5801	7.2876	8.0642	8.9161	9.8497	10.872	11.991	13.215	14.552	23.298	36.644	56.694	86.381	129.75
13	6.8858	7.6987	8.5994	9.5964	10.699	11.918	13.264	14.749	16.386	18.190	30.288	49.470	79.371	125.25	194.62
14	7.9875	9.0075	10.147	11.420	12.839	14.421	16.182	18.141	20.319	22.737	39.374	66.784	111.12	181.62	291.93
15	9.2655	10.539	11.974	13.590	15.407	17.449	19.742	22.314	25.196	28.422	51.186	90.158	155.57	263.34	437.89
16	10.748	12.330	14.129	16.172	18.488	21.114	24.086	27.446	31.243	35.527	66.542	121.71	217.80	381.85	656.84
17	12.468	14.426	16.672	19.244	22.186	25.548	29.384	33.759	38.741	44.409	86.504	164.31	304.91	553.68	985.26
18	14.463	16.879	19.673	22.901	26.623	30.913	35.849	41.523	48.039	55.511	112.46	221.82	426.88	802.83	1,477.9
19	16.777	19.748	23.214	27.252	31.948	37.404	43.736	51.074	59.568	69.389	146.19	299.46	597.63	1,164.1	2,216.8
20	19.461	23.106	27.393	32.429	38.338	45.259	53.358	62.821	73.864	86.736	190.05	404.27	836.68	1,688.0	3,325.3
21	22.574	27.034	32.324	38.591	46.005	54.764	65.096	77.269	91.592	108.42	247.06	545.77	1,171.4	2,447.5	4,987.9
22	26.186	31.629	38.142	45.923	55.206	66.264	79.418	95.041	113.57	135.53	321.18	736.79	1,639.9	3,548.9	7,481.8
23	30.376	37.006	45.008	54.649	66.247	80.180	96.889	116.90	140.83	169.41	417.54	994.66	2,295.9	5,145.9	11,223
24	35.236	43.297	53.109	65.032	79.497	97.017	118.21	143.79	174.63	211.76	542.80	1,342.8	3,214.2	7,461.6	16,834
25	40.874	50.658	62.669	77.388	95.396	117.39	144.21	176.86	216.54	264.70	705.64	1,812.8	4,499.9	10,819	25,251
26	47.414	59.270	73.949	92.092	114.48	142.04	175.94	217.54	268.51	330.87	917.33	2,447.2	6,299.8	15,688	37,877
27	55.000	69.345	87.260	109.59	137.37	171.87	214.64	267.57	332.95	413.59	1,192.5	3,303.8	8,819.8	22,748	56,815
28	63.800	81.134	102.97	130.41	164.84	207.97	261.86	329.11	412.86	516.99	1,550.3	4,460.1	12,348	32,984	85,223
29	74.009	94.927	121.50	155.19	197.81	251.64	319.47	404.81	511.95	646.23	2,015.4	6,021.1	17,287	47,827	127,834
30	85.850	111.06	143.37	184.68	237.38	304.48	389.76	497.91	634.82	807.79	2,620.0	8,128.5	24,201	69,349	191,751
35	180.31	243.50	328.00	440.70	590.67	789.75	1,053.4	1,401.8	1,861.1	2,465.2	9,727.9	36,449	130,161	444,509	1,456,110
40	378.72	533.87	750.38	1,051.7	1,469.8	2,048.4	2,847.0	3,946.4	5,455.9	7,523.2	36,119	163,437	700,038	2,849,181	11,057,332
45	795.44	1,170.5	1,716.7	2,509.7	3,657.3	5,313.0	7,694.7	11,110	15,995	22,959	134,107	732,858	3,764,971	18,262,495	83,966,617
50	1,670.7	2,566.2	3,927.4	5,988.9	9,100.4	13,781	20,797	31,279	46,890	70,065	497,929	3,286,158	20,248,916	117,057,734	637,621,500

Table B.2 Future value factor of an annuity (FVFA): future value factor of an annuity of $1: $FVFA_{i,n} = [(1 + i)^n - 1]/i$; $FVA = PMT$ or annuity $\times (FVFA_{i,n})$

Period	1%	2%	3%	4%	5%	6%	7%	8%	9%	10%	11%	12%	13%	14%	15%
1	1.0000	1.0000	1.0000	1.0000	1.0000	1.0000	1.0000	1.0000	1.0000	1.0000	1.0000	1.0000	1.0000	1.0000	1.0000
2	2.0100	2.0200	2.0300	2.0400	2.0500	2.0600	2.0700	2.0800	2.0900	2.1000	2.1100	2.1200	2.1300	2.1400	2.1500
3	3.0301	3.0604	3.0909	3.1216	3.1525	3.1836	3.2149	3.2464	3.2781	3.3100	3.3421	3.3744	3.4069	3.4396	3.4725
4	4.0604	4.1216	4.1836	4.2465	4.3101	4.3746	4.4399	4.5061	4.5731	4.6410	4.7097	4.7793	4.8498	4.9211	4.9934
5	5.1010	5.2040	5.3091	5.4163	5.5256	5.6371	5.7507	5.8666	5.9847	6.1051	6.2278	6.3528	6.4803	6.6101	6.7424
6	6.1520	6.3081	6.4684	6.6330	6.8019	6.9753	7.1533	7.3359	7.5233	7.7156	7.9129	8.1152	8.3227	8.5355	8.7537
7	7.2135	7.4343	7.6625	7.8983	8.1420	8.3938	8.6540	8.9228	9.2004	9.4872	9.7833	10.089	10.405	10.730	11.067
8	8.2857	8.5830	8.8923	9.2142	9.5491	9.8975	10.260	10.637	11.028	11.436	11.859	12.300	12.757	13.233	13.727
9	9.3685	9.7546	10.159	10.583	11.027	11.491	11.978	12.488	13.021	13.579	14.164	14.776	15.416	16.085	16.786
10	10.462	10.950	11.464	12.006	12.578	13.181	13.816	14.487	15.193	15.937	16.722	17.549	18.420	19.337	20.304
11	11.567	12.169	12.808	13.486	14.207	14.972	15.784	16.645	17.560	18.531	19.561	20.655	21.814	23.045	24.349
12	12.683	13.412	14.192	15.026	15.917	16.870	17.888	18.977	20.141	21.384	22.713	24.133	25.650	27.271	29.002
13	13.809	14.680	15.618	16.627	17.713	18.882	20.141	21.495	22.953	24.523	26.212	28.029	29.985	32.089	34.352
14	14.947	15.974	17.086	18.292	19.599	21.015	22.550	24.215	26.019	27.975	30.095	32.393	34.883	37.581	40.505
15	16.097	17.293	18.599	20.024	21.579	23.276	25.129	27.152	29.361	31.772	34.405	37.280	40.417	43.842	47.580
16	17.258	18.639	20.157	21.825	23.657	25.673	27.888	30.324	33.003	35.950	39.190	42.753	46.672	50.980	55.717
17	18.430	20.012	21.762	23.698	25.840	28.213	30.840	33.750	36.974	40.545	44.501	48.884	53.739	59.118	65.075
18	19.615	21.412	23.414	25.645	28.132	30.906	33.999	37.450	41.301	45.599	50.396	55.750	61.725	68.394	75.836
19	20.811	22.841	25.117	27.671	30.539	33.760	37.379	41.446	46.018	51.159	56.939	63.440	70.749	78.969	88.212
20	22.019	24.297	26.870	29.778	33.066	36.786	40.995	45.762	51.160	57.275	64.203	72.052	80.947	91.025	102.44
21	23.239	25.783	28.676	31.969	35.719	39.993	44.865	50.423	56.765	64.002	72.265	81.699	92.470	104.77	118.81
22	24.472	27.299	30.537	34.248	38.505	43.392	49.006	55.457	62.873	71.403	81.214	92.503	105.49	120.44	137.63
23	25.716	28.845	32.453	36.618	41.430	46.996	53.436	60.893	69.532	79.543	91.148	104.60	120.20	138.30	159.28
24	26.973	30.422	34.426	39.083	44.502	50.816	58.177	66.765	76.790	88.497	102.17	118.16	136.83	158.66	184.17
25	28.243	32.030	36.459	41.646	47.727	54.865	63.249	73.106	84.701	98.347	114.41	133.33	155.62	181.87	212.79
26	29.526	33.671	38.553	44.312	51.113	59.156	68.676	79.954	93.324	109.18	128.00	150.33	176.85	208.33	245.71
27	30.821	35.344	40.710	47.084	54.669	63.706	74.484	87.351	102.72	121.10	143.08	169.37	200.84	238.50	283.57
28	32.129	37.051	42.931	49.968	58.403	68.528	80.698	95.339	112.97	134.21	159.82	190.70	227.95	272.89	327.10
29	33.450	38.792	45.219	52.966	62.323	73.640	87.347	103.97	124.14	148.63	178.40	214.58	258.58	312.09	377.17
30	34.785	40.568	47.575	56.085	66.439	79.058	94.461	113.28	136.31	164.49	199.02	241.33	293.20	356.79	434.75
35	41.660	49.994	60.462	73.652	90.320	111.43	138.24	172.32	215.71	271.02	341.59	431.66	546.68	693.57	881.17
40	48.886	60.402	75.401	95.026	120.80	154.76	199.64	259.06	337.88	442.59	581.83	767.09	1,013.7	1,342.0	1,779.1
45	56.481	71.893	92.720	121.03	159.70	212.74	285.75	386.51	525.86	718.90	986.64	1,358.2	1,874.2	2,590.6	3,585.1
50	64.463	84.579	112.80	152.67	209.35	290.34	406.53	573.77	815.08	1,163.9	1,668.8	2,400.0	3,459.5	4,994.5	7,217.7

Period	16%	17%	18%	19%	20%	21%	22%	23%	24%	25%	30%	35%	40%	45%	50%
1	1.0000	1.0000	1.0000	1.0000	1.0000	1.0000	1.0000	1.0000	1.0000	1.0000	1.0000	1.0000	1.0000	1.0000	1.0000
2	2.1600	2.1700	2.1800	2.1900	2.2000	2.2100	2.2200	2.2300	2.2400	2.2500	2.3000	2.3500	2.4000	2.4500	2.5000
3	3.5056	3.5389	3.5724	3.6061	3.6400	3.6741	3.7084	3.7429	3.7776	3.8125	3.9900	4.1725	4.3600	4.5525	4.7500
4	5.0665	5.1405	5.2154	5.2913	5.3680	5.4457	5.5242	5.6038	5.6842	5.7656	6.1870	6.6329	7.1040	7.6011	8.1250
5	6.8771	7.0144	7.1542	7.2966	7.4416	7.5892	7.7396	7.8926	8.0484	8.2070	9.0431	9.9544	10.946	12.022	13.188
6	8.9775	9.2068	9.4420	9.6830	9.9299	10.183	10.442	10.708	10.980	11.259	12.756	14.438	16.324	18.431	20.781
7	11.414	11.772	12.142	12.523	12.916	13.321	13.740	14.171	14.615	15.073	17.583	20.492	23.853	27.725	32.172
8	14.240	14.773	15.327	15.902	16.499	17.119	17.762	18.430	19.123	19.842	23.858	28.664	34.395	41.202	49.258
9	17.519	18.285	19.086	19.923	20.799	21.714	22.670	23.669	24.712	25.802	32.015	39.696	49.153	60.743	74.887
10	21.321	22.393	23.521	24.709	25.959	27.274	28.657	30.113	31.643	33.253	42.619	54.590	69.814	89.077	113.33
11	25.733	27.200	28.755	30.404	32.150	34.001	35.962	38.039	40.238	42.566	56.405	74.697	98.739	130.16	171.00
12	30.850	32.824	34.931	37.180	39.581	42.142	44.874	47.788	50.895	54.208	74.327	101.84	139.23	189.73	257.49
13	36.786	39.404	42.219	45.244	48.497	51.991	55.746	59.779	64.110	68.760	97.625	138.48	195.93	276.12	387.24
14	43.672	47.103	50.818	54.841	59.196	63.909	69.010	74.528	80.496	86.949	127.91	187.95	275.30	401.37	581.86
15	51.660	56.110	60.965	66.261	72.035	78.330	85.192	92.669	100.82	109.69	167.29	254.74	386.42	582.98	873.79
16	60.925	66.649	72.939	79.850	87.442	95.780	104.93	114.98	126.01	138.11	218.47	344.90	541.99	846.32	1,311.7
17	71.673	78.979	87.068	96.022	105.93	116.89	129.02	142.43	157.25	173.64	285.01	466.61	759.78	1,228.2	1,968.5
18	84.141	93.406	103.74	115.27	128.12	142.44	158.40	176.19	195.99	218.04	371.52	630.92	1,064.7	1,781.8	2,953.8
19	98.603	110.28	123.41	138.17	154.74	173.35	194.25	217.71	244.03	273.56	483.97	852.75	1,491.6	2,584.7	4,431.7
20	115.38	130.03	146.63	165.42	186.69	210.76	237.99	268.79	303.60	342.94	630.17	1,152.2	2,089.2	3,748.8	6,648.5
21	134.84	153.14	174.02	197.85	225.03	256.02	291.35	331.61	377.46	429.68	820.22	1,556.5	2,925.9	5,436.7	9,973.8
22	157.41	180.17	206.34	236.44	271.03	310.78	356.44	408.88	469.06	538.10	1,067.3	2,102.3	4,097.2	7,884.3	14,962
23	183.60	211.80	244.49	282.36	326.24	377.05	435.86	503.92	582.63	673.63	1,388.5	2,839.0	5,737.1	11,433	22,443
24	213.98	248.81	289.49	337.01	392.48	457.22	532.75	620.82	723.46	843.03	1,806.0	3,833.7	8,033.0	16,579	33,666
25	249.21	292.10	342.60	402.04	471.98	554.24	650.96	764.61	898.09	1,054.8	2,348.8	5,176.5	11,247	24,041	50,500
26	290.09	342.76	405.27	479.43	567.38	671.63	795.17	941.46	1,114.6	1,319.5	3,054.4	6,989.3	15,747	34,860	75,752
27	337.50	402.03	479.22	571.52	681.85	813.68	971.10	1,159.0	1,383.1	1,650.4	3,971.8	9,436.5	22,047	50,548	113,628
28	392.50	471.38	566.48	681.11	819.22	985.55	1,185.7	1,426.6	1,716.1	2,064.0	5,164.3	12,740	30,867	73,296	170,443
29	456.30	552.51	669.45	811.52	984.07	1,193.5	1,447.6	1,755.7	2,129.0	2,580.9	6,714.6	17,200	43,214	106,280	255,666
30	530.31	647.44	790.95	966.71	1,181.9	1,445.2	1,767.1	2,160.5	2,640.9	3,227.2	8,730.0	23,222	60,501	154,107	383,500
35	1,120.7	1,426.5	1,816.7	2,314.2	2,948.3	3,755.9	4,783.6	6,090.3	7,750.2	9,856.8	32,423	104,136	325,400	987,794	2,912,217
40	2,360.8	3,134.5	4,163.2	5,529.8	7,343.9	9,749.5	12,937	17,154	22,729	30,089	120,393	466,960	1,750,092	6,331,512	22,114,663
45	4,965.3	6,879.3	9,531.6	13,203	18,281	25,295	34,971	48,302	66,640	91,831	447,019	2,093,876	9,412,424	40,583,319	167,933,233
50	10,436	15,090	21,813	31,515	45,497	65,617	94,525	135,992	195,373	280,256	1,659,761	9,389,020	50,622,288	260,128,295	1,275,242,998

Table B.3 Present value factor of $1: $PVF_{i,n} = 1/(1+i)^n$; $PV = FV \times (PVF_{i,n})$

Period	1%	2%	3%	4%	5%	6%	7%	8%	9%	10%	11%	12%	13%	14%	15%
1	0.9901	0.9804	0.9709	0.9615	0.9524	0.9434	0.9346	0.9259	0.9174	0.9091	0.9009	0.8929	0.8850	0.8772	0.8696
2	0.9803	0.9612	0.9426	0.9246	0.9070	0.8900	0.8734	0.8573	0.8417	0.8264	0.8116	0.7972	0.7831	0.7695	0.7561
3	0.9706	0.9423	0.9151	0.8890	0.8638	0.8396	0.8163	0.7938	0.7722	0.7513	0.7312	0.7118	0.6931	0.6750	0.6575
4	0.9610	0.9238	0.8885	0.8548	0.8227	0.7921	0.7629	0.7350	0.7084	0.6830	0.6587	0.6355	0.6133	0.5921	0.5718
5	0.9515	0.9057	0.8626	0.8219	0.7835	0.7473	0.7130	0.6806	0.6499	0.6209	0.5935	0.5674	0.5428	0.5194	0.4972
6	0.9420	0.8880	0.8375	0.7903	0.7462	0.7050	0.6663	0.6302	0.5963	0.5645	0.5346	0.5066	0.4803	0.4556	0.4323
7	0.9327	0.8706	0.8131	0.7599	0.7107	0.6651	0.6227	0.5835	0.5470	0.5132	0.4817	0.4523	0.4251	0.3996	0.3759
8	0.9235	0.8535	0.7894	0.7307	0.6768	0.6274	0.5820	0.5403	0.5019	0.4665	0.4339	0.4039	0.3762	0.3506	0.3269
9	0.9143	0.8368	0.7664	0.7026	0.6446	0.5919	0.5439	0.5002	0.4604	0.4241	0.3909	0.3606	0.3329	0.3075	0.2843
10	0.9053	0.8203	0.7441	0.6756	0.6139	0.5584	0.5083	0.4632	0.4224	0.3855	0.3522	0.3220	0.2946	0.2697	0.2472
11	0.8963	0.8043	0.7224	0.6496	0.5847	0.5268	0.4751	0.4289	0.3875	0.3505	0.3173	0.2875	0.2607	0.2366	0.2149
12	0.8874	0.7885	0.7014	0.6246	0.5568	0.4970	0.4440	0.3971	0.3555	0.3186	0.2858	0.2567	0.2307	0.2076	0.1869
13	0.8787	0.7730	0.6810	0.6006	0.5303	0.4688	0.4150	0.3677	0.3262	0.2897	0.2575	0.2292	0.2042	0.1821	0.1625
14	0.8700	0.7579	0.6611	0.5775	0.5051	0.4423	0.3878	0.3405	0.2992	0.2633	0.2320	0.2046	0.1807	0.1597	0.1413
15	0.8613	0.7430	0.6419	0.5553	0.4810	0.4173	0.3624	0.3152	0.2745	0.2394	0.2090	0.1827	0.1599	0.1401	0.1229
16	0.8528	0.7284	0.6232	0.5339	0.4581	0.3936	0.3387	0.2919	0.2519	0.2176	0.1883	0.1631	0.1415	0.1229	0.1069
17	0.8444	0.7142	0.6050	0.5134	0.4363	0.3714	0.3166	0.2703	0.2311	0.1978	0.1696	0.1456	0.1252	0.1078	0.0929
18	0.8360	0.7002	0.5874	0.4936	0.4155	0.3503	0.2959	0.2502	0.2120	0.1799	0.1528	0.1300	0.1108	0.0946	0.0808
19	0.8277	0.6864	0.5703	0.4746	0.3957	0.3305	0.2765	0.2317	0.1945	0.1635	0.1377	0.1161	0.0981	0.0829	0.0703
20	0.8195	0.6730	0.5537	0.4564	0.3769	0.3118	0.2584	0.2145	0.1784	0.1486	0.1240	0.1037	0.0868	0.0728	0.0611
21	0.8114	0.6598	0.5375	0.4388	0.3589	0.2942	0.2415	0.1987	0.1637	0.1351	0.1117	0.0926	0.0768	0.0638	0.0531
22	0.8034	0.6468	0.5219	0.4220	0.3418	0.2775	0.2257	0.1839	0.1502	0.1228	0.1007	0.0826	0.0680	0.0560	0.0462
23	0.7954	0.6342	0.5067	0.4057	0.3256	0.2618	0.2109	0.1703	0.1378	0.1117	0.0907	0.0738	0.0601	0.0491	0.0402
24	0.7876	0.6217	0.4919	0.3901	0.3101	0.2470	0.1971	0.1577	0.1264	0.1015	0.0817	0.0659	0.0532	0.0431	0.0349
25	0.7798	0.6095	0.4776	0.3751	0.2953	0.2330	0.1842	0.1460	0.1160	0.0923	0.0736	0.0588	0.0471	0.0378	0.0304
26	0.7720	0.5976	0.4637	0.3607	0.2812	0.2198	0.1722	0.1352	0.1064	0.0839	0.0663	0.0525	0.0417	0.0331	0.0264
27	0.7644	0.5859	0.4502	0.3468	0.2678	0.2074	0.1609	0.1252	0.0976	0.0763	0.0597	0.0469	0.0369	0.0291	0.0230
28	0.7568	0.5744	0.4371	0.3335	0.2551	0.1956	0.1504	0.1159	0.0895	0.0693	0.0538	0.0419	0.0326	0.0255	0.0200
29	0.7493	0.5631	0.4243	0.3207	0.2429	0.1846	0.1406	0.1073	0.0822	0.0630	0.0485	0.0374	0.0289	0.0224	0.0174
30	0.7419	0.5521	0.4120	0.3083	0.2314	0.1741	0.1314	0.0994	0.0754	0.0573	0.0437	0.0334	0.0256	0.0196	0.0151
35	0.7059	0.5000	0.3554	0.2534	0.1813	0.1301	0.0937	0.0676	0.0490	0.0356	0.0259	0.0189	0.0139	0.0102	0.0075
40	0.6717	0.4529	0.3066	0.2083	0.1420	0.0972	0.0668	0.0460	0.0318	0.0221	0.0154	0.0107	0.0075	0.0053	0.0037
45	0.6391	0.4102	0.2644	0.1712	0.1113	0.0727	0.0476	0.0313	0.0207	0.0137	0.0091	0.0061	0.0041	0.0027	0.0019
50	0.6080	0.3715	0.2281	0.1407	0.0872	0.0543	0.0339	0.0213	0.0134	0.0085	0.0054	0.0035	0.0022	0.0014	0.0009

Period	16 %	17 %	18 %	19 %	20 %	21 %	22 %	23 %	24 %	25 %	30 %	35 %	40 %	45 %	50 %
1	0.8621	0.8547	0.8475	0.8403	0.8333	0.8264	0.8197	0.8130	0.8065	0.8000	0.7692	0.7407	0.7143	0.6897	0.6667
2	0.7432	0.7305	0.7182	0.7062	0.6944	0.6830	0.6719	0.6610	0.6504	0.6400	0.5917	0.5487	0.5102	0.4756	0.4444
3	0.6407	0.6244	0.6086	0.5934	0.5787	0.5645	0.5507	0.5374	0.5245	0.5120	0.4552	0.4064	0.3644	0.3280	0.2963
4	0.5523	0.5337	0.5158	0.4987	0.4823	0.4665	0.4514	0.4369	0.4230	0.4096	0.3501	0.3011	0.2603	0.2262	0.1975
5	0.4761	0.4561	0.4371	0.4190	0.4019	0.3855	0.3700	0.3552	0.3411	0.3277	0.2693	0.2230	0.1859	0.1560	0.1317
6	0.4104	0.3898	0.3704	0.3521	0.3349	0.3186	0.3033	0.2888	0.2751	0.2621	0.2072	0.1652	0.1328	0.1076	0.0878
7	0.3538	0.3332	0.3139	0.2959	0.2791	0.2633	0.2486	0.2348	0.2218	0.2097	0.1594	0.1224	0.0949	0.0742	0.0585
8	0.3050	0.2848	0.2660	0.2487	0.2326	0.2176	0.2038	0.1909	0.1789	0.1678	0.1226	0.0906	0.0678	0.0512	0.0390
9	0.2630	0.2434	0.2255	0.2090	0.1938	0.1799	0.1670	0.1552	0.1443	0.1342	0.0943	0.0671	0.0484	0.0353	0.0260
10	0.2267	0.2080	0.1911	0.1756	0.1615	0.1486	0.1369	0.1262	0.1164	0.1074	0.0725	0.0497	0.0346	0.0243	0.0173
11	0.1954	0.1778	0.1619	0.1476	0.1346	0.1228	0.1122	0.1026	0.0938	0.0859	0.0558	0.0368	0.0247	0.0168	0.0116
12	0.1685	0.1520	0.1372	0.1240	0.1122	0.1015	0.0920	0.0834	0.0757	0.0687	0.0429	0.0273	0.0176	0.0116	0.0077
13	0.1452	0.1299	0.1163	0.1042	0.0935	0.0839	0.0754	0.0678	0.0610	0.0550	0.0330	0.0202	0.0126	0.0080	0.0051
14	0.1252	0.1110	0.0985	0.0876	0.0779	0.0693	0.0618	0.0551	0.0492	0.0440	0.0254	0.0150	0.0090	0.0055	0.0034
15	0.1079	0.0949	0.0835	0.0736	0.0649	0.0573	0.0507	0.0448	0.0397	0.0352	0.0195	0.0111	0.0064	0.0038	0.0023
16	0.0930	0.0811	0.0708	0.0618	0.0541	0.0474	0.0415	0.0364	0.0320	0.0281	0.0150	0.0082	0.0046	0.0026	0.0015
17	0.0802	0.0693	0.0600	0.0520	0.0451	0.0391	0.0340	0.0296	0.0258	0.0225	0.0116	0.0061	0.0033	0.0018	0.0010
18	0.0691	0.0592	0.0508	0.0437	0.0376	0.0323	0.0279	0.0241	0.0208	0.0180	0.0089	0.0045	0.0023	0.0012	0.0007
19	0.0596	0.0506	0.0431	0.0367	0.0313	0.0267	0.0229	0.0196	0.0168	0.0144	0.0068	0.0033	0.0017	0.0009	0.0005
20	0.0514	0.0433	0.0365	0.0308	0.0261	0.0221	0.0187	0.0159	0.0135	0.0115	0.0053	0.0025	0.0012	0.0006	0.0003
21	0.0443	0.0370	0.0309	0.0259	0.0217	0.0183	0.0154	0.0129	0.0109	0.0092	0.0040	0.0018	0.0009	0.0004	0.0002
22	0.0382	0.0316	0.0262	0.0218	0.0181	0.0151	0.0126	0.0105	0.0088	0.0074	0.0031	0.0014	0.0006	0.0003	0.0001
23	0.0329	0.0270	0.0222	0.0183	0.0151	0.0125	0.0103	0.0086	0.0071	0.0059	0.0024	0.0010	0.0004	0.0002	0.0001
24	0.0284	0.0231	0.0188	0.0154	0.0126	0.0103	0.0085	0.0070	0.0057	0.0047	0.0018	0.0007	0.0003	0.0001	0.0001
25	0.0245	0.0197	0.0160	0.0129	0.0105	0.0085	0.0069	0.0057	0.0046	0.0038	0.0014	0.0006	0.0002	0.0001	0.0001
26	0.0211	0.0169	0.0135	0.0109	0.0087	0.0070	0.0057	0.0046	0.0037	0.0030	0.0011	0.0004	0.0002	0.0001	0.0000
27	0.0182	0.0144	0.0115	0.0091	0.0073	0.0058	0.0047	0.0037	0.0030	0.0024	0.0008	0.0003	0.0001	0.0000	0.0000
28	0.0157	0.0123	0.0097	0.0077	0.0061	0.0048	0.0038	0.0030	0.0024	0.0019	0.0006	0.0002	0.0001	0.0000	0.0000
29	0.0135	0.0105	0.0082	0.0064	0.0051	0.0040	0.0031	0.0025	0.0020	0.0015	0.0005	0.0002	0.0001	0.0000	0.0000
30	0.0116	0.0090	0.0070	0.0054	0.0042	0.0033	0.0026	0.0020	0.0016	0.0012	0.0004	0.0001	0.0001	0.0000	0.0000
35	0.0055	0.0041	0.0030	0.0023	0.0017	0.0013	0.0009	0.0007	0.0005	0.0004	0.0001	0.0000	0.0000	0.0000	0.0000
40	0.0026	0.0019	0.0013	0.0010	0.0007	0.0005	0.0004	0.0003	0.0002	0.0001	0.0000	0.0000	0.0000	0.0000	0.0000
45	0.0013	0.0009	0.0006	0.0004	0.0003	0.0002	0.0001	0.0001	0.0001	0.0000	0.0000	0.0000	0.0000	0.0000	0.0000
50	0.0006	0.0004	0.0003	0.0002	0.0001	0.0001	0.0000	0.0000	0.0000	0.0000	0.0000	0.0000	0.0000	0.0000	0.0000

Table B.4 Present value factor of an annuity (PVFA): present value factor of an annuity of $1: $PVFA_{i,n} = [1 - 1/(1 + i)^n]/i$; $PVA = PMT$ or annuity $\times (PVFA_{i,n})$

Period	1%	2%	3%	4%	5%	6%	7%	8%	9%	10%	11%	12%	13%	14%	15%
1	0.9901	0.9804	0.9709	0.9615	0.9524	0.9434	0.9346	0.9259	0.9174	0.9091	0.9009	0.8929	0.8850	0.8772	0.8696
2	1.9704	1.9416	1.9135	1.8861	1.8594	1.8334	1.8080	1.7833	1.7591	1.7355	1.7125	1.6901	1.6681	1.6467	1.6257
3	2.9410	2.8839	2.8286	2.7751	2.7232	2.6730	2.6243	2.5771	2.5313	2.4869	2.4437	2.4018	2.3612	2.3216	2.2832
4	3.9020	3.8077	3.7171	3.6299	3.5460	3.4651	3.3872	3.3121	3.2397	3.1699	3.1024	3.0373	2.9745	2.9137	2.8550
5	4.8534	4.7135	4.5797	4.4518	4.3295	4.2124	4.1002	3.9927	3.8897	3.7908	3.6959	3.6048	3.5172	3.4331	3.3522
6	5.7955	5.6014	5.4172	5.2421	5.0757	4.9173	4.7665	4.6229	4.4859	4.3553	4.2305	4.1114	3.9975	3.8887	3.7845
7	6.7282	6.4720	6.2303	6.0021	5.7864	5.5824	5.3893	5.2064	5.0330	4.8684	4.7122	4.5638	4.4226	4.2883	4.1604
8	7.6517	7.3255	7.0197	6.7327	6.4632	6.2098	5.9713	5.7466	5.5348	5.3349	5.1461	4.9676	4.7988	4.6389	4.4873
9	8.5660	8.1622	7.7861	7.4353	7.1078	6.8017	6.5152	6.2469	5.9952	5.7590	5.5370	5.3282	5.1317	4.9464	4.7716
10	9.4713	8.9826	8.5302	8.1109	7.7217	7.3601	7.0236	6.7101	6.4177	6.1446	5.8892	5.6502	5.4262	5.2161	5.0188
11	10.368	9.7868	9.2526	8.7605	8.3064	7.8869	7.4987	7.1390	6.8052	6.4951	6.2065	5.9377	5.6869	5.4527	5.2337
12	11.255	10.575	9.9540	9.3851	8.8633	8.3838	7.9427	7.5361	7.1607	6.8137	6.4924	6.1944	5.9176	5.6603	5.4206
13	12.134	11.348	10.635	9.9856	9.3936	8.8527	8.3577	7.9038	7.4869	7.1034	6.7499	6.4235	6.1218	5.8424	5.5831
14	13.004	12.106	11.296	10.563	9.8986	9.2950	8.7455	8.2442	7.7862	7.3667	6.9819	6.6282	6.3025	6.0021	5.7245
15	13.865	12.849	11.938	11.118	10.380	9.7122	9.1079	8.5595	8.0607	7.6061	7.1909	6.8109	6.4624	6.1422	5.8474
16	14.718	13.578	12.561	11.652	10.838	10.106	9.4466	8.8514	8.3126	7.8237	7.3792	6.9740	6.6039	6.2651	5.9542
17	15.562	14.292	13.166	12.166	11.274	10.477	9.7632	9.1216	8.5436	8.0216	7.5488	7.1196	6.7291	6.3729	6.0472
18	16.398	14.992	13.754	12.659	11.690	10.828	10.059	9.3719	8.7556	8.2014	7.7016	7.2497	6.8399	6.4674	6.1280
19	17.226	15.678	14.324	13.134	12.085	11.158	10.336	9.6036	8.9501	8.3649	7.8393	7.3658	6.9380	6.5504	6.1982
20	18.046	16.351	14.877	13.590	12.462	11.470	10.594	9.8181	9.1285	8.5136	7.9633	7.4694	7.0248	6.6231	6.2593
21	18.857	17.011	15.415	14.029	12.821	11.764	10.836	10.017	9.2922	8.6487	8.0751	7.5620	7.1016	6.6870	6.3125
22	19.660	17.658	15.937	14.451	13.163	12.042	11.061	10.201	9.4424	8.7715	8.1757	7.6446	7.1695	6.7429	6.3587
23	20.456	18.292	16.444	14.857	13.489	12.303	11.272	10.371	9.5802	8.8832	8.2664	7.7184	7.2297	6.7921	6.3988
24	21.243	18.914	16.936	15.247	13.799	12.550	11.469	10.529	9.7066	8.9847	8.3481	7.7843	7.2829	6.8351	6.4338
25	22.023	19.523	17.413	15.622	14.094	12.783	11.654	10.675	9.8226	9.0770	8.4217	7.8431	7.3300	6.8729	6.4641
26	22.795	20.121	17.877	15.983	14.375	13.003	11.826	10.810	9.9290	9.1609	8.4881	7.8957	7.3717	6.9061	6.4906
27	23.560	20.707	18.327	16.330	14.643	13.211	11.987	10.935	10.027	9.2372	8.5478	7.9426	7.4086	6.9352	6.5135
28	24.316	21.281	18.764	16.663	14.898	13.406	12.137	11.051	10.116	9.3066	8.6016	7.9844	7.4412	6.9607	6.5335
29	25.066	21.844	19.188	16.984	15.141	13.591	12.278	11.158	10.198	9.3696	8.6501	8.0218	7.4701	6.9830	6.5509
30	25.808	22.396	19.600	17.292	15.372	13.765	12.409	11.258	10.274	9.4269	8.6938	8.0552	7.4957	7.0027	6.5660
35	29.409	24.999	21.487	18.665	16.374	14.498	12.948	11.655	10.567	9.6442	8.8552	8.1755	7.5856	7.0700	6.6166
40	32.835	27.355	23.115	19.793	17.159	15.046	13.332	11.925	10.757	9.7791	8.9511	8.2438	7.6344	7.1050	6.6418
45	36.095	29.490	24.519	20.720	17.774	15.456	13.606	12.108	10.881	9.8628	9.0079	8.2825	7.6609	7.1232	6.6543
50	39.196	31.424	25.730	21.482	18.256	15.762	13.801	12.233	10.962	9.9148	9.0417	8.3045	7.6752	7.1327	6.6605

Period	16%	17%	18%	19%	20%	21%	22%	23%	24%	25%	30%	35%	40%	45%	50%
1	0.8621	0.8547	0.8475	0.8403	0.8333	0.8264	0.8197	0.8130	0.8065	0.8000	0.7692	0.7407	0.7143	0.6897	0.6667
2	1.6052	1.5852	1.5656	1.5465	1.5278	1.5095	1.4915	1.4740	1.4568	1.4400	1.3609	1.2894	1.2245	1.1653	1.1111
3	2.2459	2.2096	2.1743	2.1399	2.1065	2.0739	2.0422	2.0114	1.9813	1.9520	1.8161	1.6959	1.5889	1.4933	1.4074
4	2.7982	2.7432	2.6901	2.6386	2.5887	2.5404	2.4936	2.4483	2.4043	2.3616	2.1662	1.9969	1.8492	1.7195	1.6049
5	3.2743	3.1993	3.1272	3.0576	2.9906	2.9260	2.8636	2.8035	2.7454	2.6893	2.4356	2.2200	2.0352	1.8755	1.7366
6	3.6847	3.5892	3.4976	3.4098	3.3255	3.2446	3.1669	3.0923	3.0205	2.9514	2.6427	2.3852	2.1680	1.9831	1.8244
7	4.0386	3.9224	3.8115	3.7057	3.6046	3.5079	3.4155	3.3270	3.2423	3.1611	2.8021	2.5075	2.2628	2.0573	1.8829
8	4.3436	4.2072	4.0776	3.9544	3.8372	3.7256	3.6193	3.5179	3.4212	3.3289	2.9247	2.5982	2.3306	2.1085	1.9220
9	4.6065	4.4506	4.3030	4.1633	4.0310	3.9054	3.7863	3.6731	3.5655	3.4631	3.0190	2.6653	2.3790	2.1438	1.9480
10	4.8332	4.6586	4.4941	4.3389	4.1925	4.0541	3.9232	3.7993	3.6819	3.5705	3.0915	2.7150	2.4136	2.1681	1.9653
11	5.0286	4.8364	4.6560	4.4865	4.3271	4.1769	4.0354	3.9018	3.7757	3.6564	3.1473	2.7519	2.4383	2.1849	1.9769
12	5.1971	4.9884	4.7932	4.6105	4.4392	4.2784	4.1274	3.9852	3.8514	3.7251	3.1903	2.7792	2.4559	2.1965	1.9846
13	5.3423	5.1183	4.9095	4.7147	4.5327	4.3624	4.2028	4.0530	3.9124	3.7801	3.2233	2.7994	2.4685	2.2045	1.9897
14	5.4675	5.2293	5.0081	4.8023	4.6106	4.4317	4.2646	4.1082	3.9616	3.8241	3.2487	2.8144	2.4775	2.2100	1.9931
15	5.5755	5.3242	5.0916	4.8759	4.6755	4.4890	4.3152	4.1530	4.0013	3.8593	3.2682	2.8255	2.4839	2.2138	1.9954
16	5.6685	5.4053	5.1624	4.9377	4.7296	4.5364	4.3567	4.1894	4.0333	3.8874	3.2832	2.8337	2.4885	2.2164	1.9970
17	5.7487	5.4746	5.2223	4.9897	4.7746	4.5755	4.3908	4.2190	4.0591	3.9099	3.2948	2.8398	2.4918	2.2182	1.9980
18	5.8178	5.5339	5.2732	5.0333	4.8122	4.6079	4.4187	4.2431	4.0799	3.9279	3.3037	2.8443	2.4941	2.2195	1.9986
19	5.8775	5.5845	5.3162	5.0700	4.8435	4.6346	4.4415	4.2627	4.0967	3.9424	3.3105	2.8476	2.4958	2.2203	1.9991
20	5.9288	5.6278	5.3527	5.1009	4.8696	4.6567	4.4603	4.2786	4.1103	3.9539	3.3158	2.8501	2.4970	2.2209	1.9994
21	5.9731	5.6648	5.3837	5.1268	4.8913	4.6750	4.4756	4.2916	4.1212	3.9631	3.3198	2.8519	2.4979	2.2213	1.9996
22	6.0113	5.6964	5.4099	5.1486	4.9094	4.6900	4.4882	4.3021	4.1300	3.9705	3.3230	2.8533	2.4985	2.2216	1.9997
23	6.0442	5.7234	5.4321	5.1668	4.9245	4.7025	4.4985	4.3106	4.1371	3.9764	3.3254	2.8543	2.4989	2.2218	1.9998
24	6.0726	5.7465	5.4509	5.1822	4.9371	4.7128	4.5070	4.3176	4.1428	3.9811	3.3272	2.8550	2.4992	2.2219	1.9999
25	6.0971	5.7662	5.4669	5.1951	4.9476	4.7213	4.5139	4.3232	4.1474	3.9849	3.3286	2.8556	2.4994	2.2220	1.9999
26	6.1182	5.7831	5.4804	5.2060	4.9563	4.7284	4.5196	4.3278	4.1511	3.9879	3.3297	2.8560	2.4996	2.2221	1.9999
27	6.1364	5.7975	5.4919	5.2151	4.9636	4.7342	4.5243	4.3316	4.1542	3.9903	3.3305	2.8563	2.4997	2.2221	1.9999
28	6.1520	5.8099	5.5016	5.2228	4.9697	4.7390	4.5281	4.3346	4.1566	3.9923	3.3312	2.8565	2.4998	2.2222	2.0000
29	6.1656	5.8204	5.5098	5.2292	4.9747	4.7430	4.5312	4.3371	4.1585	3.9938	3.3317	2.8567	2.4999	2.2222	2.0000
30	6.1772	5.8294	5.5168	5.2347	4.9789	4.7463	4.5338	4.3391	4.1601	3.9950	3.3321	2.8568	2.4999	2.2222	2.0000
35	6.2153	5.8582	5.5386	5.2512	4.9915	4.7559	4.5411	4.3447	4.1644	3.9984	3.3330	2.8571	2.5000	2.2222	2.0000
40	6.2335	5.8713	5.5482	5.2582	4.9966	4.7596	4.5439	4.3467	4.1659	3.9995	3.3332	2.8571	2.5000	2.2222	2.0000
45	6.2421	5.8773	5.5523	5.2611	4.9986	4.7610	4.5449	4.3474	4.1664	3.9998	3.3333	2.8571	2.5000	2.2222	2.0000
50	6.2463	5.8801	5.5541	5.2623	4.9995	4.7616	4.5452	4.3477	4.1666	3.9999	3.3333	2.8571	2.5000	2.2222	2.0000

Note

1. One could also use the RATE financial function, which will be discussed in the upcoming section on how to solve for the interest rate of a loan, by inserting 7 for Nper value, setting the patient revenue value of 20X0 equal to Pv and patient revenue value of 20X7 equal to Fv. You will also need to convert one of the patient revenue values to a negative number.

CHAPTER 7

THE INVESTMENT DECISION

Capital investment decisions involve large monetary investments expected to achieve long-term benefits for an organization. Such investments, common in health care, fall into three categories:

- **Strategic decisions:** Capital investment decisions designed to increase a health care organization's strategic (long-term) position (e.g., purchasing physician practices to increase horizontal integration)

- **Expansion decisions:** Capital investment decisions designed to increase the operational capability of a health care organization (e.g., increasing examination space in a group practice to accommodate increased volume)

- **Replacement decisions:** Capital investment decisions designed to replace older assets with newer, cost-saving ones (e.g., replacing a hospital's existing cost-accounting system with a newer, cost-saving one)

A capital investment decision has two components: determining if the investment is worthwhile, and determining how to finance the investment. Although these two decisions are interrelated, they should be separated. This chapter focuses on the first component: determining whether a capital investment should be undertaken. It is organized around three factors important to analyzing capital investment decisions: the objectives of capital investment analysis, three techniques to analyze capital investment decisions, and technical concerns in capital budgeting. Chapter Eight focuses on capital financing alternatives. Perspectives 7.1 and 7.2 offer some examples of capital investments.

LEARNING OBJECTIVES

- Explain the financial objectives of health care providers.

- Evaluate various capital investment alternatives.

- Calculate and interpret net present value (NPV).

- Calculate and interpret the internal rate of return (IRR).

Capital Investment Decision
A decision involving a high-dollar investment expected to achieve long-term benefits for an organization.

Strategic Decision
A capital investment decision designed to increase a health care organization's strategic (long-term) position.

Expansion Decision
A capital investment decision designed to increase the operational capability of a health care organization.

Caution: Although the issues of whether an investment is worthwhile and how to finance that investment are interrelated, they should be considered separately.

Replacement Decision

A capital investment decision designed to replace older assets with newer (often cost-saving) ones.

Objectives of Capital Investment Analysis

A capital investment is expected to achieve long-term benefits for the organization that generally fall into three categories: nonfinancial benefits,

PERSPECTIVE 7.1 TYPES OF CAPITAL BUDGETING DECISIONS TO BE MADE IN THE FUTURE UNDER HEALTH REFORM

A managing director for Navigant consulting firm observes that a health care system will require some capital investment in the plant and equipment of its hospitals in order to improve patient outcomes and patient safety, which are critical elements of health reform requirements. He notes that a health care system that renovates and redesigns the physical layout of its hospitals to achieve technology integration as well as process improvement will do a better job in coordinating care, especially among its critical services such as emergency department care, diagnostics, and therapeutic services. Strategically, he notes that health care systems will more than likely invest more in ambulatory care services while investing less in inpatient services. However, the external planning of these decisions will require financial analysis to support them.

The consultant also believes that health care systems' strategic growth initiatives going forward will include the following:

1. Growing ambulatory care offerings while scaling back on inpatient services

2. Renovating an inefficient hospital in its current location or building a newer one with higher capital investment but greater long-term operational benefits

3. Eliminating or consolidating duplicative services to reduce costs

4. Optimizing locations by identifying and developing a retail orientation, which will include having more ambulatory settings to make preventive and primary care more accessible, which will in turn reduce costs

However, to finance these capital decisions, health care systems and hospitals will need capital. The consultant also underscores that hospitals without access to capital may need to find capital partners through mergers, affiliations, joint ventures, or other third-party sources.

Source: Adapted from L. Dunn, Don't overlook facilities' role in meeting health reform's imperatives, *Becker's Hospital Review*, November 22, 2011, www.beckershospitalreview.com/hospital-management-administration/dont-overlook-facilities-role-in-meeting-health-reforms-imperatives.html.

PERSPECTIVE 7.2 CONSTRUCTION SURVEY GIVES INSIGHT ON FUTURE HOSPITAL REVENUE AND NONREVENUE CAPITAL PROJECTS

The 2012 annual construction survey by *Healthcare Facilities Management* and the American Society for Healthcare Engineering provides insight on the type of capital investments hospitals will be making in the future. The survey found that only 19 percent of the 531 hospitals completing the survey are planning on new hospital construction. However, 26 percent of the responding hospitals also indicated that these plans are being reevaluated; 19 percent of the responding hospitals are less likely to proceed and 23 percent of the hospitals will definitely not proceed. In addition, almost 75 percent of the hospitals indicated that they will revise, review, or possibly not go ahead with capital projects for facility renovation. This downturn in capital investment stems from the uncertainty associated with health care reform and a downturn in profit margins. In addition, hospitals have indicated that they are placing a greater emphasis on the return on investment of their projects. As one respondent hospital stated, in its capital decisions it is putting "more focus on ROI and justification of all costs." In terms of future capital allocation, hospitals are allocating just 16 percent for new construction, which is half of what they did in the prior year, and 21 percent for renovation projects.

A greater allocation is being budgeted for non-revenue-generating capital projects related to infrastructure, such as chillers, boilers, and air handlers, because equipment of this nature is deteriorating and its use is being extended beyond its expected life. In terms of revenue-generating building projects, hospitals are focused on constructing interventional suites, which combine surgery and imaging, as well as tech-laden emergency departments. They are also focused on capital investments in laboratories, as science and technology are playing an increasingly strong role in medicine. Projecting allocation out by type of capital expenditures: 17 percent of responding hospitals mentioned emergency departments, 16 percent medical office expansion, and 16 percent primary care clinics. The hiring of physicians, especially specialists, is an underlying reason for the construction of medical office buildings.

Source: Adapted from D. Carpenter and S. Hoppszallern, Time to build? Reform uncertainties drive financial scrutiny for new projects, *Health Facilities Management*, 2012;25:2:12–18, 20, www.unboundmedicine.com/medline/citation/22413615/Time_to_build_Reform_uncertainties_drive_financial_scrutiny_for_new_projects.

financial returns, and the ability to attract more funds in the future (see Exhibit 7.1). Clearly, these three objectives are highly interrelated. In the following discussion, it is important to keep in mind that *investors* are not just those external to an organization. When an organization purchases new assets or starts a new program, it is also an investor: it is investing in itself.

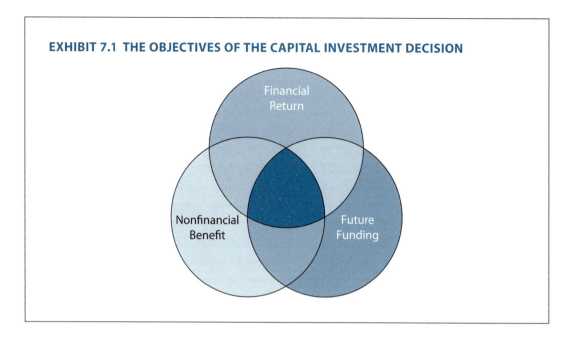

EXHIBIT 7.1 THE OBJECTIVES OF THE CAPITAL INVESTMENT DECISION

Financial Return

Nonfinancial Benefit

Future Funding

Nonfinancial Benefits

How well an investment enhances the survival of the organization and supports its mission, patients, employees, and the community is a primary concern in many capital investment decisions. A particularly interesting movement in health care is the increasing number of governmental agencies with taxing authority asking for proof of community benefit. Community benefits include increased access to different types of care, higher quality of care, lower charges, the provision of charity care, and the employment of community members, as illustrated in Perspective 7.3.

Financial Returns

Direct financial benefits are a primary concern not only to health care organizations but also to many—if not all—investors who invest in health care organizations and their projects. Direct financial benefits to investors can take two forms. The first is periodic payments in the form of dividends to stockholders or interest to bondholders, or both. (Bonds are discussed in Chapter Eight.) *Dividends* represent the portion of profit that an organization distributes to equity investors, whereas *interest* is a payment to creditors, those who have loaned the organization funds or otherwise extended credit.

PERSPECTIVE 7.3 MAYO CLINIC: AN EXAMPLE OF COMMUNITY BENEFIT IN CAPITAL DECISIONS

The CFO of the Mayo Clinic presents his perspective on the clinic's nonprofit mission and its capital decisions on how to expend its profits in terms like these: "As a humanitarian not-for-profit organization, Mayo Clinic is not in the business of making money for money's sake," and, "All earnings are reinvested into programs and initiatives that are aimed at advancing our mission." Over the next five years Mayo is expected to spend $700 million per year in capital projects. Sixty percent of its capital dollars are earmarked for internal renewal and replacement projects and 40 percent for external strategic efforts. It is noteworthy that some projects in prior years were not viewed as ones that would generate a return on investment. Mayo has started building two proton beam therapy facilities, which are experimental cancer treatment centers that intend to target cancer cells without affecting healthy tissue. Critics argue that a project of this nature is expensive and the proton beam therapy's clinical benefits are unproven. However, the CEO of Mayo supported the investment, stating that the proton beam therapy facility is "motivated by the best interests of our patients, not 'profit' or competitiveness."

Source: Adapted from B. Herman, Mayo Clinic earnings rise 18 percent, large capital project plans announced, *Becker's Hospital Review*, February 23, 2012, www.beckershospitalreview.com/racs-/-icd-9-/-icd-10/mayo-clinic -earnings-rise-18-large-capital-project-plans-announced.html.

The second type of benefit to an investor comes in the form of *retained earnings*, the portion of the profits the organization keeps in-house to use for growth and to support its mission. This describes the plowing back or investing of funds (including retained earnings) into capital projects that appreciate in value. *Capital appreciation* takes place whenever an investment is worth more when it is sold than when it was purchased. For investor-owned organizations, this appreciation in value increases the value of investors' stock.

Although almost all organizations can make periodic payments to their investors in the form of interest, by law only investor-owned health care organizations can distribute dividends outside the organization.

Retained Earnings
The portion of profits an organization keeps for itself to use for growth and to support its mission.

Capital Appreciation
A gain that occurs when an asset is worth more when sold than when purchased. Common examples of assets that may produce capital appreciation are land, property, and stocks.

Ability to Attract Funds in the Future

Without new capital funds, many health care organizations would be unable to offer new services, support medical research, or subsidize unprofitable services. Therefore, another objective of capital investment is to invest in profitable projects or services that will attract debt (borrowing) and equity financing in the future by external investors. (Capital financing is discussed at length in Chapter Eight. Capital financing includes funds from a variety of sources, such as governmental entities, foundations, and community-based organizations.)

Analytical Methods

An investment decision involves many factors (see Perspectives 7.4 and 7.5). Three commonly used financial techniques to analyze capital investment decisions for health care organizations are

- Payback method
- Net present value method
- Internal rate of return method

 Key Point Until now, this book has stressed the accrual method of accounting. However, the techniques introduced in this chapter—payback, net present value (NPV), and the internal rate of return (IRR)—use only cash flows. Therefore, when only accrual information is available (such as information from financial statements), accrual items must be converted into cash flows. An example is shown in the discussion of net present value.

Suppose Marquee Valley Hospital has $1 million available to invest in a new business (Exhibit 7.2, rows 1 and 3). After examining the market-

---

PERSPECTIVE 7.4 EXAMPLE OF A REPLACEMENT PROJECT WITH COST SAVINGS AND PAYBACK

A hospital in Queens, New York, installed an energy efficient central chiller plant. In addition, the new chiller system was intended to produce an overall improvement in the efficiency of the hospital's air-conditioning system. The previous chiller had an annual utility cost of $500,000, while the newer, efficient version costs $350,000 to operate, which results in a cash savings of $150,000 in utility costs. In addition, the hospital expects to achieve maintenance savings of $15,000 per year. To purchase and install the new system was expected to require a capital outlay of $1.9 million. Taking into account the operational savings, along with an energy rebate from the state, this New York hospital expected a payback period of just over ten years.

Source: New York Hospital Queens, Chiller replacement project 2011, www.nyhq.org/oth/Page.asp?PageID =OTH001604.

PERSPECTIVE 7.5 PUBLICLY TRADED HOSPITAL MANAGEMENT COMPANY JOINT VENTURES WITH AN ACADEMIC MEDICAL CENTER TO HELP BOTH COMPANIES EXPAND STRATEGICALLY

On January 2011, LifePoint Hospitals, Inc., a publicly traded hospital management company on the New York Stock Exchange, developed a joint venture arrangement with Duke University Health System to own and operate community hospitals. The Duke-LifePoint partnership is willing to consider an array of arrangements with hospitals, ranging from full ownership to joint ventures and shared governance.

Partnering hospitals will have access to the clinical expertise of world-renowned physicians and specialists from Duke and the operational and management expertise of LifePoint, which focuses on nonurban facilities. More importantly Duke can depend upon capital funding from LifePoint to finance replacement facilities and renovations of older facilities as well as the purchase of new health care technology and imaging equipment, such as 64-slice CT machines, MRI machines, and digital mammography machines. In terms of type of hospitals, LifePoint seeks to acquire ones located outside major urban markets, in areas with a growing population base and diversified employment base.

For example, for one hospital acquisition, Duke and LifePoint's capital investment called for building an outpatient surgery center and comprehensive cancer center. In addition, the partnership's capital plans included renovating to create private rooms and investing in new IT infrastructure, especially in emergency departments, so patients would be treated with the proper care and the department would achieve accurate coding and charges for services.

Source: Adapted from Investment Weekly News, Duke LifePoint Healthcare: Marquette General signs memorandum of understanding with Duke LifePoint, *Investment Weekly News*, March 24, 2012, www.verticalnews.com/article.php?articleID=6696017.

place, the hospital has narrowed its possibilities to two promising options, each of which would expend the full amount of money available: it could buy an existing physician practice, or it could build its own small satellite clinic. If it buys the physician practice, it would expect to generate new net cash inflows of $333,333 each year for six years (Exhibit 7.2, row 2). By investing in its own satellite clinic, Marquee Valley could expect to generate net cash flows of $200,000, $250,000, $300,000, $350,000, $450,000, and $650,000 over the next six years (Exhibit 7.2, row 4).

Key Point The term *cash flow* is used interchangeably with *net cash flow*. Net cash flow is the result of subtracting *cash outflows* from *cash inflows*.

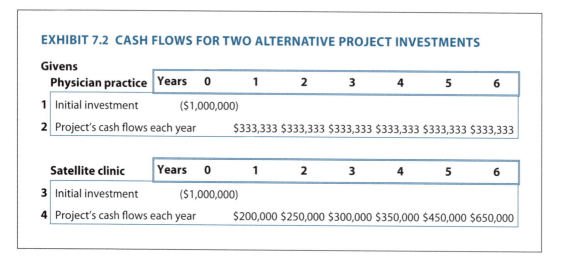

EXHIBIT 7.2 CASH FLOWS FOR TWO ALTERNATIVE PROJECT INVESTMENTS

Givens

Physician practice	Years	0	1	2	3	4	5	6
1 Initial investment		($1,000,000)						
2 Project's cash flows each year			$333,333	$333,333	$333,333	$333,333	$333,333	$333,333

Satellite clinic	Years	0	1	2	3	4	5	6
3 Initial investment		($1,000,000)						
4 Project's cash flows each year			$200,000	$250,000	$300,000	$350,000	$450,000	$650,000

Payback Method

Payback Method
A method to evaluate the feasibility of an investment by determining how long it would take to recover the initial investment, disregarding the time value of money.

One way to analyze these investments is to calculate the time needed to recoup each investment. This is called the *payback method*, and it is illustrated in Exhibit 7.3, which builds on Exhibit 7.2.

Analysis

Exhibit 7.3 shows four rows for each investment: the initial investment, the beginning balance for each year, the cash flow for each year, and the cumulative cash flow for each year, in rows A through D, respectively. Although the satellite clinic begins the fourth year with a $250,000 deficit (row B), it has a positive net cash flow of $350,000 during the year (row C), resulting in a cumulative cash flow by the end of the fourth year of $100,000. Thus, as shown in row D, during the fourth year, the hospital would have recouped its investment. By bringing in $333,333 each year, the physician practice recoups its $1 million investment by the end of the third year. Under either scenario, the hospital would be tying up its money for at least three years.

The actual month that breakeven occurs can be obtained by dividing the deficit at the end of the year before breaking even by the average monthly inflow in the break-even year. For example, the deficit at the end of the third year for the satellite clinic is $250,000, with an average monthly inflow during the fourth year of $29,167 ($350,000 / 12). Thus, Marquee Valley would break even midway through September ($250,000 / $29,167 = 8.6 months) of the fourth year. If it bought the physician practice, it would break even at the end of the third year because it ends year 3 with no deficit.

EXHIBIT 7.3 CALCULATION OF PAYBACK YEAR FOR TWO ALTERNATIVE INVESTMENTS

Physician practice

	Years	0	1	2	3	4	5	6
A	Initial investment[a]	($1,000,000)						
B	Beginning of year balance[b]		($1,000,000)	($666,667)	($333,333)	($0)	$333,333	$666,667
C	Project's cash flows each year[c]		$333,333	$333,333	$333,333	$333,333	$333,333	$333,333
D	Cumulative cash flow (A + B + C)	($1,000,000)	($666,667)	($333,333)	**($0)**	$333,333	$666,667	$1,000,000

[a]Exhibit 7.2, row 1.
[b]Balance from end of previous year, row D.
[c]Exhibit 7.2, row 2.
Break-even year = year 3.

Satellite clinic

	Years	0	1	2	3	4	5	6
A	Initial investment[d]	($1,000,000)						
B	Beginning of year balance[e]		($1,000,000)	($800,000)	($550,000)	($250,000)	$100,000	$550,000
C	Project's cash flows each year[f]		$200,000	$250,000	$300,000	$350,000	$450,000	$650,000
D	Cumulative cash flow (A + B + C)	($1,000,000)	($800,000)	($550,000)	($250,000)	**$100,000**	$550,000	$1,200,000

[d]Exhibit 7.2, row 3.
[e]Balance from end of previous year, row D.
[f]Exhibit 7.2, row 4.
Break-even year = year 4.

If net cash inflows are equal each year (as with the physician practice), the number of years for an investment to break even simply equals the initial investment divided by the annual net cash flows resulting from the investment, and use of a more detailed analysis, such as in Exhibit 7.3, is unnecessary. Thus the payback time for the physician practice would be $1,000,000 / $333,333, which equals three years, the same answer derived in Exhibit 7.3.

Key Point The formula to calculate the break-even point in years when cash flows are equal each year is: Initial Investment / Annual Cash Flows.

Strengths and Weaknesses of the Payback Method

The strengths of the payback method are that it is simple to calculate and easy to understand (see Exhibit 7.4). There are three major weaknesses of the payback method, however: it gives an answer in years, not dollars; it disregards cash flows after the payback time; and it does not account for the time value of money. Each of these is discussed briefly in this section.

- *The payback is in years, not dollars.* Knowing that a project has a payback of three years does not provide certain key financial information, such as the size of the dollar impact on the organization in future years.

- *The payback method disregards cash flows after the payback time.* For example, the physician practice has equal annual cash inflows and a

---

EXHIBIT 7.4 STRENGTHS AND WEAKNESSES OF THE PAYBACK METHOD

Strengths

- Simple to calculate.

- Easy to understand.

Weaknesses

- Answers in years, not dollars.

- Disregards cash flows after payback.

- Does not account for the time value of money.

payback of three years, whereas the satellite clinic has unequal annual cash inflows and does not reach payback until year 4. Thus the physician practice, with its shorter payback, would appear to be the better investment. However, the satellite clinic has better cash flows in later years, and by the end of year 6, it brings in $200,000 more than does the physician practice. Hence, in addition to time until payback, it is important to consider the cash flows after the payback date when making an investment.

- *The payback method does not account for the time value of money.* Chapter Six demonstrated that a dollar received sometime in the future is not worth the same as a dollar received today. The two evaluation methods discussed in the remainder of this chapter, net present value and internal rate of return, take the time value of money into account, whereas the payback method does not.

Net Present Value

Because of the deficiencies of the payback method, a preferred alternative for analyzing capital investments is a net present value analysis. *Net present value* (NPV) is the difference between the initial amount paid for an investment and its associated future cash flows that have been adjusted (discounted) by the cost of capital. The cost of capital includes two costs: first, investors (bondholders and stockholders) are being asked to delay the consumption of their funds by investing in the project (time value of money); and second, these investors face a risk that the investment may not generate the revenues and net cash flows anticipated, leaving them with an inadequate rate of return, or the project may fail altogether, leaving the investors with perhaps nothing other than a tax loss.

On the one hand, if the sum of the *discounted cash flows* resulting from the investment is greater than the initial investment itself, then the NPV is positive. Thus, from a purely financial standpoint, the project is acceptable, all else being equal. On the other hand, if the sum of the discounted cash flows resulting from the investment is less than the initial investment, then over time the investment brings in less than what was initially paid out, the NPV is negative, and the investment should be rejected.

Example of a Net Present Value Analysis: The Satellite Clinic

In the example used earlier the annual cash flows were provided (Exhibit 7.3), but in real-world situations, organizations may not always have such information readily available. Therefore, in the following example (Exhibit 7.5), the same annual cash flows are used as in the previous example

Net Present Value
The difference between the initial amount paid for an investment and the future cash inflows the investment brings in, adjusted for the cost of capital.

Discounted Cash Flows
Cash flows adjusted to account for the cost of capital.

Cost of Capital
The rate of return required to undertake a project; the cost of capital accounts for both the time value of money and risk (also called the *hurdle rate* or *discount rate*).

EXHIBIT 7.5 COMPUTATION OF NPV FOR THE SATELLITE CLINIC

	Years	0	1	2	3	4	5	6
1	Initial investment	($1,000,000)						
2	Net revenue		$400,000	$550,000	$800,000	$900,000	$1,100,000	$1,370,000
3	Cash operating expense		$200,000	$300,000	$500,000	$550,000	$650,000	$850,000
4	Annual depreciation		$145,000	$145,000	$145,000	$145,000	$145,000	$145,000
5	Salvage value (end of year 6)							$130,000
6	Cost of capital	10%						

		Years	0	1	2	3	4	5	6
A	Initial investment	Given 1	($1,000,000)						
B	Net revenue	Given 2		$400,000	$550,000	$800,000	$900,000	$1,100,000	$1,370,000
C	Less: cash operating expenses	Given 3		200,000	300,000	500,000	550,000	650,000	850,000
D	Less: depreciation expense	Given 4		145,000	145,000	145,000	145,000	145,000	145,000
E	Net operating income	B − C − D		55,000	105,000	155,000	205,000	305,000	375,000
F	Add: depreciation expense	Given 4		145,000	145,000	145,000	145,000	145,000	145,000
G	Net operating cash flows	E + F		200,000	250,000	300,000	350,000	450,000	520,000
H	Add: sale of salvage value	Given 5							130,000
I	Project cash flows	G + H		$200,000	$250,000	$300,000	$350,000	$450,000	$650,000
J	Cost of capital	Given 6		10%	10%	10%	10%	10%	10%
K	Present value interest factors[a]	$1/(1+i)^n$		0.9091	0.8264	0.7513	0.6830	0.6209	0.5645
L	Annual PV of cash flows	I × K		$181,818	$206,612	$225,394	$239,055	$279,415	$366,908
M	PV of cash flows	Sum L	$1,499,202						
N	Net present value	A + M	$499,202						

[a]Present value interest factors in the exhibit have been calculated by formula, but are necessarily rounded for presentation. Therefore, there may be a difference between the number displayed and that calculated manually.

($200,000, $250,000, $300,000, $350,000, $450,000, and $650,000), but these numbers had to be derived using additional information commonly found in a budget forecast (revenues, expenses, depreciation, etc).

Key Point The following terms are used interchangeably: *cost of capital, discount rate,* and *hurdle rate.*

To calculate the net present value (NPV) of the satellite clinic alternative (Exhibit 7.5), follow these steps:

Step 1. Identify the initial cash outflow.

Step 2. Determine revenues and expenses (net operating income):

    a. Identify annual net revenues.

    b. Identify annual cash operating expenses and depreciation expense.

    c. Compute annual net income.

Step 3. Add depreciation expense back in to get net operating cash flows.

Step 4. Add (subtract) any nonannual cash flows.

Step 5. Adjust for working capital.

Step 6. Determine the present value of each year's cash flow.

Step 7. Sum the present values of all cash flows.

Step 8. Determine the net present value of the project.

    a. Identify the initial cash outflow (row A).

      • The initial investment in the satellite clinic is $1,000,000.

    b. Determine net operating income (rows B, C, D, and E):

      • Identify annual cash inflows (revenues). Use net revenues rather than gross revenues, to account for discounts and allowances that will not be collected.

      • Identify annual cash operating expenses and depreciation expense.

      • Compute annual net operating income.

    c. Add depreciation back in to compute net operating cash flows (rows F and G).

        The annual expenses (Step 2b) include depreciation expenses, estimated at $145,000 annually. However, depreciation is an expense that does not require any cash outflow. Therefore, to calculate actual cash flows, an amount equal to

Salvage Value
The amount of cash to be received when an asset (e.g., equipment) is sold, usually at the end of its useful life (also called *terminal value, residual value,* or *scrap value*).

depreciation expense is added back into net income, resulting in a higher cash flow.

d.　Add (subtract) any nonannual cash flows (rows H and I).

At times, various nonannual cash flows may occur during a project. In this example, the only nonannual cash flow is a cash inflow in year 6 resulting from selling some assets of the investment project. The *salvage value* is estimated to be $130,000.

Key Point　In deriving the annual cash flows from pro forma operating statements that include depreciation expense, the depreciation expense, and/or any other noncash expense (e.g., amortization of *goodwill*), is added back to the bottom line (operating income).

Key Point　Interest expense should not be included as a cash flow because it is part of financing flows and is included in the discount rate. Therefore, if interest expense is included in the operating expenses, then for the nontaxpaying entity, it should be added back into revenues in excess of expenses or earnings.

Goodwill
The value of intangible factors such as brand reputation, customer or supplier relationships, employee competencies, and the like that are expected to affect an entity's future earning power. An acquiring entity may pay cash and assume liabilities in excess of the fair value of the assets acquired in order to account for this value.

e.　Adjust for working capital.

Some projects affect working capital, and to the extent that this effect is material, it must be considered. This particular example assumes there are no material working capital effects. (This concept is discussed in depth in Appendix D at the end of this chapter.)

f.　Determine the present value of each year's cash flow (rows I, J, K, and L).

Steps 1 through 5 estimate cash flows that will occur each year. Step 6 discounts these cash flows with an assumed discount rate of 10 percent, using the methods discussed in Chapter Six. The $200,000 received at the end of year 1 (row I) is worth $181,818 in today's dollars (row L). The $250,000 received two years from now (row I) is worth only $206,612 today (row L). The cash flows received in years 3 through 6 are discounted similarly.

g.　Sum the present values of all cash flows (row M).

h.　Determine the net present value of the project (rows A, M, and N).

The net present value of the project is the difference between the discounted annual cash flows and the initial investment. The net present value (NPV), $499,202, is computed by adding the initial investment, $1,000,000, a cash outflow, to the present value of the annual cash flows, $1,499,202. If this were the only investment alternative, because the NPV is positive, this investment would be accepted based only on financial criteria.

Key Point The terms *present value* and *net present value* should not be confused. Whereas present value is the sum of discounted future cash flows, net present value is equal to the present value net (less) the cost of the initial investment. Hence, the outcome shown in Exhibit 7.5. Although the present value of the cash flows is $1,499,202 (the sum of the cash flows for years 1 through 6), the net present value is only $499,202 (the cash flows from years 1 through 6 less the cost of the initial $1,000,000 investment).

It is also possible to calculate the NPV of the physician practice introduced in Exhibit 7.2. Because the cash flows from this investment are equal in both amount and timing, they can be treated as an ordinary annuity of $333,333 for six years at 10 percent. The present value factor for this ordinary annuity is 4.3553. Thus the present value of the cash flows is $1,451,765 (4.3553 × $333,333), and the net present value of the physician practice would be $451,765 ($1,451,765 − $1,000,000).

Decision Rules When Using NPV
As noted in Exhibit 7.5, the net present value of the satellite clinic investment, after adjusting for depreciation and salvage value, is $499,202.

- The general decision rule when using NPV is
  - If NPV > 0, accept the project.
  - If NPV < 0, reject the project.
  - If NPV = 0, then accept or reject.

Given this rule, the satellite clinic should be purchased because it has a positive NPV of $499,202. This rule applies in most cases; however, the rule is modified for two other possible situations.

- If two or more mutually exclusive projects are being considered, the one with the higher or highest positive NPV should be chosen. Thus, if a second project were being considered, such as the purchase of the physician practice, the satellite clinic project would be selected for having the higher NPV ($499,202 versus $451,765). Only if the physician practice NPV were higher than the $499,202 would that project be selected instead.

- If two or more mutually exclusive projects are being considered and one must be selected regardless of NPV, then the one with the higher or highest NPV should be chosen, even if its NPV is negative. Suppose a health care organization is considering developing either a burn unit or a school-based education program. An analysis determines that one project has an NPV of –$4,000,000, whereas the other has an NPV of –$1,500,000. If it had been decided in advance that one of the two projects will be undertaken, then the one with the higher NPV (lesser loss) should be chosen. In this case, –$1,500,000 would be the better choice.

Using Spreadsheets to Calculate NPV

Any popular spreadsheet is an ideal platform to calculate net present value because most, if not all, spreadsheets have built-in functions that simplify the determination of NPV. Exhibit 7.6 shows how the NPV function in Excel can be used to compute the present value, $1,499,202, of the annual

EXHIBIT 7.6 USING EXCEL TO CALCULATE THE NET PRESENT VALUE (NPV) OF UNEQUAL ANNUAL CASH FLOWS, ASSUMING A 10 PERCENT DISCOUNT RATE

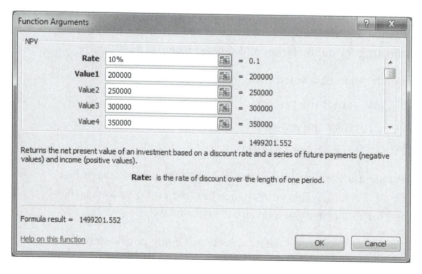

cash flows in Exhibit 7.5 (cash flows for all six years are entered, although only cash flows for the first four years are shown). Excel's NPV function is similar to its PV function, but allows the use of unequal cash flows. Finally, the initial investment, −$1,000,000, must be added outside the NPV function formula, which computes the present value of the annual project cash flows, $1,499,202, to obtain the NPV of $499,202. (A common mistake among users of the NPV function is to include the initial investment as a value in the NPV function formula. The initial investment must be added outside the function and needs to represent the negative outflow for the initial investment.)

 Key Point When using the Excel NPV function, the initial investment value must be added to the NPV function result and not entered as a value within the function itself.

Strengths and Weakness of the NPV Method

The NPV method has a number of strengths and weaknesses (Exhibit 7.7). Its strengths are that it provides an answer in dollars, not years; it accounts for all cash flows in the project, including those beyond the payback period; and it discounts the cash flows by the cost of capital. Its main difficulties are developing estimates of cash flows and the discount rate.

Conceptually, NPV is strong because it accounts for all cash flows in a project and discounts at the cost of capital. However, the cost of capital can be difficult to determine, as discussed in Appendix C.

EXHIBIT 7.7 STRENGTHS AND WEAKNESSES OF AN NPV ANALYSIS

Strengths

- Answers in dollars, not years.
- Accounts for all the cash flows in the project.
- Discounts at the cost of capital.

Weaknesses

- Cash flow estimates may be difficult to develop.
- Discount rate may be difficult to determine.

Internal Rate of Return

The rate of return on an investment that makes the net present value equal to $0, after all cash flows have been discounted at the same rate. It is also the *discount rate* at which the discounted cash flows over the life of the project exactly equal the initial investment.

Internal Rate of Return

The *internal rate of return* (IRR) on an investment can be defined and interpreted several ways. It can mean the discount rate at which the discounted cash flows over the life of the project exactly equal the initial investment, the discount rate that results in a net present value equal to zero, or the percentage return on the investment. (In contrast, NPV is the dollar return on the investment.) The method used to solve for the IRR depends on whether the cash flows are equal or unequal.

Equal Cash Flows

When the cash flows are equal in each period, the IRR can be determined by first finding the present value factor for an annuity and then converting the answer to a discount rate depending on the number of years. Because the physician practice example used earlier has equal cash flows in each period, its IRR can be found by

- Computing the present value factor for an annuity (PVFA) (see Chapter Six):

$$PV = Annuity \times PVFA_{i,n}$$

$$\$1,000,000 = \$333,333 \times PVFA_{i,6}$$

$$PVFA_{i,6} = 3.0$$

- Finding the interest rate that yields this PVFA factor for six periods. In the present value of an annuity table (Appendix B, Table B.4), in the row for six time periods (because the investment is over six years), the column heading for the number closest to 3.0 (the PVFA factor) is the IRR. In this case, the PVFA factor of 3.0 lies somewhere between the 24 percent and 25 percent columns; thus the IRR is approximately 24.5 percent.

Unequal Cash Flows

Business calculators and computer programs make finding the IRR for unequal cash flows relatively easy. Excel's function is called IRR (see Exhibit 7.8). Either all the operating cash flow values of the project, including the initial investment, are entered individually or an array of cells containing these values is referenced (the initial investment must be a negative value in either case because it is a cash outflow). As shown in Exhibit 7.8, the IRR appears at the bottom of the box.

EXHIBIT 7.8 USING EXCEL TO CALCULATE THE IRR FOR A $1 MILLION INVESTMENT WITH UNEQUAL OPERATING CASH FLOWS RECEIVED AT THE END OF EACH OF SIX SUCCESSIVE YEARS

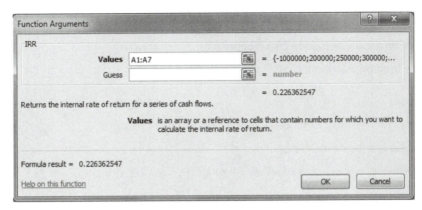

Note: The values in the array A1:A7 = -1000000; 200000; 250000; 300000; 350000; 450000; 650000.

Key Point In contrast to Excel's NPV function, Excel's IRR function requires the initial investment as one of the entries in the function.

Decision Rules When Using the IRR

When an organization chooses a project according to the IRR method, its financial decision depends on the value of the IRR relative to the *required rate of return on the investment* (which is also called the *cost of capital* or *hurdle rate*).

Required Rate of Return
The minimal internal rate of return on any investment that will justify that investment (also called *cost of capital* or *hurdle rate*).

- If the IRR is greater than the required rate of return, the project should be accepted.

- If the IRR is less than the required rate of return, the project should be rejected.

- If the IRR is equal to the required rate of return, the facility should be indifferent about accepting or rejecting the project.

Strengths and Weaknesses of IRR Analysis

IRR has three major strengths as a decision criterion (Exhibit 7.9): it considers all the relevant cash flows related to the investment project, it is a time value of money–based approach, and managers are accustomed to

---

EXHIBIT 7.9 STRENGTHS AND WEAKNESSES OF THE IRR ANALYSIS

Strengths

- Considers all relevant cash flows of the investment project.
- Takes a time value of money–based approach.
- Widely used by practitioners and easily understood.

Weaknesses

- Assumes reinvestment of proceeds at the internal rate of return.
- Estimates may be difficult to develop.
- Can generate multiple rates of return if future cash flows are estimates.

---

evaluating projects by their respective rates of return. IRR also has three weaknesses as a decision criterion: it assumes that proceeds are reinvested at the internal rate of return, which may or may not be equal to the cost of capital; developing estimates of cash flows is difficult; and the IRR sometimes generates multiple rates of return, if future cash flows are estimates. Still, this method is widely used in industry as the preferred way to make responsible investment decisions.

Using an NPV Analysis for a Replacement Decision

The previous analyses have focused on situations in which an organization was interested in either expanding its existing services or offering a new service altogether. However, a common and more complicated analysis is the *replacement decision*, which must be made by an organization when it contemplates replacing an older, existing asset with a newer, more cost-efficient one. There are two ways to undertake this problem, both using a net present value (NPV) approach and both yielding the same result. The first approach is to compare the NPV of continuing as is with the NPV of the replacement alternative, with the preferred investment alternative being the one yielding the higher NPV. The second approach is to perform a single NPV analysis using the *incremental differences* brought about by replacing an asset. If the single NPV is positive, then the replacement alternative is preferred.

Example

Assume that a radiology department in a not-for-profit hospital is considering renovating its X-ray processing area with new equipment that is faster and produces better, more reliable images. The existing equipment was purchased five years ago for $1,150,000 and is being depreciated on a *straight-line* basis over a ten-year life to a $150,000 salvage value. The old equipment can be sold now for its current book value of $650,000 ($1,150,000 original cost less $500,000 in accumulated depreciation).

Straight-Line Depreciation
A depreciation method that depreciates an asset an equal amount each year until it reaches its salvage value at the end of its useful life.

The new equipment can be purchased for $1,500,000 and is estimated to have a five-year life. It would be depreciated on a straight-line basis to a $750,000 salvage value. The radiology department is a revenue-producing center. Presently, forty-five patients per day, 260 days per year, can be screened by one radiology technologist at an average reimbursement of $75 per test, but a significant portion of these patients must be given a second test at no additional charge because the first image is inconclusive. The new equipment, because it is not only faster but produces images of better quality, can process sixty patients per day. (The hospital believes that sufficient demand exists to fully utilize the higher capacity of the new equipment.) An in-depth discussion of how to estimate future cash flows is found in Appendix C.

The old equipment costs $60,000 per year in utilities and maintenance. The new equipment would cost $30,000 per year in utilities and maintenance. The annual labor expenses will not change because one radiology technologist is needed to operate either piece of equipment. Cost of capital for this organization is 9 percent.

Solution

Exhibits 7.10a and 7.10b present the *comparative approach* to solving this problem. This approach employs the same eight steps outlined in Exhibit 7.5. An NPV is calculated for each alternative, and then the NPVs are compared to determine which is higher. Exhibit 7.11 uses an alternative method, the *incremental approach*, to solve the same problem. Instead of calculating two NPVs and comparing them, this approach calculates a single NPV based on marginal differences for each cash flow. The results are exactly the same.

Using the comparative approach, the net present value (NPV) over the next five years for the new equipment, $4,071,651 (Exhibit 7.10b, row N), is higher than that of the old equipment, $3,277,280 (Exhibit 7.10a, row N). Therefore, the decision in this case would be to renovate the X-ray department with the new equipment. Similarly, using the incremental

EXHIBIT 7.10a NPV COMPARATIVE ANALYSIS OF A REPLACEMENT DECISION: OLD EQUIPMENT

Cash Flows with the Old Equipment

Givens

1 Initial investment	$0
2 Annual revenues[a]	$877,500
3 Annual cash operating expenses	$60,000
4 Annual depreciation[b]	$100,000
5 Salvage value at 10 years (5 years hence)	$150,000
6 Cost of capital	9%

[a]$75 per Exam × 45 Exams per day × 260 Operating days per year.
[b]($1,150,000 Initial cost − $150,000 Salvage value) / 10 years.

	Years	0	1	2	3	4	5
A Initial investment	Given 1	$0					
B Net revenues	Given 2		$877,500	$877,500	$877,500	$877,500	$877,500
C Less: cash operating expenses	Given 3		60,000	60,000	60,000	60,000	60,000
D Less: depreciation expense	Given 4		100,000	100,000	100,000	100,000	100,000
E Operating income	B − C − D		717,500	717,500	717,500	717,500	717,500
F Add: depreciation expense	Given 4		100,000	100,000	100,000	100,000	100,000
G Net operating cash flows	E + F		817,500	817,500	817,500	817,500	817,500
H Add: sale of salvage	Given 5						150,000
I Project cash flows	G + H		$817,500	$817,500	$817,500	$817,500	$967,500
J Cost of capital	Given 6		9%	9%	9%	9%	9%
K Present value interest factors	$1/(1 + i)^n$		0.9174	0.8417	0.7722	0.7084	0.6499
L Annual PV of cash flows[c]	I × K		$750,000	$688,073	$631,260	$579,138	$628,809
M PV of cash flows	Sum L	$3,277,280					
N Net present value	A + M	$3,277,280					

[c]Present value interest factors in the exhibit have been calculated by formula, but are necessarily rounded for presentation. Therefore, there may be a difference between the number displayed and that calculated manually.

EXHIBIT 7.10b NPV COMPARATIVE ANALYSIS OF A REPLACEMENT DECISION: NEW EQUIPMENT

Cash Flows with the New Equipment

Givens

1	Initial investment amount[a]	($850,000)
2	Annual revenues[b]	$1,170,000
3	Annual cash operating expenses	$30,000
4	Annual depreciation[c]	$150,000
5	Salvage value (5 years hence)	$750,000
6	Cost of capital	9%

[a] −$1,500,000 Initial cost + $650,000 Sale of old equipment.
[b] $75 per Exam × 60 Exams per day × 260 Operating days per year.
[c] ($1,500,000 Initial cost − $750,000 Salvage value) / 5 years.

		Years	0	1	2	3	4	5
A	Initial investment	Given 1	($850,000)					
B	Net revenues	Given 2		$1,170,000	$1,170,000	$1,170,000	$1,170,000	$1,170,000
C	Less: cash operating expenses	Given 3		30,000	30,000	30,000	30,000	30,000
D	Less: depreciation expense	Given 4		150,000	150,000	150,000	150,000	150,000
E	Operating income	B − C − D		990,000	990,000	990,000	990,000	990,000
F	Add: depreciation expense	Given 4		150,000	150,000	150,000	150,000	150,000
G	Net operating cash flows	E + F		1,140,000	1,140,000	1,140,000	1,140,000	1,140,000
H	Add: sale of salvage value	Given 5						750,000
I	Project cash flows	G + H		$1,140,000	$1,140,000	$1,140,000	$1,140,000	$1,890,000
J	Cost of capital	Given 6		9%	9%	9%	9%	9%
K	Present value interest factors	$1/(1+i)^n$		0.9174	0.8417	0.7722	0.7084	0.6499
L	Annual PV of cash flows[d]	I × K		$1,045,872	$959,515	$880,289	$807,605	$1,228,370
M	PV of cash flows	Sum L	$4,921,651					
N	**Net present value**	**A + M**	**$4,071,651**					

[d] Present value interest factors in the exhibit have been calculated by formula, but are necessarily rounded for presentation. Therefore, there may be a difference between the number displayed and that calculated manually.

EXHIBIT 7.11 NPV INCREMENTAL ANALYSIS OF A REPLACEMENT DECISION

Cash Flows

Givens	Old Equipment	New Equipment	Incremental Difference (New − Old)	
1 Initial investment		($850,000)	($850,000)	
2 Annual revenues[a]	$877,500	$1,170,000	$292,500	Incremental net revenues
3 Annual cash operating expenses	($60,000)	($30,000)	$30,000	Incremental operating cash savings
4 Annual depreciation[b]	$100,000	$150,000	$50,000	Incremental depreciation expenses
5 Salvage value	$150,000	$750,000	$600,000	Incremental salvage value
6 Cost of capital			9%	

[a]Old: $75 per Exam × 45 Exams per day × 260 Operating days per year. New: $75 per Exam × 60 Exams per day × 260 Operating days per year.
[b]Old: ($1,150,000 Initial cost − $150,000 Salvage value) / 10 years.
New: ($1,500,000 Initial cost − $750,000 Salvage value) / 5 years.

		Years	0	1	2	3	4	5
A	Initial investment	Given 1	($850,000)					
B	Incremental net revenues	Given 2		$292,500	$292,500	$292,500	$292,500	$292,500
C	Incremental operating cash savings	Given 3		30,000	30,000	30,000	30,000	30,000
D	Incremental depreciation expenses	Given 4		50,000	50,000	50,000	50,000	50,000
E	Incremental net operating income	$(B + C) - D$		272,500	272,500	272,500	272,500	272,500
F	Add: incremental depreciation	Given 4		50,000	50,000	50,000	50,000	50,000
G	Incremental net operating cash flow	$E + F$		322,500	322,500	322,500	322,500	322,500
H	Add: incremental salvage value	Given 5						600,000
I	Project incremental cash flows	$G + H$		$322,500	$322,500	$322,500	$322,500	$922,500
J	Cost of capital	Given 6		9%	9%	9%	9%	9%
K	Present value interest factors	$1 / (1 + i)^n$		0.9174	0.8417	0.7722	0.7084	0.6499
L	Annual PV of incremental cash flows[c]	$I \times K$		$295,872	$271,442	$249,029	$228,467	$599,562
M	PV of incremental cash flows	Sum L	$1,644,371					
N	Net present value	$A + M$	$794,371					

[c]Present value interest factors in the exhibit have been calculated by formula, but are necessarily rounded for presentation. Therefore, there may be a difference between the number displayed and that calculated manually.

approach, the NPV is $794,371 (Exhibit 7.11, row N). Thus, because the NPV is positive, the replacement decision should be made. Incidentally, note that the $794,371 NPV using the incremental method is exactly the difference between the two alternatives ($4,071,651 – $3,277,280) using the comparative approach. Thus the results are the same using either method; it is just the method of calculation that differs.

Before the hospital makes a final decision, however, several issues must be considered:

• The purchase of a new asset typically requires a large up-front expenditure, which may not always be feasible.

• Future cash flows are difficult to determine and may not always be accurate, especially in the salvage value.

• The exact cost of capital is difficult to determine.

• Although not the case here, replacement of an old asset with a new asset may be more expensive (i.e., $NPV_{New} < NPV_{Old}$), but replacement may be necessary for other reasons, such as to remain competitive by being able to offer the latest technology to consumers.

Summary

This chapter introduced three methods to evaluate large-dollar, multiyear investment decisions: payback, net present value, and internal rate of return. The payback method measures how long it will take to recover the initial investment. The strengths of the payback method are that it is simple to calculate and easy to understand. Its major weaknesses are that it does not account for the time value of money; it provides an answer in years, not dollars; and it disregards cash flows after the payback.

The NPV method overcomes the weaknesses of the payback method by accounting for cash flows after payback and discounting these cash flows by the project's cost of capital. The project's cost of capital is the rate of return that compensates investors for the time value of money and for the risk of the investment. The NPV measures the difference between the present value of the operating cash flows generated by the investment and the initial cost of that investment. The NPV technique measures the dollar return on the investment.

The general decision rule regarding NPV is: if $NPV > 0$, accept the project; if $NPV < 0$, reject the project; if $NPV = 0$, then accept or reject. If two or more mutually exclusive projects are being considered, then the one with the higher or highest positive NPV should be chosen. If two or more mutually exclusive projects are being considered and one must be undertaken regardless of the NPV, then the one with the higher or highest NPV should be chosen, even if the NPV is negative.

The strengths of the NPV method of capital investment analysis are that it provides an answer in dollars, not years; it accounts for all cash flows from the project, including those beyond the payback period; and it discounts these cash flows at the cost of capital. The major weakness of the NPV method is that the discount rate is often difficult to determine and may be hard to justify. NPV can be calculated by following these eight steps:

Step 1.   Identify the initial cash outflow.

Step 2.   Determine revenues and expenses (net income):

      a.   Identify annual net revenues.

      b.   Identify annual cash operating expenses and depreciation expense.

      c.   Compute annual net income.

Step 3.   Add depreciation expense back in to get net operating cash flows.

Step 4.   Add (subtract) any nonannual cash flows.

Step 5.   Adjust for working capital.

Step 6.   Determine the present value of each year's cash flow.

Step 7.   Sum the present values of all cash flows.

Step 8.   Determine the net present value of the project.

The IRR method determines the actual percentage return on the investment. When an organization chooses a project according to the IRR method, its decision depends on the value of the IRR relative to the required rate of return on the investment (also called the cost of capital or hurdle rate).

- If the IRR is greater than the required rate of return, the project should be accepted.

- If the IRR is less than the required rate of return, the project should be rejected.

- If the IRR is equal to the required rate of return, the facility should be indifferent about accepting or rejecting the project.

KEY TERMS

a. Beta

b. Cannibalization

c. Capital appreciation

d. Capital investment decisions

e. Capital investments

f. Cost of capital

g. Discount rate

h. Discounted cash flows

i. Dividends

j. Expansion decision

k. Goodwill

l. Hurdle rate

m. Incremental cash flows

n. Interest

o. Internal rate of return

p. Internal rate of return method

q. Net present value

r. Net present value method

s. Nonregular cash flows

t. Operating cash flows

u. Opportunity costs

v. Payback method

w. Regular cash flows

x. Replacement decision

y. Required rate of return

z. Residual value

aa. Retained earnings

bb. Salvage value

cc. Scrap value

dd. Straight-line depreciation

ee. Strategic decision

ff. Sunk costs

gg. Terminal value

hh. Weighted average cost of capital

Key Equation

Payback in years if cash flows are equal each year:

Initial Investment / Annual Cash Flows

REVIEW QUESTIONS AND PROBLEMS

Note that these questions and problems ask readers to use materials from Appendices C, D, E, and F, which are to be found at the end of this chapter.

nitions. Define the key terms listed previously.

ıment on the following statement: When a not-for-profit facility receives a contribution from a member of the community, the cost of capital is inconsequential when
deciding how to use this contribution because it is, in effect, free money.

3. From a capital investment point of view, what are the goals of a health care facility?

4. What are the primary drawbacks of the payback method as a capital budgeting
technique?

5. When using the IRR approach, when can the internal rate of return be determined simply
by dividing the initial outlay by the cash flows?

6. Why do pro forma income statements adjust for depreciation expense when developing
projected cash flows for a project?

7. If a hospital were considering a new women's health initiative, what spillover cash flows
might result?

8. When performing a capital budgeting analysis, what costs should be included and what
costs should be excluded as part of an initial investment?

9. Why are financing flows such as interest expense and dividend payments excluded from
the computation of cash flows?

10. Would a decision that is based on NPV ever change if it were based on IRR instead? Why
or why not?

11. Alameda Hospital is expecting its new cancer center to generate the following cash flows:

Givens	Years	0	1	2	3	4	5
Initial investment		($30,000,000)					
Net operating cash flows			$6,000,000	$8,000,000	$16,000,000	$20,000,000	$30,000,000

a. Determine the payback for the new cancer center.

b. Determine the net present value using a cost of capital of 15 percent.

c. Determine the net present value at a cost of capital of 20 percent, and compute the
internal rate of return.

d. At a 15 percent cost of capital, should the project be accepted? At a 20 percent cost
of capital, should the project be accepted? Explain.

12. Washington Community is expecting its new dialysis unit to generate the following cash
flows:

Givens	Years	0	1	2	3	4	5
Initial investment		($15,000,000)					
Net operating cash flows			$2,000,000	$4,000,000	$5,000,000	$8,000,000	$16,000,000

a. Determine the payback for the new dialysis unit.

b. Determine the NPV using a cost of capital of 15 percent.

c. Determine the NPV at a cost of capital of 20 percent and compute the IRR.

d. At a 15 percent cost of capital, should the project be accepted? At a 20 percent cost of capital, should the project be accepted? Explain.

13. St. Rose Hospital expects Projects A and B to generate the following cash flows:

Givens (in '000s)	Years	0	1	2	3	4	5
1 Initial investment		($3,500)					
2 Net operating cash flows for Project A			$2,500	$2,000	$1,500	$1,000	$600
3 Net operating cash flows for Project B			$600	$1,000	$1,500	$2,000	$2,500

*project θ outgoe
or pick higher
NPV*

a. Determine the NPV for both projects using a cost of capital of 20 percent.

b. Determine the NPV for both projects using a cost of capital of 10 percent.

c. At a 10 percent cost of capital, which project should be accepted? At a 20 percent cost of capital, which project should be accepted? Explain. *if mutally exclusive or indept both could be accepted*

14. Valley Care Medical Center expects Projects X and Y to generate the following cash flows:

Givens (in '000s)	Years	0	1	2	3	4	5
1 Initial investment		($7,500)					
2 Net operating cash flows for Project X			$7,000	$5,000	$3,000	$2,000	$1,500
3 Net operating cash flows for Project Y			$1,500	$2,000	$3,000	$5,000	$7,000

and "dr" are both aka interest

*same as COC
= COC ?*

a. Determine the NPV for both projects using a cost of capital of 17 percent.

b. Determine the NPV for both projects using a cost of capital of 12 percent.

c. At a 12 percent discount rate, which project should be accepted? At a 17 percent discount rate, which project should be accepted? Explain.

15. Kaiser Oakland Practice expects Projects 1 and 2 to generate the following cash flows:

Project 1 (in '000s)

Givens	Years	0	1	2	3	4	5
1 Initial investment		($2,800)					
2 Net operating cash flows			$300	$500	$800	$1,200	$2,000

Project 2 (in '000s)

Givens	Years	0	1	2	3	4	5
1 Initial investment		($5,000)					
2 Net operating cash flows			$1,300	$1,300	$1,300	$1,300	$1,300

a. Determine the payback for both projects.

b. Determine the IRR.

c. Determine the NPV at a cost of capital of 12 percent.

16. Colusa Regional Medical Center expects Alpha Project and Beta Project to generate the following:

Alpha Project (in '000s)

Givens	Years	0	1	2	3	4	5
1 Initial investment		($20,000)					
2 Net operating cash flows			($10,000)	$8,000	$12,000	$15,000	$26,000

Beta Project (in '000s)

Givens	Years	0	1	2	3	4	5
1 Initial investment		($28,000)					
2 Net operating cash flows			$8,000	$8,000	$8,000	$8,000	$8,000

a. Determine the payback for both projects.

b. Determine the IRR.

c. Determine the NPV at a cost of capital of 20 percent.

17. Biggs-Gridley Memorial Hospital, a nontaxpaying entity, is starting a new inpatient heart center on its third floor. The expected patient volume demands will generate $5,000,000 per year in revenues for the next five years. The new center will incur operating expenses, excluding depreciation, of $3,000,000 per year for the next five years. The initial cost of building and equipment is $7,000,000. Straight-line depreciation is used to estimate depreciation expense, and the building and equipment will be depreciated over a five-year life to their salvage value. The expected salvage value of the building and equipment at year five is $800,000. The cost of capital for this project is 10 percent.

a. Compute the NPV and IRR to determine the financial feasibility of this project.

b. Compute the NPV and IRR to determine the financial feasibility of this project if this were a tax-paying entity with a tax rate of 30 percent. (*Hint*: see Appendix E. Because the hospital is depreciating to the salvage value, there is no tax effect on the sale of the asset.)

18. Marshall Healthcare System, a nontaxpaying entity, is planning to purchase imaging equipment, including an MRI and ultrasonogram equipment, for its new imaging center. The equipment will generate $3,000,000 per year in revenues for the next five years. The expected operating expenses, excluding depreciation, will increase expenses by $1,200,000 per year for the next five years. The initial capital investment outlay for the imaging equipment is $5,500,000, which will be depreciated on a straight-line basis to its salvage value. The salvage value at year five is $800,000. The cost of capital for this project is 12 percent.

a. Compute the NPV and IRR to determine the financial feasibility of this project.

b. Compute the NPV and IRR to determine the financial feasibility of this project if this were a taxpaying entity with a tax rate of 40 percent. (*Hint*: see Appendix E. Because the organization is depreciating to the salvage value, there is no tax effect on the sale of the asset.)

19. Due to rising utility costs, Los Medanos Community Hospital wants to replace its existing computer-controlled heating, ventilation, and air-conditioning (HVAC) system with a more efficient version. The existing system was purchased three years ago for $240,000 and is being depreciated on a straight-line basis over an eight-year life to a salvage value of $0. Although the current book value for the existing system is $150,000, this system could be sold for only $80,000 today. The new system would cost $600,000 and would be depreciated on a straight-line basis over a five-year life to a salvage value of $0. The new heating and cooling system would reduce utility costs by $200,000 per year for five years and would not affect the level of net working capital. The economic life of the new system is five years, and the required rate of return on the project is 8 percent.

a. Should the existing HVAC system be replaced? Use the incremental NPV approach to evaluate the decision; assume the hospital is a not-for-profit facility.

b. If the facility were a taxpaying entity with a tax rate of 30 percent, should the existing HVAC system be replaced? Use the incremental NPV approach to evaluate the decision. (*Hint*: see Appendix F.)

20. Because of its inability to control film and personnel costs in its radiology department, Sanger General Hospital wants to replace its existing picture archive and communication (PAC) system with a newer version. The existing system, which has a current book value of $2,250,000, was purchased three years ago for $3,600,000 and is being depreciated on a straight-line basis over an eight-year life to a salvage value of $0. This system could be sold for $800,000 today. The new PAC system would reduce the need for staff by eight people per year for five years at a savings of $40,000 per person per year, and it would reduce film costs by $2,000,000 per year. The project would not affect the level of net working capital. The new PAC system would cost $9,000,000 and would be depreciated on a straight-line basis over a five-year life to a salvage value of $0. The economic life of the new system is five years, and the required rate of return on the project is 7 percent.

a. Should the existing PAC system be replaced? Use the incremental NPV approach to evaluate the decision; assume the hospital is a not-for-profit facility.

b. If the facility were a taxpaying entity with a tax rate of 30 percent, should the existing PAC system be replaced? Use the incremental NPV approach to evaluate the decision. (*Hint*: see Appendix F.)

21. Calexico Hospital plans to invest in a new MRI. The cost of the MRI is $1,800,000. The machine has an economic life of five years, and it will be depreciated over a five-year life to a $200,000 salvage value. Additional revenues attributed to the new machine will amount to $1,500,000 per year for five years. Additional operating costs, excluding

depreciation expense, will amount to $1,000,000 per year for five years. Over the life of the machine, net working capital will increase by $30,000 per year for five years.

a. Assuming that hospital is a nontaxpaying entity, what is the project's NPV at a discount rate of 8 percent, and what is the project's IRR? Is the decision to accept or reject the same under either capital budgeting method, or does it differ?

b. Assuming that this hospital is a taxpaying entity and its tax rate is 30 percent, what is the project's NPV at a cost of capital of 8 percent, and what is the project's IRR? Is the decision to accept or reject the same under either capital budgeting method, or does it differ? (*Hint*: see Appendices C, D, and E.)

22. Glenn Medical Center has seen a growth in patient volume since its primary competitor decided to relocate to a different area of the city. To accommodate this growth, a consultant has advised Glenn Medical to invest in a positron-emission tomography (PET) scanner. The cost to implement the unit would be $4,000,000. The useful life of this equipment is typically about six years, and it will be depreciated over a six-year life to a $400,000 salvage value. Additional patient volume will yield $3,000,000 in new revenues the first year. These first-year total revenues will increase by $600,000 each year thereafter, but the unit is expensive to operate. Additional staff and variable costs, excluding depreciation expense, will come to $2,200,000 the first year, but these expenses are expected to rise by $400,000 each year thereafter. Over the life of the machine, net working capital will increase by $18,000 per year for six years.

a. Assuming that Glenn Medical Center is a nontaxpaying entity, what is the project's NPV at a discount rate of 9 percent, and what is the project's IRR? Depending on the method used, what is the investment decision?

b. Assuming that Glenn Medical Center is a taxpaying entity and its tax rate is 40 percent, what is the project's NPV at a discount rate of 9 percent, and what is the project's IRR? Depending on the method used, what is the investment decision? (*Hint*: see Appendices C, D, and E.)

23. Long-Term Acute-Care Hospital (LTAC) owns an abandoned warehouse. The after-tax value of the land is $800,000. The furniture and fixtures of the warehouse have been fully depreciated to an after-tax market value of $70,000. The two options LTAC faces are either to sell the land and furniture and fixtures or to convert the building into a forty-bed, free-standing new facility. To refurbish and renovate the facility would cost $4,500,000. The new building and equipment would be depreciated on a straight-line basis over a ten-year life to a $700,000 salvage value. At the end of ten years, the land could be sold for an after-tax value of $3,500,000. The new rehab facility's pro forma income statement for the next ten years is shown below. Net working capital will increase at a rate of $20,000 per year over the life of the project. LTAC has a 30 percent tax rate and a required rate of return of 7 percent. Use both the NPV technique and IRR method to evaluate this project. (*Hint*: see Appendices C, D, and E.)

Pro Forma Income Statement	Years 1–5	Years 6–10
Net Patient Revenues / Year	$8.5 million / Year	$10.0 million / Year
Operating Expenses (excludes depreciation expense) / Year	$8.0 million / Year	$9.0 million / Year

24. Heart Hospital is in possession of a nonoperational, fifty-bed hospital. The after-tax value of the land is $2,500,000. The equipment and the building are fully depreciated and have an after-tax market value of $3,500,000. The hospital could either sell off its property or convert it into a new state-of-the-art acute-care hospital. An analysis of the market reveals that the facility could attract 9,000 discharges per year, a number expected to increase at a rate of 3 percent per year. Projected net patient revenue per discharge is $10,000 for the first year, increasing annually by 4 percent thereafter. Projected operating expense per discharge is $8,400 for the first year, increasing annually by 6 percent thereafter. Renovation costs to create a plush facility would be $45,000,000. The new facility would be depreciated on a straight-line basis over a ten-year life to a $12,000,000 salvage value. At the end of ten years, the land is expected to be sold for an after-tax value of $6,000,000. Net working capital will increase at a rate of $3,000,000 per year over the life of the project. Heart Hospital has a 35 percent tax rate and a required rate of return of 9 percent. Use the NPV technique and IRR method to evaluate this project. (*Hint*: see Appendices C, D, and E.)

25. Kern Valley Hospital, a taxpaying entity, wants to replace its current labor-intensive tele-medicine system with a new automated version that would cost $3,500,000 to purchase. This new system has a five-year life and would be depreciated on a straight-line basis to a salvage value of $350,000. The current telemedicine system was purchased five years ago for $1,600,000, has five years remaining on its useful life, and would be depreciated similarly to a salvage value of $300,000. This current system could be sold in the market-place now for $350,000. The new telemedicine system has annual labor operating costs of $185,000, whereas the current system has annual labor operating costs of $1,000,000. Neither system will change patient revenues. The hospital has a 40 percent tax rate and a required rate of return of 7 percent. The financial analysis will be projected over a five-year period. Use the NPV approach to determine if the new telemedicine system should be selected. (*Hint*: see Appendix F.)

26. Topping Medical Center, a for-profit institution, wants to replace its film-based mammog-raphy equipment with new digital models. The cost of the new digital models is $3,500,000. The current models were purchased three years ago for $1,400,000. The new digital models have a five-year life and will be depreciated on a straight-line basis to a salvage

value of $600,000. The current models have five years remaining on their useful lives and will be depreciated on a straight-line basis to a salvage value of $400,000. The current models could be sold in the marketplace for $1,200,000. The new models are expected to generate annual cash cost savings on film of $400,000 per year relative to the current models. Neither system will change patient revenues. The imaging center has a 40 percent tax rate and required rate of return of 5 percent. The financial analysis will be projected over a five-year period. Use the NPV approach to determine if the new digital model should be selected. (*Hint*: see Appendix F.)

27. Sutter Lakeside Hospital, a taxpaying entity, is considering a new ambulatory surgical center (ASC). The building and equipment for the new ASC will cost $5,500,000. The equipment and building will be depreciated on a straight-line basis over the project's five-year life to a $2,500,000 salvage value. The new ASC's projected net revenue and expenses are as follows. Net revenues are expected to be $5,000,000 the first year and will grow by 9 percent each year thereafter. The operating expenses, which exclude interest and depreciation expenses, will be $4,500,000 the first year and are expected to grow annually by 3 percent for every year after that. Interest expense will be $700,000 per year, and principal payments on the loan will be $1,000,000 a year. In the first year of operation, the new ASC is expected to generate additional after-tax cash flows of $600,000 from radiology and other ancillary services, which will grow at an annual rate of 5 percent per year for every year after that. Starting in year 1, net working capital will increase by $350,000 per year for the first four years, but during the last year of the project, net working capital will decrease by $250,000. The tax rate for the hospital is 40 percent, and its cost of capital is 15 percent. Use both the NPV and IRR approaches to determine if this project should be undertaken. (*Hint*: see Appendices C, D, and E.)

28. Garfield Medical System, a taxpaying entity, is considering a new orthopedic center. The building and equipment for the new center will cost $7,500,000. The equipment and building will be depreciated on a straight-line basis over its five-year life to a $2,500,000 salvage value. The new orthopedic center's projected net revenue and expenses are listed below. The project will be financed partially by debt capital. Interest expense is expected to be $600,000 per year, and principal payments on the bank loan are expected to be $1,250,000 per year for the first five years of the loan. The new orthopedic center is expected to take away after-tax cash profits of $1,000,000 per year from inpatient ortho-pedic services. The tax rate for the institution is 40 percent, and its cost of capital is 10 percent. Two years ago, a $100,000 financial feasibility study was conducted and paid for. Pro forma working capital projections are listed below. These are the permanent account balances for inventory, accounts receivable, and accounts payable. Use the NPV and IRR approaches to determine if this project should be undertaken. (*Hint*: see Appendices C and E.)

Pro forma income statement accounts for the Orthopedic Center (in 000's)

Years	0	1	2	3	4	5
Net revenues		$6,500	$9,500	$12,000	$14,000	$16,000
Operating expenses before dep. and int.		$6,000	$6,500	$7,000	$7,500	$8,500
Annual interest expense		$600	$600	$600	$600	$600
Annual depreciation expense		$1,000	$1,000	$1,000	$1,000	$1,000

Pro forma working capital accounts for the Orthopedic Center (in 000's)

Working capital: inventory, A/R		$2,500	$3,500	$4,000	$3,000	$2,000
Working capital: accounts payable		$700	$1,100	$1,600	$2,000	$1,400

Appendix C: Technical Concerns in Calculating Net Present Value

This appendix addresses three commonly asked questions about performing a net present value analysis:

- How does an organization determine the amount of the initial investment?
- How does an organization determine the annual cash flows?
- How does an organization determine a discount rate?

How Does an Organization Determine the Amount of the Initial Investment?

Included Costs

Expenditures for plant, property, and equipment are usually the primary initial investment items in a capital project. The amount recorded for these items is the purchase price plus all costs related to making the investment "ready to go," including costs of labor, renovation of space, rewiring, and transportation, and any investment in working capital (cash, inventory).

Along with these relatively tangible costs, the initial investment amount should include any planning costs incurred specifically for the project after it has been selected. General planning costs incurred to decide which capital project to undertake are not included because they are *sunk costs* (costs incurred before a specific project has been selected).

Sunk Costs
Costs incurred in the past. (They should not be included in NPV-type analyses.)

Opportunity Cost

Proceeds lost by forgoing or delaying opportunities other than the opportunity chosen.

The final cost category to include in the initial cost estimate is the *opportunity cost*, which is proceeds lost by forgoing other opportunities in order to pursue a particular project. For example, suppose a health care facility has a plot of land which it could either sell for $150,000 or build a long-term care facility. If it builds on the land, it will be earning a profit from the new facility; even though no cash is changing hands, yet losing the chance to collect that $150,000 from the sale of the land. Thus $150,000 would be included as part of the initial outlay, as an opportunity cost or a cash outflow, if the organization chose to build the new facility.

Excluded Costs

In an NPV analysis, several cost categories explicitly should not be included as initial investment costs. For example, though the purchase price of assets should be included in the initial cost, interest paid as a result of borrowing money to finance those assets should not be included because interest costs are financing flows and are reflected in the cost of capital.

Costs that have already occurred in the past are sunk costs and should not be included in the analysis. For example, $50,000 already spent by the health care organization to renovate a building should not be included as part of the cost for a new project. The initial investment should include only the cost of plant, property, and equipment; investment in working capital; additional planning costs; and opportunity costs (see Exhibit C.1).

EXHIBIT C.1 INITIAL COSTS OF AN INVESTMENT

Included Costs

- Plant, property, and equipment, and related preparation costs
- Additional planning costs
- Opportunity costs

Excluded Costs

- Interest costs
- Sunk costs

How Does an Organization Determine the Annual Cash Flows?

An NPV analysis evaluates the relationship between an initial investment and the *incremental cash flows* in the future resulting from that investment. There are three types of incremental cash flows: operating, spillover, and nonregular.

Incremental Cash Flows
Cash flows that occur solely as a result of a particular action, such as undertaking a project.

Operating Cash Flows

Incremental operating cash flows are the new, ongoing cash flows that occur solely as a result of undertaking a project. They include payments received for services rendered and expenditures for such things as labor, materials, marketing, utilities, and taxes. Excluded from NPV analyses are principal and interest payments made on loans to finance the project and any dividends that may result from the project. The purpose of maintaining this separation is to assess whether a project can generate enough positive cash flows from operations on its own merits to pay off its financing costs (interest, principal payments, and dividends).

Key Point Operating flows are kept separate from financing flows. Operating cash flows include revenues, labor and supply expenses, and so forth. Financing cash flows include interest expenses, principal payments, and dividends.

To realize these flows under the cash basis of accounting, the revenue and expense accounts are converted to a cash basis by changes in the net working capital. These adjustments are discussed under the example of computing cash flows in Appendix D.

Key Point If a health care provider is a for-profit organization, a project's positive net cash flows also entail tax payments according to the organization's tax rate. Therefore, operating cash flows are calculated *after tax*. Appendix E provides a detailed example of how to generate appropriate cash flows for taxable entities.

Spillover Cash Flows

Spillover cash flows, which can be classified into two types, are increases or decreases in cash flows that occur elsewhere in an organization once a project is undertaken. The first type occurs when a new service produces additional cash flow to other departments. For example, if a facility were expanding its emergency department, additional revenues could be generated by ancillary support services, such as radiology or laboratory. The

Cannibalization

What occurs when a new service or product decreases the revenues from other services or product lines; this result is considered a cash outflow.

Operating Cash Flows

Cash flows that occur on a regular basis, often following implementation of a project (also called *regular cash flows*).

second type occurs when a new service diminishes cash flow elsewhere, sometimes called *cannibalization*. For example, if a facility were evaluating the development of an outpatient diagnostic center, it would have to consider the expected loss in cash flow for the existing inpatient diagnostic center. This loss in cash profits for inpatient services is a cash outflow.

Non-regular Cash Flows and Terminal Value Cash Flows

As opposed to *operating cash flows*, which by definition occur on a regular basis, *non-regular cash flows* are incremental cash flows that occur on an irregular basis, typically at the end of the life of a project. One of the most common nonregular cash flows is salvage value, the money received from selling an asset at the termination of a project. Another typical cash flow at the end of a project's life is recovery of working capital, typically a cash inflow. Exhibit C.2 describes cash flows to be included or excluded, and Appendix D discusses the recovery of working capital.

EXHIBIT C.2 THE COMPONENTS OF INCREMENTAL CASH FLOWS

Included items	Excluded items
Operating cash flows	*Existing cash flows not affected by the project being considered*
• Revenues in the form of payments (inflows)	• Revenues already being generated by an existing service
• Cash payments for labor, supplies, utilities, marketing, and taxes (outflows)	
Spillover cash flows	*Financing-related items*
• Effects of a new service on other departments, such as ancillary services (inflows)	• Interest
	• Principal payments
	• Dividends
• Effects of a new service's cannibalizing similar existing services (outflows)	**Adjusted items**
Non-regular cash flows (terminal value cash flows)	*Accrual-based items*
	• Revenues earned but not received in cash
• Salvage value of equipment that will be sold at the end of a project (inflow)	• Expenses recognized but no cash expended (i.e., depreciation, accrued expenses)
• Recovery of working capital (inflow)	
	Other
	• Changes in net working capital

Accuracy of Cash Flow Estimates

Because cash flows occur at some point in the future, they cannot be measured precisely. Expected revenues or projected cost savings can only be estimated, based on a market analysis and the current operations of the organization. On the one hand, unforeseeable events, such as new competition or an unexpected rise in energy prices, could significantly cut back on positive cash inflow. On the other hand, an investment such as a convenient new visitor parking deck may be so popular that it draws in unexpected patient volume, which would increase revenues. Given that the future cash flows must be present to offset the cost of the initial investment, marked variation in these cash flows could alter the final NPV decision.

Nonregular Cash Flows
Cash flows that occur sporadically or on an irregular basis. A common nonregular cash flow is salvage value, the receipt of funds following a one-time sale of an asset at the end of its useful life.

How Does an Organization Determine a Discount Rate?

Although commonly thought of as an adjustment for the time value of money, the discount rate also accounts for capital project risk. The discount rate, or cost of capital, marks the required rate of return for investors who fund the project to compensate them for the risk of the investment opportunity and the temporary loss of these funds being used for the project. Investors who provide primary sources of debt financing for health care providers include bondholders and private lenders such as banks. Investors who provide sources of equity financing for health care providers are stockholders. For-profit health care providers have stockholders who expect a return on the providers' stock. Nonprofit health care providers do not have stockholders; however, they should operate as if their community expects returns, or benefits, in the form of higher quality health care, lower charges, and the provision of charity care. Operating under this assumption will force nonprofits to accept capital projects that can generate positive cash flow not only to pay the interest expense on debt but also, and more importantly, to earn additional cash flows to fund future capital expenditures and support these community benefits.

To estimate the required rate of return for capital projects, with risk similar to the current risk associated with the health care organization, a facility can use its current cost of capital, calculated in terms of its *weighted average cost of capital*, or WACC. For example, if a hospital plans to build a replacement hospital, the WACC can be used because the risk associated with this project is similar to the operating risk for the hospital. However, if the hospital were investing in a health insurance company, the operating risk for that business would not be the same as the hospital's risk, and the WACC would not be used. Instead the cost of capital for insurance companies would be used in the NPV analysis. The WACC formula defines a hospital's cost of capital as the sum of its cost of debt (Kd) and its cost of equity (Ke); these costs are weighted by their respective proportions of debt (D / V) and equity (E / V):

$$WACC = Kd(D / V) + Ke(E / V)$$

The cost of equity, or the return that stockholders should expect to earn when investing in a share of stock, has three components. This analysis will focus only on common stock (and not on preferred stock). The first component is the risk-free rate (Rf), which typically is measured by the long-term, thirty-year U.S. Treasury bond and represents the floor. Since stocks are riskier than government securities, stock investors expect to earn more on stocks than they would on the risk-free asset. The second component is the added premium, or expected return, that accounts for the risk of investing in the general stock market, which is called the *market risk premium*. This risk premium is the difference between the return on the entire stock market (Rm) and the risk-free rate of return ($Rm - Rf$). The historical performance of a specific stock market index, such as Standard & Poor's index, is used to project future returns on the stock market. Using historical data, Standard & Poor's index projects an expected return between 8 percent and 11 percent. If the risk-free rate equals 4 percent, then the market risk premium, or the added return for investing in the stock market, equals 4 percent (8% − 4%). The final component, beta, measures the risk potential of the individual company relative to the risk potential of the overall stock market. The beta of the market, or the average company risk, is 1, so a company with a beta of 2 is considered twice as risky as the market in general. Thus, if the stock market increases by 10 percent, then the return on this company may increase by 20 percent. Recently, hospital management companies' betas ranged from .87 for Life-Point, Inc., to 1.84 for Community Health Systems, Inc. A health care company's beta is influenced by the risk for the hospital industry in general and the individual company's amounts of fixed operating costs and debt. Health care companies with higher fixed costs (or greater operating risk) and higher amounts of debt (or greater financial risk) will incur greater variability in the earnings and produce higher beta values. It is beyond the scope of this textbook to discuss the details of how beta is measured. Web sites such as Value Pro (www.valuepro.net) and That's WACC! (thatswacc.com) tell investors the specific beta value for a company's stock and its WACC. For nonprofit hospitals and health systems, which have no stock and thus no beta, one could use the average beta for all hospital management companies as a proxy for this component of the WACC.

Combining all the components results in the final model, called the *capital asset pricing model* (CAPM), which can be used to find the expected return on equity or stock (*Ke*), as follows:

$$Ke = (Rf) + (Rm - Rf)\, beta$$

Given this model, Community Health System's stock return can be estimated, which is equal to the risk-free rate (4 percent) and its market risk premium (4.0 percent) times its beta value of 1.84. Given these values, Community Health System's expected stock or equity return is 11.4 percent:

$$Ke = (Rf) + (Rm - Rf)\, beta$$

$$Ke = 4\% + (8\% - 4\%)\, 1.84$$

$$Ke = 11.4\%$$

For the weighted average cost of capital, the weights can be estimated from the market or balance sheet value of debt and equity, while total value (*V*) can be estimated from total assets, or the sum of the market values of debt and equity. Market value of equity equals total shares outstanding times current share price, while market value of debt equals the hospital's market value of any outstanding debt borrowings. Proxy measures for the cost of debt can be based on interest rates for its expected bond rating or the market rates of existing debt.

The cost of debt for tax deduction of interest expense is also adjusted if the hospital is a taxpaying entity. For example, assuming a cost of debt of 6 percent and a debt weight of 60 percent, and given a corporate tax rate of 40 percent, the cost of debt will be adjusted to 3.6 percent and accounts for the after-tax cost of debt. Given the Community Health System's cost equity of 11.4 percent and equity weight of 40 percent, its WACC equals 6.72 percent:

$$WACC = Kd(1 - t)(D/V) + Ke(E/V)$$

$$6.72\% = 6\%(1 - .4) \times 60\% + 11.4\% \times 40\%$$

Key Point The *discount rate* is also called the *opportunity cost of capital* to the company undertaking the capital investment project. It is the cost of the next best alternative, those returns the company would be forgoing by making this investment as opposed to another. From the lenders' or investors' points of view, it is the return they forgo by investing their money in this project rather than alternative projects of similar risk. For example, if an investor-owned hospital chain were issuing stock to purchase a health insurance business, investors considering buying this stock would expect at least the return on the stocks of other publicly held health insurance companies, such as Cigna or Aetna.

Appendix D: Adjustments for Net Working Capital

To the extent that new projects affect working capital, adjustments in cash flows must be made. If working capital increases, then the organization has invested additional resources in working capital: that is, the project requires the organization to increase both its current asset accounts, which result in cash outflows, and current liability accounts, which are cash inflows, because they delay the use of cash (see the example below). The difference between current assets and current liabilities is called *net working capital*, as discussed in Chapter Five. The effects of changes in net working capital must be accounted for each year. If there is an increase in net working capital, the amount is subtracted from net operating cash flows; likewise, for a decrease, the amount is added to net operating cash flows.

Key Point Increases in net working capital mean cash outlays. Decreases in net working capital mean cash inflows.

Exhibit D.1, continuing the example of building a satellite hospital, illustrates how to adjust for changes in net working capital. Assume that the organization had balance sheet results as shown in rows 7 to 9 of Exhibit D.1. In row 9, its net working capital (Current assets – Current liabilities) is shown as $1,000, $1,300, $1,800, $600, $400, and $300 in years 1 through 6, respectively.

The change in net working capital is the difference between the current year's net working capital and that from the previous year (row 10). For example, the change in net working capital the first year was $1,000 ($1,000 in year 1 – $0 in year 0). The second year's change in net working capital was $300 ($1,300 in year 2 – $1,000 in year 1). The same procedure is followed for years 3 through 6. As noted earlier, if net working capital increases, then cash decreases, which must be subtracted from the cash flows. If net working capital decreases, then cash increases, and that amount must be added to cash flows. Because net working capital increased by $1,000 in year 1 (row 10), $1,000 (row I) is subtracted from the net operating cash flows (row G). This process is continued for the remaining years.

EXHIBIT D.1 COMPUTATION OF NET PRESENT VALUE FOR A SATELLITE HOSPITAL, INCLUDING WORKING CAPITAL ADJUSTMENTS

	Givens	Years 0	1	2	3	4	5	6
1	Initial investment	($1,000,000)						
2	Net revenues		$400,000	$550,000	$800,000	$900,000	$1,100,000	$1,370,000
3	Cash operating expenses		200,000	300,000	500,000	550,000	650,000	850,000
4	Depreciation expense		145,000	145,000	145,000	145,000	145,000	145,000
5	Sale of assets							130,000
6	Cost of capital	10%						
7	Current assets		$2,200	$4,800	$7,400	$1,400	$1,300	$1,200
8	Current liabilities		$1,200	$3,500	$5,600	$800	$900	$900
9	Net working capital	Given 7 − Given 8 $0	$1,000	$1,300	$1,800	$600	$400	$300
10	Change in net working capital	a $1,000	$1,000	$300	$500	($1,200)	($200)	($100)

[a]Net working capital (current year) − Net working capital (previous year)

Net Present Value for Satellite Hospital, Adjusting for Depreciation, Working Capital, and Salvage Value

		Years 0	1	2	3	4	5	6
A	Initial investment	Given 1 ($1,000,000)						
B	Net revenues	Given 2	$400,000	$550,000	$800,000	$900,000	$1,100,000	$1,370,000
C	Less: cash operating expenses before depreciation	Given 3	200,000	300,000	500,000	550,000	650,000	850,000
D	Less: depreciation expense	Given 4	145,000	145,000	145,000	145,000	145,000	145,000
E	Operating income	B − C − D	55,000	105,000	155,000	205,000	305,000	375,000
F	Add: depreciation expense	Given 4	145,000	145,000	145,000	145,000	145,000	145,000
G	Net operating cash flows	E + F	200,000	250,000	300,000	350,000	450,000	520,000
H	Add: sale of assets	Given 5						130,000
I	Adjustments for changes in working capital	−Given 10	(1,000)	(300)	(500)	1,200	200	100
J	Recapture of net working capital	−Sum I						300
K	Project cash flows	G + H + I + J	$199,000	$249,700	$299,500	$351,200	$450,200	$650,400
L	Cost of capital	Given 6	10%	10%	10%	10%	10%	10%
M	Present value interest factors	$1/(1+i)^n$	0.9091	0.8264	0.7513	0.6830	0.6209	0.5645
N	Annual PV of cash flows[b]	K × M	$180,909	$206,364	$225,019	$239,874	$279,539	$367,134
O	PV of cash flows	Sum N	$1,498,838					
P	Net present value	A + O	$498,838					

[b]Present value interest factors in the exhibit have been calculated by formula, but are necessarily rounded for presentation. Therefore, there may be a difference between the number displayed and that calculated manually.

Key Point Increases in net working capital are cash *outflows*. Decreases in net working capital are cash *inflows*.

In the first three years, cash outflows occurred, and net working capital for the project increased (row 10). But in year 4 and thereafter, the decreases in net working capital constituted cash inflows for those years. The facility is no longer investing cash in current assets and current liabilities. It is decreasing its investment in cash, collecting at a higher rate on its receivables, or reducing its outstanding payables (or all of these).

Once the changes in net working capital have been calculated, they are entered into the NPV calculation to adjust for changes in cash flows due to changes in net working capital (rows I and J).

 Key Point Interest-bearing, short-term debt (notes payable) should be excluded from calculations of changes in net working capital because it represents financing flows and is accounted for in the cost of capital.

When a project ends, it is assumed that the total amount of net working capital investment has been recaptured and accounted for as a cash inflow, and that plant and equipment will be sold or disposed of. In regard to the recapture of net working capital, typically all project receivables are collected, all project inventory gets sold, and all project payables are paid. The recapture of changes in net working capital is the sum of all the changes in net working capital during the life of the project. In the case of the satellite hospital, this amount is −$300 [($1,000) + ($300) + ($500) + $1,200 + $200 + $100]. The negative $300 indicates an ending excess balance of $300 in net working capital to sell off; therefore, $300 in net working capital becomes a cash inflow that can be recaptured or recovered (see Exhibit D.1, row J).

Appendix E: Tax Implications for For-Profit Entities in a Capital Budgeting Decision and the Adjustment for Interest Expense

This appendix introduces an NPV analysis for a for-profit entity. The total number of for-profit hospitals in the United States at the turn of the century represented less than 15 percent of the total number of short-term community hospitals. In contrast, there were more than 7,000 skilled- and intermediate-care nursing homes nationwide, of which more than two-thirds were for-profit entities. Also, more than two-thirds of the managed care insurers were tax-paying entities. Therefore, it is imperative to consider the tax effects that can take place in a for-profit investment analysis. Appendix C discussed the separation of financing flows from the operating cash flow analysis for an NPV analysis. When computing a cash flow analysis from a projected income statement for a for-profit entity, interest expense needs to be taken out in order to adjust for the tax effect. The following analysis shows what the calculations would be if the satellite hospital project were a for-profit endeavor.

The two most important tax adjustments that must be made for for-profit entities are accounting for the effect of taxes on operating income and accounting for the tax effect from the gains or losses resulting from the sale of assets at the expected end of the project's life. This example focuses only on the first adjustment because gains and losses, like most other tax effects, are complicated and therefore only introduced in this text.

As shown in Exhibit E.1, the analysis looks nearly identical to that for not-for-profit entities (Exhibit D.1), except for the tax expense and interest expense accounts and the inclusion of a new line for payment of taxes (Exhibit E.1, row G, which assumes that the organization has a 40 percent tax rate on its net income). In year 1, the organization had earnings before taxes of $30,000 (row F). Because the tax rate is 40 percent, it must pay an additional $12,000 in taxes ($30,000 × 0.40). In year 2, it pays $32,000 in taxes on earnings before tax of $80,000 (rows F and G). A similar analysis is conducted for years 3 through 6.

At this point, an adjustment must be made for interest because interest expense affected net income (and thus the amount of taxes paid), but interest expense is not itself an operating cash flow. Thus, interest expense must be added back at the amount of (1 − Tax rate) to determine true cash outflows. This is done in row J, where $15,000 is added back [$25,000 × (1 − 0.40)]. In effect, the interest expense provided a tax deduction of $10,000 ($25,000 × 0.40 saved), which represents a cash inflow. Thus the true cash outflow is only $15,000 ($25,000 − $10,000), which matches the value in row J. For nonprofit entities with interest expense in the projected income statement, the full amount of the interest expense is added back in because the tax rate is zero. The remainder of the analysis remains the same. Overall, the NPV for the hospital as a taxpaying entity equals $181,116 (row T), versus $498,838 as a not-for-profit hospital (Exhibit D.1, row P); so the NPV for the for-profit is much less than that for the not-for-profit.

EXHIBIT E.1 NPV DECISION ASSUMING SATELLITE HOSPITAL IS FOR-PROFIT

Givens	Years	0	1	2	3	4	5	6
1	Initial investment	($1,000,000)						
2	Net revenues		$400,000	$550,000	$800,000	$900,000	$1,100,000	$1,370,000
3	Cash operating expenses		$200,000	$300,000	$500,000	$550,000	$650,000	$850,000
4	Depreciation expense		$145,000	$145,000	$145,000	$145,000	$145,000	$145,000
5	Interest expense		$25,000	$25,000	$25,000	$25,000	$25,000	$25,000
6	Sale of assets							$130,000
7	Cost of capital	10%						
8	Tax rate	40%						
9	Current assets		$2,200	$4,800	$7,400	$1,400	$1,300	$1,200
10	Current liabilities		$1,200	$3,500	$5,600	$800	$900	$900
11	Net working capital	Given 9 – Given 10	$0	$1,000	$1,300	$1,800	$600	$400	$300
12	**Change in net working capital**	a		$1,000	$300	$500	($1,200)	($200)	($100)

aNet working capital (current year) – Net working capital (previous year)

Net Present Value for Satellite Hospital, Adjusting for Depreciation, Interest, Working Capital, and Salvage Value

			Years 0	1	2	3	4	5	6
A	Initial investment	Given 1	($1,000,000)						
B	Net revenues	Given 2		$400,000	$550,000	$800,000	$900,000	$1,100,000	$1,370,000
C	Less: cash operating expenses before dep. and int.	Given 3		200,000	300,000	500,000	550,000	650,000	850,000
D	Less: depreciation expense	Given 4		145,000	145,000	145,000	145,000	145,000	145,000
E	Less: interest expense	Given 5		25,000	25,000	25,000	25,000	25,000	25,000
F	Earnings before taxes	B – C – D – E		30,000	80,000	130,000	180,000	280,000	350,000
G	Less: tax expense (40% tax rate)	Given 8 × F		12,000	32,000	52,000	72,000	112,000	140,000
H	Earnings after tax	F – G		18,000	48,000	78,000	108,000	168,000	210,000
I	Add: depreciation expense	Given 4		145,000	145,000	145,000	145,000	145,000	145,000
J	Add: interest expense (1 – tax rate)	(1 – Given 8) × E		15,000	15,000	15,000	15,000	15,000	15,000
K	Net operating cash flow	H + I + J		178,000	208,000	238,000	268,000	328,000	370,000
L	Add: sale of assets[b]	Given 6							130,000
M	Adjustments for changes in working capital	–Given 12	(1,000)	(300)	(500)	1,200	200	100	
N	Recapture of net working capital	–Sum M							300
O	Project cash flows	K + L + M + N		$177,000	$207,700	$237,500	$269,200	$328,200	$500,400
P	Cost of capital	Given 7		10%	10%	10%	10%	10%	10%
Q	Present value interest factors	$1/(1+i)^n$		0.9091	0.8264	0.7513	0.6830	0.6209	0.5645
R	Annual PV of cash flows[c]	O × Q		$160,909	$171,653	$178,437	$183,867	$203,786	$282,463
S	PV of cash flows	Sum R	$1,181,116						
T	Net present value	A + S	$181,116						

[b] There is no tax effect from selling the asset, because it was depreciated to the salvage value; therefore, salvage value equals book value.

[c] Present value interest factors in the exhibit have been calculated by formula, but are necessarily rounded for presentation. Therefore, there may be a difference between the number displayed and that calculated manually.

Appendix F: Comprehensive Capital Budgeting Replacement Cost Example

Assume that a cardiology laboratory is considering replacing its manual electrocardiography (EKG) management information system (MIS) with a new, more efficient product. The new system automatically stores EKG and stress records online. The existing system was purchased five years ago for $70,000 and is being depreciated over a ten-year life to a salvage value of $10,000. The old system can be sold now at a market price of $20,000 and has a book value of $40,000 ($70,000 Original cost − $30,000 Accumulated depreciation). The new system can be purchased for $100,000 and is esti-mated to have a five-year life. It can be depreciated to a salvage value of $20,000. Because the organization is paid on a per procedure basis, there are no new revenues directly associated with the improved EKG system. Thus the focus becomes the cash savings in operational expenses. Annual labor expenses will drop from $50,000 for the old system to $15,000 for the new system, resulting in a labor cash savings of $35,000. Purchasing the new system will increase net working capital by $1,000 each year, com-pared with a $300 annual increase for the old system, starting in year 1. This appendix provides comparative and incremental NPV analyses of this situation, first assuming that the lab is not-for-profit and then assuming that it is investor owned. In both cases the cost of capital is 5 percent.

Comparative Approach: Not-for-Profit Analysis

As its name implies, the comparative approach compares the cash flows resulting from continuing with the existing alternative to those that would result if the equipment were replaced. The comparative approach does this by separately calculating each of these cash flows and then com-paring the end results (Exhibit F.1).

Were the organization to continue with the existing system, there would be no investment at year 0 (it has already been made), and the oper-ating loss would be $56,000 a year (row D), which includes operating expenses (row B) and depreciation expense (row C). However, because operating loss contains depreciation, and depreciation is an expense that does not require a cash outlay, depreciation must be added back in order to derive cash flows from operations. This is done in row F by adding $6,000 (row E) back to the $56,000 operating loss (row D). Although the same result ($50,000, row F) can be derived without first subtracting and then adding back depreciation expense, this approach makes it easier to compare the not-for-profit and for-profit analyses. Because the change in net working capital increases by $300 each year, the resultant cash outflow must be accounted for (row G). However, as explained in Appendix D, this will be recovered at the end of the project (row I). The only other cash flow to account for is the $10,000 salvage value that results in a cash inflow in year 5 (row H). Finally, the cash flows are computed for each of the five years (row J), and then discounted using the cost of capital (rows K and L). This information forms the basis for calculating the NPV of the cash flows attributable to the existing machine: $208,762 (row O).

The initial outlay, expenses, depreciation, salvage value, and working capital effects differ for the purchase of the replacement system (Exhibit F.1, lower half). The initial outlay is computed in row A. Although the new equipment costs $100,000, the organization has to pay only $80,000 from its existing funds because it can allocate $20,000 from the sale of the existing equipment.

Because net working capital increases by $1,000 each year, the resulting cash outflow must be accounted for (rows G and I). The remaining steps in the replacement analysis are the same as those in the previous analysis, and only the amounts differ. Using the comparative approach, the NPV of the replacement alternative is –$129,683 (row O). Thus, because the replacement alternative has the higher NPV (–$129,683 versus –$208,762), the replacement alternative should be undertaken.

Comparative Approach: For-Profit Analysis

The for-profit analysis is exactly the same as that for the not-for-profit analysis, with the two exceptions shown in Exhibit F.2, rows E and F, which arise as a result of the effects of taxes on cash flows and, ultimately, affect NPV. As in the not-for-profit analysis, earnings (or loss) before tax is calculated in row D. Because earnings get taxed at 40 percent, the resulting tax savings would be $22,400 for the existing alternative as compared with $12,400 for the replacement alternative, respectively (row E, both sections). Because earnings before tax is negative, the organization is losing money but will not be incurring negative taxes. However, the tax expense becomes a positive value because this tax loss can be either carried forward to offset future income or carried back to offset prior income to result in a tax refund. This has the same effect as a cash inflow: for each additional $1.00 in expenses, the organization pays $0.40 less in taxes. Therefore these tax savings get added back into the loss in row D. Taking into account the tax effects, the NPV of the existing alternative is –$111,782, and the NPV of the replacement alternative is –$67,998. Again, showing a smaller loss, or a savings of $43,784 (row R, bottom table), the replacement alternative should be undertaken, all else being equal.

EXHIBIT F.1 COMPARATIVE APPROACH TO ANALYZING A CAPITAL BUDGETING DECISION: NOT-FOR-PROFIT ENTITY

Existing equipment

Givens	Years	0	1	2	3	4	5
1 Initial outlay		$0					
2 Operating expenses			($50,000)	($50,000)	($50,000)	($50,000)	($50,000)
3 Depreciation expense			($6,000)	($6,000)	($6,000)	($6,000)	($6,000)
4 Change in net working capital			$300	$300	$300	$300	$300
5 Salvage value							$10,000
6 Cost of capital	5%						

	Years	0	1	2	3	4	5
A Initial outlay	Given 1	$0					
B Operating expenses before depreciation	Given 2		($50,000)	($50,000)	($50,000)	($50,000)	($50,000)
C Depreciation expense	Given 3		(6,000)	(6,000)	(6,000)	(6,000)	(6,000)
D Operating income (loss)	B + C		(56,000)	(56,000)	(56,000)	(56,000)	(56,000)
E Add: depreciation expense	-Given 3		6,000	6,000	6,000	6,000	6,000
F Net operating cash flow	D + E		(50,000)	(50,000)	(50,000)	(50,000)	(50,000)
G Change in net working capital	-Given 4		(300)	(300)	(300)	(300)	(300)
Terminal value changes							
H Salvage value	Given 5						10,000
I Recovery of net working capital	-Sum G						1,500
J Change in net cash flow	F + G + H + I		($50,300)	($50,300)	($50,300)	($50,300)	($38,800)
K Cost of capital	Given 6		5%	5%	5%	5%	5%
L Present value interest factor	$1/(1+i)^n$		0.9524	0.9070	0.8638	0.8227	0.7835
M Annual PV of cash flows[a]	J × L		($47,905)	($45,624)	($43,451)	($41,382)	($30,401)
N Sum of PV of cash flows	Sum M	($208,762)					
O Net present value	A + N	($208,762)					

[a]Present value interest factors in the exhibit have been calculated by formula, but are necessarily rounded for presentation. Therefore, there may be a difference between the number displayed and that calculated manually.

EXHIBIT F.1 (CONTINUED)

Replacement equipment

Givens		Years 0	1	2	3	4	5
1	Initial outlay	($80,000) b					
2	Operating expenses		($15,000)	($15,000)	($15,000)	($15,000)	($15,000)
3	Depreciation expense		($16,000)	($16,000)	($16,000)	($16,000)	($16,000)
4	Change in net working capital		$1,000	$1,000	$1,000	$1,000	$1,000
5	Salvage value						$20,000
6	Cost of capital	5%					

			Years 0	1	2	3	4	5
A	Initial outlay	Given 1	($80,000)					
B	Operating expenses before depreciation	Given 2		($15,000)	($15,000)	($15,000)	($15,000)	($15,000)
C	Depreciation expense	Given 3		(16,000)	(16,000)	(16,000)	(16,000)	(16,000)
D	Operating income (loss)	B + C		(31,000)	(31,000)	(31,000)	(31,000)	(31,000)
E	Add: depreciation expense	–Given 3		16,000	16,000	16,000	16,000	16,000
F	Net operating cash flow	D + E		(15,000)	(15,000)	(15,000)	(15,000)	(15,000)
G	Change in net working capital	–Given 4		(1,000)	(1,000)	(1,000)	(1,000)	(1,000)
	Terminal value changes							
H	Salvage value	Given 5						20,000
I	Recovery of net working capital	–Sum G						5,000
J	Change in net cash flow	F + G + H + I	($80,000)	($16,000)	($16,000)	($16,000)	($16,000)	$9,000
K	Cost of capital	Given 6		5%	5%	5%	5%	5%
L	Present value interest factor	$1/(1+i)^n$		0.9524	0.9070	0.8638	0.8227	0.7835
M	Annual PV of cash flows[a]	J × L	($80,000)	($15,238)	($14,512)	($13,821)	($13,163)	$7,052
N	Sum of PV of cash flows	Sum M	($49,683)					
O	**Net present value**	**A + N**	**($129,683)**					
P	**NPV difference**	c	**$79,079**					

b—$100,000 Purchase of new equipment + $20,000 Sale of old equipment.

c—(−$129,683 Replacement system) − (−$208,762 Existing system) = $79,079.

EXHIBIT F.2 COMPARATIVE APPROACH TO ANALYZING A CAPITAL BUDGETING DECISION: FOR-PROFIT ENTITY

Existing equipment

	Givens	Years	0	1	2	3	4	5
1	Initial outlay		$0					
2	Operating expenses			($50,000)	($50,000)	($50,000)	($50,000)	($50,000)
3	Depreciation expense			($6,000)	($6,000)	($6,000)	($6,000)	($6,000)
4	Change in net working capital			$300	$300	$300	$300	$300
5	Salvage value							$10,000
6	Cost of capital	5%						
7	Tax rate	40%						

	Years		0	1	2	3	4	5
A	Initial outlay	Given 1	$0					
B	Operating expenses before depreciation	Given 2		($50,000)	($50,000)	($50,000)	($50,000)	($50,000)
C	Depreciation expense	Given 3		(6,000)	(6,000)	(6,000)	(6,000)	(6,000)
D	Earnings (loss) before tax	B + C		(56,000)	(56,000)	(56,000)	(56,000)	(56,000)
E	Taxes at 40%	Given 7 × D		22,400	22,400	22,400	22,400	22,400
F	Earnings after tax	D + E		(33,600)	(33,600)	(33,600)	(33,600)	(33,600)
G	Add: depreciation expense	−Given 3		6,000	6,000	6,000	6,000	6,000
H	Net operating cash flow	F + G		(27,600)	(27,600)	(27,600)	(27,600)	(27,600)
I	Change in net working capital	−Given 4		(300)	(300)	(300)	(300)	(300)
	Terminal value changes							
J	Salvage value	Given 5						10,000
K	Recovery of net working capital	− Sum I						1,500
L	Change in net cash flow	H + I + J + K		($27,900)	($27,900)	($27,900)	($27,900)	($16,400)
M	Cost of capital	Given 6		5%	5%	5%	5%	5%
N	Present value interest factor	$1/(1+i)^n$		0.9524	0.9070	0.8638	0.8227	0.7835
O	Annual PV of cash flows[a]	L × N		($26,571)	($25,306)	($24,101)	($22,953)	($12,850)
P	Sum of PV of cash flows	Sum O	($111,782)					
Q	**Net present value**	A + P	**($111,782)**					

[a]Present value interest factors in the exhibit have been calculated by formula, but are necessarily rounded for presentation. Therefore, there may be a difference between the number displayed and that calculated manually.

EXHIBIT F.2 (CONTINUED)

Replacement equipment

Givens

		Years 0	1	2	3	4	5
1	Initial outlay	($72,000)[b]					
2	Operating expenses		($15,000)	($15,000)	($15,000)	($15,000)	($15,000)
3	Depreciation expense		($16,000)	($16,000)	($16,000)	($16,000)	($16,000)
4	Change in net working capital		$1,000	$1,000	$1,000	$1,000	$1,000
5	Salvage value						$20,000
6	Cost of capital	5%					
7	Tax rate	40%					

			Years 0	1	2	3	4	5
A	Initial outlay	Given 1	($72,000)					
B	Operating expenses before depreciation	Given 2		($15,000)	($15,000)	($15,000)	($15,000)	($15,000)
C	Depreciation expense	Given 3		(16,000)	(16,000)	(16,000)	(16,000)	(16,000)
D	Earnings before tax (loss before tax)	B + C		(31,000)	(31,000)	(31,000)	(31,000)	(31,000)
E	Taxes at 40%	Given 7 × D		12,400	12,400	12,400	12,400	12,400
F	Net income or earnings after tax	D + E		(18,600)	(18,600)	(18,600)	(18,600)	(18,600)
G	Add: depreciation expense	– Given 3		16,000	16,000	16,000	16,000	16,000
H	Net operating cash flow	F + G		(2,600)	(2,600)	(2,600)	(2,600)	(2,600)
I	Change in net working capital	–Given 4		(1,000)	(1,000)	(1,000)	(1,000)	(1,000)
	Terminal value changes							
J	Salvage value	Given 5						20,000
K	Recovery of net working capital	–Sum I						5,000
L	Change in net cash flow	H + I + J + K		($3,600)	($3,600)	($3,600)	($3,600)	$21,400
M	Cost of capital	Given 6		5%	5%	5%	5%	5%
N	Present value interest factor	$1/(1+i)^n$		0.9524	0.9070	0.8638	0.8227	0.7835
O	Annual PV of cash flows[a]	L × N		($3,429)	($3,265)	($3,110)	($2,962)	$16,767
P	Sum of PV of cash flows	Sum O	$4,002					
Q	**Net present value**	**A + P**	**($67,998)**					
R	**NPV difference**	c	**43,784**					

[b] —$100,000 Purchase of new equipment + $20,000 Sale of old equipment + $8,000 in Tax savings from loss on sale of existing equipment (0.40 Tax rate × $20,000 Loss)

[c] (−$67,998) − (−$111,782) = $43,784

353

Incremental Approach: Not-for-Profit Analysis

Exhibit F.3 analyzes the same replacement decision using the incremental approach. It looks at the savings (or lack thereof) for each item that would result if the decision were made to replace the old EKG system with a new product. To make this decision, several aspects of cash flows must be taken into account.

Though the new MIS system costs $100,000, the facility receives $20,000 from the sale of the old system. Thus the initial outlay is $80,000 (row A). The change in operating cash flows produces a net operating cash flow savings of $35,000 per year (row B, $15,000 replacement equipment labor expense versus $50,000 in labor expenses for the existing equipment).

As with the comparative analysis, in this nontaxpaying example, depreciation expense could be disregarded altogether because it has no effect on cash flow. However, to compare the not-for-profit and for-profit examples, operating income (needed to compute taxes in the for-profit example) is first computed by subtracting the $10,000 in depreciation expense (row C) and then adding it back to show that net operating cash flows do not change as a result of depreciation (rows E and F).

The effects of changes in working capital and the salvage value must be added to the analysis as well. Because net working capital increases by $700 annually ($300 for the existing system versus $1,000 for the replacement system), cash flows decrease by $700 each year (rows 5 and G). In year 5, the year in which the investment is assumed to end, salvage value increases by $10,000 (row H, sale of assets), which equals the incremental difference between the salvage value of the new system, $20,000, and the salvage value of the old system, $10,000. Because the project presumably ends at this time, it is also necessary to recapture $3,500 in net working capital (row I: 5 Years × $700 per year).

To determine the NPV, the cash flows each year are discounted at 5 percent and summed (rows J through O), and then the initial outlay (row A) is added. Because the NPV equals $79,079, which represents a positive return due to replacement, from a financial perspective the new EKG system should be purchased. Note that this NPV is the same as the NPV difference derived in Exhibit F.1 (bottom section, row P), as it should be.

Incremental Approach: For-Profit Analysis

Exhibit F.4 presents a similar incremental analysis, but for a for-profit, taxpaying organization. In this case, the new initial outlay is still reduced from $100,000 to $80,000 by the additional $20,000 from the sale of the

EXHIBIT F.3 INCREMENTAL APPROACH TO ANALYZING A CAPITAL BUDGETING DECISION: NOT-FOR-PROFIT ENTITY

Givens

1	Initial outlay[a]	($80,000)
2	Cost of capital	5%

Change in annual operating expenses and depreciation expense	Old MIS	New MIS	Change (New—Old)
3 Operating expenses (labor)	($50,000)	($15,000)	$35,000
4 Depreciation expense[b]	($6,000)	($16,000)	($10,000)
5 Net working capital	($300)	($1,000)	($700)
6 Salvage value	$10,000	$20,000	$10,000

[a]_$100,000 Purchase of new equipment + $20,000 Sale of old equipment.
[b]Old MIS: ($70,000 − $10,000) / 10 years = $6,000 per year. New MIS: ($100,000 − $20,000) / 5 years = $16,000 per year.

	Years	0	1	2	3	4	5
A	Initial outlay	Given 1	($80,000)					
B	Cash savings due to decreased operating expenses	Given 3		$35,000	$35,000	$35,000	$35,000	$35,000
C	Increase in depreciation expense	Given 4		(10,000)	(10,000)	(10,000)	(10,000)	(10,000)
D	Change in operating income	B + C		25,000	25,000	25,000	25,000	25,000
E	Add: increase in depreciation expense	−Given 4		10,000	10,000	10,000	10,000	10,000
F	Change in net operating cash flow	D + E		35,000	35,000	35,000	35,000	35,000
G	Change in net working capital	Given 5		(700)	(700)	(700)	(700)	(700)
	Terminal value changes							
H	Salvage value	Given 6						10,000
I	Recovery of net working capital	−Sum G						3,500
J	Change in net cash flow	F + G + H + I		$34,300	$34,300	$34,300	$34,300	$47,800
K	Cost of capital	Given 2		5%	5%	5%	5%	5%
L	Present value interest factor	$1 / (1 + i)^n$		0.9524	0.9070	0.8638	0.8227	0.7835
M	Annual PV of cash flows[c]	J × L		$32,667	$31,111	$29,630	$28,219	$37,453
N	Sum of PV cash flows	Sum M	$159,079					
O	**Net present value**	A + N	**$79,079**					

Note: MIS = management information system.

[c]Present value interest factors in the exhibit have been calculated by formula, but are necessarily rounded for presentation. Therefore, there may be a difference between the number displayed and that calculated manually.

EXHIBIT F.4 INCREMENTAL APPROACH TO ANALYZING A CAPITAL BUDGETING DECISION: FOR-PROFIT ENTITY

Givens

1 Initial outlay[a]	($72,000)
2 Cost of capital	5%
3 Tax rate	40%

Change in annual operating expenses and depreciation expense	Old MIS	New MIS	Change (New — Old)
4 Operating expenses (labor)	($50,000)	($15,000)	$35,000
5 Depreciation expense[b]	($6,000)	($16,000)	($10,000)
6 Net working capital	($300)	($1,000)	($700)
7 Salvage value	$10,000	$20,000	$10,000

[a]($100,000) Purchase of new equipment + $20,000 Sale of old equipment + $8,000 (0.40 × $20,000) Tax savings (due to sale at a loss).
[b]Old MIS: ($70,000 − $10,000) / 10 years = $6,000 per year. New MIS: ($100,000 − $20,000) / 5 years = $16,000 per year.

	Years	0	1	2	3	4	5
A	Initial outlay	Given 1	($72,000)					
B	Cash savings due to decreased operating expenses	Given 4		$35,000	$35,000	$35,000	$35,000	$35,000
C	Increase in depreciation expense[c]	Given 5		(10,000)	(10,000)	(10,000)	(10,000)	(10,000)
D	Change in earnings before tax	B + C		25,000	25,000	25,000	25,000	25,000
E	Less: increased tax expense	Given 3 × D		10,000	10,000	10,000	10,000	10,000
F	Increase in net income or earnings after tax	D − E		15,000	15,000	15,000	15,000	15,000
G	Add: increase in depreciation expense	−Given 5		10,000	10,000	10,000	10,000	10,000
H	Change in net operating cash flow	F + G		25,000	25,000	25,000	25,000	25,000
I	Change in net working capital	Given 6		(700)	(700)	(700)	(700)	(700)
	Terminal value changes							
J	Change in salvage value	Given 7						10,000
K	Recovery of net working capital	−Sum I						3,500
L	Change in net cash flow	H + I + J + K		$24,300	$24,300	$24,300	$24,300	$37,800
M	Cost of capital	Given 2		5%	5%	5%	5%	5%
N	Present value interest factor	$1/(1+i)^n$		0.9524	0.9070	0.8638	0.8227	0.7835
O	Annual PV of cash flows[d]	L × N		$23,143	$22,041	$20,991	$19,992	$29,617
P	Sum of PV cash flows	Sum O	$115,784					
Q	**Net present value**	A + P	**$43,784**					

[c]In row C, depreciation expense increased. However, it is an expense and must be deducted from cash savings.
[d]Present value interest factors in the exhibit have been calculated by formula, but are necessarily rounded for presentation. Therefore, there may be a difference between the number displayed and that calculated manually.

old system, but it is also reduced another $8,000 (to $72,000) by the tax effect of that sale (row 1). This tax benefit arises because the organization sells a system with a $40,000 book value for $20,000, incurring a $20,000 loss. Assuming a 40 percent tax rate, it will pay $8,000 less in taxes (0.40 × $20,000) than it would have if it had not sold the machine.

Taxes also affect operating income and represent a real cash outflow. Because the change in earnings before tax is $25,000 (row D), assuming a 40 percent tax rate, taxes will increase by $10,000 (row E), thereby reducing the change in net income to $15,000 (row F). However, reflected in this $15,000 net income is the $10,000 in depreciation expense that does not require a cash outflow. Therefore this $10,000 must be added back in, and cash flow becomes $25,000 (rows G and H). The remainder of the analysis remains the same as for the not-for-profit analysis, adjusting for the change in net working capital and the terminal value.

After accounting for the sale of the new system at its termination date and discounting at the cost of capital, the decision to make this investment results in a positive NPV of $43,784 (row Q). Because the NPV is positive, the investment should be made. Again, this value expectedly equals that shown in row R in the bottom section of Exhibit F.2.

Appendix Summary

This appendix provided both a comparative and an incremental NPV analysis of purchasing a new EKG MIS system. The analysis was conducted for

---

EXHIBIT F.5 RESULTS OF THE COMPARATIVE AND INCREMENTAL NPV ANALYSES OF REPLACING AN EXISTING EKG SYSTEM

	Not-for-Profit Institution	For-Profit Institution
Replace equipment	($129,683)[a]	($67,998)[b]
Keep existing equipment	($208,762)[a]	($111,782)[b]
Difference (replace – keep)	$79,079	$43,784
Incremental approach	$79,079[c]	$43,784[d]

[a]Exhibit F.1, comparative approach.
[b]Exhibit F.2, comparative approach.
[c]Exhibit F.3, incremental approach.
[d]Exhibit F.4, incremental approach.

both a not-for-profit and a for-profit entity. The summary of results presented in Exhibit F.5 shows that the comparative and incremental approaches provide exactly the same answer. Thus the method used depends only on preference and has no effect on the final result. In this case, though tax effects are considerable, they do not change the decision.

CHAPTER 8

CAPITAL FINANCING FOR HEALTH CARE PROVIDERS

In Chapters Two and Three, the basic accounting equation was defined as Assets = Liabilities + Net Assets. Because liabilities are debts and net assets represent the community's equity in a not-for-profit health care organization, in terms of the sources of financing, the basic accounting equation can also be thought of as

$$\text{Assets} = \text{Debt} + \text{Equity}$$

This equation shows that any increase in assets must be balanced by a similar increase in debt or equity, or both. The structuring of debt relative to equity is called the *capital structure decision* and is becoming increasingly important to both for-profit and not-for-profit providers. This was not always the case: in the 1970s and early 1980s, the cost of capital was never a major concern for health care providers. As with other operational costs, health care organizations simply passed on the costs of debt and equity financing to third-party payors. Hospitals had no trouble accessing capital markets because they were virtually guaranteed any income needed to cover debts. In today's environment, however, health policymakers need to recognize that cutbacks in Medicare and Medicaid reimbursement resulting from governmental policy, the implementation of at-risk prospective payment systems, industry changes stemming from the increased usage of outpatient services, and the rise in competition among physician and free-standing surgical centers can limit the access to debt and equity financing among hospital industry entities. For example, a hospital system with a poor bond credit rating due to an increase in Medicaid volume

LEARNING OBJECTIVES

- Describe the types of equity and debt financing.

- Define various bond terminology.

- Compare tax-exempt with taxable financing.

- Explain lease financing.

and lower Medicaid payments may experience a downgrade in its credit rating, which in turn may increase its cost of capital, thereby restricting its ability to purchase or replace plant and equipment. A hospital system unable to maintain and update its facilities could experience a reduction in its ability to attract and retain physicians and patients, which in turn might reduce patient volume and result in further financial distress. The lingering economic recession and uncertainty about health care reform continue to cause hospitals to delay capital project investments. As a result, hospitals are retaining their cash flow in the form of cash and investments, paying down existing debt, focusing on operational efficiency improvements, and moving their clinical services into lower-cost outpatient settings.

Perspective 8.1 provides an example of how strong cash flow and a dominant market position can improve the credit rating of a health care system. Conversely, Perspective 8.2 offers insight into how capital from for-profit entities is causing capital-starved nonprofit systems to change their ownership status to for profit.

PERSPECTIVE 8.1 KEY MARKET AND FINANCIAL FACTORS DRIVE UPGRADE IN RATING

Fitch Ratings upgraded Blanchard Valley Health System (BVHS) in Findlay, Ohio, to A from A–. BVHS owns two acute-care hospitals, a 150-bed hospital in Findlay and a 25-bed hospital twenty miles southwest in Bluffton; a multispecialty medical group; a foundation; and several other affiliates.

The key credit strengths behind the rating improvement were strong operating cash flow, a high liquidity position, and an improved market position.

- *Operating cash flow.* In 2011, BVHS generated a strong 9.2 percent operating margin and a 16.6 percent operating EBITDA margin, compared to a 9.1 percent operating margin and a 16.1 percent operating EBITDA margin in 2010. Fitch takes a favorable view of health care systems with operating margins above 10 percent, which leaves sufficient cash flow to cover debt service, finance capital projects, and/or build liquidity.

- *Liquidity.* BVHS possesses $184.2 million in unrestricted cash and investments, which equals 318.4 days cash on hand and 119.5 percent cash to debt, comparable to Fitch's A category medians of 194.1 days cash on hand and 113.8 percent cash to debt. Since 2008, BVHS has continued to build its liquidity position 20 percent per year via strong cash flow, revenue cycle management, and improved asset valuation.

- *Market position.* BVHS holds a leading market position within its primary service area, as reflected by 75.8 percent market share. Further, BVHS has developed a collaborative relationship with local employers and payors.

Key credit weaknesses that Fitch views as a concern to the health care system are as follows:

- *Debt position.* BVHS's debt ratios are high for the A rating category. BVHS has debt to capitalization of 46.4 percent and its maximum annual debt service (MADS) is 4.8 percent of revenue. These ratios are unfavorable when compared with Fitch's A category medians of 41.9 percent and 2.9 percent, respectively.

- *Limited operating capacity.* BVHS facilities are located within a limited geographical area in Ohio. In addition, its small revenue size presents a potential risk to its revenue base, and it makes the health system susceptible to changes in payor mix or physician complement.

Source: Fitch Ratings, Fitch Ratings has upgraded to 'A' from 'A–' the ratings on the following Hancock County, Ohio bonds issued on behalf of Blanchard Valley Regional Medical Center (d/b/a Blanchard Valley Health System, BVHS), March 5, 2012, www.fitchratings.com/creditdesk/press_releases/detail.cfm?pr_id=744395.

PERSPECTIVE 8.2 ACCESS TO FOR-PROFIT EQUITY CAPITAL FUNDS NONPROFIT SYSTEMS

In November 2010, the $895 million purchase of a six-hospital system owned by Caritas Christi Health Care of Boston by New York private-equity firm Cerberus Capital Management was approved by the Vatican and the Archdiocese of Boston. The underlying operational reason for this sale was the system's need for capital; it had faced a capital shortfall throughout the previous decade. Another driving factor in this sale, which other nonprofit hospitals across the country were also facing, was declining operating margins. The cash infusion of $895 million from Cerberus consisted of $200 million to pay off existing system debt, $295 million to make the pension fund solvent again, and $400 million to fund capital projects, from fixing leaky roofs to building a new medical office building. Caritas viewed the change in ownership as a change in tax status but not mission status, in that the system is now serving the community by paying taxes as well, which are expected to be $20 million a year. For now, the health care system, renamed Steward Health Care System, is retaining its Catholic ethical and religious directives, unless that becomes 'materially burdensome' for the system. If Cerberus decides to change these directives, it would be required to donate $25 million to a charity of the church chosen by the archdiocese.

Source: Adapted from J. Carlson, Keeping the doors open, *Modern Healthcare*, 2010;40(46):8.

The first section of this chapter briefly examines equity financing. The remaining sections focus on the issuance of bonds, the main source of debt financing for many health care organizations, and on lease financing, which is similar to debt financing.

Equity Financing

The primary sources of equity financing for not-for-profit health care organizations are internally generated funds, philanthropy, governmental grants, and sale of real estate including medical office buildings, whereas the primary sources of equity financing for for-profit organizations are internally generated funds and stock issuances. Unfortunately, internally generated funds—those funds retained from operations (retained earnings)—are shrinking. As discussed in Chapter One, financial pressures have lowered revenues and eroded earnings for health care organizations, especially hospitals. Therefore these organizations must be able to generate new sources of capital in order to survive.

Because the equity account on the balance sheet represents the claim on assets, as earnings increase an organization builds its asset base. Typically, health care organizations use their most liquid assets on a balance sheet (i.e., cash, marketable securities, and long-term investments) to finance small capital purchases. But by doing so, an organization incurs an opportunity cost, which represents the lost financial returns from not putting these funds into short- and long-term investments. Assuming these funds are not invested in tax-exempt debt funds, the financial returns from these short- and long-term investments are higher than the interest cost on tax-exempt debt. Because tax-exempt debt financing is a cheaper source of capital than equity financing, nonprofit health care organizations try to minimize their cost of capital by using more debt than equity in their financing decisions. As a result, nonprofit hospitals are motivated to enhance the liquidity of their organization so that bond rating agencies will assign them a higher credit rating, which in turn will lower their cost of debt. The opposite is true for for-profit hospitals because they are driven to enhance stockholder wealth; they seek to maximize cash flow and use the cash they retain to invest in capital projects and to return the capital to stockholders in the form of dividends or stock buybacks, or both.

 Key Point Equity financing for not-for-profits is derived from retained earnings, governmental grants, sale of assets, and contributions. Equity financing for for-profits comes from issuing stock as well as from retained earnings.

The Tax Reform Act of 1986 was seen as a major setback for health care providers because it lowered the tax deduction available to private individuals who wanted to make philanthropic donations. Nevertheless, charitable giving remains a major source of capital for certain health care providers. Although individuals who make contributions do not receive a direct monetary return, they expect nonmonetary benefits for the community in terms of greater access to or increased quality of care. As health care providers reach their debt limits, equity financing becomes their only source of new funds. In addition to externally generated equity, such as grants and appropriations that are available to all health care organizations, for-profit organizations (commonly referred to as *investor-owned*) can also issue stock. Exhibit 8.1 lists selected advantages and disadvantages of issuing stock versus debt financing.

The stock markets generally require a higher rate of return on equity financing (issuing stock) relative to debt financing (issuing bonds). This is due to the greater uncertainty associated with equity relative to debt: organizations are legally required to pay back debt, but there is no legal obligation on an issuer's part to pay back equity.

EXHIBIT 8.1 COMPARISON OF STOCK AND DEBT FINANCING

	Stock	Debt Financing
Ownership	Ownership rights given to investors.	No ownership rights given up.
Tax implications	Dividends are not tax deductible.	Interest on debt is deductible.
Set payments	Dividends are not required to be paid.	Debt service payments are legally required to be made.
Amount of payments	Dividend payment amount is at the organization's discretion.	Debt service payments are legally specified as to amount.
Time limit of payments	No limit.	Time limit is part of borrowing agreement.
Restrictions on other actions	Indirect—through giving up of ownership.	Restrictions may be placed on operations and capital acquisition.

Debt Financing

The major alternative to equity financing is debt financing: borrowing money from others at a cost. The remainder of this chapter describes several types of debt financing and then the process of issuing bonds. Hospitals continue to depend on tax-exempt debt as their primary source of capital, a decision attributable to low interest rates since the year 2000. Perspective 8.3 provides insight on how a large health system issued tax-exempt debt to refinance a newly acquired system's debt as well as to fund its capital purchases. Certainly, system-affiliated hospitals have greater access to capital than other hospitals, given their diversity of services, the geographical diversity of their market areas, and their overall financial strength.

Term Loan

A loan, typically issued by a bank, that has a maturity of one to ten years.

Bond

A form of long-term financing whereby an issuer receives cash from a lender (an *investor*), and in return issues a promissory note (a *bond*) agreeing to make principal or interest payments on specific dates.

Sources of Debt Financing by Maturity

The general rule of thumb is to borrow short term for short-term needs and long term for long-term needs. Short-term borrowing was discussed in Chapter Five, on working capital. There are two important types of long-term financing: *term loans*, which typically must be paid off within ten years, and *bonds*, which typically have a maturity of twenty to thirty-five years. Bonds are the primary source of long-term financing for many

---

PERSPECTIVE 8.3 USING TAX-EXEMPT DEBT TO REFINANCE EXISTING DEBT AND FUND NEW CAPITAL PROJECTS

Ascension Health Care System, a St. Louis–based hospital network, plans to issue $600 million in bonds, in part to refinance $425 million of outstanding bonds previously issued by Alexian Brothers Health Systems of Illinois, which Ascension recently acquired. The refinancing would help to lower interest payments, and thus Alexian's operating costs, as well as improve its operating margin, which stands at 2.4 percent. Ascension is the nation's largest Catholic health care system, with $15.6 billion in revenue (sixteen times Alexian's revenue), and has an operating margin of 3.5 percent. Its strong credit rating enables it to borrow money at low interest rates. To help the newly acquired Alexian system compete in its suburban Chicago market areas, Ascension plans to use the remaining $175 million of the bond proceeds to upgrade Alexian's facilities.

Source: Adapted from K. Schorsch, Alexian's new parent eyes $600 million bond issue, *Crain's Chicago Business*, February 9, 2012, www.chicagobusiness.com/article/20120209/NEWS03/120209781/alexians-new-parent-eyes -600-million-bond-issue.

tax-exempt health care entities. Term loans, such as bank loans, conventional mortgages, and mortgages backed by the Federal Housing Administration (FHA), require the borrower to pay off or amortize the principal value of the loan over its life. The amortization of a loan requires equal periodic payments for principal and interest obligations. (Appendix G provides a detailed analysis of the computation and development of a loan amortization schedule.) In contrast, the payment of a bond can require the payment of the principal at maturity, at which time the bondholder receives the face value of the bond, and interest payments can be paid either periodically or all at once at maturity, along with the principal.

In contrast to a bank, which lends funds, the issuer of a bond receives funds from the purchasers of the bond, typically the public. However, bond payments may be structured so that the issuer can make early repayments of the principal or equal payments over the life of the bond through a *sinking fund*. In the latter case, the issuer makes payments to the bond trustee, who then uses the funds to retire a portion of the debt.

Sinking Fund
A fund in which monies are set aside each year to ensure that a bond can be liquidated at maturity.

Key Point *Short-term financing* typically refers to a wide range of financing, from debt that must be paid back almost immediately to debt that may not have to be paid off for a year. *Long-term financing* typically refers to debt that will be paid off in a period longer than one year.

Sources of Debt Financing by Type of Interest Rate

Fixed and Variable Interest

Fixed interest rate debt describes a security whose rate does not change during the lifetime of the bond; conversely, *variable interest rate debt* describes a security whose rate changes based on market conditions and can fluctuate on a daily, weekly, or monthly basis. Thus, when hospitals borrow on a variable basis, they are exposed to changes in interest rates; this exposure is called *interest rate risk*. As a result, some hospitals are attracted to fixed rate debt because of the predictability of future payments, but the generally higher cost of fixed rate debt may encourage other hospitals to borrow on the lower-cost, variable basis. Types of variable rate bonds include *variable rate demand bonds* and *auction rate securities*. Variable rate demand bonds allow the investor to *put*, which means to *sell*, the bonds back to a remarketing agent within a short time, typically thirty days, who will then attempt to sell, or remarket, the bonds. This ability of investors to sell back these bonds is called the *put risk*. Typically, these bonds are supported by a bank letter of credit, whereby the bond trustee can draw upon a bank to repurchase the bonds in case all the bonds are not resold by the agent. This potential inability to resell the bonds is called the *remarketing risk*. Another major risk with variable rate demand bonds is that the hospital may not be able to renew its letter of credit from a bank, a renewal that typically occurs every one to three years. Hospitals that experience a decline in their credit position due to declining patient revenues, greater competition, and so forth, may not be able to renew their letter of credit with the bank, and the potential for this is called the *renewal risk*. Also, lower credit standards in the banking industry, as happened during the credit crises of 2008 and 2009, can cause banks to stop offering a line of credit, which in turn may make it difficult for hospitals to renew an existing line of credit or to secure a new one.

Unlike demand variable rate bonds, auction variable rate bonds allow the bondholders to resell the bonds through an auction process rather than the put feature of the variable rate debt. As a result, the hospital does not need to establish and pay for a letter of credit from a bank. In 2008, the downgrading of bond insurers, as a result of their insuring of subprime mortgage securities, resulted in no buyers for auction rate securities and essentially forced health care systems and hospitals from this market.

The primary concern with variable interest rates is that these rates may increase, which could cause an unanticipated demand for cash flow. However, throughout the last decade, the average fixed rate for tax-exempt debt was 5.13 percent compared to 1.89 percent for variable rate tax-exempt debt. This low rate makes variable rate debt appealing, by allowing hospitals to lower their overall cost of capital. However, variable rates can also rise. Exhibit 8.2a summarizes the advantages and disadvantages of fixed and variable rate debt. Perspective 8.4 provides an explanation of the economic credit crisis of 2008 and the ways it affected interest rates for the hospital industry.

Hedging
The art of offsetting high variable rate debt payments with returns from variable rate investments.

Health care providers may use variable rate debt if they have sufficient cash flows and cash investment accounts to hedge against changes in interest rates (*interest rate risk*). The concept of *hedging* is that as variable interest rates increase, so too will the returns on the facility's investments, thereby offsetting increased interest payments. As a result, hospital issuers with strong liquidity and cash flow may opt to use a mix of fixed and variable rate debt, such as 40 percent and 60 percent, respectively.

Interest Rate Swap

Hospitals continually look for financial mechanisms to lower their cost of debt, especially when interest rates decline. One approach is to refinance the bond by issuing new debt to retire the old debt. To avoid the issuance costs of new debt or refunding its existing debt, a hospital can use an

EXHIBIT 8.2a SELECTED ADVANTAGES AND DISADVANTAGES OF FIXED AND VARIABLE RATE DEBT

Advantages

Fixed rate debt

1. Fixed debt service payments.

2. Fixed interest rate; no risk related to interest rate changes (*interest rate risk*).

3. No risk that investors will sell bonds back (*put risk*).

4. No letter of credit required from bank.

Variable rate debt

1. Lower up-front issuance costs.

2. Lower initial interest rate.

3. Greater call or refund flexibility for issuer.

4. Greater matching or hedging between interest income from investments and interest expense from variable debt.

Disadvantages

Fixed rate debt

1. Higher up-front or issuance expenses.

2. Market conditions may result in low variable rate debt over the life of the fixed rate loan; this may result in paying higher interest cost over life of loan.

3. Typically, for the first 10 years, the issuer cannot *call* or refund bonds back, unless the issuer uses advance refunding, which can only be done once.

4. Can result in a negative arbitrage situation, whereby income earned from investments is less than the interest cost of fixed debt.

Variable rate debt

1. Higher interest costs if interest rates increase (*interest rate risk*).

2. Unstable debt service payments.

3. Decline in cash flow if interest rates increase.

4. Bondholders can sell, or put, the bonds back (*put risk*).

5. Requires liquidity to pay off bondholders if unable to find buyers. Hospitals typically pay for a bank letter of credit rather than use their own liquidity.

6. Banks require a renewed letter of credit every 3 to 5 years (*renewal risk*). High-credit-risk hospitals may have trouble renewing letter of credit.

PERSPECTIVE 8.4 THE MOVEMENT AWAY FROM VARIABLE RATE DEBT AND THE HISTORY OF THE CREDIT CRISIS

In 2011, only 43 percent of the bonds issued by nonprofit hospitals were used to fund capital projects; the remaining 57 percent of the bond issues were used to refund existing bonds. The forces behind the movement to refund bonds were lower interest rates and a shift by hospitals to more conservative, fixed rate debt. From 2000 to 2007, hospitals were issuing primarily variable rate debt because of low variable rates, the availability of bond insurance, and demand by bond investors for variable rate securities. By 2005 and 2006, variable rate debt accounted for 60 percent to 70 percent of all hospital bond issues.

One variable rate product issued by hospitals was the insured auction rate security (ARS). However, in late 2007 and early 2008, the market for auction rate securities collapsed, due to lower credit ratings for the bond insurers. Bond insurers experienced a downgrade in their credit ratings from insuring subprime mortgage securities. The other variable rate security issued by hospitals was the variable rate demand bond (VRDB), a security backed by letters of credit from banks. However, the rates on VRDBs rose as well because banks also suffered credit rating downgrades during the financial crisis. Given these risk factors, new investors were no longer buying variable rate hospital debt, which resulted in an illiquid position for those investors who already owned these variable rate securities. As a result, the boards, CEOs, and CFOs of hospitals and health care systems decided to repurchase or refinance their variable rate bonds by issuing fixed rate debt. By 2009, the bond market had shifted back to fixed rate debt, with over 70 percent of debt issued using this type of interest rate. Current market conditions have resulted in low fixed interest rates, which continue to support the issuance of fixed rate debt, and only large, financially strong health care systems are returning to the variable rate mode of interest.

Source: Adapted from G. Huang, The rise, fall, and future of not-for-profit hospital debt issuance, *MuniNet Guide*, February 16, 2012, www.muninetguide.com/articles/hospital-debt-issuance-trends-489.

Interest Rate Swap

An exchange, or swap, of interest rates (from fixed to variable rate or from variable to fixed rate) between a hospital borrower and another party, typically a bank or investment banking firm, with the intent of securing a more favorable rate.

interest rate swap, whereby the hospital borrower exchanges, or *swaps*, interest rates with another party, typically a bank or investment banking firm. One type of swap involves switching fixed rate debt to floating, or variable, rate debt (a *fixed to floating rate swap*). Under this type of swap, a hospital that is paying a fixed interest rate to its bondholders decides to exchange, or swap, to a variable interest rate. To carry out this swap, the hospital will pay a variable interest rate to the bank over the life of the swap, and the bank will pay a fixed interest rate to the hospital, which the hospital will use to pay the current bondholders their fixed interest rate. A hospital would consider using this type of swap or exchange in interest rates if the variable, or floating, rate for tax-exempt debt is below the fixed rate the hospital is paying to its current bondholders, which in turn allows the facility to achieve a lower cost of debt. However, it is important for hospitals to have the cash and investment hedge to offset any unexpected rise in interest rates. From the bondholders' perspective, it is important to remember that they are not affected by the interest rate swap. The hospital is still obligated to pay them their fixed rate interest rate. The hospital borrower could also exchange, or swap, from a floating or variable rate to a fixed rate. This *floating to fixed rate swap* can be considered when the hospital wants to avoid the risk of rising variable rates and to lock into a fixed rate without issuing new debt. Again, it is important to remember that the current bondholders are not affected by this exchange and will still receive their variable or floating rate.

For a further understanding of how a swap works, Exhibit 8.2b presents two examples for St. Mary's Hospital, an entity that is currently paying a 3 percent variable rate to its existing bondholders, which is based on the market rate index for tax-exempt bonds (Exhibit 8.2b, row A). St. Mary's wants to avoid the risk of rising variable interest rates, and it locks into a fixed rate by entering into a floating to fixed rate swap agreement, called a *fixed payor* swap agreement. The hospital contracts with a local bank, or *counterparty*, to pay St. Mary's a variable rate of 3 percent, based on the variable market rate index for tax-exempt bonds (see row B). The hospital uses this variable rate payment to pay the 3 percent to its existing variable rate bondholders. The net difference (see row C) is zero because the variable rate it receives from the bank is equivalent to the variable rate it needs to pay its existing bondholders. Because St. Mary's is exchanging or swapping to a fixed rate, it needs to pay the bank, or counterparty, a fixed rate of 5 percent (see row D), which is the going market rate for a thirty-year, fixed rate swap. The total interest rate cost to St. Mary's is 5 percent (row E), which is the sum of the fixed rate (row D) and the net difference (0 percent, row C), which is the difference between what St. Mary's needs to pay the existing variable rate bondholders and what it receives from the bank. In short, St. Mary's is able to lock into a fixed rate of 5 percent without issuing new debt, while its existing bondholders continue to receive their variable rate.

For some floating to fixed rate swap agreements, the hospital's interest rate to existing bondholders (row A) may be higher than the interest rate it receives from the counterparty, because the hospital is a higher credit risk or the maturity of the swap is less than the maturity of the bond. Using the previous example, the hospital may be paying 1 percentage point above

EXHIBIT 8.2b   EXPLANATION OF FIXED PAYOR AND FIXED RECEIVER INTEREST RATE SWAPS

St. Mary's Hospital Enters into a *Fixed Payor* Swap Agreement with a Bank (a *Counterparty*)

Givens

1	Interest rate on hospital's existing variable rate debt.	3%
2	Counterparty, or bank, contracts to pay hospital a variable interest rate.	3%
3	Hospital contracts with counterparty to pay a fixed interest rate.	5%
4	Maturity of bond and swap.	30 years

Total Interest Cost to St. Mary's Hospital When Entering into a Floating to Fixed Rate Swap Agreement

A	Hospital pays variable rate debt for existing debt.	Given 1	3%
B	Counterparty, or bank, pays hospital variable rate for existing bondholders.	Given 2	3%
C	Net difference between hospital variable rate and bank variable rate.	A − B	0%
D	Hospital pays fixed coupon rate to counterparty.	Given 3	5%
E	Total interest rate cost to St Mary's Hospital.	C + D	5%

St. Mary's Hospital Enters into an *Fixed Receiver* Swap Agreement with a Bank (a *Counterparty*)

Givens

5	Interest rate on hospital's existing fixed rate debt.	5%
6	Counterparty, or bank, contracts to pay hospital a fixed interest rate.	4%
7	Hospital contracts with counterparty to pay a variable interest rate.[a]	2%
8	Maturity of bond.	30 years
9	Maturity of swap.	20 years

Total Interest Cost to St. Mary's Hospital When Entering into a Fixed to Floating Rate Swap Agreement

F	Hospital pays fixed rate debt for existing debt.	Given 5	5%
G	Counterparty, or bank, pays hospital fixed rate for existing bondholders.	Given 6	4%
H	Net difference between hospital's fixed rate and bank's fixed rate.	F − G	1%
I	Hospital pays variable rate to counterparty.[a]	Given 7	2%
J	Total interest rate cost to St. Mary's Hospital.	H + I	3%

[a]Assumes market variable rate index declined to 2 percent from 3 percent under the fixed payor swap case.

the variable market rate index for tax-exempt bonds (4% = 3% + 1%) to its current bondholders. Under this scenario, St. Mary's total interest rate cost is 6 percent, which is the sum of the fixed rate it pays the bank, 5 percent, and the net difference, 1 percent (1% = 4% − 3%), between what the hospital needs to pay the existing bondholders, 4 percent, and what St. Mary's receives from the bank, 3 percent.

Exhibit 8.2b also includes an example of a *fixed receiver* swap agreement. In this case, St. Mary's Hospital is currently paying a 5 percent fixed rate to its existing bondholders (row F). St. Mary's wants to diversify the interest rates on its debt by paying a portion of it on a variable rate basis. It is able to achieve this outcome by entering into a fixed to floating (i.e., variable) rate swap agreement with existing debt, rather than issuing new variable rate debt. The hospital contracts with a local bank, or counterparty, to pay St. Mary's a fixed rate of 4 percent, which is the going market rate for a twenty-year, fixed payor swap (row G). The hospital uses this fixed rate payment to pay most of the 5 percent for its existing fixed rate bondholders, which is a thirty-year bond rate. The net difference (row H) is 1 percent, because the fixed rate it receives from the bank (4%) is for a twenty-year swap, whereas the fixed rate it needs to pay its existing bondholders (5%) is for a thirty-year bond; therefore, the earlier maturity date or length of the swap results in a lower rate. As part of its swap contract, St. Mary's also needs to pay a 2 percent variable rate, which is based on an updated market variable rate index of 2 percent to the counterparty (row I). The total interest rate cost to St. Mary's is therefore 3 percent (row J), which is the sum of the variable rate, 2 percent (row I), and the net difference of 1 percent (row H). Overall, St. Mary's is able to access lower-cost, variable rate debt by entering into a fixed receiver swap without issuing new variable rate debt. It is beyond the scope of this textbook to address the other facets of interest rate swaps and the types of risk hospitals face when entering into an interest rate swap contract.[1]

Selected Types of Health Care Debt Financing

This section discusses further several specific types of debt financing: bank loans, conventional mortgages, pooled equipment financing, FHA program loans, and bonds.

Bank Term Loans

Loans traditionally issued by banks with maturities of one to ten years are defined as *term loans*. These loans are usually paid off in equal, or *level*, amounts over the life of the loan.

Conventional Mortgages

Collateral

An asset with clear value (such as land or buildings) that is pledged against a loan to reduce risk to the lender. If the loan is not paid off satisfactorily, the lender has a legal claim to seize the pledged asset.

Under a *conventional mortgage*, the health care facility pledges its land or building(s) as *collateral* for a loan. Typical lenders include commercial banks, insurance companies, and savings and loan institutions. The term of the loan is normally twenty years. Unfortunately, the lender may allow the borrower to finance only a portion of the purchase, requiring a down payment on the rest.

Pooled Equipment Financing

To create greater access to tax-exempt debt financing for less expensive loans, a program of *pooled equipment financing* was developed. Given the high fixed issuance costs of borrowing, pooled financing spreads these costs over a number of health care borrowers, who each receive a portion of the loan. State or regional hospital associations typically sponsor pooled equipment financing programs.

FHA Program Loans

To improve marketability and encourage lower interest rates, the government-sponsored FHA provides mortgage insurance for health care facilities' loans. The insurance guarantees the principal and interest on a loan, which reduces risk to the bondholders. The disadvantages are the fees charged and the time it takes to have a loan approved. Many FHA-insured loans can take a year or more to implement.

Bonds

A *bond* is a long-term contract whereby on specific dates a borrower agrees to make principal or interest payments (or both) to the holder of the bond, that is, the entity who lent the funds. The section below describes key terms used in the rest of this chapter as they relate to bonds and the bond issuance process.

- *Indenture and covenant.* A legal document that states the conditions and terms of a bond is called an *indenture*. It is usually a lengthy document—often one hundred pages or more—and discusses the interest mode (daily, weekly, or long-term rates), payment provisions, call features, and repayment years of the debt. It also lists the numerous covenants of the bond. A loan covenant is a legal provision stated in the bond that the issuer must follow, addressing such matters as the security backing the bond, the amount of future debt that can be offered, and acceptable ranges for liquidity and debt service coverage ratios. Covenants protect the claims of bondholders on the facility's assets in case of default.

- *Debenture.* A *debenture* is an unsecured bond; that is, it is not backed by specific assets of the organization.

- *Subordinated debenture.* A *subordinated debenture* is an unsecured bond that is junior to debenture bonds. In the case of default, debenture bondholders are paid first. A subordinated debenture is more risky to the investor and thus pays a higher interest rate.

- *Par value.* The *par value* of a bond is the security's face value, such as $1,000 or $5,000. This is the amount that a bondholder is paid at the time of the bond's maturity.

- *Coupon rate and coupon payment.* The *coupon rate* is the stated interest rate on the bond, as promised by the issuer. The *coupon payment* is the amount the holder of the coupon receives periodically, usually semiannually. It equals the coupon rate times the face value of the bond payment. For example, if the coupon rate is 10 percent for a bond with a $1,000 par value, the coupon payment is $100 annually or $50 semiannually.

- *Callable bonds.* *Callable bonds* may be redeemed by the issuer before they mature. An issuer may call a bond because its coupon rate is higher than the presently prevailing interest rates for bonds, or because the issuer wants to eliminate restrictions caused by having the bond outstanding. To attract investors, most callable bonds guarantee a certain coupon payment for ten years (the *call protection period*) and contain a call price feature that equals par value plus a call premium, usually equal to 1 to 2 percent of the outstanding balance.

- *Zero coupon bonds.* The term *coupon* refers to the amount of interest that will be paid by the issuer to the bondholders. Bonds issued with no coupon at all are called *zero coupon bonds*. The trade-off made by the issuer for not making any coupon payments over the lifetime of a bond is that the bond must be issued at a deep discount, that is, at less than face value, which means that the issuer receives less initially in bond proceeds. Investors are attracted to these bonds not only because of their bigger discount rates but also because investors need not concern themselves with managing and reinvesting coupon payments (although they still must pay annual taxes on portions of taxable bonds).

- *Serial bonds.* The term *serial bonds* refers to a portion of a fixed rate bond issue that matures during the early due dates of the issue, typically during the first ten to fifteen years, and that has its own interest rate. Bonds of this nature allow the investor to purchase bonds with shorter maturities in addition to investing in bonds with longer maturities. In contrast, *term bonds* make up the remaining larger portion and have longer maturities (between twenty and thirty years).

- *Basis points.* Security traders discuss the changes in a bond's interest rate in terms of basis points. A *basis point* is 1/100th of 1 percent. Thus 100 basis points is equal to 1 percent, and one bond yielding 5.75 percent and another bond yielding 5.65 percent have a *spread* of 10 basis points. Traders also consider the basis point spread between different types of bonds. For example, the spread between taxable and tax-exempt bonds may be 300 basis points, or there may be a spread of 30 basis points between AAA and A– rated bonds (bond ratings are discussed more later).

- *Sinking fund.* A bond contract, i.e., a covenant, may establish that part of the principal be paid back each year out of a fund earmarked for the orderly retirement or the redemption of bonds before maturity. This fund is called a *sinking fund*, and monies for the fund are paid periodically to the trustee who maintains the fund for the health care provider. This contractual process is analogous to the principal repayment of a mortgage.

- *Secondary market. Secondary markets* deal in buying and selling bonds that have already been issued.

- *Debt service reserve fund. Debt service reserve funds*, typically equivalent to one year of principal and interest payments, are set aside with a trustee to act as a safeguard against default during the life of the loan period.

Tax-Exempt Bonds

Tax-exempt bonds are bonds whose interest payments to the investor are exempt from federal income taxes, and in some cases state and local income taxes as well; thus the interest payments are typically lower than those from bonds that do not have tax-exempt status (such as taxable municipal or corporate bonds). The lower interest payments of tax-exempt financing have made it the primary choice of debt financing for not-for-profit health care organizations. These bonds can be issued only by an organization that has been designated a tax-exempt organization by the Internal Revenue Service, such as a state, city, or local government and its respective agencies, and the funds must be used for projects that qualify as *exempt uses*. Rather than having assets as collateral, these bonds are backed by either the issuer's general obligations or specific revenues; the latter are called *tax-exempt revenue bonds*.

For most health care organizations, the issuance of a tax-exempt revenue bond will require the security of a *mortgage*, meaning the health care provider will pledge its real property and equipment as security, or collateral, in the case of default. In today's market, health care providers with an A or higher bond rating normally are not required to pledge their fixed assets as collateral; in the unlikely case of default, creditors are secured by the pledge of the health care provider's revenues. However, creditors can enhance their security indirectly by requiring a negative pledge on a health care provider's real estate. A *negative pledge* prohibits the health care provider from giving a lien (claim) on its real estate to any other creditor.

Another advantage to the issuer of tax-exempt bonds other than lower interest rates is their long maturity to term, often thirty to thirty-five years, as compared with the seven to twenty years typical of taxable bonds. One disadvantage is the higher issuance cost due to documentation fees for the issuing authority, bond counsel fees, and other documentation required to achieve tax-exempt status on the issue. Slower issuance is another drawback. Because the facility must act through a governmental authority, the bureaucratic approval and issuance process increases the time it takes to bring the security to market.[2]

Key Point Tax-exempt bonds have lower interest rates than do taxable bonds because investors in tax-exempt bonds do not have to pay taxes on the interest income they receive.

Taxable Bonds

Taxable bonds differ from tax-exempt bonds primarily in that the coupon payments must be reported as taxable income by the investor, resulting in a higher interest rate for the health care issuer. Taxable bonds typically have a shorter maturity (twenty years) and do not have restrictions on the use of proceeds. As noted earlier, the proceeds of tax-exempt debt can benefit only the tax-exempt entity; therefore, projects that involve partnering with a taxpaying entity, such as a physician practice or specific medical office buildings or parking garages used by physician offices, can be financed only with taxable debt and do not qualify for tax-exempt debt.

Bond Issuance Process

Before a bond can be issued, it must be sold by either public or private placement. Health care providers, whether they are issuing a taxable or a

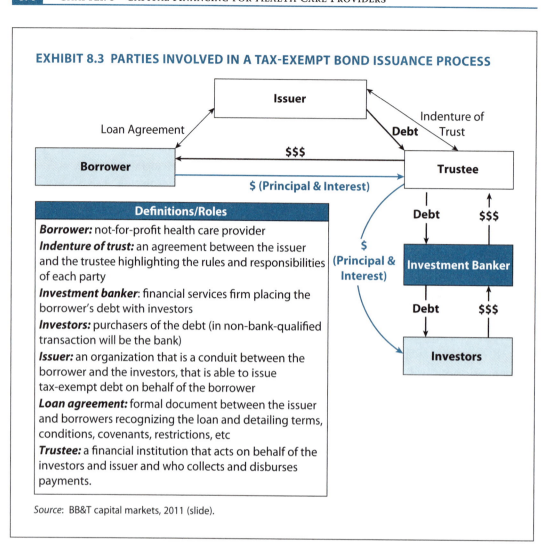

EXHIBIT 8.3 PARTIES INVOLVED IN A TAX-EXEMPT BOND ISSUANCE PROCESS

Definitions/Roles

Borrower: not-for-profit health care provider

Indenture of trust: an agreement between the issuer and the trustee highlighting the rules and responsibilities of each party

Investment banker: financial services firm placing the borrower's debt with investors

Investors: purchasers of the debt (in non-bank-qualified transaction will be the bank)

Issuer: an organization that is a conduit between the borrower and the investors, that is able to issue tax-exempt debt on behalf of the borrower

Loan agreement: formal document between the issuer and borrowers recognizing the loan and detailing terms, conditions, covenants, restrictions, etc

Trustee: a financial institution that acts on behalf of the investors and issuer and who collects and disburses payments.

Source: BB&T capital markets, 2011 (slide).

tax-exempt bond, must select between public or private placement. In a *public offering*, a bond is sold to the investing public through an *underwriter*, sometimes called an *investment banker*. *Private placements* are sold to a particular institution or group of institutions (banks, pension funds, or insurance companies), also with the assistance of an underwriter. Exhibit 8.3 introduces the key parties involved in the bond issuance process, which is discussed in more detail below.

Public versus Private Placement

The advantage of private over public placement is primarily that the issuer avoids public disclosure in the form of a bond rating, credit enhancement, and official statement (OS) at the time of issuance as well as after the issuance. Removing these parts from the issuance process also lowers the costs and shortens the time required to issue the bonds. Although there is no OS, there is a private placement memorandum, which is limited in scope compared to an OS and is circulated to all buyers of the private placement. The primary disadvantage of private placement is that because of the bonds' reduced liquidity in this narrower market, buyers demand higher interest rates. If a buyer desires to resell the bonds, there is no public secondary market, only other qualified institutional buyers. In the past most health care facilities selected public placement because the lower interest cost differential over the lifetime of the bonds offsets the front-end savings of a private placement. However, in today's market, hospitals are finding private placement attractive because they can match the length of the project with the length of the financing, particularly when it comes to projects related to medical and information technology equipment.

Public offering of a bond by a tax-exempt health care institution requires supplying an official statement (OS) to investors. Tax-exempt bond issuers do not have to file this statement with the Securities and Exchange Commission (SEC). Underwriters are required to submit the OS to the Municipal Securities Rulemaking Board (MSRB). As well as annual updates of financial information (audited financials and key ratios related to bond covenants) to its repository database called electronic municipal market access (EMMA). In contrast, stock or bond issues offered by for-profit corporations have stiffer disclosure requirements for investors and require registration with the SEC and annual and quarterly reports to stockholders. The OS must fully disclose information about the obligated organization (i.e., the one that promises to pay) and the project for which the bonds are issued. This information allows investors to assess the risk of the issue, and includes the financial state of the facility (audited financial statements), operational background (medical and management staff, service area, services offered, sources of revenues), the terms of the issue, and in some cases, a *feasibility study* of the project being financed.[3]

Feasibility Study
A preliminary study undertaken by an organization and compiled by a third party to determine and document a project's financial viability. Depending on the results of this study, a decision will be made whether or not to proceed with the project.

Steps in the Bond Issuance Process

An organization considering issuing bonds as its source of capital must go through a long and arduous process before it actually receives any cash. The bond-issuing process for not-for-profit organizations using public markets, which can take twelve to eighteen months before any cash is received, is described in this section.

1. The health care borrower updates its capital plan, measures its *debt capacity,* **and attempts to 'get its house in order.'**

Over a year before actually starting the bond issuance process, a health care provider needs to 'get its house in order' if it is to receive an investment grade bond rating. For example, it may attempt to build up cash reserves, decrease receivables, or liquidate some existing debt—or all three. In addition, it may update its strategic and capital plan and improve its information system or other parts of its infrastructure. The provider may also conduct a financial feasibility study of the project (see Chapter Seven regarding NPV and IRR), as well as assess its debt borrowing capacity. Exhibit G.4 in Appendix G, at the end of the chapter, presents an example of how debt capacity is measured. A hospital may spend $750,000 on plans for a $55 million project, only to find out later that its cash flow and liquidity limit its debt capacity to $35 million.

2. The health care borrower identifies and selects the key parties involved in the bond issuance process.

The bond issuance process involves a host of parties vital to the issuance of tax-exempt financing. The primary members of this group are an underwriter or investment banker, the issuing authority, and a bond *trustee.* Other members include lawyers, accountants, financial advisors, and feasibility consultants, if needed. The underwriters, sometimes referred to as investment bankers, are the main coordinators of the bond issuance process, though in some cases an independent financial advisor is hired for this role. They provide advice during the capital planning stage, assist in identifying the debt structure (for example, the use of fixed versus variable rate debt), oversee the purchase of credit insurance, select rating agencies and bond insurers, participate in the writing of the bond documents, organize the key members, and plan the timetable of the bond deal. At the time of the bond issuance, the primary role of the underwriter is to purchase the bonds from the hospital via the governmental authority and then market and sell the bonds to investors.

To spread the risk, the leading investment banker may invite other investment bankers to help sell the bonds. The comanagers or selling group, or both, may consist of local investment banking firms (to enhance marketability and lower the interest rate through state tax deductions as well) or national investment banking firms, such as JP Morgan Chase, Goldman Sachs, or Merrill Lynch.

The trustee, typically a bank, acts as an agent for the bondholders and performs two important functions. First, the trustee collects the principal and interest payments from the health care providers and makes these payments to the bondholders. Second, the trustee ensures that the health

Debt Capacity

The amount of total debt that an organization can be reasonably expected to take on and pay off in a timely manner.

Trustee

An agent for bondholders who ensures that the health care facility is making timely principal and interest payments to the bondholders and complies with legal covenants of the bond.

care provider complies with the legal covenants of the bond. For example, if the health care provider were required to maintain a debt service coverage ratio above 2.5 and debt to total capital of less than 50 percent, the trustee would monitor its performance with respect to these ratios. If the health care provider did not comply, it would be in default on the bond.

3. **The health care borrower is evaluated by a credit rating agency.**

When issuing either tax-exempt or taxable bonds to the public, health care providers turn to bond rating agencies to objectively evaluate their creditworthiness. They normally seek a credit rating from two out of the three rating agencies: Fitch Ratings, Moody's, and Standard & Poor's (S&P). *Creditworthiness* measures the borrower's ability to make interest and principal payments at the contracted times over the life of the bond. Rating agencies consider a range of factors to evaluate a borrower's credit risk, including financial, market, physician, utilization, and management data. They also assess any capital budgeting or financial feasibility studies related to the financed project. However, if the health care borrower does not expect its facility to receive a quality rating, it may forgo disclosure of the rating and issue a nonrated bond. (For conventional mortgage loans, a commercial bank performs the evaluation.)

Financial Evaluation

From a financial standpoint, the lender or rating agency is primarily interested in evaluating a health care provider's ability to pay. This can be measured by the debt service coverage ratio, as discussed in Chapter Four:

$$\text{Debt Service Coverage} = (\text{Net Income} + \text{Interest} + \text{Depreciation} + \text{Amortization}) / \text{Maximum Annual Debt Service Payments}$$

The numerator represents the health care provider's operating cash flow before its interest payments, depreciation, and amortization expenses, and it is divided by the maximum annual loan payments of principal and interest required over the life of the bond. Lenders or rating agencies expect a minimum debt service coverage ratio of 1.2. They also measure ability to pay using several other financial ratios, such as days cash on hand, operating margin, cash and investments to long-term debt, and long-term debt to total capital.

 Key Point Debt service coverage ratio is one of the primary financial ratios used to evaluate a health care provider's ability to meet debt service payments.

Market Evaluation

In this step, the lender or rating agency evaluates the demand for the investment project. A wide range of factors are considered in this step, including local demographics (population growth, income levels, unemployment rate in the market area), competition from other health care providers, penetration of managed care, the industrial base of the local economy, and last, the borrower's market share for key service lines, such as cardiology, orthopedics, and oncology.

Physician and Management Evaluation

Because physicians are responsible for admissions, lenders pay particular attention to the characteristics of the staff, including the number of medical staff members by specialties, their ages, the percentage of admissions by staff members, the number of board-certified physicians, and the recruitment and retention of staff.

The lender or credit rating agency also examines the health care provider's management staff for such things as background and experience, how they are organized, and how they relate to the medical staff. Any recent turnover of management staff and its effect on the organization would be scrutinized closely.

4. The bond is rated by a credit rating agency.

Rating agencies visit the facility to gain further insight into the operation of the hospital and the relationship among management staff, board members, and medical staff. After reviewing quantitative data and performing an on-site assessment, the rating analysts recommend a final rating, which can be appealed by the borrower. The rating assesses the organization's creditworthiness, or the likelihood of default on a bond. The higher the rating, the lower the interest rate the organization has to pay (a higher rating implies less risk of default to investors but also means a lower coupon rate). The three primary rating agencies are Fitch Ratings, Moody's, and Standard & Poor's (S&P). The rating assigned to an issue affects the interest rate and marketability of the bond. Depending on the size and complexity of the issue, simply getting a rating can cost the issuer from $1,000 to $50,000. The assigned ratings used by all agencies are listed in Exhibit 8.4. *Investment grade* ratings range from AAA to BBB (S&P and Fitch) or Aaa to Baa (Moody's), of which the highest are called *quality* ratings. *Junk bonds* are rated BB and below by S&P and Ba and below by Moody's. Within the junk bond category are *substandard* and *speculative* bonds, both of which are considered risky investments. Some providers may choose not to have their bonds rated because their organizations are relatively small or they expect to receive a *below investment grade* rating.

EXHIBIT 8.4 COMPARISON OF MOODY'S, FITCH'S, AND S&P'S BOND RATINGS

Moody's	Fitch and S&P	Interpretation	Grade of the Bond
Aaa	AAA	Judged to be the best quality.	Quality
Aa	AA	High quality, smaller amount of protection than AAA.	Quality
A	A	Many favorable investment attributes.	Investment grade
Baa	BBB	Medium grade; neither highly protected nor poorly secured.	Investment grade
Ba	BB	Speculative elements; future cannot be considered as well assured.	Substandard junk bonds
B	B	Generally lack characteristics of desirable investment.	Substandard junk bonds
Caa	CCC	Poor standing; may be in default or have elements of danger.	Speculative junk bonds
Ca, C	CC,C	Very speculative; often in default; very poor prospects.	Speculative junk bonds
DDD	D	Bond in default	Speculative junk bonds

Key Point Investment grade bonds are at or above S&P's BBB rating or Moody's Baa rating. Bonds below this rating from either agency may be considered junk bonds.

Typically, a health care provider is unable to achieve the top AAA or Aaa rating unless it purchases a credit enhancement via bond insurance. Health care providers in the AA or Aa rating category not only have excellent financial strength but are more likely to be health care systems with strong management, large bed size, and a superior medical staff. These hospitals tend to rely less on Medicare and Medicaid revenues, exhibit low debt ratios, generate strong profits, and possess large cash reserves. Health care providers in the BBB or Baa and substandard categories are normally smaller facilities located in competitive or rural markets and serve a high proportion of Medicare and Medicaid patients. Furthermore, their cash reserves tend to be low, and they possess a high amount of debt. Exhibit

---

EXHIBIT 8.5 SELECTED MEDIAN RATIO VALUES FOR NOT-FOR-PROFIT HOSPITALS AND HEALTH SYSTEMS, 2010

	Bond Rating		
Measure	**AA**	**A**	**BBB**
Debt service coverage ratio	5.4	3.6	2.6
Operating margin	4.1%	2.5%	0.9%
Total profit margin	6.4%	3.7%	2.6%
Nonoperating revenue as % of total revenue	2.1%	1.4%	1.2%
Age of plant, years	9.2	10.1	12.2
Days cash on hand	230	158	127
Days in accounts receivable	44	45	47
Average payment period, days	65	59	66
Long-term debt to total capital	31%	43%	64%
Cash and investment to total debt	165%	100%	74%

Source: 2010 Nonprofit health care system medians by rating category, August 8, 2011, Standard & Poor's Rating Agency.

8.5 lists three S&P bond ratings for not-for-profit hospitals and offers a sample of their respective financial ratios. Perspective 8.5 discusses the process that the Fitch rating agency follows in rating a health care provider's bond.

A health care provider can strengthen its credit rating, and thereby lower its interest rate and increase its marketability, through either bond insurance or a letter of credit. For a fee of 0.07 to 2 percent of the bond's total value, a facility can obtain bond insurance that guarantees the timely payments of principal and interest to bondholders in the unlikely event of default by the health care provider. The rating then assigned to the bond is a function of the credit strength of the bond insurance company. During the credit and mortgage crisis of 2008, major bond insurers such as AMBAC and MBIA lost their AAA credit ratings because they branched out from the municipal bond market and insured high-risk, mortgage-backed securities. In 2010 AMBAC filed for bankruptcy, as did the parent company of bond insurer FGIC. In 2012, there was one bond insurer left, Assured Guaranty, which had an Aa rating from Moody's.

PERSPECTIVE 8.5 HEALTH CARE RATING PROCESS

Fitch Ratings considers both quantitative and qualitative factors in rating a health care provider. The rating agency makes an *opinion* regarding how timely the hospital will be in the payment of its principal and interest. The rating process takes the following steps: collecting financial and operational information on the hospital, meeting with management and/or making a visit to the facility, presenting the collected information to a credit committee, and reaching a rating decision based on the findings of the credit committee. Various characteristics are assessed in the rating process, ranging from board governance to service area to operational performance to financial performance. In terms of board governance, a hospital is viewed favorably if it maintains a written investment policy, reports its financial statements in a timely manner, and retains a stable management and diverse board of directors, including members from the medical staff. Since financial performance is affected by the demand for health care services, market factors are critical indicators in the rating process as well. Being located in a diversified economic region with high per capita income, low unemployment, and a growing population adds to a hospital's credit strength. In addition, the degree to which a hospital has penetrated the market suggests its ability to capture market share as well as its negotiating leverage with health insurers. How effectively management makes future financial projections is analyzed by a rating agency as well. The rating agency will focus on the assumptions that influence the projected financial results and how they relate to environmental changes and project plans. Projections that assume high volume growth, large market share improvements, higher reimbursement rates, and/or a reduction in expenses will be assessed in a conservative manner by the rating agency and may require sensitivity analyses to adjust these assumptions and their financial outcomes.

Source: J. LeBuhn and E. Wong, Nonprofit hospitals and health systems rating criteria, Fitch Ratings, August 12, 2011, www.fitchratings.com/creditdesk/reports/report_frame.cfm?rpt_id=648836.

Obtaining a *letter of credit* through a bank is another option to enhance the rating of an issuer's bond. The cost is an initial fee plus an ongoing percentage, typically between .50 percent and 1 percent, of the outstanding amount remaining on the issue each year. Again, the bond's rating is dependent on the strength of the bank. The recent effects of the recession that ended in 2009 and Europe's sovereign debt crisis put the credit ratings of two large banks at risk, Bank of America and Citigroup. When a bank's bond rating is downgraded, an associated hospital's rating declines as well because a downgraded bank is then supporting payment obligations on the bonds.

The rating of a bond issue traded in the marketplace, called an *outstanding bond issue*, is reviewed on a periodic basis and can be either upgraded or downgraded, depending on the issuer's present financial or operational conditions. For example, S&P lowered the rating of a hospital in North Carolina from BBB to BB after it had issued debt to pay for a replacement hospital. The agency cited decreased patient volume, loss of key physicians, and poor economic conditions in the market area that contributed to a lower debt service coverage ratio of 1.0, an operating margin of −1.6 percent, and declines in other key financial ratios. Typically, hospital and health system bonds rated above investment grade demonstrate improved financial and utilization indicators. These improvements range from higher profitability and cash flow, higher returns from investments, and a stronger liquidity position to operational changes related to the return of the hospital to its core business of patient care and an overall gain in hospital efficiency. Perspective 8.6 lists specific factors affecting the downgrade in the credit rating of a tax-exempt hospital bond.

   5. **The health care borrower enters into a loan agreement with the governmental authority, the issuer of the bonds.**

   The hospital borrower issues its bonds through a governmental authority, which may be a city, county, or state entity. A loan agreement that is equivalent to the bond payments establishes this relationship and specifies that the hospital borrower, not the issuer, is responsible for the debt payments.

   6. **The underwriters sell the bonds to bondholders at the public offering price, and the trustee provides the health care provider with the *net proceeds from the bond issuance*.**

   The issuance process actually begins several weeks before the official pricing date of the bonds, when the underwriters (there may be only one underwriter) issue a preliminary official statement (POS) to prospective buyers approximately two weeks before pricing. This document allows investors to assess the borrower's creditworthiness. After assessing the market for current interest rates, the underwriters construct a prepricing scale of interest rates for various maturities. The underwriters' primary objective is to achieve the lowest interest rate for the borrower that will still attract investors to purchase the bond. Thus the objective of the underwriters is to achieve an equilibrium interest rate that ensures marketability yet avoids oversubscription of the issue. If on the pricing date oversubscription occurs, this indicates that the interest rate is set too high and thus is unfavorable to the borrower (health care provider). In this case the underwriters will lower the interest rate, which will decrease the number of bond orders and make the interest rate fairer to the borrower.

   Once the final interest rates for given maturities have been set, an agreement is signed by the issuer and the leading underwriter. Shortly

Bond Insurance

Insurance that protects against default and helps a hospital borrower to lower its cost of debt and improve bond marketability.

Outstanding Bond Issue

A bond that trades in the marketplace.

Net Proceeds from a Bond Issuance

Gross proceeds less the underwriters' and others' issuance fees.

Preliminary Official Statement (POS)

A statement offered to prospective buyers of a bond by the underwriters to help determine a fair market price for the bond (also called a *red herring*).

PERSPECTIVE 8.6 FACTORS AFFECTING CREDIT DOWNGRADE IN RATING A HOSPITAL BOND

The following key factors contributed to the downgraded rating of a hospital by Fitch Ratings from BBB to BBB–. The facility is a 124-bed, acute-care hospital with total operating revenues of $96.2 million and is located in Texas.

Decrease in utilization. The hospital successfully recruited five physicians but still experienced a decline in patient volume. Acute admissions dropped to 4.5 percent in 2011, and September admissions were down by 15 percent as compared to the prior time period.

Decline in cash flow and debt service coverage. In September 2011, its net revenues were down by 12 percent as compared to the same time period in 2010. This decline in revenues lowered the hospital's profitability as well as its cash flow to meet debt service payments. Cash flow margin was 5.1 percent at the end of the quarter for September 2011 compared to Fitch's BBB median value of 8.5 percent.

The credit strengths of the facility included the following:

Strong balance sheet position. The hospital's days cash on hand on September 30, 2011, was 298.7 and its cash to debt ratio was 109 percent, which exceeded the respective Fitch medians of 128.6 days and 79.8 percent, respectively. The hospital's debt to capitalization was favorable as well with a ratio value of 38.1 percent compared to Fitch's BBB median value of 48.4 percent.

New facility. The hospital is a fairly new facility with a replacement building built in 2008, resulting in an extremely low average age of plant of 5.6 years for 2011. As a new facility, the hospital also has modest capital expenditures going forward.

Source: Fitch Ratings, Fitch downgrades Peterson Regional Medical Center (TX) revs to 'BBB–', November 16, 2011, www.fitchratings.com/creditdesk/press_releases/detail.cfm?pr_id=733653.

thereafter, the underwriters purchase the bonds and sell them to investors at the predetermined price. The bond issuance process closes approximately two weeks later when the underwriters transfer the proceeds to the health care provider via the trustee. In short, the pricing period allows the underwriters to obtain indications of market interest rates from institutional buyers to reduce their own risk before buying the bonds.

The cost of the issuance process includes service payments for legal, accounting, feasibility, and underwriting or investment banking services; financial advisors; the trustee; and any credit enhancement (bond insurance or letter of credit). The fees may vary from 1 to 2 percent of the total amount issued.

After the issuance process has been completed, the health care provider makes monthly interest and principal payments to the trustee, who in turn pays the investors or bondholders on a semiannual basis for interest payments and on an annual basis (or as directed by the maturity schedule) for the principal payments.

Bank-Qualified, or Direct Private Placement, Loans

As previously mentioned, investors holding variable rate tax-exempt bonds can put, or sell, their bonds back to a remarketing agent. The agent uses its best effort to resell the bonds. When the bonds cannot be resold, variable rate bonds are secured by a letter of credit from a bank, so that the bond trustee can draw upon that letter of credit to pay off the principal and interest on the unsold bonds. If the bank holds the bonds for a defined period of time, typically ninety days, and is unable to sell the bonds, the bank typically charges a higher interest rate, typically 12 percent, and shortens the term or maturity of the bonds from thirty years to one to three years. As a result of the bank's holding the bonds, the hospital incurs higher debt service payments and a shorter time frame (i.e., maturity) in which to pay off the bonds.

To avoid this put and remarketing risk, hospitals and health care systems are now using a *direct, tax-exempt loan bond purchase* by a bank. As banks improved financially from the credit crisis of 2008 and 2009, they viewed these loans as a way to expand to a more profitable line of business. There are several advantages to a direct debt purchase by a bank as compared to variable rate demand bonds backed by a letter of credit. The first advantage is that a direct debt purchase is less time consuming and cheaper to issue versus an offering of bonds to the general public. The second advantage is that a loan does not require a credit rating by a rating agency, unlike a tax-exempt bond. The third advantage, as noted above, is that the loan avoids remarketing and put risks since the bank is buying the bonds directly. A potential fourth advantage depends on whether the hospital's private placement can be considered *bank qualified* by the issuing municipality. If the loan does qualify, then the bank can deduct 80 percent of its interest costs, which could result in a lower interest rate for the hospital. One disadvantage to these bank loans for the hospital is that the bank has the right after a comparatively short period of time (between five and ten years) to assess the credit risk of the hospital and call in the bonds. At that time the hospital can either find another bank to take on the debt or refinance the debt with a new bond offering. A second disadvantage of these bank loans is that they are accompanied by more restrictive covenants than bonds issued in the public bond market. For example, a bank loan may require a hospital to maintain a days cash on hand ratio of 150 days, whereas a public bond issuance may require only 100 days.

Lease Financing

As health care facilities find it more difficult to acquire capital to finance equipment, many consider lease arrangements as a necessary and viable alternative. Leasing now accounts for 20 to 25 percent of all health care provider equipment spending. A lease involves two parties: the *lessor*, who owns the asset, and the *lessee*, who pays the lessor for the use of the asset but does not own it. A health care provider may decide to enter into a lease arrangement for several reasons:

Lessor
An entity that owns an asset that is then leased out.

Lessee
An entity that negotiates the use of another's asset via a lease.

1. *To avoid the bureaucratic delays of capital budget requests.* Because of the longer, closer scrutiny given capital budgeting requests by top management and the board, an administrator may find it more convenient to lease a piece of medical equipment than to request it in the capital budget. This is especially true for state- or city-owned facilities whose capital purchases require governmental approval.

Key Point The lessor owns the asset, and the lessee makes lease payments to the lessor for the use of the asset.

2. *To avoid technological obsolescence.* Given the rapid changes in health care technology, lessees can avoid paying for high-tech equipment that may become outdated shortly. By leasing, a facility can continually upgrade its equipment; the risk of technological obsolescence then shifts to the lessor.

3. *To receive better maintenance services.* Most full-service leases include maintenance for the equipment. Some believe that because the lessor owns the equipment, the maintenance is better.

4. *To allow for convenience.* If an asset is to be used for only a short time, leasing is less time consuming and costly than buying and then selling shortly thereafter. Because leasing constitutes 100 percent financing, leasing companies advertise that it frees cash for other purposes. A facility may also avoid a cash down payment by borrowing enough to cover the full cost of the lease, which is less than buying the asset outright. Thus, from a financial perspective, lease financing appears equivalent to debt financing, with the only major difference being that a facility never actually owns a leased asset.

Operating Lease

A lease for a period shorter than the useful life of the leased asset (one year or less). This type of leasing arrangement can be canceled at any time without penalty, but there is no option to purchase the asset once the lease has expired.

Operating Lease

An *operating lease* is used for service equipment leased for periods shorter than the equipment's economic life, usually between a few days and a year. The lessor's aim is to lease for less than the equipment's full cost but to recover the cost by leasing the same asset many times over its economic life. The usual types of assets covered by operating leases are computers, copier machines, and vehicles. The lessor incurs all the ownership costs of maintenance, service, and insurance on the leased equipment.

A second characteristic of operating leases is a cancellation clause, which gives the lessee the option to return the leased asset to the lessor with little or no penalty at any time during the life of the lease. Finally, if the operating lease complies with specific accounting standards (e.g., no automatic transfer of title), it can be treated as *off balance sheet financing*. This means that the lease is not reported on the balance sheet under long-term debt but instead is reflected on the income statement as an operating expense. The Financial Accounting Standards Board (FASB) has specific conditions that define an operating versus a capital lease.[4]

Capital Lease

A lease that lasts for an extended period, up to the life of the leased asset. This type of lease cannot be canceled without penalty, and at the end of the lease period, the lessee may have the option to purchase the asset (also called a *financial lease*).

Capital Lease

In a *capital lease*, also called a *financial lease*, the lessor aims to lease the asset for virtually all of its economic life. In return, the lessee is committed to lease payments for the entire lease period. The lessee does not have the option to cancel a capital lease immediately without a substantial penalty but does have an option to buy the leased asset at the end of the lease agreement. The latter option tends to be more expensive than if the facility had initially bought the equipment outright because the lessor always operates with a margin for profit; however, the lessee may not be in a financial position initially to afford the full cost of the asset.

Financial Lease

See the definition of *capital lease*.

Sale and Leaseback Arrangement

A type of capital lease whereby an institution sells an owned asset and simultaneously leases it back from the purchaser. The selling institution retains the right to use the asset and also benefits from the immediate acquisition of cash from the sale.

One type of capital lease used by the health care industry is the *sale and leaseback arrangement*, whereby a health care provider sells an owned asset (such as a clinic) to a third party and simultaneously leases it back from the purchaser. By selling the owned asset, the facility is able to obtain immediate capital while still retaining use of the asset.

From a financial management perspective, a capital lease has implications similar to buying an asset and financing it with debt. Buying through borrowing and negotiating a capital lease are similar in that both require contractual payments (debt or lease payments) over the life of the asset, and both options incur the costs of operating the asset. In addition, the capital lease, just like a debt obligation, is reported in the balance sheet under long-term debt obligations. The primary difference occurs at the end of the asset's life, when the lease provisions require the asset to be returned to the lessor (the owner), unless the contract stipulates an option to buy or renew. In contrast, under the buy-borrow option, the owner may either sell or continue to use an asset at any point.

A final note on the topic of capital leases is that for the past several years, the Financial Accounting Standards Board (FASB) has been working to unite the FASB standards with the International Financial Accounting Standards (IFRS). One aspect of this process has been to revisit lease accounting. Many entities structure their leases for plant and equipment in such a way as to avoid capitalizing the assets; therefore, on the majority of leases, rent expense for the payment will be reflected on the operating statement. The FASB has been deliberating on how to best reflect the properties of leases that extend beyond one year into several years, which has led to significant controversy around the issue as the matter awaits settlement. Regardless of the mechanics, however, the probable outcome will be to require entities to record leased assets as *right of use* assets, which will equal the present value of the minimum lease payments. The liability account for the leased assets would then be called *liability under lease*. But the methodology by which these assets and the corresponding liability are to be amortized remains to be determined.

Right of Use Asset
The recorded value of a leased asset, which is equal to the present value of the lease payments.

 Key Point In contrast to an operating lease, a capital lease has attributes similar to owning an asset. The latter type of leasing arrangement may also provide the option to buy the asset.

Analysis of the Lease versus Purchase Decision

One of the most common financial decisions made by a health care organization is whether to buy or lease a needed asset. The usual approach is to compare the present value cost of a buy decision with the present value cost of a lease decision over a specified time. From a purely financial standpoint, the option with the lower present value cost is preferable. In making this assessment, several factors must be considered. Taxpaying entities realize either an effective lower net lease payment from the tax deduction of the lease payment or an interest and depreciation tax shield from buying the asset. The cost of ownership includes the outflow of cash to maintain the asset offset by the inflow of cash from its salvage value. Interest and depreciation expenses act as *tax shields* because they are tax-deductible expenses, which reduce the taxes paid to the government. Last, the cash flows under the lease option are discounted back at the after-tax cost of debt rather than at the cost of capital.

Tax Shield
An investment for a for-profit entity that reduces the amount of income tax to be paid, often because interest and depreciation expenses are tax deductible.

Suppose Five-Star General Hospital is undecided about purchasing a $10 million piece of equipment or leasing it. If it decides to buy the asset, it can borrow the full amount from its local bank at a rate of 10 percent; the equipment would be depreciated at a rate of $2 million per year over its five-year life to a zero salvage value. Under the lease arrangement, the gross lease payments would be $3 million per year, starting one year from now. Assuming the organization is a taxpaying entity with a 30 percent tax rate, which is the better alternative from an economic standpoint?

Exhibit 8.6 presents the analysis of this purchasing versus leasing decision. Because the present value sum of the financing flows for purchasing is the higher of the two options (i.e., less of a loss), −$7,540,000 versus −$8,610,000, purchasing the asset is the desired alternative to leasing.

• A loan amortization schedule (similar to the one in Exhibit G.3) is presented in columns A through D in the purchasing arrangement section of Exhibit 8.6. The loan amortization amount ($2,638,000, Given 1) is calculated by dividing the initial investment amount ($10 million) by the present value factor for an annuity at 10 percent interest for five years (3.7908). Column A represents the only cash outflows, which are the loan payments.

• Columns E and F present cash inflows from interest and depreciation expense tax shields. The interest expense tax shield was computed by multiplying the interest expense in column B by the tax rate of 30 percent (Given 4). The depreciation tax shield inflow ($600,000) was computed by multiplying the annual depreciation expense, $2 million, by the same tax rate, 30 percent (Givens 3 and 4).

• The net cash outflow, column G, equals the annual loan payment from column A less the tax shield amounts in columns E and F. Finally, the net cash outflow is discounted back at the net after-tax cost of debt: $10\% \times (1 - 0.30) = 7\%$. Because the cash flows are net of taxes, the calculations should be based on the net after-tax cost of debt as well. Column H gives the present value factors at 7 percent, and column I shows the net present value of the decision to purchase the asset, −$7,540,000.

• The lower section of Exhibit 8.6 shows the calculations for the leasing alternative. Cash outflows, column L, are also examined net of taxes; thus the net payment equals only $2.1 million per year [$3 million $\times (1 - 0.30)$]. These net payments are also discounted back at the same net after-tax cost of debt rate of 7 percent. Column N shows the present value of the leasing decision, −$8,610,000.

EXHIBIT 8.6 COMPARISON OF PURCHASING ARRANGEMENT WITH LEASING ARRANGEMENT FOR FIVE-STAR GENERAL HOSPITAL

Givens (in '000s)

1	Annual annuity payment[a]	$2,638
2	Interest rate	10%
3	Annual depreciation expense[b]	$2,000
4	Tax rate	30%
5	Depreciation expense tax shield[c]	$600
6	After-tax cost of debt[d]	7%
7	Before-tax lease payments	$3,000

[a] PVFA, 10%, 5 yrs = 3.7908. $10,000 initial investment / 3.7908
[b] $10,000 purchase price / 5 years useful life = $2,000 depreciation expense per year
[c] $2,000 depreciation expense per year × 30% tax rate = $600 tax shield per year
[d] (Interest Rate) × (1 − Tax Rate) = 10% × (1 − 30%) = 7%

Purchasing Arrangement

	A	B	C	D	E	F	G	H	I
		Interest			Interest	Depreciation	Net Cash		PV of Net Cash
	Annuity	Expense	Principal	Remaining	Expense Tax	Expense Tax	Outflow	PV Factor	Outflows
	Payment	(D* ×	Payment	Balance	Shield (B ×	Shield	(if owned)	from	(if owned)
Year	(Given 1)	Given 2)	(A − B)	(D* − C)	Given 4)	(Given 5)	[A − (E + F)]	(Given 6)	(G × H)
0				$10,000					
1	$2,638	$1,000	$1,638	8,362	$300	$600	$1,738	0.9346	$1,624
2	2,638	836	1,802	6,560	251	600	1,787	0.8734	1,561
3	2,638	656	1,982	4,578	197	600	1,841	0.8163	1,503
4	2,638	458	2,180	2,398	137	600	1,901	0.7629	1,450
5	2,638	240	2,398	0	72	600	1,966	0.7130	1,402
Total									$7,540

Note: D* is the previous year's Column D value.

Leasing Arrangement

	J	K	L	M	N
			Net after Lease		PV of Net Cash
	Before-Tax Lease	Lease Tax Shield	Payments	PV Factor from	Outflows (if leased)
Year	Payments (Given 7)	(J × Given 4)	(J − K)	(Given 6)	(L × M)
0					
1	$3,000	$900	$2,100	0.9346	$1,963
2	3,000	900	2,100	0.8734	1,834
3	3,000	900	2,100	0.8163	1,714
4	3,000	900	2,100	0.7629	1,602
5	3,000	900	2,100	0.7130	1,497
Total					$8,610

Note: All dollar figures are expressed in thousands.

If Five-Star General were a nontaxpaying entity, there would be no tax shield benefits. In that case, the analysis would be simplified by comparing only the present value of the loan payments with the present value of the lease payments, but the cost of debt would be 10 percent, not 7 percent. Although normally it would be necessary to go through these calculations if the payments differed each year, it can easily be seen here that with flat payments every year under both options ($2.638 million borrowing versus $3.0 million leasing), purchasing would be less costly than leasing. Therefore the present value of the loan of $10 million would be less than the present value of the lease, and the decision would be to borrow the funds and buy the asset.

Caution: The salvage, or residual, value of an asset should also be considered in the buy-or-borrow evaluation. Residual values are a cash inflow. Because the cash flow of the residual value is less certain than the debt and lease cash flows, some financial analysts may use a higher rate than the after-tax cost of debt to discount this cash flow.

Summary

There are three ways to finance assets: by using debt (liabilities), equity, or a combination of the two.

> Assets = Debt + Equity

Any increase in assets must be balanced by a similar increase in debt or equity, or both. The structuring of debt relative to equity is called the *capital structure decision* and is increasingly important to both for-profit and not-for-profit providers. In today's environment characterized by prospective and capitated payments, the increased use of managed care and outpatient services, and increasing cutbacks caused by competition, obtaining debt and equity financing is a much more complicated undertaking than in the past. Both types of financing have advantages and disadvantages.

The primary sources of equity financing for not-for-profit health care organizations are internally generated funds, philanthropy, and governmental grants, whereas for-profit facilities rely primarily on internally generated funds and stock issuances. Unfortunately, internally generated funds—funds retained from operations (retained earnings)—are shrinking.

A rule of thumb is to borrow short term for short-term needs and long term for long-term needs. Short-term financing typically refers to a wide range of financing, from debt that must be paid back almost immediately to debt that may not have to be paid off for up to a year. Long-term financing typically refers to debt that must be paid off in a period longer than a year. The two major types of long-term financing are term loans, which must be paid off in one to ten years, and bonds, which may have a final maturity of up to twenty to thirty-five years. Bonds are the primary source of long-term financing for tax-exempt health care entities.

Types of debt financing available to not-for-profit health care organizations include bank term loans, conventional mortgages, FHA-insured mortgages, tax-exempt financing (available only to not-for-profit organizations), and taxable bonds.

Organizations that decide to issue bonds generally go through a series of six steps:

Step 1. The health care borrower updates its capital plan, measures its debt capacity, and attempts to "get its house in order."

Step 2. The health care borrower selects the key parties involved in the bond issuance.

Step 3. The health care borrower is evaluated by a credit rating agency.

Step 4. The bond issue is rated by the credit rating agency.

Step 5. The health care borrower enters into a loan agreement with the governmental authority, the issuer of the bonds.

Step 6. The underwriters sell the bonds to bondholders at the public offering price, and the trustee provides the health care provider with the net proceeds.

Bonds can be issued with either fixed rate or variable rate interest, each of which has advantages and disadvantages.

An alternative to traditional equity and debt financing is leasing. Leasing is undertaken for four reasons: to avoid the bureaucratic delays of capital budget requests, to avoid technological obsolescence, to receive better maintenance services, and to allow for convenience.

There are two types of leases: operating and capital. An operating lease is used for service equipment leased for periods shorter than the equipment's economic life, usually between a few days and a year. Under a capital lease, the lessor aims to lease the asset for virtually all of its economic life.

KEY TERMS

a. Amortization

b. Bank-qualified loan

c. Bond

d. Bond issuance

e. Capital lease	**t.** Operating lease
f. Collateral	**u.** Outstanding bond issue
g. Debt capacity	**v.** Par value
h. Discount	**w.** Preliminary official statement (POS)
i. Feasibility study	
j. Financial lease	**x.** Premium
k. Fixed income security	**y.** Rating of bond
l. Hedging	**z.** Required market rate
m. Interest rate swap	**aa.** Right of use asset
n. Lessee	**bb.** Sale and leaseback arrangement
o. Lessor	
p. Letter of credit	**cc.** Sinking fund
q. Market value	**dd.** Tax shield
r. Net proceeds from a bond issuance	**ee.** Term loan
	ff. Trustee
s. Off balance sheet financing	**gg.** Yield to maturity

Key Equations

• Bond valuation (annual coupon payments):

$$\text{Market Value} = (\text{Coupon Payment}) \times \text{PVFA}(k, n) + (\text{Par Value}) \times \text{PVF}(k, n)$$

• Bond valuation (semiannual periods for coupon payments):

$$\text{Market Value} = (\text{Coupon Payment} / 2) \times \text{PVFA}(k / 2, n \times 2) + (\text{Par Value}) \times \text{PVF}(k / 2, n \times 2)$$

REVIEW QUESTIONS AND PROBLEMS

1. **Definitions.** Define the key terms listed above.

2. **Equity position.** What avenues are available for for-profit and not-for-profit health care providers to increase their equity position?

3. **Debt versus equity financing**. What are the advantages and disadvantages to a taxpaying entity in issuing debt as opposed to equity?

4. **Debt financing**. Does adding debt increase or decrease the flexibility of a health care provider? Why?

5. **Basis points**. How much is a basis point? How many basis points are there between 6 5/8 percent and 6 3/4 percent?

6. **Debentures**. Explain the difference between subordinated debentures and debentures.

7. **Bonds**. Name at least two factors that might cause a facility to call in its bond.

8. **Bonds**. What are the advantages and disadvantages of a taxable bond relative to a tax-exempt bond? Who is the issuer of tax-exempt bonds?

9. **Bonds**. What party acts on behalf of bondholders to ensure that the issuing facility not only is complying with the covenants of the bond but also is making timely principal and interest payments to the bondholders?

10. **Investment bankers**. Why would an investment banker syndicate a bond issue with other investment bankers?

11. **Bonds**. Compare private placement bond issues with public placement bond issues.

12. **Credit ratings**. Identify two ways that a health care provider can strengthen its credit rating. What are some of the ramifications of these options?

13. **Credit ratings**. What can cause a health care provider's credit rating to be downgraded?

14. **Market rates**. What impact do required market rate changes have on bonds of longer maturities?

15. **Leasing**. What are the potential new names of the asset and liability accounts for a leased asset, and how are leases with terms greater than twelve months treated under the new accounting regulations?

16. **Leasing**. Why might an organization enter into a leasing arrangement?

17. **Bond valuation**. If a $ 1,000 zero coupon bond with a 30-year maturity has a market price of $412, what is its rate of return? (*Hint*: see Appendix G.)

18. **Bond valuation**. If a $1,000 zero coupon bond with a 10-year maturity has a market price of $508.30, what is its rate of return? (*Hint*: see Appendix G.)

19. **Bond valuation**. A tax-exempt bond was recently issued at an annual 10 percent coupon rate and matures 15 years from today. The par value of the bond is $1,000. (*Hint*: see Appendix G.)

    a. If required market rates are 10 percent, what is the market price of the bond?

    b. If required market rates fall to 5 percent, what is the market price of the bond?

  c. If required market rates rise to 14 percent, what is the market price of the bond?

  d. At what required market rate (10 percent, 5 percent, or 14 percent) does the above bond sell at a discount? At a premium?

20. **Bond valuation.** A tax-exempt bond was recently issued at an annual 8 percent coupon rate and matures 20 years from today. The par value of the bond is $5,000. (*Hint*: see Appendix G.)

  a. If required market rates are 8 percent, what is the market price of the bond?

  b. If required market rates fall to 4 percent, what is the market price of the bond?

  c. If required market rates rise to 12 percent, what is the market price of the bond?

  d. At what required market rate (8 percent, 4 percent, or 12 percent) does the above bond sell at a discount? At a premium?

21. **Bond valuation.** Assuming that the bond in problem 19 matures in 5 years, what would be the market prices under the various required market interest rate changes? (*Hint*: see Appendix G.)

22. **Bond valuation.** Assuming that the bond in problem 20 matures in 10 years, what would be the market prices under the various required market interest rate changes? (*Hint*: see Appendix G.)

23. **Bond valuation.** Hanover County Hospital plans to issue a tax-exempt bond at an annual coupon rate of 6 percent with a maturity of 20 years. The par value of the bond is $1,000. (*Hint*: see Appendix G.)

  a. If required market rates are 6 percent, what is the value of the bond?

  b. If required market rates fall to 3 percent, what is the value of the bond?

  c. If required market rates fall to 10 percent, what is the value of the bond?

  d. At what required market rate (6 percent, 3 percent, or 10 percent) does the above bond sell at a discount? At a premium?

24. **Bond valuation.** Assuming that the bond in problem 23 matures in 10 years, what would be the market prices under the various required interest rate changes? (*Hint*: see Appendix G.)

25. **Bond valuation.** A $1,000 par value bond with an annual 8 percent coupon rate will mature in 10 years. Coupon payments are made semiannually. What is its market price if the required annual market rate is 6 percent? (*Hint*: see Appendix G.)

26. **Bond valuation.** A $1,000 par value bond with an annual 12 percent coupon rate will mature in 15 years. Coupon payments are made semiannually. What is the market price if the required annual market rate is 10 percent? (*Hint*: see Appendix G.)

27. **Bond valuation**. Currently, Sentaria Hospital's tax–exempt bond issuance is selling for $619.70 per bond and has a remaining maturity of 15 years. If the par value is $1,000 and the coupon rate is 5 percent, what is the yield to maturity? (*Hint*: see Appendix G.)

28. **Bond valuation**. Harbor Hospital's tax-exempt bond is currently selling for $803.64 and has a remaining maturity of 20 years. If the par value is $1,000 and the coupon rate is 6 percent, what is the yield to maturity? (*Hint*: see Appendix G.)

29. **Loan amortization**. The Johns Hopkington Hospital needs to borrow $3 million to purchase an MRI. The interest rate for the loan is 6 percent. Principal and interest payments are equal debt service payments, made on an annual basis. The length of the loan is 5 years. The CFO of Johns Hopkington wants to develop a loan amortization schedule for this debt borrowing for tomorrow morning's meeting. Prepare such a schedule. (*Hint*: see Appendix G.)

30. **Loan amortization**. Laurel Regional Hospital needs to borrow $80 million to finance its new facility. The interest rate is 8 percent for the loan. Principal and interest payments are equal debt service payments, made on an annual basis. The length of the loan is 10 years. The CEO would like to develop a loan amortization schedule for this debt issuance. Prepare such a schedule. (*Hint*: see Appendix G.)

31. **Purchase versus lease**. Lower Merion Medical Center, a taxpaying entity, has made the decision to purchase a new laser surgical device. The device costs $1,200,000 and will be depreciated on a straight-line basis over 5 years to a zero salvage value. Lower Merion could borrow the full amount at a 6 percent rate for 5 years, which is also the implied borrowing rate for the lease. The after-tax cost of debt equals 4 percent. Alternatively, it could lease the device for 5 years. The before-tax lease payments per year would be $350,000. The tax rate for this center is 40 percent. From a financial perspective, should Lower Merion lease the surgical device or borrow the money to purchase it?

32. **Purchase versus lease**. Hopewell Health System wants either to borrow money to purchase a hospital or to enter into a lease agreement with the city of Hopewell. The purchase price of the hospital is $55 million. Assuming 100 percent financing, the interest rate is 8 percent for the loan, with an after-tax cost of debt of 5 percent. The 8 percent interest rate on the loan is also the implied borrowing rate for the lease. The length both of the loan and of the lease is 5 years. The before-tax lease payments are expected to be $15 million per year. The tax rate is 40 percent for Hopewell Health System. Should Hopewell Health lease or borrow the money to purchase the hospital?

33. **Purchase versus lease**. Penn Medical Center, a taxpaying entity, is considering the purchase of a 64-slice computed tomography scanner. The cost of the scanner is $4 million. The scanner would be depreciated over 10 years on a straight-line basis to a zero salvage value. The tax rate is 40 percent. The financing options include either borrowing for the full cost of the scanner or leasing a scanner. The lease option is a 5-year lease with equal

before-tax lease payments of $950,000 per year. The borrowing alternative is a 5-year loan covering the entire cost of the scanner at an interest rate of 5 percent, which is also the implied lease rate. The after-tax cost of debt is 3 percent. Should Penn Medical lease the scanner or borrow the full amount to purchase it?

34. **Purchase versus lease**. Maryland General Hospital, a taxpaying entity, is considering a leasing arrangement for its ambulance fleet. The fleet of ambulances costs $375,000 and will be depreciated over a 10-year life to a salvage value of $75,000. Maryland General could finance the entire fleet with equal annual debt and principal payments at a before-tax cost of debt of 9 percent and an after-tax cost of debt at 6 percent for 10 years. The implied lease rate is also 9 percent. Alternatively, it could lease the fleet for 10 years. The before-tax lease payments are $45,000 per year for 10 years. Maryland General's tax rate is 40 percent. From a financial perspective, should Maryland General lease or borrow the money to buy the ambulances?

35. **Debt capacity**. Northwest Hospital is considering a new replacement hospital and plans to issue long-term bonds to finance the project. Before it meets with its investment bankers, the hospital wants to estimate how much additional debt it can take on. Currently, the hospital has annual debt service payments of $3 million, and its cash flow available to meet debt service payment is $65 million per year. For its new debt issuance, the hospital plans to issue fixed rate debt for 20 years. It also assumes that Fitch Ratings will assign it an A rating. Fitch's median debt service coverage ratio for A rated bonds is 4.4x. The expected fixed interest rate for a 20-year, A rated, tax-exempt bond is 5 percent. Using Fitch's median debt service coverage ratio for an A rated bond along with the prior information, how much additional debt could Northwest Hospital take on? (*Hint*: see Appendix G.)

36. **Debt capacity**. Shore Health System is considering developing full-service imaging centers across its service area and plans to issue long-term debt to finance these centers. Before it meets with its investment bankers, it wants to estimate how much additional debt it can take on. Currently, Shore Health System has annual debt service payments of $7 million, and its cash flow available to meet debt service payment is $30 million per year. For its new debt issuance, it plans to issue fixed rate debt for 30 years. It also assumes Fitch Ratings will assign it a BBB rating. Fitch's median debt service coverage ratio for BBB rated large health care systems is 2.90x. The expected fixed rate for a 30-year, BBB rated long-term bond is 7 percent. Using Fitch's median debt service coverage ratio for a BBB rated bond along with the prior information, how much additional debt could Shore take on? (*Hint*: see Appendix G.)

Appendix G: Bond Valuation, Loan Amortization, and Debt Borrowing Capacity

A facility plans to market bonds at the lowest possible interest rate, but to do so, it first must carefully scrutinize the current market's relationship between bond prices and yield to maturity. Because many bonds have a call feature as well, the facility must also examine how this will affect interest rates. The facility must understand the process of paying off its debt.

Fixed Income Security
A bond that pays fixed amounts of interest at regular periodic intervals, usually semiannually.

Market Value
What a bond would sell for in today's open market.

Par Value
The face value amount of a bond; it is the amount the bondholder is paid at maturity, and it does not include any coupon payments.

Bond Valuation for Yield to Maturity

Most bonds are *fixed income securities*, which means the investor receives a fixed amount of interest periodically, usually semiannually, over the lifetime of the bond. With fixed interest rate securities, the coupon payment does not change from year to year, even though the market interest rate may change. A bond's *market value* is the price at which a bond can be bought or sold today in the open market. Although market value should not be confused with *par value* (a bond's face value), a bond may be issued with an equal market value and par value.

The *yield to maturity* (YTM), or *required market rate* of a bond, is used by analysts to determine the return on the bond. The YTM is the rate at which the market value of a bond is equal to the bond's present value of future coupon payments plus par value. The bond valuation formula is defined as

$$MV = \left[\sum_{t=1}^{n} CP_t \times (1+k)^t \right] + PV/(1+k)^n$$

where *MV* is the market value (price) of the bond, *CP* represents the coupon payment on the bond, *PV* is the bond's par value, *n* is the number of periods to maturity, *t* represents 1, 2, 3, . . . n periods, and *k* indicates the yield to maturity (required market rate).

Fortunately, it is not necessary to use this formula in its present form, which can get lengthy and complicated. In fact, the first part of the formula after the summation sign is simply the calculation for the present value of an annuity; the latter part of the formula reduces to a basic present value term. In line with the terms discussed in Chapter Six, the formula can be simplified to:

Yield to Maturity
The rate at which the market value of a bond is equal to the bond's present value of future coupon payments plus par value.

Required Market Rate
The market interest rate on bonds of similar risk.

$$\text{Market value} = (\text{Coupon Payment}) \times \text{PVFA}(k, n) + (\text{Par Value}) \times \text{PVF}(k, n)$$

EXHIBIT G.1a EXAMPLE OF HOW TO USE THE BOND VALUATION FORMULA WHERE COUPON RATE EQUALS REQUIRED MARKET RATE

Givens

1	Par value	$5,000
2	Market rate (k)	8%
3	Time horizon in years (n)	20
4	Coupon rate	8%
5	Coupon payment[a]	$400

[a] Coupon Payment = (Coupon Rate) × (Par Value)

Market Value = (Coupon Payment) × PVFA(k,n) + (Par Value) × PVF(k,n)
Market Value = $400 × PVFA(0.08, 20) + $5,000 × PVF(0.08, 20)
Market Value = $400 × 9.8181 + $5,000 × 0.2145
Market Value = $3,927 + $1,073 = $5,000

Exhibit G.1a shows how to use the formula by proving that when the coupon rate equals the required market rate, market value equals par value. Suppose a hospital wants to issue $100,000 worth of bonds with a twenty-year maturity date. The present market interest rate is 8 percent, and the hospital sets its coupon rate at 8 percent to equal the required market rate. Bonds are sold in denominations of $1,000 or $5,000 each, which is the par value.

As with the techniques to find the internal rate of return (IRR), trial and error is used to find the yield to maturity (k). For example, if the coupon rate is 9 percent, par value is $1,000, market price is $1,200, and the time to maturity is twenty years, what is the yield to maturity? Solving for k through trial and error yields a value of about 7 percent:

$1,200 = $90×PVFA(k, 20)+$1,000×PVF(k, 20)
$1,211=($90×10.594)+($1,000×0.258) when k = exactly 0.07

Alternatively, the IRR function can be used to solve for market rate, k (see Exhibit G.1b).

Bond Valuation for Market Price

The formula also can be used to solve for the market value of a bond. It shows that market value equals the present value of the cash flows in the form of principal and interest payments, discounted back at the required

EXHIBIT G.1b USING EXCEL'S IRR FORMULA TO SOLVE FOR A BOND'S YIELD TO MATURITY, OR MARKET RATE (K)

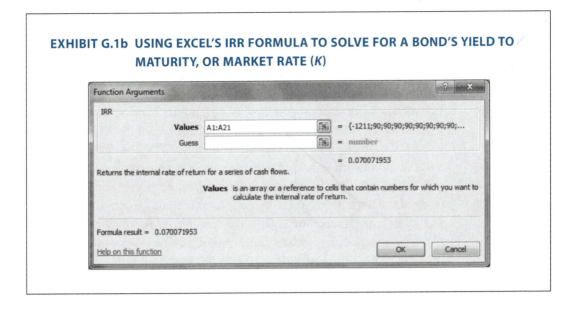

market rate. The required market rate is estimated by examining market rates from publicly traded bonds of similar risk and maturity. This market rate also indicates how the market perceives the issuer's financial condition, the loan covenants, and a bond's collateral. (A more complete discussion of how market rates change is presented in the next section.)

There is an inverse relationship between market value and required market rate: when the required market rate is higher than a bond's coupon rate, the market value is less than par value; when the required market rate is lower, the market value is higher. And as stated before, when the coupon rate and the required market rate are equal, the market value will be equal to the par value.

When the required market rate is higher than the coupon rate, a bond is said to be selling at a *discount* from its par value. The reason lies with the action of the market: no one will pay par value for a bond with 9 percent coupon payments if the market rate is 10 percent. Consequently, the price of the outstanding bond must fall to the point that produces an effective market rate of 10 percent with the same coupon payment.

Conversely, when the required market rate is lower than the coupon rate, a bond is said to be selling at a *premium*. Market factors again are the reason for this: if the present market rate is only 8 percent but the coupon payments are at 9 percent, investors will be willing to pay more for the bonds than their par value, which pushes up the market price.

Although the focus to this point has been on the effect of changing interest rates in the marketplace, the time to maturity can have a significant

Discount
When the market rate is higher than the coupon rate, a bond is said to be selling at a discount from its par value (also see the definition of *premium*).

Premium
When the market rate is lower than the coupon rate, a bond is said to be selling at a premium (also see the definition of *discount*).

impact as well. If the required market rate equals the coupon rate, then regardless of maturity date, market value will always be equal to par value. However, when these two rates differ, maturity date has an effect. When a bond is selling at a discount (determined by interest rates), a bond of longer maturity will sell at a lesser price than a bond of shorter maturity will. Conversely, when a bond is selling at a premium, a longer maturity bond will sell for more than one with a shorter maturity. Exhibit G.2a shows the impact of both required market rates and maturity on the market value for a $1,000 bond with 9 percent annual coupon payments, and Exhibit G.2b shows how the NPV function in Excel can be used to compute the market price of the bond for a 9 percent coupon rate bond, required market rate of 10 percent, par value of $1,000, and maturity of twenty years.

A longer maturity makes bond prices more sensitive to changes in required market interest rates. Thus, in response to interest rate changes, the prices of longer maturity bonds change more than do those of shorter maturity bonds. When the coupon rate and the market rate are equal, the market price of a bond equals its face value, regardless of maturity.

Bond Valuation for Other Payment Periods

Many bonds pay interest semiannually—in some cases, quarterly. If so, the bond valuation formula can be adjusted to account for any number of payment periods within a year (q), using the following formula:

$$MV = \left[\sum_{t=1}^{n} (CP_t / q) \times (1 + k/q)^t \right] + PV / (1 + k/q)^{nq}$$

EXHIBIT G.2a EFFECT OF MARKET RATES AND MATURITY ON A BOND'S MARKET VALUE

Par value: $1,000
Coupon rate: 9%

	k = 0.08	k = 0.09	k = 0.10
Maturity = 10 years	$1,067	$1,000	$939
Maturity = 20 years	$1,099	$1,000	$915
Maturity = 30 years	$1,112	$1,000	$905

Note: k = market interest rate.

EXHIBIT G.2b USING EXCEL'S NPV FUNCTION TO SOLVE FOR A BOND'S MARKET VALUE

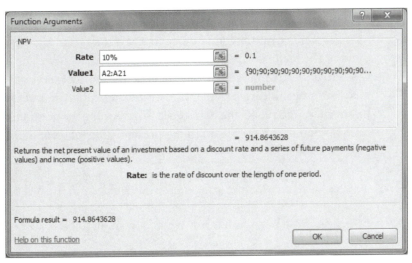

Function Arguments

NPV

Rate	10%	= 0.1
Value1	A2:A21	= {90;90;90;90;90;90;90;90;90;90;90...
Value2		= number

= 914.8643628

Returns the net present value of an investment based on a discount rate and a series of future payments (negative values) and income (positive values).

    Rate: is the rate of discount over the length of one period.

Formula result = 914.8643628

Help on this function   OK   Cancel

Note: Coupon payments of $90 per year for 20 years plus an additional $1,000 at year 20 for the par value, discounted back to the present value at 10 percent, result in a market price of $915.

where *MV* is the market value (price) of the bond, *CP* is the coupon payment on the bond, *PV* represents the bond's par value of the bond, *n* indicates the number of periods to maturity, *t* represents 1, 2, 3, . . . *n* periods, *k* is the yield to maturity (required market rate), and *q* is the number of payment periods per year. For example, suppose the previously described bond, which had an annual coupon rate of 9 percent, required payments semiannually instead of annually. If the term or maturity of the bond were fifteen years, the required market rate 8 percent, and the par value $1,000, the market value of the bond would be computed as follows:

Market Value $= ($Coupon Payment$/2) \times$PVFA$(k/2, n \times 2) + ($Par Value$) \times$PVF$(k/2, n \times 2)$

$MV = ($\$90$/2) \times$PVFA$(0.08/2, 15 \times 2) + $\$1,000 \times$PVF$(0.08/2, 15 \times 2)$

$MV = $\$45 \times$PVFA$(0.04, 30) + $\$1,000 \times$PVF$(0.04, 30)$

$MV = $\$45 \times 17.292 + $\$1,000 \times 0.308 = $\$1,086.14$

Amortization of a Term Loan

The *amortization* of a term loan is the gradual process of paying off the debt through a series of equal periodic payments. Each payment covers a

Amortization

The gradual process of paying off debt through a series of equal periodic payments. Each payment covers a portion of the principal plus current interest. The periodic payments are equal over the lifetime of the loan, but the proportion going toward the principal gradually increases. The amount of a payment can be determined by using the formula to calculate the present value of an annuity.

portion of the principal plus current interest. The periodic payments are equal over the lifetime of the loan, but the proportion going toward the principal gradually increases. For most long-term debt, health care providers opt for this form of level debt service. This option is usually not available for short-term financing. Some short-term debt loans require equal interest payments over the life of the loan and a total principal payment at the end of the loan.

To illustrate how an issuer computes its level debt service requirement, assume a health care provider borrows $1 million at an interest rate of 10 percent for ten years. The first step is to determine the periodic debt service requirements, which equate to the present value of an annuity:

$$\$1,000,000 = (\text{Annuity Payment}) \times \text{PVFA}(0.10, 10)$$

The present value interest factor for an annuity at 10 percent for 10 years is 6.1446.

$$\$1,000,000 = \text{Annuity Payment} \times 6.1446$$
$$\$1,000,000 / 6.1446 = \text{Annual Payment}$$
$$\$162,745 = \text{Annual Payment}$$

Thus, the annual loan payment amount from the health care provider is $162,745 for ten years. One could also use the Excel PMT function to arrive at annual payments, as was discussed in Chapter Six. As noted earlier, each payment is composed of both principal and interest. The loan amortization schedule for this example is given in Exhibit G.3.

Debt Borrowing Capacity

A hospital or health system can estimate its debt borrowing capacity, specifically how much additional debt it can take on, by selecting a capital structure ratio value for a given bond rating. Hospitals can reference any of the three credit rating agencies' annual reports (from Fitch Ratings, Moody's, or Standard & Poor's) that publish the median ratio values for their rated bonds. In these reports, the agencies list key capital structure ratio values by each bond rating category. The key ratios include debt service coverage ratio, cash to total debt, long-term debt to total capital, and so forth.

For example, a hospital expecting to issue additional debt to fund a renovation might assume that its bond rating from Fitch would be BBB.

EXHIBIT G.3 LOAN AMORTIZATION SCHEDULE FOR A $1 MILLION LOAN AT 10 PERCENT INTEREST OVER 10 YEARS

Givens

1	Annuity payment	$162,745
2	Interest rate	10%

	A	B	C	D
	Annuity Payment	**Interest Expense**	**Principal Payments**	**Remaining Balance**[a,b]
Year	**(Given 1)**	**(Given 2 × D*)**	**(A − B)**	**(D* − C)**
0				$1,000,000
1	$162,745	$100,000	$62,745	937,255
2	162,745	93,725	69,020	868,235
3	162,745	86,823	75,922	792,313
4	162,745	79,231	83,514	708,799
5	162,745	70,880	91,866	616,933
6	162,745	61,693	101,052	515,881
7	162,745	51,588	111,157	404,724
8	162,745	40,472	122,273	282,451
9	162,745	28,245	134,500	147,950
10	$162,745	$14,795	$147,950	$0

[a]D* is the previous year's value of column D.
[b]Columns may not total due to rounding.

Exhibit G.4 shows that with a BBB rating, the median ratio value for the debt service coverage ratio is 2.50. Currently, the hospital has $30 million in cash flow available to fund the debt service payments. To estimate its new projected debt service payments, the facility first divides the $30 million of cash available for debt service payments by the debt service coverage ratio value of 2.50, arriving at $12 million:

Debt Service Payments = Cash Available for Debt Service Payments / Debt Service Coverage
Debt Service Payments = $30,000,000 / 2.50
Debt Service Payments = $12,000,000

EXHIBIT G.4 STEPS TO COMPUTE ADDED DEBT CAPACITY BASED ON DEBT SERVICE COVERAGE (DSC) RATIO

Given

1	Cash flow available for debt service payments[a]	$30,000,000
2	Debt service coverage at given rating of BBB	2.50
3	Current debt service payments	$4,000,000
4	Maturity of new bond, years	30
5	Fixed interest rate for new bond	6%
6	Assumed bond rating	BBB

[a]Cash Flow Available for Debt Service = Net Income + Interest Expense + Depreciation Expense

A	Cash flow available for debt service payments	Given 1	$30,000,000
B	Debt service coverage at given rating of BBB	Given 2	2.50
C	Projected debt service payments	A / B	$12,000,000
D	Current debt service payments	Given 3	$4,000,000
E	Additional debt service payments	C − D	$8,000,000
F	Maturity of new bond, years	Given 4	30
G	Fixed interest rate for new bond	Given 5	6%
H	Present value annuity factor	PVFA(0.06, 30)	13.76
I	Additional debt borrowings	E × H	$110,118,649

An alternative option is to use the present value function to compute the value of the loan.

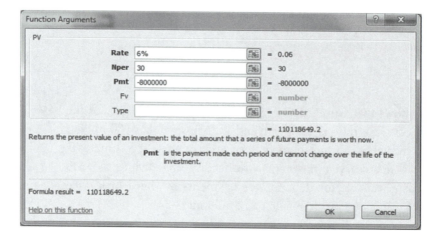

This $12 million is the total amount that the hospital could afford to pay per year toward its overall debt obligations However, assume that the hospital already has current debt service payments of $4 million. In this scenario, the hospital would be able to afford additional annual debt service payments of only $8 million ($12,000,000 − $4,000,000). See Exhibit G.4, rows A through E.

Assuming a 6 percent fixed rate for tax-exempt debt for a thirty-year bond with additional annual debt service payments of $8 million, the hospital can compute its additional debt borrowing capacity. The additional total debt can be computed by identifying the present value factor for an annuity at 6 percent interest for thirty years (13.76) and then multiplying this value by $8 million.

$$\text{Present Value of Loan} = \text{Annuity Payment} \times \text{PVFA}(0.06, 30)$$
$$\text{Present Value of Loan} = \$8,000,000 \times 13.76$$
$$\text{Present Value of Loan} = \$110,118,649$$

One could also use Excel's present value function to solve for the value of the loan (see Exhibit G.4). Given these assumptions, the hospital could borrow an additional $110 million over thirty years, assuming its financial status remained intact during the loan period. The hospital could also estimate its additional debt borrowing capacity based on other key financial ratios, such as long-term debt to total capital and cash to total debt ratios, from the credit rating agencies' median ratio value for the rating selected.

Notes

1. To learn more about these risk issues, refer to D. L. Taub, Understanding municipal derivatives, *Government Finance Review*, August 2005, www.sifma .org/capital_markets/docs/UnderstandingMuniDerivatives.pdf; to learn more about swaps, visit www.youtube.com/watch?v=vzRnT-tpfmQ.

2. To learn more about tax-exempt bonds and the issuance process, go to the Electronic Municipal Market Access Education Center website, www.emma .msrb.org/EducationCenter/EducationCenter.aspx.

3. For electronic access to official statements for tax-exempt health care provider bond issues, visit www.munios.com.

4. Further discussion of operating versus capital leases is beyond the scope of this textbook; see FASB statement number 13 for a detailed explanation of these conditions, www.fasb.org/pdf/fas13.pdf.

CHAPTER 9

USING COST INFORMATION TO MAKE SPECIAL DECISIONS

From time to time, administrators face such decisions as these:

- Should we offer a particular service or group of services?

- What volume of services do we need to provide to break even?

- How much must we charge or be reimbursed for a service to be financially viable?

- Should we offer a service in-house or should we contract with another organization?

- Should we replace equipment?

Questions such as these are called *special decisions* because they are made on an as-needed basis as opposed to a standard schedule. This chapter provides tools to help health care organizations answer these and similar questions. It begins with a discussion of break-even analysis and the role of fixed and variable costs in decision making. It then turns to the related topics of the break-even chart, contribution margin, and product margin.

Key Point When the special decisions discussed in this chapter involve multiyear periods, the time value of money must be considered, as discussed in Chapters Six and Seven.

Although this chapter focuses primarily on financial concerns, nonfinancial criteria also must be considered when making special decisions. In certain cases, nonfinancial criteria may even outweigh the results of a financial

LEARNING OBJECTIVES

- Define fixed and variable costs.

- Compute price, fixed cost, variable cost per unit, or quantity, given the others.

- Construct and interpret a break-even chart.

- Apply the concepts of contribution margin and product margin to the following types of decisions: make or buy, adding or dropping a service, and expanding or reducing a service.

EXHIBIT 9.1 RELATIONSHIP BETWEEN FINANCIAL AND NONFINANCIAL CRITERIA AND DECISION MAKING

Meets Financial Criteria

	Yes	No
Yes (Meets Nonfinancial Criteria)	Proceed	?
No	?	Don't Proceed

analysis. For instance, even when a financial analysis shows that a project meets the financial criterion of breaking even, management may decide not to undertake the project because it does not sufficiently meet the organization's community service goals. Conversely, a money-losing program may be retained because it provides a strategic benefit; for example, not all transplant services generate a positive margin, but a hospital may elect to provide all services nonetheless to be able to demonstrate that it has a comprehensive transplant program. As shown in Exhibit 9.1, the course of action is clear only when a project meets or fails to meet both the financial and the nonfinancial criteria.

Break-Even Analysis

Break-Even Analysis
A technique to analyze the relationship among revenues, costs, and volume (also called *cost-volume-profit analysis*, or *CVP analysis*).

A fundamental financial criterion used to make special decisions is whether or not a service's future revenues will be sufficient to cover its ongoing costs. To answer such a question, management must understand the relationship among revenues, costs, and volume. *Break-even analysis*, also called *cost-volume-profit (CVP) analysis*, provides tools to study these relationships. The remainder of this section explores break-even analysis and how it can be used to help answer numerous questions facing health care organizations.

Using the Break-Even Approach to Determine Prices, Charges, and Reimbursement

Suppose a home health director wants to know how much her agency must be reimbursed per visit for her commercial home health service line to break even. Assuming for the moment that the only costs for this service line are $200,000 for staffing (two RNs and one nursing assistant), then to break even, revenues must also equal $200,000.

$$\text{Revenues} = \text{Costs}$$
$$\$200,000 = \$200,000$$

Although knowing that $200,000 is necessary to cover costs, the director still does not know how much she must be reimbursed *for each visit* to reach her $200,000 target. The fewer the visits, the higher the reimbursement needs to be per visit; conversely, the higher the number of visits, the lower that reimbursement needs to be per visit to earn the $200,000. Thus, to determine the necessary per visit reimbursement to break even, she must know the number of visits.

Key Point The formula to determine total revenues when price and quantity are known is Total Revenues = Price × Quantity.

Key Point The terms *quantity, volume,* and *activity* are often used interchangeably when referring to the number of visits, number of patients, number of services, or the activities of providers and patients related to the delivery or receipt of health care goods and services.

As shown in Exhibit 9.2, if only 1,000 visits were made, she would have to receive $200 per visit (column D, $200,000 / 1,000). However, with 5,000 visits, she would need to receive only $40 per visit ($200,000 / 5,000). This inverse relationship between price and volume to obtain a specified amount of revenue (i.e., $200,000) is summarized in the equation:

$$\text{Total Revenues} = \text{Price} \times \text{Quantity}$$

where *quantity* is used generically to represent number of visits, number of patients, number of services, or another relevant number. Because price

EXHIBIT 9.2 ILLUSTRATION OF HOW PRICE AND FIXED COST PER VISIT VARY WITH VOLUME, HOLDING TOTAL REVENUE AND TOTAL FIXED COSTS CONSTANT

A	B	C	D	E
Number of Visits (Given)	**Total Revenues (Given)**	**Total Fixed Costs (Given)**	**Price/Visit (B / A)**	**Fixed Cost/Visit (C / A)**
1,000	$200,000	$200,000	$200	$200
2,000	$200,000	$200,000	$100	$100
3,000	$200,000	$200,000	$67	$67
4,000	$200,000	$200,000	$50	$50
5,000	$200,000	$200,000	$40	$40

EXHIBIT 9.3 USING THE CONCEPT OF BREAKEVEN TO DEVELOP THE BREAK-EVEN EQUATION

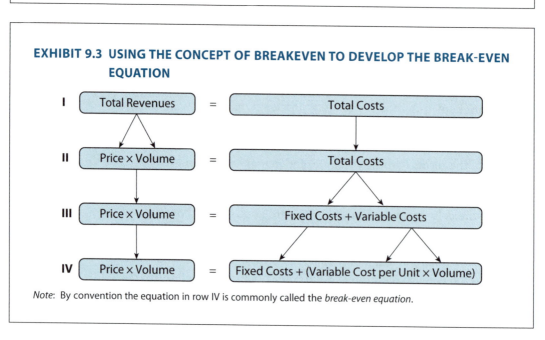

Note: By convention the equation in row IV is commonly called the *break-even equation*.

times quantity equals total revenues, and total revenues equal total costs, the basic break-even formula can be restated as:

$$(\text{Price} \times \text{Quantity}) = \text{Total Costs}$$

This is shown in row II in Exhibit 9.3.

Caution: For simplification purposes, the terms *price* and *reimbursement* are used interchangeably in the following discussion. To the extent they differ in any particular situation, an adjustment should be made.

Break-Even Analysis: The Role of Fixed Costs

Just as price per visit varies inversely with volume if total revenue remains constant, the average fixed cost per visit is also inversely related to volume as long as total fixed cost remains constant (Exhibit 9.2, column E). If the fixed costs remain at $200,000 and only 1,000 visits are delivered, the average fixed cost per visit is $200 ($200,000 / 1,000 visits). But at 5,000 visits, the average fixed cost per visit drops to $40 ($200,000 / 5,000 visits).

This example illustrates the two major attributes of fixed costs:

- Fixed costs stay the same in total as volume increases; hence, the term *fixed* (in Exhibit 9.2 they remained at $200,000).

- Fixed costs per unit change inversely with volume (in Exhibit 9.2 they decreased from an average of $200 per visit to $40 per visit as volume increased from 1,000 to 5,000 visits).

Key Point The term *cost per unit* is shorthand for *average cost per unit*. Thus the terms *average fixed cost per unit* and *fixed cost per unit* are used interchangeably. Similarly, the terms *average variable cost per unit* and *variable cost per unit* are used interchangeably. (Variable costs will be discussed shortly.)

Although fixed cost per unit decreases as volume increases, it does so at a decreasing rate. Exhibit 9.4 shows that cost per visit drops quickly at

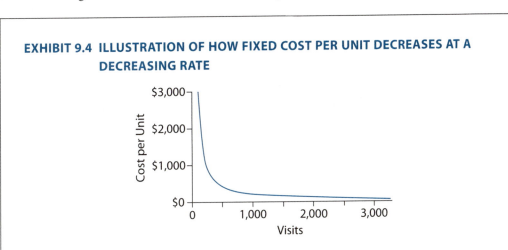

EXHIBIT 9.4 ILLUSTRATION OF HOW FIXED COST PER UNIT DECREASES AT A DECREASING RATE

first, but as the number of visits increases toward capacity, each additional visit decreases the per unit cost at a gradually decreasing rate. In other words, fixed assets provide the capacity to provide service, and if these assets are being used inefficiently (low volume relative to capacity), considerable gains can be made in per unit cost by increasing volume. However, if these assets are already being used efficiently (high volume relative to capacity), the per unit cost decreases by a lesser amount for each additional unit of service provided. Perspective 9.1 illustrates how organizations supplying services to the health care industry have been forced to cut their fixed costs.

Of course, at some point the capacity of the assets is reached, and there is a need to expand (for instance, by buying new equipment or hiring new staff). In such a case, fixed costs would no longer remain fixed at $200,000 but would step up to a new level. When the lower or upper limits

PERSPECTIVE 9.1 PRIVATE PRACTITIONERS LEARN ON THE JOB

A common concern among physicians, particularly those who try to go into private practice, is that the financial aspects of running a business are not being taught in medical school. As a result, physicians are oftentimes forced to learn on the job the hard way. Start-up costs can be significant, reimbursements oftentimes are fixed, and billing and collections is a mystery.

"Overhead continues to go up, but your ability to raise prices is very limited," said Dr. J. Fred Ralston Jr., past president of the American College of Physicians and an internist with Fayetteville Medical Associates, a group practice in Tennessee.

Given fixed Medicare payments and nonnegotiable managed care contracts, it is difficult to move the dial on revenue. So physicians looking to maintain profits often turn to controlling costs. Interviews with business-minded doctors indicate that a medical practice can become a cost-efficient machine if managers control human resource expenses, spread out fixed costs as much as possible, exploit information technology, and carefully track business metrics.

"Personnel is clearly the biggest place you can save," said Dr. Jack Flyer, a physician with CardioCare in Chevy Chase, Maryland. Another quick fix is to stretch fixed costs across more physicians or expanded office hours. At Hopewell Dental Care outside Columbus, Ohio, the four partners see patients most evenings until 7 p.m. and on Saturdays, to spread the cost of office space over as much time as possible.

Source: Adapted from K. Reynolds Lewis, Medical practices work on ways to serve patients and bottom line, *New York Times*, September 7, 2011, www.nytimes.com/2011/09/08/business/smallbusiness/medical-practices-keep-eye-on-the-business-side.html?pagewanted=all.

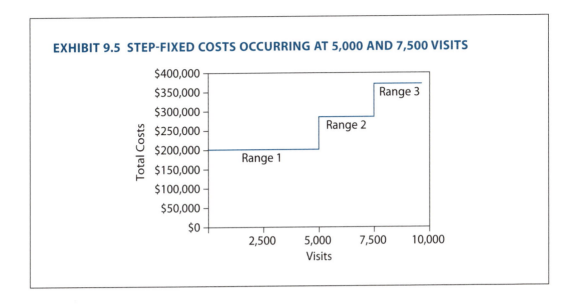

EXHIBIT 9.5 STEP-FIXED COSTS OCCURRING AT 5,000 AND 7,500 VISITS

of capacity are reached, and it becomes necessary to add or drop capacity (e.g., full-time staff), the organization is said to be going beyond the *relevant range* of its *fixed costs*. However, within the relevant range, fixed costs remain fixed.

Exhibit 9.5 shows that the fixed costs of $200,000 in labor for the home health service are considered fixed up to 5,000 visits (relevant range 1). Then, assuming an additional full-time RN would be needed if volume exceeded 5,000 visits, the fixed costs would take a step up to $285,000 (assuming that each new RN costs $85,000). The fixed costs then would remain at this level (relevant range 2) until visits reached 7,500, at which point they would step up to $370,000 (relevant range 3), when yet another full-time RN would have to be hired. To the extent that there are *step-fixed costs*, the break-even formula can become complicated. Thus, it is strongly suggested that break-even analyses with step-fixed costs be done on electronic spreadsheets.

Relevant Range
The range of activity over which *total fixed costs* or *per unit variable cost* (or both) do not vary.

Fixed Costs
Costs that stay the same in total over the relevant range but change inversely on a per unit basis as activity changes.

Step-Fixed Costs
Costs that increase in total over wide, discrete steps.

Caution: There are two major errors that must be avoided when using fixed cost information to make decisions: (1) assuming that cost per unit does not change when volume changes, and (2) using fixed cost per unit derived at one level to forecast total fixed costs at another level.

In regard to the first type of error noted in the caution, the way that fixed cost per unit changes with a change in volume was just illustrated.

In regard to the second type of error, suppose that the home health agency, which has $200,000 in fixed costs, made 4,000 visits this year (Exhibit 9.6, second row). Using this information, the administrator correctly calculates the average fixed cost per visit to be $50 ($200,000 / 4,000 visits). The next year the agency plans to make 5,000 visits (third row). The administrator would be making an error if she assumed that the average fixed cost per visit would remain at $50. Because volume increases from 4,000 visits to 5,000, and total fixed cost remains at $200,000 (it's fixed!), the average fixed cost per visit decreases from $50 per visit ($200,000 / 4,000 visits) to $40 per visit ($200,000 / 5,000 visits). Thus, if the administrator were trying to set her price to cover her fixed cost, she might set it too high (at $50) if she failed to recognize that cost has decreased (to $40) because of increased volume. Conversely, as shown in Exhibit 9.6, if the administrator were using the $50 per visit derived at 4,000 visits to estimate her fixed cost at 3,000 visits, her estimate would be too low.

Break-Even Analysis: The Role of Variable Costs

Thus far, it has been assumed that all costs are fixed or step-fixed. Now assume instead that a home health agency pays employees an average of

EXHIBIT 9.6 ILLUSTRATION OF THE ERROR OF USING FIXED COST PER UNIT DERIVED AT ONE LEVEL OF ACTIVITY TO CALCULATE TOTAL FIXED COST AT ANOTHER LEVEL

A	B	C	D	E
Volume (Estimated)	**Assumed per Unit Fixed Cost[a] (Given)**	**Estimated Total Fixed Cost (A × B)**	**Actual Fixed Cost (Given)**	**Overestimate (Underestimate) (C − D)**
3,000	$50	$150,000	$200,000	($50,000)[b]
4,000	$50	$200,000	$200,000	$0[c]
5,000	$50	$250,000	$200,000	$50,000[d]

[a]All three examples use the unit cost derived at 4,000 units to estimate total fixed cost.
[b]If the unit fixed cost is originally derived at a higher volume, the total fixed cost estimate will be too low.
[c]If the unit fixed cost is originally derived at the same volume, the total fixed cost estimate will be correct.
[d]If the unit fixed cost is originally derived at a lower volume, the total fixed cost estimate will be too high.

$25 a visit, rather than a salary. Thus, 100 visits would cost $2,500 (100 × $25). For 1,000 or 10,000 visits, costs would increase to $25,000 (1,000 × $25) and $250,000 (10,000 × $25), respectively. Because total cost varies *directly* with activity (in this case visits), these costs are called *variable costs*, though the cost per unit remains the same, $25.

Thus, the two major characteristics of variable costs have been identified, and they are just the opposite of those for fixed costs:

- Total variable costs change directly with a change in activity.

- Variable cost per unit stays the same with a change in activity.

The formula that describes the relationship between variable cost and activity is:

> Total Variable Cost = Variable Cost per Unit × Number of Units of Activity

Variable Costs
Costs that stay the same per unit but change directly in total with a change in activity over the relevant range: Total Variable Cost = Variable Cost per Unit × Number of Units of Activity.

As discussed earlier, when total fixed costs go beyond the relevant range, they often take the form of step-fixed costs, though it is possible to substitute variable costs for fixed costs (e.g., by paying a new home health nurse by the visit rather than hiring another full-time nurse). When variable costs per unit go beyond the relevant range, it is possible to have either an increase or a decrease in cost per unit. For instance, if volume increases significantly, an organization may be able to obtain a volume discount on supplies. Of course, if volume drops, the opposite effect may occur: the organization may lose its discounts and have an increase in variable cost per unit. As with fixed costs, as volume goes beyond the relevant range, it becomes difficult to use the break-even formula to solve break-even problems with variable costs, and using a spreadsheet model is recommended.

 Key Point By convention, when the terms *fixed costs* and *variable costs* are used, it is understood that they remain constant in total (fixed costs) or on a per unit basis (variable costs), respectively, only within a relevant range.

Exhibit 9.7 summarizes and compares the major characteristics of fixed and variable costs in relation to volume within a relevant range. Fixed costs stay the same in total but change per unit as volume changes, whereas variable costs change in total but remain constant per unit with changes in volume. Perspectives 9.2 and 9.3 discuss how focusing on value and achieving economies of scale can lower both fixed and variable unit costs.

EXHIBIT 9.7 ILLUSTRATION OF HOW FIXED AND VARIABLE COSTS ARE AFFECTED BY CHANGES IN VOLUME

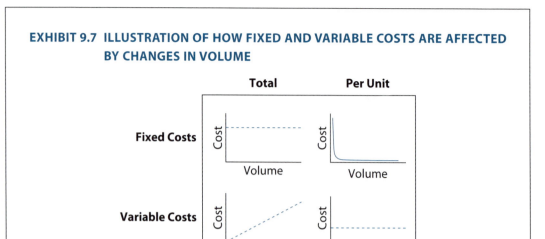

PERSPECTIVE 9.2 VALUE-BASED RETURN ON INVESTMENT

"Each year, I can point to thousands of Intermountain patients who would have died but did not. . . . We have also taken well over $150 million in variable costs out of Intermountain in the last couple of years. That's a massive ROI."

This quote comes from an interview I did with Brent James, MD, chief quality officer at Intermountain Healthcare. The quote demonstrates the significant benefits of a value focus.

Historically, improved quality (measured by reduced harm, improved outcomes, and enhanced patient experience) was assumed to increase costs. In fact, many healthcare leaders and purchasers believed that higher cost was a proxy for higher quality. However, a majority of outcomes and comparative effectiveness research has found little relationship between the quality of a service and its cost. And much of the research has found that increased services often reduce quality. Given these research findings, purchasers (employers, government, and consumers) increasingly are focused on the value they receive from services by measuring both quality and payment (or cost). . . .

The focus on value promotes improved clinical and administrative processes, which improves outcomes and the patient experience. Another benefit is reduction in variation and unnecessary, non-value-added activities, which in turn reduces variable costs and some fixed costs. Increased value potentially increases a healthcare provider's volume of patients and purchasers, resulting in lower per-unit total costs as the remaining fixed cost is spread over a larger base. By driving value, providers will improve quality, reduce cost, and increase the volume of patients associated with them. This is the value ROI.

Source: Excerpted from R. L. Clark, The value ROI, ReadPeriodicals.com, March 1, 2012, www.readperiodicals .com/201203/2623044611.html.

PERSPECTIVE 9.3 ECONOMIES OF SCALE TO REDUCE UNIT COSTS

Economies of scale (EOS) is the core principle that makes our modern world possible. The miracle of the EOS principle is that despite the high cost of investment, millions of consumers can afford goods which are high quality and conveniently accessible. The health care industry does not effectively leverage the economy of scale principle. The health care provider, consultant, or business executive that is armed with the knowledge of the basics of this powerful principle can consistently make sound investment and operational decisions.

To simplify, we can think of fixed costs as those costs which we have to pay regardless of how many units are produced. Variable costs are those costs which scale with the number of units produced. Cost per unit decreases as the number of units increases. It is this principle which makes feasible blockbuster drugs, modern air travel, automobiles, iPhones, and cities; basically, any product whose significant capital costs can be spread out over a large number of units produced.

There are four fundamental methods to apply economy of scale principles to affect health care, as demonstrated in Table 9.1. Together these methods provide the strategic framework to leverage EOS principles in health care.

Source: Adapted from R. Bond, Economies of scale and the accountable care organization, May 2012, ACODatabase.com. Reproduced by permission of the author.

Using the Break-Even Equation

The break-even formula can now be expanded and modified to include variable costs (Exhibit 9.3, row 3), as shown in row 4 in Exhibit 9.3:

$$\text{Price} \times \text{Volume} = \text{Fixed Cost} + \text{Variable Cost}$$

Expanding this equation to address the points in the previous discussion yields the basic break-even equation:

$$\text{Price} \times \text{Volume} = \text{Fixed Cost} + (\text{Variable Cost per Unit} \times \text{Volume})$$

Exhibit 9.8 illustrates how the break-even formula can be used to find the price, quantity (volume), fixed cost, or variable cost per unit needed to break even when each of the other factors is known. In situation 1 of Exhibit 9.8, price is unknown; in situation 2, quantity (volume) is unknown; in situation 3, total fixed cost is unknown; and in situation 4, variable cost per unit is unknown.

Table 9.1 Four methods of applying EOS principles

How	Description	Example
Scale up Volume	The economic principle is to spread out the design and delivery costs of a care process over a large number of patients. This method implies the creation of processes focused on treating a particular disease condition (e.g., heart disease, cancer) as scale requires uniform processes for efficiency.	**Specialty hospitals** – (e.g., heart hospitals, cancer centers)
Reduce Costs	The obvious way to reduce costs is to, well, reduce costs. A particularly promising area is the application of information technology to reduce the cost and time to develop protocols for evidence-based medicine and standards of care. Studies to develop protocols could potentially be shorter in duration, involve smaller study sizes, and be disseminated to the point of care more rapidly.	**Development of new Standard of Care Protocols** – Electronic medical records can make studies less costly
Alter Fixed and Variable Cost Structure	Technology can particularly have a dramatic impact on cost structure. For example, the introduction of cloud computing and software as a service (SaaS) has transformed information technology costs from a fixed to a variable cost. Cloud computing and Saas makes it possible to spread the cost of information technology over a large number of consumers.	**SaaS delivery of Care Coordination Software** – Information technology which spreads development costs over many providers
Innovate Business Model	The application of business model design in healthcare is currently far underutilized. Business model innovations can change both the level of cost and the proportions of fixed to variable cost.	**Behavioral Health** – Group and internet based therapy can match care delivery with needs of patients

Source: R. Bond, Economies of scale and the accountable care organization, May 2012, ACODatabase.com. Reproduced by permission of the author.

EXHIBIT 9.8 APPLYING THE BREAK-EVEN FORMULA

	A	B	C	D	E
Givens				**Total**	**Variable**
	Situation	**Price**	**Quantity**[a]	**Fixed Cost**	**Cost per Unit**[b]
	Situation 1	?	4,000	$200,000	$25
	Situation 2	$100	?	$200,000	$25
	Situation 3	$100	4,000	?	$25
	Situation 4	$100	4,000	$200,000	?

[a]For example, number of visits.
[b]For example, cost of supplies per visit.

Situation 1. Finding the break-even *price*, given quantity, total fixed cost, and variable cost per unit

				Total Fixed		**Variable Cost**		
Setup:	**Price**	×	**Quantity** =	**Cost**	+	**per Unit**	×	**Quantity**
	Price	×	4,000 =	$200,000	+	$25	×	4,000
Solution:	**Price**	×	4,000 =	$200,000	+		$100,000	
	Price	×	4,000 =	$300,000				
	Price		=	$75				

Situation 2. Finding the break-even *quantity*, given price, total fixed cost, and variable cost per unit

			Total Fixed		**Variable Cost**		
Setup:	**Price** × **Quantity** =	**Cost**	+	**per Unit**	×	**Quantity**
	$100 × **Quantity** =	$200,000	+	$25	×	Quantity
Solution:	$75 × **Quantity** =	$200,000				
	Quantity =	$2,667				

Situation 3. Finding the break-even *total fixed* cost, given price, quantity, and variable cost per unit

			Total Fixed		**Variable Cost**		
Setup:	**Price** × **Quantity** =	**Cost**	+	**per Unit**	×	**Quantity**
	$100 × 4,000 =	TFC	+	$25	×	4,000
Solution:	$400,000 =	TFC	+		$100,000	
	$300,000 =	TFC				

Situation 4. Finding the break-even *variable cost per unit*, given price, quantity, and total fixed cost

			Total Fixed		**Variable Cost**		
Setup:	**Price** × **Quantity** =	**Cost**	+	**per Unit**	×	**Quantity**
	$100 × 4,000 =	$200,000	+	VCU	×	4,000
Solution:	$400,000 =	$200,000	+	VCU	×	4,000
	$200,000 =			VCU	×	4,000
	$50 =			VCU		

Expanding the Break-Even Equation to Include Indirect Costs and Required Profit

For simplicity, up to this point revenues have exactly matched those costs that the organization can directly associate with a service, such as the costs for the two RNs and nursing assistant and miscellaneous variable costs such as supplies and transportation. However, it is often desirable that revenues cover other costs, such as overhead, and perhaps provide a *margin* (profit). As discussed in more detail in Chapter Twelve, *direct costs* are those that an organization can measure or trace to a particular patient or service (e.g., the time a nurse or nursing assistant spends with a client), whereas *indirect costs* are those that the organization is not able to associate with a particular patient or service (e.g., the cost of the billing clerk or computer system). Exhibit 9.9 extends the break-even equation shown in Exhibit 9.3 to account for indirect costs and profit, and Exhibit 9.10 expands the example from Exhibit 9.8 to illustrate how to use the extended equation. These examples assume that both indirect costs and profits are fixed amounts (which is usually the case), though the equation can be modified to account for other instances.

In situations 1 to 3 of Exhibit 9.10, price is unknown, and various combinations of indirect costs and desired profit are added to the information originally provided in Exhibit 9.8. Such analyses are used when an

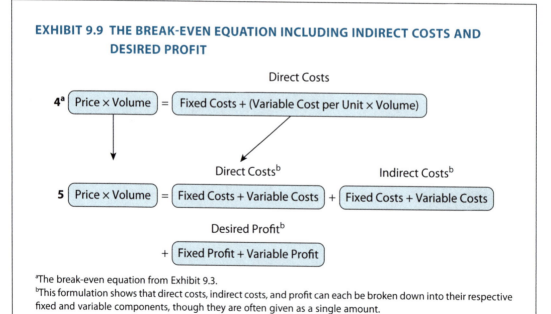

EXHIBIT 9.9 THE BREAK-EVEN EQUATION INCLUDING INDIRECT COSTS AND DESIRED PROFIT

[a]The break-even equation from Exhibit 9.3.
[b]This formulation shows that direct costs, indirect costs, and profit can each be broken down into their respective fixed and variable components, though they are often given as a single amount.

EXHIBIT 9.10 APPLYING THE BREAK-EVEN EQUATION TO SITUATIONS WITH INDIRECT COSTS OR DESIRED PROFIT (OR BOTH)

Givens Situation	Price	Quantity[a]	Total Fixed Cost	Variable Cost per Unit[b]	Indirect Costs	Desired Profit
1	?	4,000	$200,000	$50	$24,000	$0
2	?	4,000	$200,000	$50	$0	$20,000
3	?	4,000	$200,000	$50	$24,000	$20,000
4	$100	4,000	?	$50	$24,000	$20,000

[a] For example, number of visits.
[b] For example, cost of supplies per visit.

Situation 1. Finding the break-even *price*, given quantity, total fixed cost, variable cost per unit, and indirect costs

Setup:	Price × Quantity	=	Total Fixed Cost	+	Variable Cost per Unit			+	Indirect Costs	+	Desired Profit
Solution:	Price × 4,000	=	$200,000	+	$50	×	4,000	+	$24,000	+	$0
	Price × 4,000	=	$200,000	+			$200,000	+	$24,000		
	Price × 4,000	=	$424,000								
	Price	=	$106								

Situation 2. Finding the break-even *price*, given quantity, total fixed cost, variable cost per unit, and desired profit

Setup:	Price × Quantity	=	Total Fixed Cost	+	Variable Cost per Unit			+	Indirect Costs	+	Desired Profit
Solution:	Price × 4,000	=	$200,000	+	$50	×	4,000	+	$0	+	$20,000
	Price × 4,000	=	$200,000	+			$200,000	+			$20,000
	Price × 4,000	=	$420,000								
	Price	=	$105								

(Continued)

EXHIBIT 9.10 (CONTINUED)

Situation 3. Finding the break-even _price_, given quantity, total fixed cost, variable cost per unit, indirect costs, and desired profit

Setup:

Price	×	Quantity	=	Total Fixed Cost	+	Variable Cost per Unit	×	Quantity	+	Indirect Costs	+	Desired Profit

Solution:

Price	×	4,000	=	$200,000	+	$50	×	4,000	+	$24,000	+	$20,000
Price	×	4,000	=	$200,000	+			$200,000	+	$44,000		
Price	×	4,000	=	$444,000								
Price			=	$111								

Situation 4. Finding the break-even _total fixed cost_, given price, quantity, variable cost per unit, indirect costs, and desired profit

Setup:

Price	×	Quantity	=	Total Fixed Cost	+	Variable Cost per Unit	×	Quantity	+	Indirect Costs	+	Desired Profit

Solution:

$100	×	4,000	=	TFC	+	$50	×	4,000	+	$24,000	+	$20,000
$100	×	4,000	=	TFC	+			$200,000	+	$44,000		
		$400,000	=	TFC	+	$244,000						
		$156,000	=	Total Fixed Cost								

organization is trying to determine whether the reimbursement it will receive is sufficient to cover its costs and desired profit for a particular service. For example, in situation 3, if the organization were not reimbursed at least $111 per visit, management could conclude that the reimbursement would be insufficient to cover its direct and indirect costs and desired margin and perhaps decide not to provide the service at this rate or try to renegotiate a higher rate.

In situation 4 of Exhibit 9.10, all the factors are given except for total fixed costs. A situation such as this occurs when an organization is given a set price (reimbursement) and must control its costs to ensure that they do not exceed that reimbursement. In this case, given the indirect costs and desired profit, the organization must ensure that its direct fixed costs do not exceed $156,000. Such an approach, called *target costing*, is common in health care, where the government is the price setter and the provider is the price taker. Perspective 9.4 illustrates the importance of knowing costs in order to understand if reimbursement will be adequate.

Target Costing
Controlling costs or decreasing profit margins (or both) to meet or beat a predetermined price or reimbursement rate.

PERSPECTIVE 9.4 KNOWING PRACTICE COSTS

The health care system in the United States has continuously evolved as it becomes increasingly apparent that reimbursements cannot keep pace with rising costs. Even in the smallest of settings, the private physician practice, challenges can be daunting.

Among the changes that will affect medical groups is a shift away from fee-for-service payment to a system in which providers are paid through bundled or global methodologies, [which] places significant risk on the provider for excessive utilization. The latest trend toward value-based purchasing ties reimbursements to outcome measures.

One of the foundations of good business is to know how much it costs to provide a service. If the procedure is performed inside the practice, it must bear a larger share of building, facility, and staffing expenses whereas a procedure performed in a hospital, ambulatory surgery center, or other location bears its share of administrative, billing, malpractice insurance, and marketing expenses but few other costs.

In addition to serving as an essential tool to manage practice overhead, knowing cost per procedure provides practice administrators with an edge when negotiating with payors, which will become an increasingly powerful skill in the evolving health care industry.

While health care may be changing, certain skills will remain essential. Knowing your practice costs is important today, and it will remain important in the future.

Source: Adapted from D. Gans, Knowing practice costs will become increasingly important, *MGMA Connexion*, January 2012:17–18.

The Break-Even Chart

A break-even chart graphically displays the relationships in the break-even equation. For instance, Exhibits 9.11a, 9.11b, and 9.11c present different ways to graph the data in Exhibit 9.8, where the revenue per visit is $100, fixed costs are $200,000, and variable cost is $25 per visit. Exhibit 9.11a

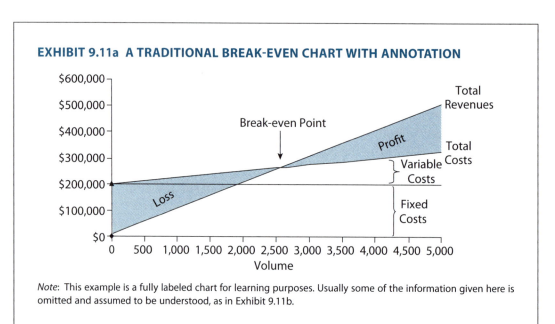

EXHIBIT 9.11a A TRADITIONAL BREAK-EVEN CHART WITH ANNOTATION

Note: This example is a fully labeled chart for learning purposes. Usually some of the information given here is omitted and assumed to be understood, as in Exhibit 9.11b.

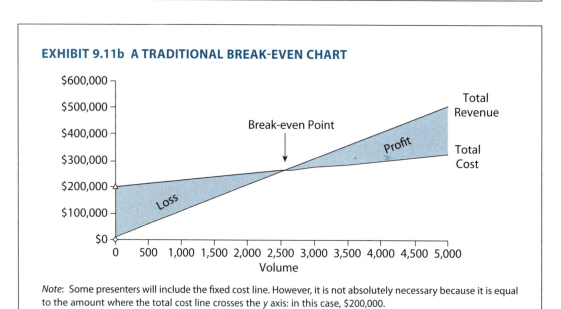

EXHIBIT 9.11b A TRADITIONAL BREAK-EVEN CHART

Note: Some presenters will include the fixed cost line. However, it is not absolutely necessary because it is equal to the amount where the total cost line crosses the *y* axis: in this case, $200,000.

EXHIBIT 9.11c A BREAK-EVEN CHART EMPHASIZING NET INCOME

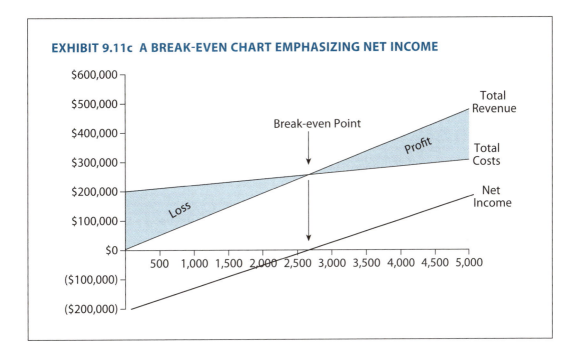

presents this information in the traditional break-even chart format but with considerable annotation. The three lines represent fixed cost, total cost, and total revenues. The total revenue line begins at $0 (the amount of revenue earned when no services are offered) and increases by $100 for each home health visit made. Because, by definition, fixed costs do not change with volume, the fixed cost line begins at $200,000 and remains at that level. Because total cost is made up of fixed cost plus variable cost, the total cost line begins at $200,000 (the level of fixed cost at zero units of service) and grows by $25 (the variable cost per unit) for each unit of service provided.

At 2,667 visits, the total revenue and total cost lines cross. Before 2,667 visits, the net income is negative, whereas after 2,667 visits, it is positive. Thus, the *break-even point*, the point at which total revenues equal total costs, is 2,667 visits. Before the break-even point, the size of the space between the *total revenue* line and the *total cost* line equals the amount of loss. After the break-even point, the size of the space between the total revenue line and the total cost line equals the amount of profit.

Because it is so difficult to visually determine how much the actual loss or profit is by using the traditional version, increasingly a newer version of this chart is being used (see Exhibit 9.11c). In addition to the information typically presented in Exhibit 9.11b, the newer version presents net income: total revenues less total costs. Note that in all three charts, breakeven is

Break-Even Point

The point where total revenues equal total costs.

Contribution Margin per Unit
Per unit revenue minus per unit variable cost.

Incremental Costs
Additional costs incurred solely as a result of an action or activity or a particular set of actions or activities.

Total Contribution Margin
Total revenues minus total variable costs.

achieved at 2,667 visits. In general, the old version should be used where detailed cost information is important, and the new version should be used in cases where the amount of profit is the essential concern.

A Shortcut to Calculating Breakeven: The Contribution Margin

Per unit revenue minus per unit variable cost is called *contribution margin per unit* because, after covering *incremental (variable) costs*, this is the amount left to contribute toward covering all other costs and desired profit. If the contribution margin is known and all other costs are fixed, a shortcut formula to calculate breakeven can be used:

Break-Even Volume = Fixed Costs / Contribution Margin per Unit

---

Assume that total fixed costs are $200,000, revenue per visit is $100, and variable cost is $25 per visit. Thus the contribution margin per unit is $75 ($100 − $25), which means that the organization makes $75 more on each visit than the incremental cost of that visit. Thus, using the above formula, to cover the $200,000 in fixed costs, there must be 2,667 visits ($200,000 / $75; see Exhibit 9.12). This is the same answer that was derived using the longer formula in Exhibit 9.8, situation 2.

Finally, even if the organization does not reach breakeven, each unit of service it delivers contributes $75 toward covering its fixed costs and overhead. This leads to the *contribution margin rule*: if the contribution

---

EXHIBIT 9.12 BREAK-EVEN EQUATION USING THE CONTRIBUTION MARGIN APPROACH

Givens:	Revenue per visit	$100
	Variable cost per visit	$25
	Contribution margin per visit	$75
	Fixed cost	$200,000

To determine the break-even quantity using the contribution margin approach:

$$\frac{\text{Fixed cost}}{\text{Contribution margin per unit}} = \frac{\$200,000}{\$75} = 2,667 \text{ Visits}$$

margin per unit is positive, then it is in the best financial interest of the organization to continue to provide additional units of that service, even if the organization is not fully covering all of its other costs, *ceteris paribus* ("with all else being the same"). Conversely, if the contribution margin is negative, it is not in the best interest of the organization to continue to provide additional units of service, *ceteris paribus*.

Key Point The contribution margin can be determined on a total or a per unit basis. *Total Contribution Margin* = Total Revenue − Total Variable Cost. *Contribution Margin per Unit* = Revenue per Unit − Variable Cost per Unit. It is the amount of profit made on each additional unit produced if all other costs remain the same.

Contribution Margin Rule

If the contribution margin per unit is positive and no other additional costs will be incurred, then it is in the best financial interest of the organization to continue to provide additional units of that service, even if the organization is not fully covering all of its other costs. Conversely, if the contribution margin is negative, it is not in the best interest of the organization to continue to provide additional units of service, *ceteris parabis*.

Effects of Capitation on Break-Even Analysis

With continual emphasis on cost control, some managed care companies have used capitation as their preferred method of payment, though value-based reimbursement and bundled service payments are now gathering increased attention. Because these payment systems are discussed in detail in Chapter Thirteen, the focus here is on how break-even analysis can be used under fixed reimbursement. Briefly, under full capitation, the insurer prepays a health care provider an agreed-on amount per member that covers a designated set of services for the insured population over a defined time period. Typically, these payments are made on a per member per month (PMPM) basis. If there are no terms to the contrary, in return for the capitated payments, the provider agrees to bear all the financial risk for the costs of services provided. If the provider's costs are below the global capitation amount, the provider keeps the difference. If the provider's costs are more than the capitation, the provider is at risk for the difference. Obviously, negotiations on both the capitated amount and any particulars of the contract (e.g., services not covered and arrangements that limit the financial risk of the provider) are critical to the provider, who must estimate the volume and type of services that may have to be performed and the amount of money needed to cover them. The following example shows a break-even analysis for a health care provider under a capitated system.

Hospital A, which has a capitation arrangement with a managed care organization, wants to negotiate a capitated contract with a multispecialty group practice to provide a major portion of the medical services that Hospital A is obligated to provide. This type of arrangement is commonly called a *subcapitation arrangement*. The population covered under this subcapitation arrangement consists of 1,400 covered lives with commercial insurance only (no Medicare or Medicaid beneficiaries).

The director of managed care contracts for the hospital clinics is under pressure to bring in new business. In weighing this opportunity, he must balance many factors, some of which will not be known until the contract is actually in effect, including the PMPM rate, the expected proportion of members needing services, and the average cost of the services that the members will actually receive. Exhibit 9.13 offers three separate scenarios, each varying one of these three factors while holding the other two constant.

EXHIBIT 9.13 AN EXAMPLE OF HOW TO PERFORM A BREAK-EVEN ANALYSIS UNDER A CAPITATED ARRANGEMENT

Givens	Number of Members	Total Fixed Cost	PMPM	Utilizaton Rate	Variable Cost per Unit
Scenario 1	1,400	$16,667	?	10%	$25
Scenario 2	1,400	$16,667	$15	?	$25
Scenario 3	1,400	$16,667	$15	10%	?

Scenario 1. Using the break-even equation to determine break-even **PMPM subcapitation rate**, given service cost and utilization rates

A. Monthly capitation amount (PMPM)	?
B. Fixed costs per month	$16,667
C. Variable costs of services per member receiving	$25
D. Percentage of members receiving services each month	10%
E. Total number of HMO capitated members	1,400

A Monthly Capitation (Estimate)	F Revenues (A × E)	G Members w/Services (D × E)	H Fixed Costs (B)	I Variable Costs (C × G)	J Total Costs (H + I)	K Net Income (F − J)
$5.00	$7,000	140	$16,667	$3,500	$20,167	($13,167)
$10.00	$14,000	140	$16,667	$3,500	$20,167	($6,167)
$14.40	**$20,167**	**140**	**$16,667**	**$3,500**	**$20,167**	**$0**
$15.00	$21,000	140	$16,667	$3,500	$20,167	$833
$20.00	$28,000	140	$16,667	$3,500	$20,167	$7,833
$25.00	$35,000	140	$16,667	$3,500	$20,167	$14,833

EXHIBIT 9.13 (CONTINUED)

Scenario 2. Using the break-even equation to determine break-even *utilization rates*, given service cost and PMPM subcapitation rates.

A. Monthly capitation amount	$15
B. Fixed costs per month	$16,667
C. Variable costs of services per member receiving	$25
D. Percentage of members receiving services each month	?
E. Total number of HMO capitated members	1,400

D	F	G	H	I	J	K
Average Util. Rate (Estimate)	Revenues (A × E)	Members w/Services (D × E)	Fixed Costs (B)	Variable Costs (C × G)	Total Costs (H + I)	Net Income (F – J)
5.00%	$21,000	70	$16,667	$1,750	$18,417	$2,583
10.00%	$21,000	140	$16,667	$3,500	$20,167	$833
12.38%	**$21,000**	**173**	**$16,667**	**$4,333**	**$21,000**	**$0**
15.00%	$21,000	210	$16,667	$5,250	$21,917	($917)
20.00%	$21,000	280	$16,667	$7,000	$23,667	($2,667)
25.00%	$21,000	350	$16,667	$8,750	$25,417	($4,417)

Scenario 3. Using the break-even equation to determine break-even *service cost*, given PMPM subcapitation rates and utilization rate

A. Monthly capitation amount	$15
B. Fixed costs per month	$16,667
C. Variable costs of services per member receiving	?
D. Percentage of members receiving services each month	10%
E. Total number of HMO capitated members	1,400

C	F	G	H	I	J	K
Variable Costs[a] (Estimate)	Revenues (A × E)	Members w/Services (D × E)	Fixed Costs (B)	Variable Costs[b] (C × G)	Total Costs (H + I)	Net Income (F – J)
$15.00	$21,000	140	$16,667	$2,100	$18,767	$2,233
$20.00	$21,000	140	$16,667	$2,800	$19,467	$1,533
$25.00	$21,000	140	$16,667	$3,500	$20,167	$833
$30.00	$21,000	140	$16,667	$4,200	$20,867	$133
$30.95	**$21,000**	**140**	**$16,667**	**$4,333**	**$21,000**	**$0**
$35.00	$21,000	140	$16,667	$4,900	$21,567	($567)

[a]Per visit.
[b]Total.

In keeping with the same example used throughout the chapter, assume that fixed costs equal $200,000 and that the variable cost per unit equals $25. However, the fixed cost figure represents the *annual* amount, whereas capitation is being paid here on a *monthly* basis (PMPM). Thus, annual fixed costs must be converted into equivalent monthly amounts, or $16,667 ($200,000 / 12 months). Variable costs remain the same and do not need to be converted.

In the first scenario (Exhibit 9.13), only the capitation rate is unknown. The clinic either gains or loses depending on whether the capitation amount is above or below $14.40 PMPM. Note that in this scenario, total costs remain constant (columns H, I, and J), regardless of the capitation amount, but total revenues vary based on the capitation rate to be paid (column A). Although Exhibit 9.13 uses a spreadsheet approach to solving scenario 1, another way to solve this problem is to set it up as an equation:

$$\text{PMPM} \times \text{Enrollees} = (\text{Enrollees} \times \text{Utilization Rate} \times \text{Variable Cost per Unit}) + \text{Fixed Cost}$$
$$\text{PMPM} \times 1,400 = (1,400 \quad \times \quad 0.10 \quad \times \quad \$25) \quad + \$16,667$$
$$1,400 \times \text{PMPM} = \$20,167$$
$$\text{PMPM} \approx \$14.40$$

In the second scenario, the percentage of members each month receiving services is unknown, but capitation is held to $15 PMPM. As expected, the lower the percentage of members receiving services, the greater the net income for the clinic. Note that in this scenario, total revenues remain constant (column F), but total costs vary (columns I and J). As with the previous scenario, scenario 2 can also be set up as an equation:

$$\text{PMPM} \times \text{Enrollees} = (\text{Enrollees} \times \text{Utilization Rate}$$
$$\times \text{Variable Cost per Unit}) + \text{Fixed Cost}$$
$$\$15 \times 1,400 = (1,400 \times \text{Utilization Rate} \times \$25) + \$16,667$$
$$\$4,333 = \$35,000 \times \text{Utilization Rate}$$
$$\text{Utilization Rate} = 0.1238$$

In the final scenario, capitation and percentage of members receiving services are held constant, but the variable cost per member receiving services is unknown. As the variable cost per member receiving services rises (column C), net income falls for the clinic (column K), as would be expected. Note that in this third scenario, as in the one before it, total revenues remain constant, but total costs vary. As with the previous scenarios, scenario 3 can also be set up as an equation:

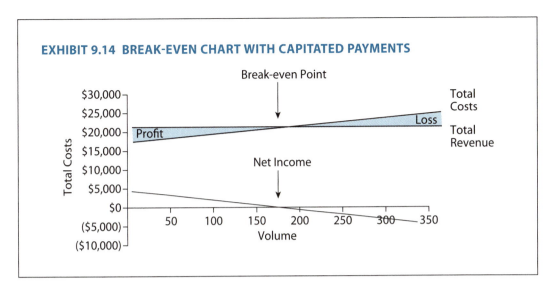

EXHIBIT 9.14 BREAK-EVEN CHART WITH CAPITATED PAYMENTS

$$PMPM \times Enrollees = (Enrollees \times Utilization\ Rate$$

$$\times Variable\ Cost\ per\ Unit) + Fixed\ Cost$$

$$\$15 \times 1,400 = (1,400 \times 0.10 \times Variable\ Cost\ per\ Unit) + \$16,667$$

$$\$4,333 = 140 \times Variable\ Cost\ per\ Unit$$

$$Variable\ Cost\ per\ Unit = \$30.95$$

As with noncapitated payments, a break-even chart can be constructed under a capitated payment environment. Exhibit 9.14 provides an illustration of this, using the same cost structure as in Exhibits 9.11a, 9.11b, and 9.11c (fixed cost = $16,667 and variable cost = $25 per visit), but revenue remains constant at $21,000 (PMPM = $15 × 1,400 patients). As opposed to the noncapitated situation where net income increases as volume increases, the more services provided here, the lower the net income. This is because revenues remain constant, but costs increase at $25 per visit.

The examples given in this chapter illustrate how a cost-volume-profit analysis can be used in both noncapitated and capitated environments. However, as the factors being considered increase, a more thorough analysis is suggested. Such an approach is presented in Chapter Ten, where such things as acuity level, payor mix, productivity, and labor force distribution are taken into account.

Product Margin

Whereas the above discussion dealt with breaking even on a single service, health care delivery is often much more complex. The following section of this chapter introduces tools and concepts applicable to situations involving multiple services. For instance, a home health agency might offer the following services: nursing assistant services, infusion therapy, physical therapy, registered dietitian services, and occupational therapy. Later in the chapter, the situation is expanded to cases involving multiple payors.

Avoidable Fixed Cost

A fixed cost that will be avoided if a service is not provided: for example, full-time nursing costs that would be saved if a service were to be closed.

Nonavoidable Fixed Cost

A fixed cost that will remain even if a particular service is discontinued: for example, full-time nursing costs in a hospital that will continue even after one of several services is dropped.

Common Costs

Costs that benefit a number of services shared by all; for example, rent, utilities, and billing (also called *joint costs*).

Multiple Services

Where multiple services are being offered, both organizational fixed costs and service-specific fixed costs must be considered. Fixed costs incurred only because a service is being provided, and not otherwise, are called *avoidable fixed costs*. For instance, continuing with the home health example, assume that of the $200,000 in fixed costs, $85,000 is to be paid for a full-time RN for just one particular service (Exhibit 9.15, row D), and if the service were not delivered, this position would be eliminated (and not just transferred to another service). In regard to the decision of whether to drop the service, the cost of this position, $85,000, is an avoidable fixed cost.

Assume that the other $115,000 of the original $200,000 of the home health agency's fixed costs will remain and must be covered whether or not the particular service is dropped (Exhibit 9.15, row E). Because these costs cannot be eliminated, they are called *nonavoidable fixed costs*. Assume in the case of the home health agency that $100,000 of the $115,000 in nonavoidable fixed costs is for salaries and benefits and $15,000 is for overhead (Exhibit 9.15, rows E1 and E2). Incidentally, overhead (i.e., rent, administration, insurance, etc.) includes many common costs, those that are not attributable to any particular service but must be covered by all of them. *Common costs* are also called *joint costs*.

Caution: Note that if an organization drops a service and the employees who delivered that service are transferred within the organization, their costs are considered nonavoidable.

Just as subtracting total variable cost from total revenue yields the total contribution margin, subtracting avoidable fixed cost from the total contribution margin yields the *product margin*. The *product margin decision rule* is this: if a service's product margin is positive, the organization will be better off financially if it continues with the service than if it drops the service, *ceteris paribus*. Conversely, if a service's product margin is negative, the organization will be better off financially if it discontinues the service, *ceteris paribus*. The product margin represents the amount that a

EXHIBIT 9.15 AN ILLUSTRATION OF THE PRODUCT MARGIN RULE

Givens

A	Net revenue per visit	$100
B	Variable cost per visit	$25
C	Contribution margin per visit (A – B)	$75
D	Avoidable fixed costs	$85,000
E	Other fixed costs	$115,000
	E1. Salaries and benefits	$100,000
	E2. Overhead costs	$15,000

F	G	H	I	J	K	L	M	N
Volume (Estimate)	Total Revenues (A × F)	Total Variable Costs (B × F)	Total Contribution Margin (G – H)	Avoidable Fixed Costs (D)	Product Margin (I – J)	Salaries and Benefits (E1)	Overhead Costs (E2)	Net Income (K – L – M)
2,000	$200,000	$50,000	$150,000	$85,000	$65,000	$100,000	$15,000	($50,000)
2,500	$250,000	$62,500	$187,500	$85,000	$102,500	$100,000	$15,000	($12,500)
2,667	**$266,700**	**$66,675**	**$200,025**	**$85,000**	**$115,025**	**$100,000**	**$15,000**	**$25**
3,000	$300,000	$75,000	$225,000	$85,000	$140,000	$100,000	$15,000	$25,000
3,500	$350,000	$87,500	$262,500	$85,000	$177,500	$100,000	$15,000	$62,500

service contributes toward covering all other costs after it has covered its own costs, those that are there solely because the service is being offered (its total variable cost and avoidable fixed cost) and that would not be there if the service were dropped. As shown in Exhibit 9.15, when an organization violates this rule and closes a service with a positive product margin (column K), the organization increases its loss by the amount of the product margin that it forgoes. Note that this rule holds for any particular service but does not work for all services taken together because common costs would not be covered.

Presume that the home health agency is trying to decide whether to continue this particular nursing service next year, and it forecasts that it will make 2,000 visits (Exhibit 9.15, column F). If the home health agency made its decision on the basis of net income, it would conclude that it should drop the service because it would conclude that it is losing $50,000 (column N). However, if it drops the service, it will be $65,000 worse off (the amount of the product margin, column K) than if it provided the 2,000 visits.

Because the product margin is the amount left over after the service has covered all of its own costs, if the service were dropped, the home health agency would lose the $65,000 to help defray its other costs (rows E1 and E2). Note also that if it dropped the service, net income would drop from −$50,000 to −$115,000.

Multiple Payors

It is possible to extend the analysis presented in Exhibit 9.15 from one payor to multiple payors. The previous example assumed that revenues were $100 per visit, but in fact, they are really an average of $100 per visit. Three scenarios are shown in Exhibit 9.16. Scenario 1 presents the basic conditions of four payors paying different rates, with a weighted average revenue of $100 ("Total" row, columns F / E). Scenario 2 explores the effect on the product margin of increasing the rate for payor 1 by 10 percent (from $110 to $121) with a corresponding drop in volume of 10 percent (from 300 visits to 270 visits). The result is that the product margin increases from $0 to $1,170 (column J). Scenario 3 shows the effect on the original conditions if all patients in payor category 1 are on a flat-fee contract fixed at $33,000, and volume increases by 10 percent. Because there are no additional revenues for these patients, the variable cost increases, but there is no change in revenue. Therefore, the product margin decreases from $0 to −$1,500. This same paradigm can be used to judge the effects of similar changes occurring with any of the four payors.

Product Margin

Total Contribution Margin — Avoidable Fixed Costs. It represents the amount that a service contributes toward covering all other costs after it has covered the costs that are there solely because the service is offered (its total variable cost and avoidable fixed costs) and that would not be there if the service were dropped.

Product Margin Decision Rule

If a service's product margin is positive, the organization will be better off financially if it continues with the service, *ceteris paribus*. Conversely, if a service's product margin is negative, the organization will be better off financially if it discontinues the service, *ceteris paribus*.

EXHIBIT 9.16 EXPANSION OF THE PRODUCT MARGIN CONCEPT TO MULTIPLE PAYORS

Scenario 1. Original conditions

Payor	A Payment per unit	B Variable cost per unit	$50
1	$110	C Avoidable fixed costs	$50,000
2	$105		
3	$101		
4	$85		

D	E	F	G	H	I	J
			Total	Total	Avoidable	
Payor		Total	Variable	Contribution	Fixed	Product
Category	Volume	Revenues	Costs	Margin	Costs	Margin
(Given)	(Given)	(A × E)	(B × E)	(F – G)	(C)	(H – I)
1	300	$33,000	$15,000	$18,000		
2	175	$18,375	$8,750	$9,625		
3	250	$25,250	$12,500	$12,750		
4	275	$23,375	$13,750	$9,625		
Total	1,000	$100,000	$50,000	$50,000	$50,000	$0

Scenario 2. Original conditions with rate for payor 1 patients increased by 10%, but payor 1 volume is decreased by 10%

Payor	A Payment per unit	B Variable cost per unit	$50
1	$121	C Avoidable fixed costs	$50,000
2	$105		
3	$101		
4	$85		

D	E	F	G	H	I	J
			Total	Total	Avoidable	
Payor		Total	Variable	Contribution	Fixed	Product
Category	Volume	Revenues	Costs	Margin	Costs	Margin
(Given)	(Given)	(A × E)	(B × E)	(F – G)	(C)	(H – I)
1	270	$32,670	$13,500	$19,170		
2	175	$18,375	$8,750	$9,625		
3	250	$25,250	$12,500	$12,750		
4	275	$23,375	$13,750	$9,625		
Total	970	$99,670	$48,500	$51,170	$50,000	$1,170

(Continued)

EXHIBIT 9.16 (CONTINUED)

Scenario 3. Original conditions with payor 1 patients being covered under a flat-fee contract in which the total payment remains $33,000, but payor 1 volume is increased by 10%.

Payor	A Payment per unit	B Variable cost per unit	$50
1	$33,000[a]	C Avoidable fixed costs	$50,000
2	$105		
3	$101		
4	$85		

D	E	F	G	H	I	J
			Total	Total	Avoidable	
Payor		Total	Variable	Contribution	Fixed	Product
Category	Volume	Revenues[a]	Costs	Margin	Costs	Margin
(Given)	(Given)	(A × E)	(B × E)	(F – G)	(C)	(H – I)
1	330	$33,000	$16,500	$16,500		
2	175	$18,375	$8,750	$9,625		
3	250	$25,250	$12,500	$12,750		
4	275	$23,375	$13,750	$9,625		
Total	1,030	$100,000	$51,500	$48,500	$50,000	($1,500)

[a]For payor 1, this formula is not used, and Total Revenues equals the fixed $33,000.

Applying the Product Margin Paradigm to Making Special Decisions

The product margin paradigm presented in Exhibits 9.15 and 9.16 can be used to address a number of special decisions, commonly categorized as make or buy, add or drop, and expand or reduce.

Make-or-Buy Decisions

Decision Rule

After comparing the product margins between the make-or-buy alternatives, the alternative with the higher product margin should be chosen.

Example

Zacharias Community Clinic (ZCC) is deciding whether to produce a portion of its laboratory tests in-house or to purchase them from a reference lab. ZCC has $200,000 in fixed costs for the lab (primarily for facilities, equipment, and staffing), all of which would remain even if ZCC purchased the tests from a reference lab. Variable cost (primarily for reagents and other supplies) is $10 per test. The reference lab has offered to do the tests for a price of $17 each. ZCC currently receives $30 per test. If 10,000 tests are performed, is ZCC better off producing them in-house (*make* alternative) or contracting with the outside lab (*buy* alternative)?

The solution is shown in Exhibit 9.17, solution 1. The product margin of the buy alternative is $70,000 less than that of the make alternative (row K). Therefore the *make* alternative is preferred. Notice that fixed costs do not have to be included in the analysis because they are the same for either alternative. However, if fixed costs do change between the two alternatives, then they would have to be considered. For instance, if $80,000 of the fixed costs were avoidable, the analysis would be as shown in solution 2 of Exhibit 9.17, row J. As a result, the *buy* alternative becomes the preferred choice. Although this option has a $70,000 lower total contribution margin (row I), it saves $80,000 in avoidable fixed costs, resulting in a positive product margin of $10,000 (row K).

Adding or Dropping a Service

Decision Rule

If a proposed new service is expected to have a positive product margin, it should be added; and if an existing service has a negative product margin, it should be dropped.

Example

Geiser HMO asked Nathaniel Clinic, a pediatric group practice, to provide 3,000 well-baby visits. Nathaniel has excess capacity to see more patients but would have to hire additional staff for $85,000. It estimates additional variable costs (such as disposable thermometers, linens, etc.) of $10 per visit. Geiser is willing to pay $65 per visit. Should Nathaniel contract with Geiser and provide the well-baby clinic?

The solution is shown in Exhibit 9.18a. Because the project has a positive product margin of $80,000, Nathaniel should agree to offer the service. But what happens now if Geiser changes the terms of the contract and will pay only $35 per visit? In this case, as shown in Exhibit 9.18b, Nathaniel would have a positive total contribution margin, $75,000 (line I) but a negative product margin, –$10,000 (line K). Nathaniel should not agree to offer the service at this price.

EXHIBIT 9.17 EXAMPLE OF A MAKE-OR-BUY DECISION

Givens			Alternative Make[a]	Buy[b]	Difference If Choose Buy Option (Buy or Make)
A	Volume of tests	(Given)	10,000	10,000	No change in volume
B	Revenue per test	(Given)	$30	$30	No change in charge
C	Variable cost per test	(Given)	$10	$17	Increase in VC/test
D	Contribution margin per test	(Given)	$20	$13	Decrease in CM
E1	Avoidable fixed cost original	(Given)	$0	$0	No change in AFC
E2	Avoidable fixed cost modified	(Given)	$80,000	$0	Decrease in AFC

Solution 1. No avoidable fixed costs

F	Volume	(A)	10,000	10,000	
G	Revenues	(A × B)	$300,000	$300,000	$0[c]
H	Variable costs	(A × C)	$100,000	$170,000	$0[d]
I	Total contribution margin	(G – H)	$200,000	$130,000	$70,000[e]
J	Avoidable fixed cost	(E1)	$0	$0	($70,000)[f]
K	Product margin	(I – J)	$200,000	$130,000	$0[g]
					($70,000)[h]

Solution 2. Avoidable fixed costs

F	Volume	(A)	10,000	10,000	
G	Revenues	(A × B)	$300,000	$300,000	$0[c]
H	Variable costs	(A × C)	$100,000	$170,000	$0[d]
I	Total contribution margin	(G – H)	$200,000	$130,000	$70,000[e]
J	Avoidable fixed cost	(E2)	$80,000	$0	($70,000)[f]
K	Product margin	(I – J)	$120,000	$130,000	($80,000)[g]
					$10,000[h]

[a]Do test in-house.
[b]Purchase tests from outside lab.
[c]Increase (decrease) in volume from choosing buy option.
[d]Increase (decrease) in revenue from choosing buy option.
[e]Increase (decrease) in variable costs by choosing buy option.
[f]Increase (decrease) in total contribution margin by choosing buy option.
[g]Increase (decrease) in avoidable fixed costs by choosing buy option.
[h]Increase (decrease) in product margin from choosing buy option.

EXHIBIT 9.18a EXAMPLE OF AN ADD-OR-DROP DECISION

		Alternative		Difference If Choose to Add Service (Do – Don't)
		Don't Add[a]	Do Add[b]	
Givens				
A	Volume	0	3,000	Increase in volume
B	Revenue per visit	$0	$65	Increase in charge
C	Cost per visit	$0	$10	Increase in VC/test
D	Contribution margin per visit	$0	$55	Increase in CM
E	Avoidable fixed cost	$0	$85,000	Increase in AFC
Solution				
F	Volume (A)	0	3,000	3,000[c]
G	Revenues (A × B)	$0	$195,000	$195,000[d]
H	Variable costs (A × C)	$0	$30,000	$30,000[e]
I	Total contribution margin (G – H)	$0	$165,000	$165,000[f]
J	Avoidable fixed costs (E)	$0	$85,000	$85,000[g]
K	Product margin (I – J)	$0	$80,000	$80,000[h]

[a]Do not open a new clinic.
[b]Open new clinic.
[c]Increase (decrease) in volume from choosing add option.
[d]Increase (decrease) in revenue from choosing add option.
[e]Increase (decrease) in variable costs by choosing add option.
[f]Increase (decrease) in avoidable fixed costs by choosing add option.
[g]Increase (decrease) in total contribution margin by choosing add option.
[h]Increase (decrease) in product margin from choosing add option.

EXHIBIT 9.18b EXAMPLE OF AN ADD-OR-DROP DECISION

Givens		Alternative		Difference If Choose to Add Service (Do – Don't)
		Don't Add[a]	Do Add[b]	
A	Volume	0	3,000	Increase in volume
B	Revenue per visit	$0	$35	Increase in charge
C	Cost per visit	$0	$10	Increase in VC/test
D	Contribution margin per visit	$0	$25	Increase in CM
E	Avoidable fixed cost	$0	$85,000	Increase in AFC
Solution				
F	Volume (A)	0	3,000	3,000[c]
G	Revenues (A × B)	$0	$105,000	$105,000[d]
H	Variable costs (A × C)	$0	$30,000	$30,000[e]
I	Total contribution margin (G – H)	$0	$75,000	$75,000[f]
J	Avoidable fixed costs (E)	$0	$85,000	$85,000[g]
K	Product margin (I – J)	$0	($10,000)	($10,000)[h]

[a] Do not open a new clinic.
[b] Open new clinic.
[c] Increase (decrease) in volume from choosing add option.
[d] Increase (decrease) in revenue from choosing add option.
[e] Increase (decrease) in variable costs by choosing add option.
[f] Increase (decrease) in avoidable fixed costs by choosing add option.
[g] Increase (decrease) in total contribution margin by choosing add option.
[h] Increase (decrease) in product margin from choosing add option.

Expanding or Reducing a Service

Decision Rule

If only one alternative *will* or *must* be chosen, then the anticipated product margin of both alternatives should be compared. The alternative with the higher anticipated product margin should be chosen.

Example

Physicians Healthcare Group (PHG) is located in the greater Barnsboro metropolitan area. One of its major revenue centers, a radiology service, receives its revenues on a capitated basis: $55 per member per year to take care of all routine radiology needs. Assume that 20 percent of the 10,000 members will receive some routine radiological service each year at an average cost of $50 per service.

PHG operates six satellite clinics that offer general and specialty medicine services to its customers. X-ray service is also available at every clinic so that patients can be examined on site immediately. This has been a successful marketing feature, as shown by the annual patient satisfaction survey, but it has been costly. Stacy Helman, the new clinic manager, has suggested centralizing the radiology operations to two locations that have the capacity to serve all six clinics. She feels this would help reduce the current fixed costs of the organization by $200,000. However, if the services were relocated, Helman predicts a 10 percent reduction in members because they would probably change HMOs. The solution is shown in Exhibit 9.19.

Given the product margin results (row K), it appears that PHG should centralize its radiology service. Even though 10 percent of the patient volume would be lost, there would be significant equipment cost savings with this option. PHG would be better off by $155,000 per year by centralizing.

Although these examples illustrate the application of the product margin paradigm, other financial analysis tools should also be employed when making these decisions. For instance, the impact of these decisions on the financial ratios of the organization should be considered (see Chapter Four). Similarly, to the extent that these decisions have multiyear implications, a more thorough analysis would discount future cash flows and assess the net present value of these decisions (see Chapters Six and Seven). Finally, these financial concerns must be weighed against nonfinancial concerns when making these decisions.

EXHIBIT 9.19 EXAMPLE OF AN EXPAND-OR-REDUCE DECISION

		Alternative		Difference If Choose to Reduce Service (Do – Don't)	
		Don't Reduce[a]	Do Reduce[b]		
Givens					
A	Members	10,000	9,000	Decrease in volume	
B	Utilization rate	20%	20%	No change in utilization rate	
C	PMPY	$55	$55	No change in PMPY	
D	Cost per test	$50	$50	No change in cost per test	
E	Avoidable fixed cost	$200,000	$0	Decrease in AFC	
Solution					
F	Members	(A)	10,000	9,000	(1,000)[c]
G	Revenues	(A × C)	$550,000	$495,000	($55,000)[d]
H	Variable costs	(A × B × D)	$100,000	$90,000	($10,000)[e]
I	Total contribution margin	(G – H)	$450,000	$405,000	($45,000)[f]
J	Avoidable fixed costs	(E)	$200,000	$0	($200,000)[g]
K	Product margin	(I – J)	$250,000	$405,000	$155,000[h]

[a]Do not reduce number of locations.
[b]Reduce number of locations.
[c]Increase (decrease) in volume from reducing locations.
[d]Increase (decrease) in revenue from reducing locations.
[e]Increase (decrease) in variable costs by reducing locations.
[f]Increase (decrease) in avoidable fixed costs by reducing locations.
[g]Increase (decrease) in total contribution margin by reducing locations.
[h]Increase (decrease) in product margin from reducing locations.

Summary

An understanding of fixed and variable costs provides a valuable tool to help make decisions of what price to charge, whether to add or drop a service, or whether to make or buy a service. Fixed costs are costs that do not vary in total but vary per unit over the relevant range. Variable costs vary in total but do not vary per unit over the relevant range. The relevant range is the range over which total fixed costs and/or per unit variable cost do not vary.

The break-even equation can be used to determine price, volume, fixed costs, or variable cost per unit when each of the other factors is known. The break-even formula is shown in equation 1 below.

The break-even point is that volume where total revenues equal total costs. The results of a break-even analysis are often presented on a break-even chart, which illustrates fixed costs, total costs, total revenues, and volume. The distance between the total cost and total revenue lines represents the amount of profit or loss the service is experiencing at any particular volume of service. An alternative form of this chart shows the difference between the total cost and total revenue lines: that is, net income.

The break-even equation can be applied to capitated situations to determine capitation rates, utilization rates, or fixed or variable costs, given the others. The break-even equation can also be extended to multipayor and multiservice situations, though the details for these situations are beyond the scope of this text. In conducting multipayor analyses that include capitated and fixed-fee patients, it is important not to adjust revenues for changes in volume, though variable costs may change. This caveat also holds for fixed-fee patients, such as those who pay on the basis of DRGs.

Per unit contribution margin is calculated by subtracting per unit variable cost from per unit revenues. It is the amount of profit made on each additional unit provided all other costs (fixed costs and overhead) remain the same. It is also the amount of incremental income from an average unit of service that is available to cover all other costs. If the contribution margin is known, a shortcut formula to calculate breakeven can be used, equation 2 below.

If (1) the decision has been made not to close down a service, (2) no other additional costs will be incurred, and (3) the contribution margin is positive, then it is in the best financial interest of the organization to continue to provide additional units of that service, even if it is not fully covering all of its other costs.

$$(\text{Price} \times \text{Volume}) = \text{Fixed Costs} + (\text{Variable Cost per Unit} \times \text{Volume}) \qquad (1)$$

$$\text{Break-Even Volume} = \text{Total Fixed Costs} / \text{Contribution Margin per Unit} \qquad (2)$$

In instances where multiple services are offered, it is likely that there are both organizational fixed costs and service-specific fixed costs. Fixed costs that are present just because the service is being provided and would not be there if the service were not offered are called avoidable fixed costs. Product margin is computed as shown in equation 3 below:

Total Revenues – Total Variable Costs – Avoidable Fixed Costs	(3)

The product margin decision rule states: if a service is covering its own variable and avoidable fixed costs, even if it does not fully cover its full share of other costs (nonavoidable fixed costs and common costs), the organization is better off delivering the service than not, all other things being equal (that is, there are no better alternatives). If the organization violates this rule and closes a service with a positive product margin, the organization increases its loss by the amount of the product margin that it forgoes. The product margin concept is useful to help answer questions related to providing a service in-house or outsourcing (make-or-buy decision), adding or dropping a service, and expanding or reducing services. In all of these analyses, sunk costs should not be considered.

Other financial analysis tools should also be employed when making these decisions. For instance, the impact on the financial ratios of the organization should be considered. Also, decisions that have multiyear implications should include a thorough analysis of future cash flows and net present value. Finally, as noted earlier, the financial concerns must be balanced with nonfinancial concerns to make these decisions.

Key Terms

a. Avoidable fixed cost

b. Break-even analysis

c. Break-even point

d. Capitation

e. Common costs

f. Contribution margin per unit

g. Contribution margin rule

h. Fixed costs

i. Incremental costs

j. Joint costs

k. Nonavoidable fixed costs

l. Product margin

m. Product margin decision rule

n. Pro forma

o. Relevant range

p. Step-fixed costs

q. Target costing

r. Total contribution margin

s. Variable costs

Key Equations

- Basic break-even equation

$$\text{Price} \times \text{Volume} = \text{Fixed Cost} + (\text{Variable Cost per Unit} \times \text{Volume})$$

- Contribution margin per unit

$$\text{Revenue per Unit} - \text{Variable Cost per Unit}$$

- Total contribution margin

$$\text{Total Revenue} - \text{Total Variable Cost}$$

- Shortcut to determine break-even volume

$$\text{Fixed Costs} / \text{Contribution Margin per Unit}$$

- Break-even equation modified to include desired profit

$$\text{Price} \times \text{Volume} = \text{Fixed Costs} + (\text{Variable Cost per Unit} \times \text{Volume}) + \text{Desired Profit}$$

- Break-even equation modified to include indirect cost and desired profit

$$\text{Price} \times \text{Volume} = \text{Direct Cost} + \text{Indirect Costs} + \text{Desired Profit}$$
$$\text{where Direct Costs} = \text{Direct Fixed Costs} + (\text{Direct Variable Cost per Unit} \times \text{Volume})$$

- Break-even equation for capitation

$$\text{PMPM} \times \text{Enrollees} = (\text{Enrollees} \times \text{Utilization Rate} \times \text{Variable Cost per Unit})$$
$$+ \text{Monthly Fixed Cost}$$

- Product margin

$$\text{Total Contribution Margin} - \text{Avoidable Fixed Costs}$$

REVIEW QUESTIONS AND PROBLEMS

1. **Definitions**. Define the previously listed key terms.

2. **Break-even formulas**. What are the formulas for

   a. The basic break-even equation?

   b. The basic break-even equation expanded to include indirect costs and desired profit?

3. **Understanding fixed and variable cost.** Briefly describe what happens to each of the following as volume increases. Assume all values stay within their relevant range.

   a. Total fixed cost?

   b. Total variable cost?

   c. Fixed cost per unit?

   d. Variable cost per unit?

4. **Step-fixed cost and the relevant range.** Explain the relationship between step-fixed costs and the relevant range.

5. **Product margin.** Based on the product margin, when is it in the best interests of an organization to continue or drop a service?

6. **Make-or-buy decision and related analyses.**

   a. What is a make-or-buy decision?

   b. What other analyses are relevant to the types of decisions discussed in this chapter?

7. **Break-even equation. Fill in the blank.** The following table contains selected data concerning several outpatient clinics in the new Ambulatory Care Center at Hope University Hospital. Fill in the missing information.

A	B	C	D	E	F
Price per Visit	**Variable Cost per Visit**	**Number of Visits**	**Contribution Margin**	**Fixed Costs**	**Net Income**
$85		3,000	$220,000		$100,000
$70	$20		$250,000	$130,000	
	$35	3,250		$165,000	$85,000
$78	$55	2,500		$60,000	

8. **Break-even equation. Fill in the blank.** Instead of the information in problem 7, assume Ambulatory Care Center's data looked like this:

A	B	C	D	E	F
Price per Visit	**Variable Cost per Visit**	**Number of Visits**	**Contribution Margin**	**Fixed Costs**	**Net Income**
$120		4,500	$350,000		$65,000
$110	$65		$135,000	$75,000	
	$45	5,300		$110,000	$90,000
$135	$75	3,800		$120,000	

9. **Expand-or-reduce decision**. Laurie Vaden is a physician with her own practi
developed contracts with several large employers to perform routine exams, fitness
duty exams, and initial screening of on-the-job injuries. She provides 200 exams per
month, charging $200 per exam. Under these contracts, she estimates her avoidable fixed
cost attributable to the exams is $1,000 per month, and she pays a lab an average of $15
per exam. She has decided she needs to increase profit, so she is considering raising her
fee to $225, even though there may be a 15 percent loss in the number of exams she
does per month. Determine the current and predicted (a) revenues, (b) variable costs, and
(c) total contribution margin. What should she be recommended to do? Why?

10. **Expand-or-reduce decision**. Janet Gilbert is director of a lab. She has some extra capacity and has contracted with some small neighboring hospitals to run some of their lab
tests. She has recently had a study conducted and has determined that her costs for these
contracts are $50,000, of which $7,000 is the variable cost of supplies. The rest is nonavoidable fixed cost. She currently charges an average of $30 per test. She is thinking of
lowering her price by 20 percent in hopes of raising her current volume of 20,000 tests
by 25 percent. If she does so, she expects her variable cost per test will go up by 5 percent.
Determine the current and predicted (a) revenues, (b) variable costs, and (c) total contribution margin and product margin. What should she be recommended to do? Why?

11. **Calculating break-even volume**. Jasmine Gonzales, administrative director of Small
Imaging Center, has been asked by the practice members to see if it is feasible to add more
staff to support the practice's mammography service, which currently has two analogue
film or screen units and two technologists. She has compiled the following information:

(handwritten: stays the same)

(handwritten: rent (same))

(handwritten: renenter ya have 2 pieces of equipment)

(handwritten: d) wifi, rent)
(handwritten: e+f) R&E (change)

Reimbursement per screen — *variable (v)*	$75
Equipment costs per month — *fixed*	$1,600
Technologist cost per mammography *(2) —v*	$20
Technologist aide per mammography *—v*	$4
Variable cost per mammography *—v*	$10
Equipment maintenance per month per machine *(2)*	$700

(handwritten: 2 techs)

(handwritten: # of screens) *(handwritten: fixed)*

a. What is the monthly patient volume needed per month to cover fixed and variable costs?

(handwritten: don't have yet or are)

b. What is the patient volume needed per month if Small Imaging Center desires to
cover its fixed and variable costs and make a $5,000 profit on this equipment to cover
other costs associated with the organization?

c. If reimbursement decreases to $55 per screen, what is the patient volume needed
per month to cover fixed and variable costs but not profit?

d. If a new technologist aide is hired, what is the patient volume needed per month at
the original reimbursement rate to cover variable costs but not profit?

12. **Calculating break-even volume.** Monica Lee, administrative director of Digital Imaging Center, has been asked by the practice members to see if it is feasible to add more staff to support the practice's mammography service, which currently has two digital units and two technologists. She has compiled the following information:

Reimbursement per mammography	$140
Equipment lease per month per machine	$12,000
Equipment maintenance per month per machine	$9,000
Technologist cost per mammography	$35
Technologist aide per mammography	$20
Variable cost per mammography	$13

a. What is the patient volume needed per month to cover fixed and variable costs?

b. What is the patient volume needed per month if Digital Imaging Center desires to cover its fixed and variable costs and make a $3,000 profit on this equipment to cover other costs associated with the organization?

c. If reimbursement decreases to $110 per screen, what is the patient volume needed per month to cover fixed and variable costs but not profit?

d. If a new technologist aide is hired, what is the patient volume needed per month at the original reimbursement rate to cover costs but not profit?

13. **Calculating break-even point and graphing.** San Juan Health Department's dental clinic projects the following costs and rates for the year 20XX.

Total fixed costs	$225,000
Variable costs	$60 per patient
Charges	$250 per patient

a. Using this information, determine the break-even point in patients.

b. Using this information, determine the break-even point in dollars.

c. Graph this scenario in a break-even chart, using a range of 0 to 3,500 patients in 500-patient increments.

d. If the clinic decides it would like to make a profit of $8,000, what is the new break-even point in patients?

e. If the clinic decides it would like to make a profit of $8,000 at 1,226 patients, what is the new break-even point in dollars?

14. **Calculating break-even point and graphing.** The North Kingstown Cancer infusion therapy division expects tremendous growth over the next year and is projecting the following cost and rate structure for the service.

Revenues	$900 per patient
Costs	
Rent	$4,200 per month
Staff	$220,000 per month
Leases	$15,000 per month
Other fixed costs	$30,000 per month
Pharmaceuticals	$700 per patient
Intravenous supplies	$45 per patient
Other patient supplies	$35 per patient

a. What volume of patients per month will it take for the center to break even?

b. What is the break-even point in dollars?

c. Graph the above scenario, using a range of 0 to 2,500 patients in 500-patient increments.

d. If the clinic needs to make a profit of $85,000 per month, what is the new break-even point in volume per month?

e. If the clinic needs to make a profit of $85,000 per month, what is the new break-even point in revenue?

15. **Determining break-even price in a reduce-or-expand decision.** QuickCare is a health care franchise that functions as a primary family health clinic, seeing unscheduled patients twenty-four hours a day. Several months after the grand opening, a corporate office management engineering study showed that the clinic was experiencing some dips in volume in the mid-afternoon hours. To increase volume, efficiency, and revenues, the clinic administrator contracted with the area high schools to provide after-school physicals for the sports teams. The initial agreement was that QuickCare would charge $150 per exam, the market average. Fixed costs were $50,000 and variable costs were $55 per physical. Although this strategy proved somewhat successful, gross profit margin lagged behind the corporate expectations. To improve its margin, the clinic is considering increasing the exam price to $175. QuickCare's administrator projects that this price increase will cause the high schools to send their athletes to other providers and that volume could drop by 33 percent. Last year QuickCare performed 1,500 examinations. The administrator feels that if the program closes down, all $50,000 in fixed costs would be saved.

a. What should QuickCare's decision be, assuming that this price increase would decrease the number of patients seen by one-third?

b. What price would QuickCare have to charge to make up for the loss of patients?

c. Using the information from the answer to question a, should QuickCare make the same decision if 40 percent of the fixed costs are avoidable? Would it be better or worse off? Why?

16. **Expand-or-reduce.** The administrator of ABC Hospital, Mr. Stevens, has just received the latest financial report, and the news is not good. The hospital has been losing money for over a year, and if things don't improve, it may lose its AA bond rating. Stevens has met with his vice president of finance, Mr. Sanger, and has asked him to identify areas for cutting costs, beginning with services that are operating at a loss. The following informa-tion is for services provided at ABC Hospital's ambulatory care clinic:

Annual volume (in patient visits)	7,000
Charge per visit	$155
Variable cost per visit	$45
Fixed costs	$700,000

   a. Suppose that all fixed costs are avoidable. What should Sanger recommend to Stevens regarding dropping the clinic?

   b. What if only $300,000 of the fixed costs were avoidable? Would this change his recommendation?

   c. Are there any other considerations that should be taken into account when making this decision?

17. **Add-or-drop decision.** The Ancome County Health Department is considering using 300 square feet of excess office space to provide a clinic for Healthchek visits. These visits are reimbursed at $75 under a Medicaid program. Variable costs per visit are $45, and provid-ing the service requires an additional physician assistant and nurse with prorated salaries of $85,000 and $65,000, respectively. The state has mandated efforts to increase the uti-lization of Medicaid eligibility, so the Department of Social Services is conducting interventions to increase eligibility awareness in the community. As a result, the health department expects 12,000 Healthchek visits in the coming year. Nonavoidable overhead costs for the health department are $300,000 per year and will be allocated to each program based on its proportional share of the health department's total office space of 2,700 square feet.

   a. What are the total contribution margin and total product margin for a Healthchek visit?

   b. Considering the total product margin, should the health department provide the service?

   c. Are there any other considerations that should be taken into account when making this decision?

18. **Add-or-drop decision.** The Midtown Women's Center offers bone densitometry scans in the office as a convenience to its patients. The clinic volume is expanding, and Sam Loch, the center's administrator, is considering dropping the bone densitometry service and

converting the space to an exam room to allow for more outpatient visits. The following information has been gathered to help with the decision.

Number of scans per year	510
Reimbursement per bone densitometry scan	$77
Bone densitometry supply cost per scan	$22
Part-time bone densitometry scan technician	$19,000
Reimbursement per office visit	$90
Supply cost per office visit	$30
Expected increase in outpatient volume if additional exam space is available	500

a. What is the contribution margin for the bone densitometry service per year?

b. Should this service continue as opposed to converting it to exam room space? Why or why not?

c. How many office visits would it take to replace the income from the bone densitometry service?

19. **Breakeven**. Sure Care Health Maintenance Organization is seeking a managed care contract with a local manufacturing plant. Sure Care estimates that the cost of providing preventive and curative care for the 500 employees and their families will be $120,000 per month. The manufacturing company offered Sure Care a premium bid of $250 per employee per month.

a. If Sure Care accepts this bid and contracts with the manufacturing firm, will Sure Care earn a profit or loss for the year? How much?

b. What premium per employee per month does Sure Care need to break even?

c. If Sure Care wants to earn $120,000 in profit for the year, what is the required premium per employee per month?

d. What concerns Sure Care in this analysis?

20. **Breakeven**. Zack Millman Clinic is seeking to provide sports-related health care services to high schools in the area. Zack Millman estimates that the cost to provide care would be $2,500 plus $15 per athlete per month on a nine-month basis. The high schools jointly offered to pay the clinic $15,000 for a nine-month contract to cover 85 athletes.

a. If the clinic accepts this bid and contracts with the high schools, will it earn a profit or loss for the year? How much?

b. What would the contract price have to be for Millman to break even?

   c. If Zack Millman Clinic wants to earn $8,000 in profit for the year, and the school system preferred to pay on a per athlete per month basis, what would the price have to be?

21. **Profit, charges, and breakeven without and with overhead.** A number of years ago, at the request of its employees, Jake Winslow and Company converted one of its small rooms to house a small pharmacy for its employees, where they can buy a few popular, prepackaged drugs. JWC only wants to break even on this service. Total cost of operating the pharmacy per year is $40,000: $2,000 a month for the contractor who operates the pharmacy and the remainder in drug costs. JWC charged $45 a month to each of 700 employees who participated last year.

   a. How much did the company make or lose during the year?

   b. In setting its rate for the coming year, how much would JWC have to charge per participating employee if it expects to break even? It estimates 700 employees per year will use this service.

   c. What if JWC also wants these employees to cover the estimated $500 overhead per month the pharmacy space costs?

   d. What would JWC have to charge if it expects drug costs to increase 10 percent per employee?

22. **Determining charges for private pay residents.** Shady Rest Nursing Home has 140 residents. The administrator is concerned about balancing the ratio of its private pay to non-private pay patients. Non-private pay sources reimburse an average of $170 per day, whereas private pay residents pay on average 100 percent of full daily charges. The administrator estimates that variable cost per resident per day is $90 for supplies, food, and contracted services, and annual fixed costs are $6,500,000.

   a. What is the daily contribution margin of each non-private pay resident?

   b. If 25 percent of the residents are non-private pay, what will Shady Rest charge the private pay patients to break even?

   c. What if non-private pay payors cover 50 percent of the residents?

   d. The owner of Shady Rest Nursing Home insists that the facility earn $1 million in annual profits. How much must the administrator raise the per day charge for the privately insured residents if 25 percent of the residents are covered by non-private pay payors?

23. **Determining charges for private pay residents.** Shady Grove Nursing Home has 250 residents. The administrator is concerned about balancing the ratio of its private pay to non-private pay patients. Non-private pay sources reimburse an average of $155 per day whereas private pay residents pay on average 90 percent of full daily charges. The administrator estimates that variable cost per resident per day is $80 for supplies, food, and contracted services, and annual fixed costs are $10 million.

a. What is the daily contribution margin of each non-private pay resident?

b. If 25 percent of the residents are non-private pay, what will Shady Grove charge the private pay patients to break even?

c. What if non-private pay payors cover 50 percent of the residents?

d. The owner of Shady Grove Nursing Home insists that the facility earn $1 million in annual profits. How much must the administrator raise the per day charge for the privately insured residents if 25 percent of the residents are covered by non-private pay payors?

24. **Add-or-drop with net present value analysis** (builds on material in Chapters Six and Seven). Franklin County Hospital, a nonprofit hospital, bought and installed a new computer system last year for $60,000. The system is designed to relay information between labs and medical units. Charlene Walker, the hospital's new computer specialist, had a meeting with Lou Campbell, vice president of finance. She said: "Lou, today I read in a journal that a new computer system has just been introduced. It costs $32,000, but I believe that by replacing our old system, we could reduce operating and maintenance costs that are now being incurred." The following are Walker's estimates:

	Present System	**New System**
Purchase and installment price	$60,000	$32,000
Useful life when purchased	6 years	5 years
Computer operating costs per year	$35,000	$15,000
Computer maintenance costs per year	$14,000	$11,000
Depreciation expenses per year	$10,000	$6,400
Cost of capital	10%	10%

a. Based on an analysis, what advice should Walker give Campbell?

b. At what price for the new computer system would Campbell be indifferent on this decision?

c. Is this a typical make-or-buy decision? Why or why not?

25. **Add-or-drop with net present value analysis** (builds on material in Chapters Six and Seven). Franklin County Hospital, a nonprofit hospital, bought and installed a new computer system last year for $90,000. The system is designed to relay information between labs and medical units. Charlene Walker, the hospital's new computer specialist, had a meeting with Lou Campbell, vice president of finance. She said: "Lou, today I read in a journal that a new computer system has just been introduced. It costs $50,000, but I believe that by replacing our old system, we could reduce operating and maintenance costs that are now being incurred." The following are Walker's estimates:

	Present System	New System
Purchase and installment price	$90,000	$50,000
Useful life when purchased	6 years	5 years
Computer operating costs per year	$35,000	$25,000
Computer operating and maintenance costs per year	$15,000	$8,000
Depreciation expenses per year	$15,000	$10,000
Cost of capital	10%	10%

a. Based on an analysis, what advice should Walker give Campbell?

b. At what price for the new computer system would Campbell be indifferent on this decision?

c. Is this a typical make-or-buy decision? Why or why not?

26. **Income statement and add-or-drop**. Lakespring Retirement Village is home to senior citizens who are fairly independent but need assistance with basic health care and occasional meals. Jill Thompson, a licensed beautician, works on salary eighteen hours a week at Lakespring. Funds at the retirement village have been getting tight due to an increase in the number of Medicaid and other low-income residents. Carl Jones, Lakespring's administrator, told Thompson that the hair salon might have to be closed. Jones is sympathetic because he knows that it will be inconvenient for many residents to get this service elsewhere, and Thompson's charges are about all the residents can afford, but he wonders how he can keep any unit open that does not break even. Jones is looking for a way to save the hair salon and has provided the following information: Jill is currently doing an average weekly business of 19 haircuts, 7 permanents, and 6 brief visits, which take half an hour, an hour, and fifteen minutes, respectively. The hair salon is currently allocated rent of $270 per month and other upkeep expenses of $60 a month. Thompson is paid $14 per hour.

	Haircuts	Permanents	Brief Visits
Charge per resident	$15.00	$25.00	$10.00
Variable costs per service performed (cleaning, styling, and setting products)	$2.00	$5.00	$4.50
Variable water expense	$0.25	$0.35	$0.35
Laundry expenses for towels, smocks, etc.	$0.15	$0.35	$0.40

a. Prepare a monthly income statement and determine the total contribution margin and total product margin for each service line. Determine net income for the service taken as a whole.

b. Should Jones close the hair salon? Why or why not?

c. Should Jones try to persuade Thompson to drop any service she now offers?

27. Practice valuation. Coffee Healthcare Associates (CHA) wants to expand its network of providers in the northwest section of the city to build its referral base for its new ambulatory surgery center. A well-respected group of three pain management physicians and one nurse practitioner have expressed interest in joining forces with CHA, but only if they can get guaranteed salaries for at least three years. Their collections have been dropping recently due to poor follow-up on denials and accounts receivable, the current secretary/receptionist is retiring, and they are ready to negotiate. The provider group has offered the following information on initial compensation requirements and payor mix and volume:

Provider	Desired Compensation
Physician 1 (owner)	$280,000
Physicians 2, 3	$235,000
Nurse practitioner	$125,000

Insurance	Annual Visit Volume
Commercial	10,900
Medicare	8,100
Medicaid	575
Self-pay	90
Other	55

Variable costs are estimated at $32 per visit, and the practice's billing expense is 9 percent of collections.

While CHA acknowledges the current payor mix, its marketing director feels that Medicaid patients will make up a much higher proportion of patients, one more closely matching the network's payor mix. Those proportions are: commercial, 45%; Medicare, 33%; Medicaid, 20%; and self-pay and other, 1% each. Additionally, due to past experience, CHA believes that overall volume will drop by 10% once the providers receive guaranteed income, despite their insistence otherwise. Last, CHA expects the providers' compensation to increase by 5 percent per year in accordance with historical network increases.

The table below shows expected reimbursements per visit over the next three years. CHA's billing expense is 9% of collections. How would CHA fare each year under this acquisition? (*Hint*: see Appendix H.)

Insurance	Average Reimbursement per Visit
Commercial	$112.50
Medicare	$84.00
Medicaid	$67.00
Self-pay	$21.75
Other	$99.00

Appendix H: Break-even Analysis for Practice Acquisition

In today's difficult health care environment, organizations try to gain a competitive edge by expanding or redefining their services, broadening their networks, engaging in joint ventures, and/or potentially buying out competitors. These decisions involve complex financial methodologies and projections to assess the long-term return, as introduced in the earlier chapters. Unless there are strategic indicators outweighing the fact that a service will lose money, the goal of any business venture would be to turn a profit, or at least break even. One common proposition is to buy out local private provider practices to broaden an institution's provider network and referral base, though as illustrated in Perspective 9.5, not all ventures prosper.

Under the current reimbursement climate, private physician practices have found it increasingly difficult to remain financially solvent. Many practices have begun to shut their doors to Medicaid and uninsured patients, forcing them to look elsewhere for needed care. At the same time, as competition for the best-paying patients intensifies, hospitals and health care systems have started to lure physician groups into their provider networks to capture their referrals for lucrative ancillary services and other profitable inpatient and surgical care. The private physicians are willing to sell their practices and lose much of their autonomy in return for stable, guaranteed incomes and the benefit of being able to offload troublesome collection efforts to the institution. Additionally, the purchasing institutions—due to their increasing clout in the marketplace from broadening their

PERSPECTIVE 9.5 EVALUATING PHYSICIAN PRACTICES

There are many reasons why expenses in medical groups acquired by a hospital or an integrated delivery system (IDS) may exceed practice revenues, including lowered provider production, the basing of provider compensation on market levels instead of on a provider's financial contribution, a different payor mix than the physician practice had before, provider-based billing, and the transfer of ancillary services from the practice to the health system.

And while the vast majority of IDS-owned medical groups operate at a loss, there are some practices that break even and others that report positive bottom lines. These practices can be considered "best of breed" in their operations and deserve a closer look.

Hospital systems attract a different payor mix than independent practices, and hospitals often employ provider-based billing and shift ancillary services to parent organizations, which can complicate comparisons with physician-owned medical groups. At the same time, an IDS-owned practice should not aim for mediocrity. IDS practices should compare provider productivity levels with private practices and examine the performance of both physician-owned and other IDS practices to evaluate their staffing and costs.

Once you examine the best-performing IDS practices, it becomes apparent that IDS medical groups do not need to lose money. Good business practices and high productivity result in an excellent bottom line, and the practices that break even or better are truly the best of breed.

Source: Adapted from D. Gans, Best of breed: what enables some hospital-owned groups to prosper? *MGMA Connexion*, May/June 2012: 21–22.

networks—oftentimes can also negotiate higher reimbursement rates from local insurers as well as cost discounts from suppliers.

Integration of physician practices can benefit both parties, but the purchasing institution must be able to accurately value the net worth of the practice in order to make a sound financial investment. In other words, can the purchase at least break even or result in a positive net return? (Some physician practices that are struggling financially owing to poor practice management may effectively view hospital purchases as a bailout.) Are there other factors involved that would still make the purchase desirable, even if it fails to reach breakeven?

Many considerations play a role in valuing a provider practice, including

- Operating revenues from the provision of services less billing fees.
- Operating expenses, both fixed and variable costs.

- Current asset valuations (book value of tangible assets, such as building, equipment, and supplies).

- Discounted value of outstanding accounts receivable.

- Estimated value of new downstream referral volumes for ancillary and inpatient or surgical services that may otherwise have been directed elsewhere to competing institutions.

Sample Analysis

Lathrop Physician Practice (LPP) is a local family practice in a respectable neighborhood. Staff consist of Dr. Lathrop, a nurse office manager, a medical assistant, and a receptionist. Over the past two years, Dr. Lathrop has been averaging twenty-four patients seen per day, and after all her expenses, her annual take-home pay in 20X0 was $150,000. She has agreed to sell her practice if she can get a guaranteed annual base salary of at least $200,000, and if her office staff, who have been loyal, are retained as part of the agreement. Exhibit H.1a is a simplified pro forma that shows actual visits and revenues for the practice in 20X0 (columns B, D), as well as collection rates by payor type (column E). There were also supplemental revenues from flu shots, shown in the lower part of the exhibit.

Pro Forma

A simplified table of categorized line items with volumes and associated revenues and expenses that are used to estimate overall financial performance.

Mabel County Hospital, which is trying to build a wide provider network, believes that LPP has a good payor mix and could generate additional downstream revenues for the hospital from referrals for ancillary, inpatient, and surgical services, which oftentimes are being sent elsewhere. Exhibit H.1b is a modified version of LPP's pro forma showing projected earnings from being included in Mabel County's provider network, which would be an incremental $66,000 from current earnings ($553,000 Projected − $487,000 Current [approximate]).

Mabel County currently outsources its billing to an outside vendor, who charges 7 percent of collections. This amount, which comes to $42,827 (7% × $611,810), must be deducted from total expected revenues as shown at the bottom of Exhibit H.1b. Also, Mabel County projects that variable costs will be the same $12 per visit, or $69,600 in total ($12 per Visit × 5,800 Visits), which must also be deducted from revenues. Last, Mabel County expects the same flu shot income of $54,000, derived on a cash basis.

LPP has $250,000 in charges tied up in outstanding accounts receivable, which would become the property of the hospital (Exhibit H.2a, columns A and B). Mabel County's calculations of the amount that collection rates diminish the longer a charge is outstanding (Exhibit H.2a, column C) yield a final collection rate of approximately 45 percent ($112,250 in

EXHIBIT H.1a CURRENT VISIT AND REVENUE STATISTICS FOR LATHROP PHYSICIAN PRACTICE IN 20X0, BEFORE ACQUISITION

A	B	C	D	E
Payor	Total 20X0 Visits	Actual Percentage of Total	Total 20X0 Collections	Average Payment per Visit
Commercial	2,850	51%	$307,800	$108.00
Medicare	2,100	38%	199,500	95.00
Medicaid	425	8%	30,600	72.00
Self-pay	120	2%	1,800	15.00
Other[a]	100	2%	10,200	102.00
Total	**5,595**	**100%**	**$549,900**	**$98.28**
		Less: billing expense (9%)	$(49,491)	
		Less: variable costs ($12 per visit)	$(67,140)	
		Net collections	**$433,269**	

[a]Workers' compensation, independent medical evaluations, union workers' contract, etc.

Additional Services	20X0 Volume	20X0 Product Margin	
Flu shots	3,600	**$54,000**	(Contribution margin of $15 each)
Total actual annual income for LPP		**$487,269**	

Payments / $250,000 in Charges, column D). After the same 7 percent billing expense, Mabel expects to net $104,393.

Last, LPP also has some tangible assets—equipment and supplies— that the hospital would acquire. These are estimated to be worth $32,000 (Exhibit H.2b). Dr. Lathrop does not own the building she practices in, but if she did, that too would constitute a significant sum that would have to be factored into the analysis (either Dr. Lathrop would continue to own the building and lease her office space to the hospital, or the hospital would have to buy the building outright).

In sum, the hospital expects that the practice acquisition would yield a pickup of $192,000 ($66,000 in improved collections, $104,000 from

EXHIBIT H.1b PROJECTED VISIT AND REVENUE STATISTICS FOR LATHROP PHYSICIAN PRACTICE IN 20X1, AFTER ACQUISITION

F	G	H	I	J
	Estimated Percentage	Projected 20X1	Network Payments	20X1 Total Expected
Payor	of Total	Visits	per Visit	Collections
Commercial	50%	2,900	$125.00	$362,500
Medicare	35%	2,030	95.00	192,850
Medicaid	10%	580	72.00	41,760
Self-Pay	3%	174	20.00	3,480
Other	2%	116	110.00	11,220
Total	100%	5,800	$105.48	$611,810

		Comments
Less: billing expense (7%)	$(42,827)	7% × $611,810
Less: variable costs ($12 per visit)	$(69,600)	$12 × 5,800 visits
Add: flu shot Income	$54,000	No change
Projected annual income for Mabel County	**$553,383**	

outstanding accounts receivable, and $32,000 in office assets). In turn, the hospital would compensate Dr. Lathrop by an additional $50,000 annually ($150,000 current pay versus. $200,000 required), and it estimates that it would need to add an additional staff person in its billing office to handle all the billing and collection efforts for the new practice (LPP currently outsources its billing services to an outside vendor). At $40,000 per year in cost for an additional biller, the increased annual outlays to acquire the practice would be $90,000 ($50,000 + $40,000, see Exhibit H.3). Given that Mabel County would have an initial pickup of $192,000 with $90,000 in new annual expenses, the hospital would be about at breakeven at the end of the second year, but would be faced with an annual operating deficit of $90,000 by the third year and each year thereafter. Therefore, the hospital would need to estimate the value of newly captured downstream referrals after two years for ancillary, inpatient, and surgical services, which would have to exceed $90,000 per year to make the practice acquisition financially viable. (Those calculations are beyond the scope of this text.)

EXHIBIT H.2a VALUATION OF CURRENT ACCOUNTS RECEIVABLE FOR LATHROP PHYSICIAN PRACTICE

A	B	C	D
	Total Outstanding Charges	**Time Lag Realization Factor**	**Factored Net Accounts Receivable**
Current	$110,000	65%	$71,500
31–60 days	75,000	40%	30,000
61–90 days	35,000	25%	8,750
91–120 days	10,000	10%	1,000
120+ days	20,000	5%	1,000
Total	**$250,000**		**$112,250**
		Less: billing expense (7%)	$(7,858)
		Projected collections of aged A/R	104,393

EXHIBIT H.2b VALUATION OF ASSETS FOR LATHROP PHYSICIAN PRACTICE

Modified book value of tangible assets (office equipment, supplies, etc.)	$32,000

EXHIBIT H.3 ADDITIONAL EXPENSES TO ACQUIRE LATHROP PHYSICIAN PRACTICE

Required base salary after acquisition	$200,000
Current base salary	150,000
Increase in base salary	50,000
Additional staff person for billing	40,000
Total additional annual expenses	**$90,000**

CHAPTER 10

BUDGETING

The budget is one of the most important documents of a health care organization and is the central document of the planning-and-control cycle. The budget serves not only as a *planning* document that identifies the revenues and resources needed for an organization to achieve its goals and objectives but also as a *control* document that allows an organization to monitor the actual revenues generated and its use of resources against what was planned.

The Planning-and-Control Cycle

As illustrated in Exhibit 10.1, the planning-and-control cycle has four major components: strategic planning, planning, implementing, and controlling. Budgeting is the central element that affects all these areas.

Strategic Planning and Planning Activities

Strategic planning and planning activities provide the basis for the organization to develop the budget. The purpose of *strategic planning* is to identify the organization's vision, mission, goals, and strategy in order to position itself for the future. The purpose of *planning* is to identify the goals, objectives, tasks, activities, and resources necessary to carry out the strategic plan over a defined time period, commonly one year. The organization's mission is usually set forth in a mission statement, which is a broad, enduring statement of its vision and purpose. The *mission statement* guides the organization into the future by identifying the unique attributes of the organization, why it exists, and what it hopes to achieve (see Perspective 10.1).

LEARNING OBJECTIVES

- State the purposes of budgeting.

- Describe the planning-and-control cycle and the five key dimensions of budgeting.

- List the major budgets and explain their relationship to each other and to the income statement and balance sheet.

- Construct each of the major budgets.

Strategic Planning
Identifying an organization's mission, goals, and strategy to best position itself for the future.

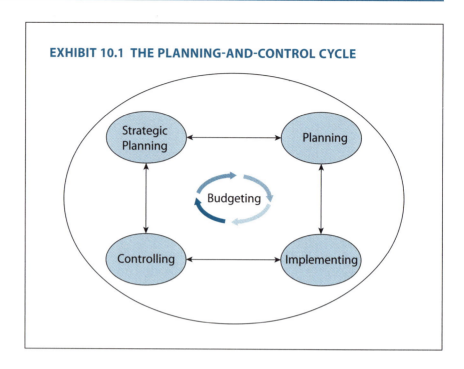

EXHIBIT 10.1 THE PLANNING-AND-CONTROL CYCLE

Planning

The process of identifying goals, objectives, tasks, activities, and resources necessary to carry out the strategic plan of the organization over the next time period, typically one year.

Mission Statement

A statement that guides the organization by identifying the unique attributes of the organization, why it exists, and what it hopes to achieve. Some organizations divide these attributes between a vision statement and a mission statement.

A major activity of the strategic planning process is to assess the organization's external and internal environments. The external environment of most health care organizations is complex, and an environmental analysis must include surveying the local, regional, national, and international environments for changes that may occur in a variety of areas, including the economy, regulation, technology, and health status of populations. Other areas of the external environment that must be examined are listed in the top part of Exhibit 10.2. Failing to thoroughly and correctly assess even one of these domains could lead to major problems for, or even the demise of, the organization. Most recently, the Patient Protection and Affordable Care Act has made significant changes to the strategy and operations of health care entities, particularly hospitals. Some of the issues that are already affecting hospitals are decreasing reimbursement due to value-based payment methodologies, the possibility of increased revenue due to expansion of Medicaid (for those states that enact it), the individual and corporate mandates for insurance coverage, and extensive IT requirements associated with producing and monitoring quality metrics that are already important and will become even more so in the value-based purchasing methodologies (see Perspective 10.2).

In addition to its external environment, a health care organization has to examine its internal environment, which includes both *tangible factors*,

PERSPECTIVE 10.1 MISSION STATEMENT OF SHRINERS HOSPITALS

The mission of any health care entity is important to help guide the entity's strategic management process. But it is probably even more important in a *not-for-profit* health care entity because it sets forth the entity's tax-exempt purpose. The IRS is scrutinizing not-for-profit health care entities because it believes that many do not provide sufficient community benefit to justify the exemption. Every initiative that a not-for-profit entity undertakes should be able to be tied back to its mission.

The mission of Shriners Hospitals for Children is to

- Provide the highest quality care to children with neuromusculoskeletal conditions, burn injuries and other special healthcare needs within a compassionate, family-centered and collaborative care environment.

- Provide for the education of physicians and other healthcare professionals.

- Conduct research to discover new knowledge that improves the quality of care and quality of life of children and families.

This mission is carried out without regard to race, color, creed, sex or sect, disability, national origin or ability of a patient or family to pay.

Its vision says:

Shriners Hospitals for Children will be the unquestioned leader, nationally and internationally, in caring for children and advancing the field in its specialty areas.

Source: Shriners Hospitals for Children, Vision and mission, www.shrinershospitalsforchildren.org/Hospitals/VisionandMission.aspx.

such as financing, staff, services, and structure, and *intangible factors*, such as its history, reputation, and the strength of its board of directors.

An important outcome of the strategic planning process is to identify goals and objectives. In the past, goals and objectives for many health care organizations were fairly narrowly restricted to the nature and scope of services the organization hoped to provide. More recently, however, they have included population impacts (e.g., to reduce low-weight births in the covered population by 15 percent over the next five years), market penetration (e.g., to capture 25 percent of the HMO market within the next five years), and financial position (e.g., to increase return on assets by 10 percent over the next three years). The goals and objectives the organization chooses to pursue affect the revenues and resources the organization will need, and these, in turn, must be reflected in its budget.

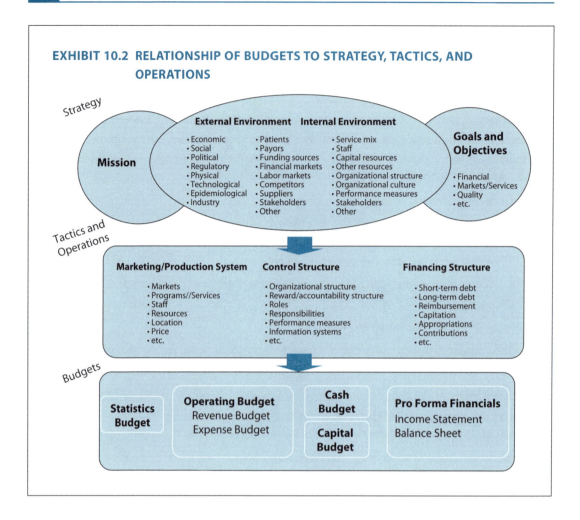

EXHIBIT 10.2 RELATIONSHIP OF BUDGETS TO STRATEGY, TACTICS, AND OPERATIONS

Whereas the organization's strategic planning process focuses on the long term, the organization also develops shorter-term plans to help it achieve its short-term objectives. Whereas the strategic plan is fairly general, *short-term plans* are more specific and identify short-term goals and objectives in more detail, primarily in regard to organizational marketing, production, control, and financing.

Short-Term Plans
Plans that identify an organization's short-term goals and objectives in detail, primarily in regard to organizational marketing, production, control, and financing.

Implementing Activities

Once the organizational plans have been defined and approved for the upcoming fiscal year, budgets need to be created for each and every department (or cost center). *Implementing activities* is the process of creating these individual budgets, which then get rolled up into service line budgets

PERSPECTIVE 10.2 EHR IMPLEMENTATION COSTS

Hospitals have always had challenges securing the initial down payment for electronic health record (EHR) implementation; a recently released poll from KPMG suggests that financing such projects remains an ongoing concern that promises to last throughout the implementation phase and beyond. . . . Forty-eight percent of those polled said they are only somewhat comfortable with the level of budgeting their organization planned for EHR deployment. Nine percent said they weren't comfortable at all with their budget plans.

With the majority of those polled expressing some level of discomfort about how they will pay for their project moving forward, Gary Anthony, principal with KPMG Healthcare, said the poll findings suggest that healthcare executives miscalculated the costs of their EHR projects. . . .

According to Anthony, recent reports that Duke University will spend $700 million to implement its EPIC EHR indicate the staggering costs of an EHR implementation project. He also said these projects are associated with maintaining and storing additional terabytes of data and providing security capabilities that adhere to Health Insurance Portability and Accountability Act (HIPAA) requirements. Additional costs come with maintaining a robust network that allows doctors and other clinicians to access the data remotely on their iPads or smartphones. . . .

Anthony estimates that salaries for employees with health IT skills have risen substantially during the last two years, which also drives up implementation cost. "There is a lack of skills in most health organizations around high-level project management disciplines. It's difficult to find people who know how to manage these very large-scale projects across the organization and who will implement the project on time and on budget," Anthony said.

Source: Excerpted from R. Lewis, EHR implementation still costs too much, *InformationWeek*, July 9, 2012, www.informationweek.com/healthcare/electronic-medical-records/ehr-implementation-still-costs-too -much/240003310.

and, eventually, the overall organizational budget. For example, the individual budgets for general medicine, cardiology, and rheumatology would all get rolled up into a combined budget for the entire Department of Medicine, and this budget would then be rolled up with the combined budget for the Department of Surgery and other budgets into the overall organizational budget.

For revenue-generating cost centers (those areas that see patients and/ or visitors and bill for their services), administrators will use historical trends, marketing projections, and revised fee schedules to estimate the volume of services that they expect to be performed and the corresponding gross revenues that they expect to generate. These revenues will be matched against projected costs for labor and general operations. Non-revenue-generating cost centers (such as Information Technology or Decision Support), will only present projected costs, and their budgets will be rolled up into the overall administration budget.

Depending upon the organizational approach to budgeting (discussed in the next section), administrative guidelines will specify how to create standardized budgets in a uniform manner that will be consistent with the organization's mission statement and goals for the upcoming time period.

Controlling Activities

Controlling Activities

Activities that provide guidance and feedback to keep the organization within its budget once that budget has been approved and is being implemented.

Planning activities provide input to the development of the budget. Once the budget has been approved and implementation begins, *controlling activities* provide guidance and feedback to keep the organization within its budget (see Exhibit 10.1). Control tools vary from organizational structure and information systems to such financial activities as supplying monthly reports to department managers regarding their expenditures against budget and giving midyear bonuses based on financial performance.

Organizational Approaches to Budgeting

Exhibit 10.3 lists five key dimensions over which organizations vary in regard to budgeting: participation, budget model, budget detail, budget forecast, and budget modifications.

EXHIBIT 10.3 KEY BUDGETING DIMENSIONS

Dimension	Approaches		
Participation	Authoritarian	←————————→	Participatory
Budget Model	Incremental/ Decremental	←————————→	Zero-Based
Budget Detail	Line-Item	←— Program —→	Performance
Budget Forecast	Annual Static	←————————→ ←————————→	Multiyear Flexible
Budget Modifications	Controlled	←————————→	Latitude

Participation

The budgeting process can vary considerably from one organization to the next in terms of the roles and responsibilities of the various organizational positions. Under an authoritarian approach, the environmental assessment and the planning of future activities are largely concentrated in a few hands at the top of the organization, and the budget is essentially dictated downward. The *authoritarian approach* is often called *top-down budgeting*. The opposite of the authoritarian approach is the *participatory approach*, in which the roles and responsibilities of the budgeting process are diffused throughout the organization. The participatory approach often begins with some general guidelines from the top, based on top management's knowledge of the environment. Within the restrictions of these general guidelines, department heads and service-line managers (e.g., women's services, emergency services, outreach services) have great latitude to develop their own budgets to submit to upper management for approval. This approach is often called a *top-down-bottom-up approach*. The roles and responsibilities of various organizational positions in the participatory approach are summarized in Exhibit 10.4. Perspective 10.3 offers an example of an institution that has been ranked as one of the best in the country, in part for including physicians in its capital decision-making processes.

Authoritarian Approach
Budgeting and decision making done by relatively few people concentrated in the highest level of the organizational structure (opposite of the *participatory approach*).

Top-Down Budgeting
See *authoritarian approach*.

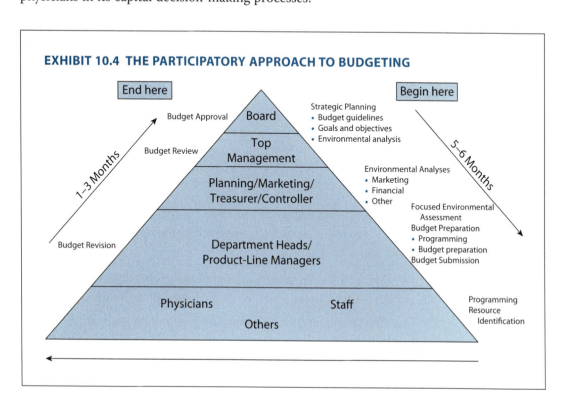

EXHIBIT 10.4 THE PARTICIPATORY APPROACH TO BUDGETING

End here

Begin here

Budget Approval   Board

Strategic Planning
• Budget guidelines
• Goals and objectives
• Environmental analysis

Budget Review   Top Management

5–6 Months

1–3 Months

Planning/Marketing/
Treasurer/Controller

Environmental Analyses
• Marketing
• Financial
• Other

Focused Environmental
Assessment
Budget Preparation
• Programming
• Budget preparation
Budget Submission

Budget Revision   Department Heads/
Product-Line Managers

Physicians   Staff

Others

Programming
Resource
Identification

PERSPECTIVE 10.3 PARTICIPATORY BUDGETING HELPS LEAD TO TOP RANKING

Providence Regional Medical Center (Everett, Wash.) . . . is the third-largest hospital in Washington, with two campuses. It is currently building a $500 million, 368-bed tower, which will double capacity. In 2008, the medical center decided to grow Providence Physician Group to about 100 members over the next three years. To reach this goal, it has increased physicians' involvement in decision-making, such as giving them half the membership in a committee establishing priorities for its capital plan. . . . [The Medical Center is part of] Providence Health System [which] has an Aa2 bond rating from Moody's Investor Services.

Source: Excerpted from L. Page, America's 50 best hospitals, *Becker's Hospital Review*, February 24, 2011, www.beckersasc.com/news-analysis/50-best-hospitals-in-america.html.

EXHIBIT 10.5 SOME KEY ADVANTAGES AND DISADVANTAGES OF THE PARTICIPATORY APPROACH TO BUDGETING

Advantages	Disadvantages
Shared understanding	Loss of control
Cooperation and competition	Time consuming
Clarified roles and responsibilities	High resource use
Motivation	Disappointment
Cost awareness	

The participatory approach to budgeting has a number of advantages beyond just forcing management to plan (see Exhibit 10.5). These advantages include

- Developing a shared understanding of the goals and objectives of the organization by those who have participated in the budgeting process
- Developing cooperation and coordination among the various departments
- Clarifying roles and responsibilities throughout the organization (thus preventing overlap)

- Motivating staff (by allowing them input into their roles, responsibilities, and accountability)

- Bringing about cost awareness as a result of being involved in resource allocation decisions

Although the participatory approach has many advantages, it has three important disadvantages:

- Participation may result in loss of control.

- Participation is time consuming and uses resources (mainly staff time) that could be devoted to other purposes.

- Participation may result in disappointment.

Budget Models

There are two basic budget models: incremental-decremental budgeting and zero-based budgeting (see Exhibit 10.3). The incremental-decremental approach begins with what exists and usually gives a slight increase, no change, or slight decrease to various line items, programs, or departments. In some cases, all programs may receive an equal increase or decrease. In other instances, management may differentially give increases or decreases.

Whereas incremental-decremental budgeting begins by asking the question, How much of an increase or decrease should each program receive?, *zero-based budgeting*, commonly called ZBB, continually questions both the need for each program and its level of funding. It asks: Why does this program or department exist in the first place?, and, What will happen as a result of changing (increasing or decreasing) its level of funding?

Although not many institutions have truly embraced zero-based budgeting, Bain, a large management consulting firm, and others are touting the concept. With today's push toward cutting costs to deal with reimbursement declines, zero-based budgeting can help to focus on priorities. In preparation for the zero-based budgeting process, each budgeting unit (department, program, or service line) prepares a budget package that provides an overall justification for the unit's work and a series of requests to show what the unit's work would look like at various levels of funding. After receiving all budget packages from all budgeting units, management chooses from among them to find the best combination of departments, programs, and service lines, and the best levels of these to meet the goals of the organization within existing resource constraints.

The following scenario illustrates what a zero-based budgeting package might look like at the general level for a small rural hospital that feels it

Participatory Approach
A method of budgeting in which the roles and responsibilities of putting together a budget are diffused throughout the organization, typically originating at the department level. There are guidelines to follow, and top-management approval must be secured (opposite of the *authoritarian approach*).

Top-Down-Bottom-Up Approach
See *participatory approach*.

Incremental-Decremental Approach
A method of budgeting that starts with an existing budget to plan future budgets.

Zero-Based Budgeting
An approach to budgeting that continually questions both the need for existing programs and their level of funding, as well as the need for new programs (often referred to as ZBB).

must establish better relationships with physician practices. In this example, the zero state is no change. The alternatives are to provide practice privileges to primary care physicians at one, two, or three physician practices. In addition to the information used in this example, many organizations would also require further detail about various line items. Such information can be found in the next section, "Budget Detail."

The Situation

San Valens Hospital wants to attract more referring primary care physicians (PCPs) into always sending their patients to San Valens, using the lure of its hospitalist service as a way for these physicians to bypass twenty-four-hour, seven-days-a-week primary care physician inpatient coverage obligations. Currently, there are three PCP groups in the local market area that have been referring their patients to a competing facility, but all these practices have expressed interest in joining the medical staff at San Valens and referring their patients there instead. Crown Colony and Westover Family Practice, on the one hand, with six and eight PCPs, respectively, have a similar mix of adult patients across all insurances and age levels; Parkland Affiliates, on the other hand, is the largest practice with eleven PCPs but, being located adjacent to a growing retirement community, tends to have a much higher proportion of elderly patients. Parkland patients also predominantly have Medicare and steady retiree incomes, and so their reimbursement is more favorable, but because of their age, they tend to utilize services at a disproportionately higher rate than is seen at the other two practices.

San Valens wants to establish itself as a regional referral center for patients and cannot discriminate based on ability to pay. However, at the same time, it wants to make financially prudent decisions and budget adequately for any changes in service capacity. Given these objectives, the hospital needs to explore the economic ramifications of gaining patients from any or all of these PCP groups as it strives to strategically position itself as the dominant area hospital. San Valens is not operating close to its full capacity.

Three alternatives are being proposed, each with considerably different costs and potential revenues, as well as different impacts on the hospital's growth, image, and political concerns (Exhibits 10.6 and 10.7a). Although the costs are fairly predictable (mainly for new staff), if volume projections are off, the revenues are not as predictable. Thus, San Valens must decide how much it wants to invest, if at all, in the three alternatives. See Exhibits 10.7a, 10.7b, 10.7c, 10.7d, and 10.7e.

EXHIBIT 10.6 SUMMARY ZERO-BASED BUDGET

	Crown Colony	Westover Family Practice	Parkland Affiliates
Practice revenues			
Initial services	$28,350	$36,800	$58,625
Follow-up services	91,350	115,200	201,000
Total	119,700	152,000	259,625
Practice expenses			
Labor expenses	162,082	202,603	330,563
Total	162,082	202,603	330,563
Hospitalist practice net income (loss)	(42,382)	(50,603)	(70,938)
Hospital income			
Net inpatient revenues (loss)	189,000	235,750	385,000
Incremental financial impact of proposal	$146,618	$185,147	$314,062
Performance measure: new admissions	900	1,150	1,750

Note: The budgets for each practice separately are considered line-item budgets. The three budgets presented altogether or in other combinations constitute a program budget. Finally, when performance targets are added to a line-item budget, it becomes a performance budget.

Concluding Remarks About Zero-Based Budgeting

Zero-based budgeting was introduced and broadly used in the mid-1960s, but it soon dropped out of favor, primarily because it was such a laborious process. Many organizations felt that too much time was being spent preparing and reviewing budget packages when in fact major changes rarely occurred. There are some signs, though, that zero-based budgeting is reemerging as health care organizations face an increasingly competitive environment, seek to implement new revenue enhancement and cost avoidance activities, and try to capture new market niches.

Budget Detail

Budgets can be classified into three categories based on the amount of detail they contain: line-item, program, and performance. A *line-item budget* has the least detail, merely listing revenues and expenses by category, such as labor, travel, and supplies. A line-item budget for the comprehensive level of care for the San Valens Hospital is shown in Exhibit 10.6.

A *program budget* not only contains the line items but also lists them by program. Exhibit 10.6 shows how the line-item budget for the three

Line-Item Budget
The least detailed budget, showing only revenues and expenses by category, such as labor or supplies.

Program Budget
An extension of the line-item budget that shows revenues and expenses by program or service lines.

EXHIBIT 10.7a INCREMENTAL REVENUE AND COST SUMMARY FOR THREE ADDITIONAL PCP PRACTICES

	Assumptions	Formula	Crown Colony	Westover Family Practice	Parkland Affiliates
	Practice profile				
A	Number of primary care physicians	(Given)	6	8	11
B	Proportion Medicare patients	(Given)	46%	51%	79%
C	Proportion Medicaid/Self-Pay patients	(Given)	10%	6%	4%
	Volume projections				
D	Annual initial service RVUs	(Given)	900	1,150	1,750
E	Annual follow-up service RVUs	(Given)	2,900	3,600	6,000
F	Average LOS per admission, days	(Given)	4.2	4.1	4.4
	Financials				
G	Incremental practice costs per year[a]		$162,082	$202,603	$330,563
H	Average reimbursement per RVU	(Given)	$31.50	$32.00	$33.50
I	Average facility profit per inpatient day	(Given)	$200	$200	$200
	Calculations				
J	Annual initial service revenues	$(D \times H)$	$28,350	$36,800	$58,625
K	Annual follow-up service revenues	$(E \times H)$	$91,350	$115,200	$201,000
L	Incremental practice costs per year[a]	(G)	$162,082	$202,603	$330,563
M	*Incremental hospitalist group income (loss)*	$(J + K - L)$	($42,382)	($50,603)	($70,938)
N	New admissions[b]	$(D / 4)$	225	288	438
O	Incremental inpatient income (loss)	$(F \times I \times N)$	$189,000	$235,750	$385,000
P	*Incremental financial impact of proposal*	$(M + O)$	$146,618	$185,147	$314,062
Q	**Performance measure: new admissions**	(N)	**225**	**288**	**438**

Note: This exhibit provides details of the summary budget found in Exhibit 10.6. The details for each of the three practices, respectively, can be found in Exhibits 10.7b through 10.7d. LOS = length of stay; RVU = relative value unit.
[a]See Exhibits 10.6 and 10.7e.
[b]Each new admission consumes 4 RVUs of service.

Performance Budget
An extension of the program budget that also lays out performance objectives.

physician practices would look as a program budget by providing detail about the three practices, which if chosen singly or in combinations would provide incremental revenues.

Finally, a *performance budget* lists revenues and expenses by line item for each program or service but adds performance measures. Exhibit 10.6 compares the level of detail shown in line-item, program, and performance budgets. Exhibit 10.7a provides additional detail to support the summary zero-based budget in Exhibit 10.6.

EXHIBIT 10.7b ZERO-BASED BUDGET PACKAGE FOR CROWN COLONY

Package: Salary, benefits, capital, and space needs
Organization: Hospitalist practice
Purpose: To provide inpatient care services for the Crown Colony patients
Method: Hospital will need an additional 0.5 FTEs of provider coverage to meet the demands of Crown Colony. This can probably be accommodated by more per diem assistance and by providing current physicians the opportunity to earn additional income by working extra shifts at the per diem rate.
Consequences of not approving this package: Crown Colony, as evidenced by its reimbursement rate, predominantly serves a working class, blue-collar community on the north side of the city, with slightly more Medicaid/Self-Pay patients than Westover. By not choosing this practice, San Valens could be seen as favoring communities who would best help the bottom line, rather than being a full provider of services for the entire region. There is no evidence of other competition for these patients, but there would be an image problem for the hospital of ignoring them.

	Assumptions		Crown Colony
	Practice profile		
A	Number of primary care physicians		6
B	Proportion Medicare patients		46%
C	Proportion Medicaid/Self-Pay patients		10%
	Volume projections		
D	Annual initial service RVUs		900
E	Annual follow-up service RVUs		2,900
F	Average LOS per admission, days		4.2
	Financials		
G	Incremental practice costs	(Exh.10.7e)	$162,082
H	Average reimbursement per RVU		$31.50
I	Average facility profit per inpatient day		$200
	Calculations		
J	Annual initial service revenues	$(D \times H)$	$28,350
K	Annual follow-up service revenues	$(E \times H)$	$91,350
L	Incremental practice costs per year	(G)	$162,082
M	*Incremental hospitalist group income (loss)*	$(J + K - L)$	($42,382)
N	New admissions[a]	(D/4)	225
O	Incremental inpatient income (loss)	$(F \times I \times N)$	$189,000
P	*Incremental financial impact of proposal*	$(M + O)$	$146,618
Q	Performance measure: new admissions	(N)	225

[a]Each new admission consumes 4 RVUs of service.

EXHIBIT 10.7c ZERO-BASED BUDGET PACKAGE FOR WESTOVER FAMILY PRACTICE

Package: Salary, benefits, capital, and space needs

Organization: Hospitalist practice

Purpose: To provide inpatient care services for the Westover Family Practice patients

Method: Hospital will need an additional 0.7 FTEs of provider coverage to meet the demands of Westover. This coverage cannot be accommodated by per diem or additional shift work alone. The hospital would have to hire another full-time physician to accommodate the workload, which would increase costs by $85,000 over what is projected.

Consequences of not approving this package: Westover Family Practice is ideally situated in an area with minimal competition for its services owing to a single bridge that discourages patients from traveling elsewhere for their primary care needs. Westover hopes to add two more physicians and three nurse practitioners over the next two years to grow its practice and ward off potential competitors. Ultimately, this would create more demand for the hospital, but San Valens would be overstaffed initially by budgeting for 1 physician FTE rather than 0.7, and there is no guarantee if or when Westover would expand.

	Assumptions		Westover Family Practice
	Practice profile		
A	Number of primary care physicians		8
B	Proportion Medicare patients		51%
C	Proportion Medicaid/Self-Pay patients		6%
	Volume projections		
D	Annual initial service RVUs		1,150
E	Annual follow-up service RVUs		3,600
F	Average LOS per admission, days		4.1
	Financials		
G	Incremental practice costs	(Exh.10.7e)	$202,603
H	Average reimbursement per RVU		$32.00
I	Average facility profit per inpatient day		$200
	Calculations		
J	Annual initial service revenues	(D × H)	$36,800
K	Annual follow-up service revenues	(E × H)	$115,200
L	Incremental practice costs per year	(G)	$202,603
M	*Incremental hospitalist group income (loss)*	(J + K − L)	($50,603)
N	New admissions[a]	(D/4)	288
O	Incremental inpatient income (loss)	(F × I × N)	$235,750
P	*Incremental financial impact of proposal*	(M + O)	$185,147
Q	Performance measure: new admissions	(N)	288

[a]Each new admission consumes 4 RVUs of service.

EXHIBIT 10.7d ZERO-BASED BUDGET PACKAGE FOR PARKLAND AFFILIATES

Package: Salary, benefits, capital, and space needs
Organization: Hospitalist practice
Purpose: To provide inpatient care services for the Parkland Affiliates patients
Method: Hospital will need an additional 1.1 FTEs of provider coverage to meet the demands of Parkland Affiliates. This coverage would require hiring a full-time physician immediately and relying on additional per diem support to accommodate the expected demand.

Consequences of not approving this package: Parkland Affiliates serves a sizeable community of well-reimbursing elderly patients who have been vocal about their desires to be able to use San Valens services. In addition, San Valens has a reputable geriatric program, but the medical director of the program has become frustrated with limited referrals of late and has threatened to build his program elsewhere unless the hospital makes a concerted effort to generate more business. He also travels to Parkland Affiliates twice per month to see patients with unique medical issues and has established close ties with all of their physicians.

	Assumptions		Parkland Affiliates
	Practice profile		
A	Number of primary care physicians		11
B	Proportion Medicare patients		79%
C	Proportion Medicaid/Self-Pay patients		4%
	Volume projections		
D	Annual initial service RVUs		1,750
E	Annual follow-up service RVUs		6,000
F	Average LOS per admission, days		4.4
	Financials		
G	Incremental practice costs	(Exh.10.7e)	$330,563
H	Average reimbursement per RVU		$33.50
I	Average facility profit per inpatient day		$200
	Calculations		
J	Annual initial service revenues	(D × H)	$58,625
K	Annual follow-up service revenues	(E × H)	$201,000
L	Incremental practice costs per year	(G)	$330,563
M	*Incremental hospitalist group income (loss)*	(J + K − L)	($70,938)
N	New admissions[a]	(D/4)	438
O	Incremental inpatient income (loss)	(F × I × N)	$385,000
P	*Incremental financial impact of proposal*	(M + O)	$314,062
Q	Performance measure: new admissions	(N)	438

[a]Each new admission consumes 4 RVUs of service.

EXHIBIT 10.7e CALCULATION OF SALARIES FOR ALL THREE PRACTICES

Basic Data

Direct annual expenses per 1.0 hospitalist FTE:

Salaries and Benefits	Cost
Salary	$200,000
Malpractice insurance	$12,000
Health and dental insurances	$17,000
LTD/Life/AD&D insurances	$1,800
CME	$3,000
6% matching 401K	$12,000
Licenses/fees/dues	$2,400
Total direct costs	$248,200
Overhead costs as percentage of direct costs: 22%	$54,604
Total costs per 1.0 new hospitalist FTEs	$302,804

	A	B	C	D	E	F	G	H
	Total Service	Hours/ RVU	Hours Needed	FTE Hours/Year	Hospitalist Efficiency	FTEs Needed	Cost to Hire FTE[c]	Performance Measure[b]
Practice Name	RVUs[a]	(Given)	(A × B)	(Given)	(Given)	[C/(D × E)]	(F x T)	(Admissions)
Crown Colony	3,800	0.25	950	2,040	87%	0.5	$162,082	225
Westover Family Practice	4,750	0.25	1,188	2,040	87%	0.7	$202,603	288
Parkland Affiliates	7,750	0.25	1,938	2,040	87%	1.1	$330,563	438

[a]From Exhibit 10.7a, rows D + E.
[b]From Exhibit 10.7a, row N: the number of projected new admissions is the performance target for each practice.
[c]Differences due to rounding.

Multiyear Budget
A budget that is forecast multiple years out, rather than just for the upcoming year.

Although virtually all organizations have annual budgets, increasingly each is part of a *multiyear budget*. Rather than forecasting revenues and expenses for just one year, organizations are finding it necessary to use multiyear budgets to forecast three to five years in advance. Because conditions change, many organizations use *rolling budgets*, which are regularly updated and extended multiyear forecasts. For example, the budget submitted for 20X1 might cover the years 20X1 through 20X5, whereas the 20X2 budget might cover years 20X2 through 20X6. In this way, the budget is always forecasting five years ahead. Some organizations *roll forward* their budgets more often than every year, updating their multiyear forecasts on a semiannual or even quarterly basis.

Single-year and multiyear budgets vary by the time horizon they forecast, whereas static and flexible budgets vary on the basis of volume projections. *Static budgets* forecast for a single level of activity, and *flexible budgets* forecast revenues and expenses for various levels of activities. For example, whereas a static budget in an ambulatory care setting might forecast revenues and expenses for 15,000 visits, a flexible budget might forecast revenues and expenses for a range of visits between 14,000 and 16,000 visits. Flexible budgets are an important tool for controlling expenses, and their use is discussed in detail in Chapter Eleven.

Rolling Budget
A multiyear budget that is updated more frequently than annually, such as semiannually or quarterly.

Static Budget
A budget that uses a single or fixed level of activity.

Flexible Budget
A budget that accommodates a range or multiple levels of activities.

Budget Modifications

In most health care organizations, criteria are established beyond which managers must request permission to make changes to their budgets. The criteria are usually set as dollar amounts or a need to move funds from one category to another (or both). For example, an administrator may be able to move amounts under $1,000 within a category (such as labor) without needing higher approval but not from one category to another (such as from labor to equipment). Particularly dramatic examples of the need for budget revisions often occur during nursing shortages, when hospitals have to continually ask their boards to approve increases in nursing salaries or contract labor in the middle of the year.

Types of Budgets

Although the term *the budget* is often used as if there were only one budget, most health care organizations develop four interrelated budgets: a statistics budget, an operating budget, a cash budget, and a capital budget. An overview of the relationship among these budgets is presented in Exhibit 10.8.

Statistics Budget

The first budget to develop is the statistics budget. The *statistics budget* identifies the amount of services that will be provided, usually listed by payor type, as in Exhibit 10.9.

- The *commercial payor* category includes a wide variety of nongovernmental entities that pay on behalf of the patient, including insurance

EXHIBIT 10.8 OVERVIEW OF THE FOUR MAJOR BUDGETS

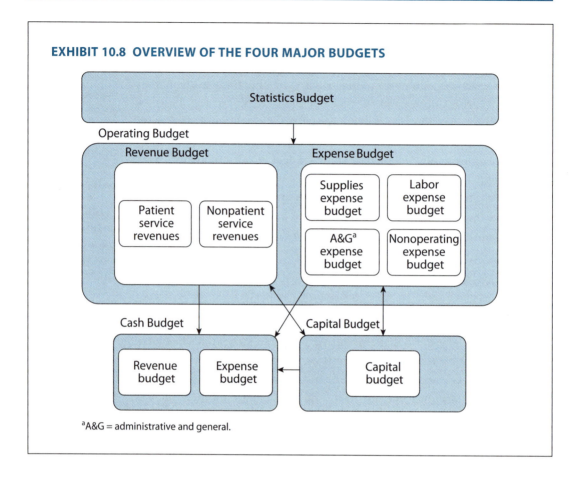

ᵃA&G = administrative and general.

EXHIBIT 10.9 STATISTICS BUDGET FOR ZMG HOSPITALIST PRACTICE (IN RVUs)

Insurance Category	Jan	Feb	Mar	Apr	May	Jun	Jul	Aug	Sep	Oct	Nov	Dec	Total
Commercial	4,730	4,420	4,768	4,428	4,232	4,342	4,440	4,568	4,398	4,652	4,472	4,918	54,368
Medicare	7,360	6,872	7,412	6,888	6,588	6,758	6,902	7,108	6,840	7,238	6,960	7,648	84,574
Medicaid/Self-Pay	1,050	982	1,060	982	940	968	988	1,018	978	1,032	992	1,092	12,082
Total	13,140	12,274	13,240	12,298	11,760	12,068	12,330	12,694	12,216	12,922	12,424	13,658	151,024

companies, PPOs, and HMOs. These organizations usually pay a pre-negotiated portion of full charges, though the amount of discount may vary considerably among payors and among procedures.

• *Medicare* is a governmental program that pays on behalf of patients older than sixty-five, patients younger than sixty-five with certain disabilities, and patients with end-stage renal disease. Medicare Part A covers hospital stays, Medicare Part B covers physician and outpatient care, and Medicare Part D covers prescriptions. Within these categories, Medicare is usually a price setter. That is, it determines what it will pay for and how much it will pay.

- *Medicaid and Self-Pay* are two types of payors often grouped together into a single category. Medicaid is a governmental program in which the federal government and state governments pay on behalf of certain low-income individuals and families who fit into an eligibility group recognized by federal and state law. Eligibility varies considerably from state to state. Medicaid typically pays considerably less than do the other two categories of payors. The Self-Pay category comprises those who pay for their own care, as opposed to the other categories in which others, called *third parties*, pay on behalf of the patient. In some cases, though an individual may be covered by a third party, that person may still have responsibility for part of the bill through copays and deductibles, as discussed in Chapter Thirteen.

Exhibit 10.9 presents the statistics budget for ZMG Hospitalist Practice, a group practice that staffs hospitals with physician internists whose specialty is inpatient care in the hospital setting. As discussed in more detail below, the statistics in this budget are stated in terms of relative value units (RVUs), which weight each type of encounter by the relative amount of resources it consumes. In the case of hospitalists, there are two main types of encounters: admissions and follow-up care (which includes discharges), with admissions consuming approximately twice the resources, mainly time, as follow-up encounters do.

Operating Budget

The *operating budget* (see Exhibit 10.10) is actually a combination of two budgets developed using the accrual basis of accounting: the revenue budget and the expense budget. Some organizations, especially those with relatively small nonoperating items, such as parking lot and gift shop revenues and expenses, include their nonoperating budget with their operating budget.

The *revenue budget* is a forecast of the operating revenues that will be earned during the budget period (see Exhibit 10.10, rows A through K). It has two components: net patient revenues (rows A through G) and nonpatient revenues (rows H through J). The *expense budget* lists all operating and nonoperating expenses that are expected to be incurred during the

---

Statistics Budget
The first budget to be prepared; one of the four major types of budgets. It identifies the amount of services that will be provided, typically categorized by payor type.

Operating Budget
One of the four major types of budgets, it comprises the revenue budget and the expense budget. The bottom line for this budget is net income.

Revenue Budget
A subset of the operating budget that is a forecast of the operating revenues that will be earned during the current budget period.

Expense Budget
A subset of the operating budget that is a forecast of the operating expenses that will be incurred during the current budget period.

EXHIBIT 10.10 OPERATING BUDGET FOR ZMG HOSPITALIST PRACTICE

		Jan	Feb	Mar	Apr	May	Jun	Jul	Aug	Sep	Oct	Nov	Dec	Total
Revenues														
A	Gross inpt. service revenues	$586,373	$547,727	$590,835	$548,798	$524,790	$538,535	$550,226	$566,470	$545,139	$576,644	$554,421	$609,488	$6,739,446
B	Gross outpt. service revenues	103,478	96,658	104,265	96,847	92,610	95,036	97,099	99,965	96,201	101,761	97,839	107,557	1,189,314
C	Total gross patient service revenues	689,850	644,385	695,100	645,645	617,400	633,570	647,325	666,435	641,340	678,405	652,260	717,045	7,928,760
D	Less: inpt. deductions & allowances	227,639	212,645	229,389	213,037	203,741	209,126	213,636	219,968	211,653	223,852	215,225	236,614	2,616,526
E	Less: outpt. deductions & allowances	40,172	37,526	40,480	37,595	35,954	36,905	37,700	38,818	37,351	39,503	37,981	41,755	461,740
F	Total deductions & allowances	267,810	250,170	269,870	250,632	239,695	246,031	251,337	258,786	249,004	263,356	253,206	278,369	3,078,266
G	Total net patient service revenues	422,040	394,215	425,230	395,013	377,705	387,539	395,988	407,649	392,336	415,049	399,054	438,676	4,850,494
H	Other operating revenues	1,182	1,238	903	901	903	901	903	903	901	903	901	903	11,440
I	Medical director appropriations	30,000	30,000	30,000	30,000	30,000	30,000	30,000	30,000	30,000	30,000	30,000	30,000	360,000
J	Program investments	—	—	—	—	—	—	—	—	—	—	—	—	—
K	**Total net revenues**	453,221	425,453	456,133	425,914	408,608	418,440	426,891	438,552	423,237	445,952	429,955	469,578	5,221,934
Expenses														
L	Provider salaries and benefits	418,667	430,167	430,167	430,167	430,167	430,167	438,600	438,600	438,600	438,600	439,600	439,600	5,203,100
M	Support staff salaries & benefits	24,583	25,344	25,344	25,344	25,344	25,813	25,813	25,813	25,813	25,813	25,813	25,813	306,646
N	Utilities	1,000	1,000	1,000	1,000	1,000	1,000	1,000	1,000	1,000	1,000	1,000	1,000	12,000
O	Supplies	600	600	600	600	600	600	600	600	600	600	600	600	7,200
P	Billing services	37,984	35,479	38,271	35,551	33,993	34,879	35,639	36,688	35,310	37,354	35,915	39,481	436,544
Q	Purchased services	—	—	—	—	—	—	—	—	—	—	—	—	—
R	General	3,593	3,590	3,587	4,180	4,175	4,170	4,363	4,357	4,350	4,344	3,838	4,331	48,879
S	Insurance	12,000	12,000	12,000	12,000	12,000	12,000	12,000	12,000	12,000	12,000	12,000	12,000	144,000
T	Depreciation	—	—	—	—	—	—	—	—	—	—	—	—	—
U	Other	10,820	10,992	11,302	11,000	10,377	10,475	10,560	10,676	10,523	10,750	10,591	10,987	129,055
V	**Total expenses**	509,247	533,528	525,626	519,842	517,656	519,103	528,574	529,734	528,196	530,462	529,856	563,893	6,335,717
X	**Excess of revenues over expenses**	($56,025)	($108,075)	($69,494)	($93,928)	($109,048)	($100,663)	($101,683)	($91,182)	($104,960)	($84,509)	($99,901)	($94,315)	($1,113,783)

PERSPECTIVE 10.4 BUDGET DEFICIT LEADS TO SCRAMBLE

Administrators at Palm Drive Hospital [in Sebastopol, California] are scrambling to put together a new financial plan in an attempt to reverse the hospital's budget deficit. The hospital at the end of February had a deficit of $864,158 and 15 days of cash on hand. "That's a very big hole," said Rick Reid, Palm Drive's interim chief executive officer and chief financial officer.

He is devising a 90-day financial plan to stem the losses. But even if it works, he still expects that the Sebastopol hospital on June 30 will have a deficit of $750,000 to carry into the next fiscal year. In contrast, the current $30.4 million budget was projected to have a surplus of $914,287 at the end of February. "Looking back, it was optimistic," Reid said. "There were certain things that had to happen and there were operational changes that were not made." . . .

Since the fiscal year began last July, Palm Drive had 789 patients who stayed 2,770 days, compared to budget expectations of 847 patients staying 3,127 days. It had 4,708 emergency room visits, compared to budget expectations of 4,985. The hospital had 22,631 outpatient visits, compared to 24,339 outpatient visits that were budgeted. "Volumes were down and a lot has to do with the economy," Reid said. "People are delaying non-emergency surgeries because they can't afford to miss work. And there has been great weather, so people are healthier than they would have been."

Source: Excerpted from B. Norberg, Palm Drive Hospital's budget deficit creating "very big hole," *The Press Democrat*, March 23, 2012, sebastopol.towns.pressdemocrat.com/2012/03/news/palm-drive-hospitals-budget-deficit-creating-very-big-hole.

budget period (see Exhibit 10.10, rows L through V). Perspective 10.4 illustrates the consequences of missing budgeted forecasts for patient volumes, while Perspective 10.5 highlights the need for health care organizations to increase their IT budgets.

Whether an item is classified as *operating* or *nonoperating* is subject to interpretation by each organization. Although this matter has received considerable attention over the years by both the accounting and health care financial management professions, there remains a lack of standardization among health care organizations in classifying specific line items.

Caution: Throughout this chapter, the numbers in the exhibits may be slightly different from those computed on a calculator and also slightly different between exhibits due to the internal rounding rules used in the computer program with which the examples were created.

PERSPECTIVE 10.5 MANAGING IT COMPLEXITIES AND COSTS

The IT departments of most healthcare organizations have expanded rapidly in recent years in response to the increasing complexities of the IT systems used to manage the growing data and communication system needs.... Healthcare organizations on every continent are making investments in EHR, mHealth, and many other clinical and nonclinical health IT systems, with investments in advanced analytics on the horizon. Other factors, such as consolidation of hospital systems in the U.S., add to the costs and complexities of IT infrastructure within healthcare organizations.

The good news is that it is possible for healthcare organizations to manage these complexities without breaking their IT budgets. Virtualization and cloud computing are two cost-effective means of reducing complexity, but healthcare organizations have been slow to adopt them....

Vendor-neutral archiving of imaging files is another strategy to reduce complexity and manage IT system costs over time. Vendor-neutral archiving greatly improves the ability of healthcare providers to find any image, no matter what vendor platform is being used, and supports simpler and cost-effective migration of imaging data in the case of a shift in PACS systems, for example.... With the average life cycle of a healthcare application at around eight years, having a strategy for data migration to a new application (and possibly vendor), becomes even more important in a world where IT systems eat up an increasing share of the budgets of healthcare organizations, yet are vital to their processes and services.

Source: Excerpted from Frost & Sullivan, *Drowning in Big Data?: Reducing Information Technology Complexities and Costs for Healthcare Organizations*, White Paper, 2012, www.emc.com/collateral/analyst-reports/frost-sullivan -reducing-information-technology-complexities-ar.pdf.

Cash Budget

One of the four major types of budgets, it displays all of the organization's projected cash inflows and outflows. The bottom line for this budget is the amount of cash available at the end of the period.

Cash Budget

Whereas the operating budget describes the expected revenues and the related resource flows, the *cash budget* (see Exhibit 10.11) represents the organization's cash inflows and outflows. The bottom line in the operating budget is the net income for the period; the bottom line in the cash budget is the amount of cash available at the end of the period (Exhibit 10.11, row O). In addition to showing cash inflows and outflows, the cash budget also details when it is necessary to borrow to cover cash shortages and when excess funds are available to invest.

Key Point The operating budget is developed using the accrual basis of accounting. Cash inflows and outflows of each line item must be estimated to convert the operating budget to the cash budget.

EXHIBIT 10.11 CASH BUDGET FOR ZMG HOSPITALIST PRACTICE

		Jan	Feb	Mar	Apr	May	Jun	Jul	Aug	Sep	Oct	Nov	Dec	Summary
A	Beginning balance	$200,000	$100,000	100,000	$100,000	$100,000	$100,000	$100,000	$100,000	$100,000	$100,000	$100,000	$100,000	$200,000
B	Net revenues	453,221	425,453	456,133	425,914	408,608	418,440	426,891	438,552	423,237	445,952	429,955	469,578	5,221,934
C	Net expenditures	(509,247)	(533,528)	(525,626)	(519,842)	(517,656)	(519,103)	(528,574)	(529,734)	(528,196)	(530,462)	(529,356)	(563,893)	(6,335,717)
D	Cash available before borrowing	143,975	(8,075)	30,506	6,072	(9,048)	(663)	(1,683)	8,818	(4,960)	15,491	99	5,685	186,217
E	Cash requirement	100,000	100,000	100,000	100,000	100,000	100,000	100,000	100,000	100,000	100,000	100,000	100,000	100,000
F	Cash excess (shortage)	43,975	(108,075)	(69,494)	(93,928)	(109,048)	(100,663)	(101,683)	(91,182)	(104,960)	(84,509)	(99,901)	(94,315)	(1,013,783)
G	Transfer excess to ST investments	43,975	—	—	—	—	—	—	—	—	—	—	—	43,975
H	Remaining deficit	—	(108,075)	(69,494)	(93,928)	(109,048)	(100,663)	(101,683)	(91,182)	(104,960)	(84,509)	(99,901)	(94,315)	(1,057,758)
I	Transfer from ST investment	—	108,075	8,573	10	10	10	10	10	10	10	10	10	116,738
J	Remaining deficit	—	—	(60,921)	(93,918)	(109,038)	(100,653)	(101,673)	(91,172)	(104,950)	(84,499)	(99,891)	(94,305)	(941,020)
K	Transfer from LT investment	—	—	113	59	58	59	58	59	59	58	59	58	641
L	Remaining deficit	—	—	(60,807)	(93,859)	(108,981)	(100,594)	(101,616)	(91,113)	(104,890)	(84,442)	(99,831)	(94,247)	(940,380)
M	Subsidy required	—	—	60,807	93,859	108,981	100,594	101,616	91,113	104,890	84,442	99,831	94,247	940,380
N	Total of transfers and subsidies	43,975	108,075	69,494	93,928	109,048	100,663	101,683	91,182	104,960	84,509	99,901	94,315	1,101,733
O	Ending balance	$100,000	$100,000	$100,000	$100,000	$100,000	$100,000	$100,000	$100,000	$100,000	$100,000	$100,000	$100,000	$100,000

EXHIBIT 10.12 CAPITAL BUDGET FOR ZMG HOSPITALIST PRACTICE

	Purchase Price	Life Years	Residual Value	Depreciation Base	Monthly Depreciation	Date of Purchase	Debt Financing	Financed from Cash
Anticipated purchases for 20X2								
Computer network	$25,000	5	$500	$24,500	$408	Apr 20X2	100%	0%
HVAC upgrade	$12,000	8	$750	$11,250	$117	Jul 20X2	90%	10%
Total	$37,000							

Capital Budget

Capital Budget
One of the four major types of budgets, it summarizes the anticipated major purchases for the year.

The *capital budget* (see Exhibit 10.12) summarizes the anticipated major purchases for the year. Capital budgets in outpatient facilities may be fairly small, but those for large systems with inpatient facilities may contain millions of dollars' worth of items.

Pro Forma Financial Statements and Ratios

Based on the information contained in these budgets, together with a small amount of additional information, an organization can develop pro forma financial statements. Pro forma financial statements are prepared to show what the organization's regular financial statements will look like if all budgets are met exactly as planned. The regular financial statements are prepared after the accounting period ends and present the actual results of the organization's activities during the period. As an example of the relationship between the budgets and financial statements, ZMG Hospitalist Practice's operating budget (see Exhibit 10.10) could serve as its statement of operations, with only a few modifications in format. Developing the balance sheet and statement of cash flows is not as straightforward, but it can be done with only a small amount of additional information.

Once the pro forma financial statements have been developed, they can be subjected to ratio analysis just as with regular financial statements.

This process is reversed in strategic financial planning, where the organization first identifies its goals in terms of the various categories of ratios (liquidity, profitability, capitalization, and activity) and then develops its budgets, over time, to meet the targets it has set for itself.

Monitoring Variances to Budget

Once the budget has been created for the upcoming time period (usually one fiscal year), it needs to be monitored on a regular basis for variances, both positive and negative (see Exhibit 10.13, which shows the status of ZMG Hospitalist Group as of June 20X1, six months into the fiscal year). A positive variance results from revenues being greater than expected or from expenses coming in less than projected (either of these outcomes would grow the bottom line), and vice versa for negative variances.

The line items in Exhibit 10.13 are identical to those shown in Exhibit 10.10, but the amounts are shown on a monthly and year-to-date (YTD) basis instead of on an annual basis. As can be seen in Exhibit 10.13, net patient service revenues, for both inpatient and outpatient services, came in slightly less than expected, $2,334,776 versus $2,401,741 (columns A through C, rows A through G). Some appropriations are fixed and known in advance, as is the case for those of the medical director of the program (row I), which show no variance at all, as would be typical in those situations. On the expense side (rows L through V), some variation can be noted. Physician salaries were $17,000 more than expected (row L), due to having to incur 17 unanticipated extra shifts at $1,000 each; this represents a negative variance to budget because the expense was more than expected. A positive variance can be noted with the billing expense in row P: since net revenues fell below the expected amount and billing expense is based on a percentage of collections, billing expense would drop proportionately. Likewise, if actual revenues exceeded budget, billing expenses would exceed the budgeted amount (for more detail on variance analysis see Chapter Eleven).

Overall for the first six months of the year, net income is down $77,881 from what was expected, an actual loss of $615,114 versus a budgeted loss of $537,233 (row X). Last, columns D through F take the year-to-date amounts and project the variances for each line item on an annual basis. The annual budgeted amounts at year end, shown in column D, match the totals in the last column of Exhibit 10.10. In column E, as June is half-way into the year, the full-year projected amounts are double those line-item amounts in column B. Column F shows the year-to-date projected variance between budgeted and actual.

EXHIBIT 10.13 VARIANCE TO BUDGET FOR ZMG HOSPITALIST PRACTICE

		A	B	C	D	E	F
		Jun 20X1 YTD Budgeted	Jun 20X1 YTD Actual	Jun 20X1 YTD Variance	20X1 Annual Budgeted	20X1 YTD Annual Projected	20X1 YTD Projected Variance
	Revenues						
A	Gross inpt. service revenues	$3,337,058	$3,245,454	($91,604)	$6,739,446	6,490,908	($248,538)
B	Gross outpt. service revenues	588,893	571,033	(17,860)	1,189,314	1,142,066	(47,248)
C	Total gross patient service revenues	3,925,950	3,816,487	109,463	7,928,760	7,632,974	(295,786)
D	Less: inpt. deductions & allowances	1,295,577	1,260,013	(35,564)	2,616,526	2,520,027	(96,500)
E	Less: outpt. deductions & allowances	228,631	221,698	(6,934)	461,740	443,395	(18,345)
F	Total deductions & allowances	1,524,209	1,481,711	(42,498)	3,078,266	2,963,422	(114,845)
G	Total net patient service revenues	2,401,741	2,334,776	(66,965)	4,850,494	4,669,552	(180,941)
H	Other operating revenues	6,027	5,904	(123)	11,440	11,808	368
I	Medical director appropriations	180,000	180,000	—	360,000	360,000	—
J	Program investments	—	—	—	—	—	—
K	**Total net revenues**	2,587,769	2,520,680	(67,089)	5,221,934	5,041,360	(180,574)
	Expenses						
L	Provider salaries and benefits	2,587,211	2,604,211	17,000	5,250,893	5,208,423	(42,470)
M	Support staff salaries & benefits	151,771	154,898	3,127	306,646	309,796	3,150
N	Utilities	6,000	5,611	(389)	12,000	11,222	(778)
O	Supplies	3,600	3,454	(146)	7,200	6,908	(292)
P	Billing services	216,157	210,130	(6,027)	436,544	420,260	(16,285)
Q	Purchased services	—	—	—	—	—	—
R	General	23,296	25,053	1,757	49,379	50,105	727
S	Insurance	72,000	72,000	—	144,000	144,000	—
T	Depreciation	—	—	—	—	—	—
U	Other	64,967	60,437	(4,530)	129,055	120,875	(8,180)
V	**Total expenses**	3,125,002	3,135,794	10,792	6,335,717	6,271,588	(64,129)
X	**Excess of revenues over expenses**	($537,233)	($615,114)	($77,881)	($1,113,783)	($1,230,228)	($116,445)

Group Purchasing Organizations

While institutions of all sizes purchase and consume supplies as part of daily operations, large organizations can incur upward of tens of millions of dollars annually in supplies expense. The most general supplies, purchased in bulk, can cost as little as pennies each (if that), while very particular items, such as the titanium screws and plates used in orthopedic surgery, can cost more than $20,000 per item.

An institution typically procures its supplies through a third-party vendor, a *middleman*, who in turn acquires the supplies directly from the manufacturers. This transfer of supplies from the manufacturer through the middleman and into the health care organization's central distribution warehouse is called a *supply chain*. In turn, the oversight of this process, including inventory storage and end-user consumption, is called *supply chain management.*

Because health care organizations generally need similar supplies, third-party vendors will contract with numerous institutions in order to be in a position to negotiate large-volume discounts from the original manufacturers (an example of economies of scale). The savings are then passed along to the health care organizations. A network of health care organizations all contracting with the same third-party vendor is called a *group purchasing organization* (GPO). GPOs offer organizations the convenience of being able to turn to one supplier for virtually all of the organization's needs, and the large-volume discounts for buying in bulk provide organizations with an essential way to manage supply costs. In return for its services, the third-party vendor charges a fee, either a fixed amount or a variable rate based on the amount of goods purchased.

Third-party vendor fees can become a sticking point in negotiations to ensure that the interests of the vendor are properly aligned with the best interests of the purchasing organizations. Under a fixed-fee arrangement, the vendor only needs to ensure that transactions occur smoothly to continue to earn its income. Fees based on a percentage of sales, in contrast, may incentivize the vendor to sell more than the organization needs or at higher rates in order to increase income. Despite this difficulty, for organizations that can find reliable and trustworthy third-party vendors who can seamlessly ensure that supplies deliveries are accurate and timely, and who can offer discounts at the same time through group purchasing, the savings outweigh the complications. Still, there is a competitive market for this middleman service, and before its annual budgeting process, the organization should evaluate its projected supplies expense for the upcoming year. As an organization drops and adds services and its supply needs

Supply Chain
The entities involved in distributing finished goods from the manufacturer to the end consumer, oftentimes including a third-party vendor, or middleman (also see the definition of *supply chain management*).

Supply Chain Management
The oversight of the supply chain process, up to and including storage and consumption by the end users (also see the definition of *supply chain*).

Group Purchasing Organization (GPO)
A network of health care organizations and a third-party vendor who are able to acquire large volumes of supplies from manufacturers at negotiated discounted rates owing to economies of scale.

change, changing to an alternative vendor who offers different pricing structures may in fact be a smart move financially.

Third-party vendors negotiate rates on thousands of items, but the negotiated rates vary across vendors, as do their fees. Depending on the combination and volume of items needed, the total overall discount obtained from one vendor can be markedly different from that offered by another, and only through careful calculations of supply needs and discounts can an organization pick the best vendor.

A simplified example to illustrate the concept is displayed in Exhibit 10.14. Assume that Mumford Regional Hospital currently has a contract with Vendor A for five key items, but Vendors B and C offer alternative prices for the same items. And while both Vendors A and C charge fixed fees for their services—of $25,000 and $30,000, respectively—Vendor B charges a variable rate of 3 percent based on total sales. With which vendor would Mumford save the most money?

As the analysis in Exhibit 10.14 shows, despite charging the highest fees, Vendor C has per unit prices competitive enough to drive its total

---

EXHIBIT 10.14 ALTERNATIVE VENDOR OPTIONS FOR MUMFORD REGIONAL

Supply	Volume of Supplies Needed	Vendor A Unit Price	Vendor A Total Cost	Vendor B Unit Price	Vendor B Total Cost	Vendor C Unit Price	Vendor C Total Cost
Item 1	88,000	$2.35	$206,800	$2.42	$212,960	$2.28	$200,640
Item 2	105,000	1.47	154,350	1.45	152,250	1.49	156,450
Item 3	65,000	3.07	199,550	3.10	201,500	3.12	202,800
Item 4	148,000	0.98	145,040	0.95	140,600	0.92	136,160
Item 5	33,000	4.47	147,510	4.39	144,870	4.40	145,200
Total costs			853,250		$852,180		$841,250
Fee		Fixed	$25,000	3% of sales	$25,565	Fixed	$30,000
Grand total			$878,250		$877,745		$871,250

costs below those of the other two vendors, making it the best option financially. On the grand scale, undertaking a complex analysis of an organization's total inventory (a process beyond the scope of this text) can result in annual cost savings amounting to hundreds of thousands of dollars or more. With a difference that significant, management must decide whether the disruption to the institution brought about by changing vendors is worth the costs. And as mentioned previously, the annual budget cycle is an ideal time to investigate whether projected supply expenses are being well contained and whether services have changed enough to warrant joining an alternative group purchasing organization to lock in better pricing agreements.

Summary

The budget is one of the most important documents of a health care organization and is the central document of the planning-and-control cycle. It identifies the revenues and resources that are needed for an organization to achieve its goals and objectives and allows the organization to monitor the actual revenues generated and its use of resources against what was planned.

The planning-and-control cycle has four major components: strategic planning, planning, implementing, and controlling. The purpose of strategic planning is to identify the organization's mission and strategy in order to position the organization for the future. A primary activity of the strategic planning process is an assessment of the organization's external and internal environments. The organization also develops specific tactical and operational plans that identify short-term goals and objectives in organizational marketing or production, control, and financing.

Five key dimensions along which organizations vary in regard to budgeting are participation, budget models, budget detail, budget forecasts, and budget modifications. Participation in the budgeting process varies from authoritarian to participatory. The authoritarian approach is often called top-down budgeting, because the budget is essentially dictated to the rest of the organization. In the participatory approach, the roles and responsibilities of the budgeting process are diffused throughout the organization. Advantages of the participatory approach include developing a shared understanding of the goals and objectives of the organization, developing cooperation and coordination, clarifying roles and responsibilities, motivating staff, and bringing about cost awareness. Its disadvantages are loss of control and excessive use of time and resources.

There are two budget models: incremental-decremental budgeting and zero-based budgeting. The incremental-decremental approach begins with what exists and gives a slight increase, no change, or a slight decrease to the various line items, programs, or departments. Zero-based budgeting continually questions both the need for each line-item, program, or department and its level of funding. In zero-based budgeting, each budgeting unit provides both an overall justification for its program and a series of requests to show what the program would look like at various levels of funding.

Based on the amount of detail they contain, budgets can be classified into three categories: line-item, program, and performance. A line-item budget has the least detail and merely lists revenues and expenses by category. A program budget not only lists the line items but also lists them by program. A performance budget lists not only line items and programs but also the performance goals that each program is expected to attain.

Because environmental conditions change, many organizations use rolling budgets, which are multiyear forecasts regularly updated and extended. Single-year and multiyear budgets vary by the time horizon they forecast; static and flexible budgets vary on the basis of volume projections. Static budgets forecast for a single level of activity; flexible budgets forecast revenues and expenses for various levels of activities.

Most health care organizations develop four interrelated budgets: a statistics budget, an operating budget, a cash budget, and a capital budget. The statistics budget identifies the amount of services that will be provided, usually by payor type.

The operating budget is a combination of two budgets developed using the accrual basis of accounting: the revenue budget and the expense budget. The revenue budget is a forecast of the operating revenues that will be earned during the budget period. It consists of net patient revenues and nonpatient revenues. The expense budget lists all operating expenses that are expected to be incurred during the budget period, both fixed and variable. Over the course of the fiscal period (typically one year), a similar month-to-date and year-to-date budget is generated to show all line-item variances and year-end projections.

The cash budget represents the organization's cash inflows and outflows. The bottom line of the cash budget is the amount of cash available at the end of the period. In addition to showing cash inflows and outflows, the cash budget also details when it is necessary to borrow when there are cash shortages and when excess funds can be invested.

The capital budget summarizes large purchases to be made during the year over a specified dollar amount. Capital budgets for outpatient facilities may be fairly small; those for large systems with inpatient facilities may contain millions of dollars' worth of items.

Using the information contained in these budgets, plus small amounts of additional information, the organization develops pro forma financial statements. Pro forma financial statements are prepared before the accounting period and present what the organization's financial statements will look like if all budgets are met exactly as planned. Once the pro forma financial statements have been developed, they can be subjected to ratio analysis just as with regular financial statements.

After the cost of labor, the largest input in a hospital's budget is the cost of supplies. One way to achieve savings in this area is to influence surgeons to use the same types of medical devices to achieve economies of scale. Another way to achieve savings through economies of scale is to contract with a group purchasing organization, which has negotiated discount rates with manufacturers. This transfer of supplies across entities is called the supply chain.

KEY TERMS

a. Authoritarian approach

b. Capital budget

c. Cash budget

d. Controlling activities

e. Expense budget

f. Fixed labor budget

g. Fixed supplies budget

h. Flexible budget

i. Gross charges

j. Group purchasing organization

k. Incremental-decremental approach

l. Labor budget

m. Line-item budget

n. Mission statement

o. Multiyear budget

p. Net charges

q. Operating budget

r. Participatory approach

s. Performance budget

t. Planning

u. Program budget

v. Relative value units (RVUs)

w. Revenue budget

x. Rolling budget

y. Short-term plans

z. Static budget

aa. Statistics budget

bb. Strategic planning

cc. Supply chain

dd. Supply chain management

ee. Top-down-bottom-up approach

ff. Top-down budgeting

gg. Variable labor budget

hh. Variable supplies budget

ii. Zero-based budgeting (ZBB)

Key Equation

Opening Inventory $+$ Purchases $-$ Cost of Goods Used $=$ Ending Inventory

REVIEW QUESTIONS AND PROBLEMS

1. **Definitions**. Define the key terms above.

2. **Budget development**. What is the purpose of the budget? Why are requests for budget revisions necessary? When should a formal request for a budget revision be submitted?

3. **Planning-and-control cycle**. What are the major components of the planning-and-control cycle?

4. **Strategic planning**. Discuss the role of strategic planning in the budgeting process. How does it differ from short-term planning?

5. **Participatory approach**. What are the advantages and disadvantages of the participatory approach to budgeting?

6. **Budget types**. What are the four major budgets of a health care organization? Briefly discuss each.

7. **Budget detail**. What are the differences among a line-item, a program, and a performance budget?

8. **Budget detail**. Using Exhibit 10.6 as an example, construct line-item, program, and performance budgets for a service or program in a health care organization.

9. **Statistics budget: forecasting encounters**. Instead of its current forecast, ZMG Hospitalist Practice now estimates that it will not obtain a major HMO contract, and its encounters for July through December are expected to rise by only 1.5% a month from the previous year. Assuming these are the only changes to Exhibit I.1a, prepare a new forecast of the number of encounters that will be made by commercial patients during the whole year. (*Hint*: see Appendix I, at the end of this chapter.)

10. **Statistics budget: forecasting encounters**. Instead of its current forecast, ZMG Hospitalist Practice now estimates that its Medicare encounters will increase by 4% a month from January through June. In July it will obtain a major contract, and its encounters from July through December will go up by 9% a month. Assuming these are the only changes to Exhibit I.1a, prepare a new forecast of the number of encounters that will be made by Medicare patients during the whole year. (*Hint*: see Appendix I, at the end of this chapter.)

11. **Statistics budget: RVU-weighted encounters**. What are RVU-weighted encounters? Why is it necessary to weight encounters by their intensity level?

12. **Statistics budget: changing intensity**. How would the estimate of Medicaid/Self-Pay encounters change if ZMG Hospitalist Practice estimated that its Medicaid/Self-Pay admissions made up 3% of the encounters and the Medicaid/Self-Pay follow-up encounters made up 9% of the encounters instead of the distribution of visits by intensity shown in Exhibit I.1b?

13. **Statistics budget: changing RVU weight**. How would the estimate of commercial weighted encounters (Exhibit I.1e) change if ZMG Hospitalist Practice estimated that its admissions had a relative value weight of 3.50 and the follow-up visits had a relative value weight of 1.75 (Exhibit I.1d)?

14. **Statistics budget: changing RVU weight**. How would the estimate of Medicare weighted encounters (Exhibit I.1e) change if ZMG Hospitalist Practice estimated that its admissions had a relative value weight of 4.25 and the follow-up visits had a relative value weight of 2.25 (Exhibit I.1d)?

15. **Revenue budget: calculating gross revenues**. Calculate ZMG Hospitalist Practice's January, February, and March Medicare gross revenues if the fee for an admission is $200 and the fee for a follow-up encounter is $100 (Exhibits I.1e and I.2a).

16. **Revenue budget: calculating gross revenues**. Calculate ZMG Hospitalist Practice's January, February, and March commercial payor gross revenues if the fee for an admission is $250 and the fee for a follow-up encounter is $125 (Exhibits I.1e and I.2a).

17. **Revenue budget: gross charges and net revenues**. What is the difference between gross charges and net revenues?

18. **Revenue budget: calculating net revenues**. Calculate ZMG Hospitalist Practice's January, February, and March Medicare net revenues if the fee for an admission is $200 and the fee for a follow-up encounter is $100 (Exhibits I.1e and I.2a). Assume that Medicare reimburses at a rate of 60% of charges.

19. **Revenue budget: calculating net revenues**. Calculate ZMG Hospitalist Practice's January, February, and March Medicaid/Self-Pay net revenues if the fee for an admission is $200 and the fee for a follow-up encounter is $100 (Exhibits I.1e and I.2a). Assume that Medicaid reimburses at a rate of 30% of charges.

20. **Labor budget: fixed and variable labor.** What is the difference between a fixed and a variable labor budget?

21. **Labor budget: calculating the fixed labor budget.** Instead of the raises stated in Exhibit I.4e, assume that all benefits are 18% and all raises are 4%, and calculate the fixed labor budget for January, February, and March. Assume that all the other assumptions in the exhibit remain the same. Explain why some salaries and benefits change from month to month and others do not.

22. **Labor budget: calculating the fixed labor budget.** Instead of the benefits stated in Exhibit I.4e, assume that all benefits are 21% and all raises are 3.5% and calculate the fixed labor budget for January, February, and March. Assume that all the other assumptions in the exhibit remain the same. Explain why some salaries and benefits change from month to month and others do not.

23. **Labor budget: variable labor.** In the variable labor budget, why is it necessary to determine how many RVUs can be handled by full-time employees?

24. **Variable labor budget: direct and indirect time.** In the variable labor budget (see Exhibit I.5b.), why is it necessary to consider efficiency?

25. **Variable labor budget: efficiency.** If the assumed efficiency of the providers changed to 85% (see Exhibit I.5c.), what would be the productive capacity for January?

26. **Variable labor budget: efficiency.** If the assumed efficiency of the providers changed to 92% (see Exhibit I.5c.), what would be the productive capacity for January?

27. **Group purchasing organizations: pricing.** Given the data in Exhibit 10.14 and retaining the same items and volumes, if Vendors A and B vowed to match Vendor C's prices, which vendor would be least expensive for Mumford Regional Hospital?

28. **Group purchasing organizations: volumes.** At the beginning of the new year, Mumford Regional's chief competitor is planning to open a brand-new Women's & Children's Hospital nearby. As a result, Mumford expects all its supply needs to decrease by 20%. Given the information in Exhibit 10.14, should Mumford continue to contract with Vendor C for its supply needs? Why or why not?

Appendix I: An Extended Example of How to Develop a Budget

This appendix shows how to develop the numbers in a budget, using ZMG Hospitalist Practice as an example. The term *the budget* is shorthand for four interrelated budgets: the statistics, operating, cash, and capital budgets.

Statistics Budget

The statistics budget is created in three steps: develop an overall volume projection, categorize volume projection by payor and encounter type, and convert encounters to weighted encounters.

- *Develop an overall volume projection.* A common approach to forecasting volume is to begin with the previous year's actual results and make adjustments for anticipated changes. In the example (Exhibit I.1a), the ZMG Hospitalist Practice makes the relatively standard assumption of 5 percent overall and monthly growth compared with the current year. Although this approach is common, to the extent that major variations can be expected, a more refined month-by-month projection would make the budget a better planning tool. (For example, the expected acquisition of a large private physician practice later on in the upcoming fiscal year would result in additional admissions to the hospitalist practice.)

- *Categorize volume projections by payor and encounter type.* As the amount of revenue earned by these encounters must eventually be estimated, the next step is to further subdivide the number of encounters just developed by the type of payor and type of patient encounter. This is done by multiplying the number of encounters developed in Exhibit I.1a by the payor and service mix information in Exhibit I.1b, which reflects ZMG's payor mix by type of encounter as it has been experienced over the past several years. The ZMG practice uses three major categories of payors: commercial insurance, Medicare, and Medicaid/Self-Pay, and categorizes its encounters into two types, admissions encounters and follow-up encounters. The result is the estimate of encounters by payor and type of encounter (Exhibit I.1c).

EXHIBIT I.1a CALCULATION OF NUMBER OF ENCOUNTERS BY PAYOR TYPE FOR THE COMING YEAR

	Jan	Feb	Mar	Apr	May	Jun	Jul	Aug	Sep	Oct	Nov	Dec	Total
Total encounters for 20X1[a]	5,007	4,676	5,044	4,686	4,480	4,596	4,697	4,833	4,653	4,923	4,734	5,202	57,531
Projected growth	5%	5%	5%	5%	5%	5%	5%	5%	5%	5%	5%	5%	5%
Total encounters for 20X2	5,257	4,910	5,296	4,920	4,704	4,826	4,932	5,075	4,886	5,169	4,971	5,462	60,408

[a]From the organization's internal records.

EXHIBIT I.1b DISTRIBUTION OF ENCOUNTERS BY PAYOR AND ENCOUNTER TYPE

	Commercial	Medicare	Medicaid/ Self-Pay	Total
Admissions	9%	14%	2%	25%
Follow-up	27%	42%	6%	75%
Total	36%	56%	8%	100%

Note: From the organization's internal records.

Relative Value Unit (RVU)

A standardized weighting that is assigned to each encounter, procedure, or surgery and that reflects resources consumed. It is also widely used by hospitals in evaluating the amounts of resources required to perform various services in a single department or across departments.

- *Convert encounters to weighted encounters.* As admissions encounters and follow-up encounters require different amounts of time, to determine staffing needs, it is necessary to convert these encounters into *weighted encounters*, commonly called *relative value units* (RVUs). An admissions encounter, when the hospitalist first encounters and examines the patient, takes about an hour, whereas a follow-up encounter takes about a half hour, Using fifteen minutes as a basic unit of measurement for an RVU (that is, 1 RVU = 15 Minutes of Work), an admissions encounter takes approximately four RVUs and a follow-up encounter takes about two RVUs (Exhibit I.1d). Multiplying the number of encounters by payor and type of encounter (Exhibit I.1c) by the relative values of each type of encounter (Exhibit I.1d) calculates the number of weighted encounters by payor and type of encounter (Exhibit I.1e). Exhibit I.1f shows how January's numbers for weighted encounters by payor and type of encounter (Exhibit I.1e) were derived.

Operating Budget

As noted earlier, the operating budget (see Exhibit 10.10) consists of two budgets developed using the accrual basis of accounting: the revenue budget and the expense budget. Development of each of these budgets for ZMG Hospitalist Practice follows.

Revenue Budget

The revenue budget has two primary parts: net patient revenues and non-patient revenues.

EXHIBIT I.1c DISTRIBUTION OF ENCOUNTERS BY PAYOR AND TYPE

	Jan	Feb	Mar	Apr	May	Jun	Jul	Aug	Sep	Oct	Nov	Dec	Total
Commercial													
Admissions	473	442	477	443	423	434	444	457	440	465	447	492	5,437
Follow-up	1,419	1,326	1,430	1,328	1,270	1,303	1,332	1,370	1,319	1,396	1,342	1,475	16,310
Total	1,892	1,768	1,907	1,771	1,693	1,737	1,776	1,827	1,759	1,861	1,789	1,967	21,747
Medicare													
Admissions	736	687	741	689	659	676	690	711	684	724	696	765	8,458
Follow-up	2,208	2,062	2,224	2,066	1,976	2,027	2,071	2,132	2,052	2,171	2,088	2,294	25,371
Total	2,944	2,749	2,965	2,755	2,635	2,703	2,761	2,843	2,736	2,895	2,784	3,059	33,829
Medicaid/Self-Pay													
Admissions	105	98	106	98	94	97	99	102	98	103	99	109	1,208
Follow-up	315	295	318	295	282	290	296	305	293	310	298	328	3,625
Total	420	393	424	393	376	387	395	407	391	413	397	437	4,833
Total encounters	5,256	4,910	5,296	4,919	4,704	4,827	4,932	5,077	4,886	5,169	4,970	5,463	60,409

Note: Computed by multiplying the projected encounters in Exhibit I.1a by the appropriate cell in Exhibit I.1b, rounded to the nearest whole number. See Exhibit I.1e for greater detail. Slight differences between Exhibits I.1a and I.1c are due to rounding.

EXHIBIT I.1d RELATIVE VALUE WEIGHTS FOR ADMISSIONS AND FOLLOW-UP ENCOUNTERS

Type of Visit	Weight
Admissions	4.00
Follow-up	2.00

Net Patient Revenues

As discussed in Chapter Two, there is a difference between gross charges and net charges. *Gross charges* are the full amount the organization bills its patients for the services rendered. *Net charges* are the amount the organization expects to receive after taking into account all discounts and allowances (except bad debt). Discounts and allowances include such items as contractual agreements between the health care provider and the payor, charity care, and sliding fee schedules.

Exhibit I.2a illustrates how the $422,040 net patient revenues for January in the operating budget (Exhibit 10.10) were determined.

- First, gross patient revenues were calculated by multiplying the number of weighted encounters for each payor by the charge for each weighted encounter, $52.50.

- Next, the amount of allowances and discounts is calculated by multiplying the gross patient revenue for each payor times the discount percentage for that payor. These discount percentages are based on historical experience and are different for each category: 30 percent, 40 percent, and 70 percent for commercial, Medicare, and Medicaid/Self-Pay, respectively. Also note in the last category, Medicaid or Self-Pay, that the 1 percent charity care allowance is treated the same way an additional discount would be but on the remaining net patient service revenue balance after the initial discount is taken.

- Finally, net patient revenues are calculated by subtracting the discount for each payor from its gross patient revenues.

Gross Charges
The full amount an organization bills its patients for rendered services.

Net Charges
The amount an organization expects to receive after accounting for discounts and allowances.

Caution: In this situation, *gross charges* and *gross revenues* are used interchangeably.

EXHIBIT I.1e WEIGHTED ENCOUNTERS BY PAYOR AND TYPE

	Jan	Feb	Mar	Apr	May	Jun	Jul	Aug	Sep	Oct	Nov	Dec	Total
Commercial													
Admissions	1,892	1,768	1,908	1,772	1,692	1,736	1,776	1,828	1,760	1,860	1,788	1,968	21,748
Follow-up	2,838	2,652	2,860	2,656	2,540	2,606	2,664	2,740	2,638	2,792	2,684	2,950	32,620
Total	4,730	4,420	4,768	4,428	4,232	4,342	4,440	4,568	4,398	4,652	4,472	4,918	54,368
Medicare													
Admissions	2,944	2,748	2,964	2,756	2,636	2,704	2,760	2,844	2,736	2,896	2,784	3,060	33,832
Follow-up	4,416	4,124	4,448	4,132	3,952	4,054	4,142	4,264	4,104	4,342	4,176	4,588	50,742
Total	7,360	6,872	7,412	6,888	6,588	6,758	6,902	7,108	6,840	7,238	6,960	7,648	84,574
Medicaid/Self-Pay													
Admissions	420	392	424	392	376	388	396	408	392	412	396	436	4,832
Follow-up	630	590	636	590	564	580	592	610	586	620	596	656	7,250
Total	1,050	982	1,060	982	940	968	988	1,018	978	1,032	992	1,092	12,082
Total	13,140	12,274	13,240	12,298	11,760	12,068	12,330	12,694	12,216	12,922	12,424	13,658	151,024

Note: Computed by multiplying the projected encounters by type and payor in Exhibit I.1c by the RVUs (4 for admissions, 2 for follow-up) in Exhibit I.1d, rounded to the nearest whole number.

EXHIBIT I.1f ILLUSTRATION OF HOW WEIGHTED ENCOUNTERS BY PAYOR TYPE (EXHIBIT I.1e) WERE DEVELOPED

	Percentage of Encounters[a]	Encounters[b]	Weights[c]	Weighted Encounters[d]
January's encounters:		5,257		
Commercial				
Admissions	9%	473	4.00	1,892
Follow-up	27%	1,419	2.00	2,838
Total	36%	1,892		4,730
Medicare				
Admissions	14%	736	4.00	2,944
Follow-up	42%	2,208	2.00	4,416
Total	56%	2,944		7,360
Medicaid/Self-Pay				
Admissions	2%	105	4.00	420
Follow-up	6%	315	2.00	630
	8%	420		1,050
Total[e]	100%	5,256		13,140

[a]Percentages of encounters can be found in Exhibit I.1b.
[b]January's encounters can be found in Exhibit I.1a. The remaining encounters are calculated by multiplying January's encounters by the corresponding percentage of encounters. The results correspond to those found in Exhibit I.1c.
[c]Original weights can be found in Exhibit I.1d.
[d]Weighted encounters are calculated by multiplying encounters by their weights. The results correspond to those in Exhibit I.1e.
[e]Slight differences are due to rounding.

Nonpatient Revenues

In addition to patient service revenues, most organizations also have nonpatient revenues. In the case of ZMG Hospitalist Practice, the nonpatient revenues are interest and consulting fees. The estimate of interest earned is developed on a separate schedule related to the cash budget (not shown here). The estimate of consulting fees is based on a review of the organization's plans for this service. The calculation of the $11,440 of nonpatient revenues ("other operating revenues") in the operating budget (see Exhibit 10.10, "Total" column, row H) is shown in the "Total" column of Exhibit I.2b.

EXHIBIT I.2a ILLUSTRATION OF HOW JANUARY'S NET PATIENT SERVICE REVENUES IN THE ZMG HOSPITALIST PRACTICE'S OPERATING BUDGET (EXHIBIT 10.10) WERE DEVELOPED

	A	B	C	D	E	F
			Gross Patient			**Net Patient**
	Weighted		**Service**	**Discount**		**Service**
	Encounters[a]	**Fees**[b]	**Revenues**	**Percentage**[b]	**Discount**[c]	**Revenues**
			(A × B)			**(C – E)**
Commercial						
Admissions	1,892	$52.50	$99,330			
Follow-up	2,838	$52.50	$148,995			
Total	4,730		$248,325	30%	$74,498	$173,828
Medicare						
Admissions	2,944	$52.50	$154,560			
Follow-up	4,416	$52.50	$231,840			
Total	7,360		$386,400	40%	$154,560	$231,840
Medicaid/Self-Pay						
Admissions	420	$52.50	$22,050			
Follow-up	630	$52.50	$33,075			
Total	1,050		$55,125	70%	$38,588	$16,538
Charity care				1%	$165	
Total	13,140		$689,850		$267,810	$422,040

[a]Exhibit I.1d.
[b]New information.
[c]The discount is computed by multiplying the total of gross charges for each payor by the discount percentage. In the case of Medicaid/Self-Pay, 1 percent of Medicaid/Self-Pay net revenues is considered charity care; therefore, this additional discount is computed by multiplying Medicaid/Self-Pay net patient service revenues by 1 percent.

EXHIBIT I.2b FORECAST OF NONPATIENT REVENUES FOR ZMG HOSPITALIST PRACTICE

	Jan	Feb	Mar	Apr	May	Jun	Jul	Aug	Sep	Oct	Nov	Dec	Total
Interest	$348	$405	$69	$68	$69	$68	$69	$69	$68	$69	$68	$69	$1,440
Consulting	833	833	833	833	833	833	833	833	833	833	833	833	10,000
Total	$1,182	$1,238	$903	$901	$903	$901	$903	$903	$901	$903	$901	$903	$11,440

Note: From the organization's internal records.

EXHIBIT I.3 OVERVIEW OF THE OPERATING EXPENSE BUDGET

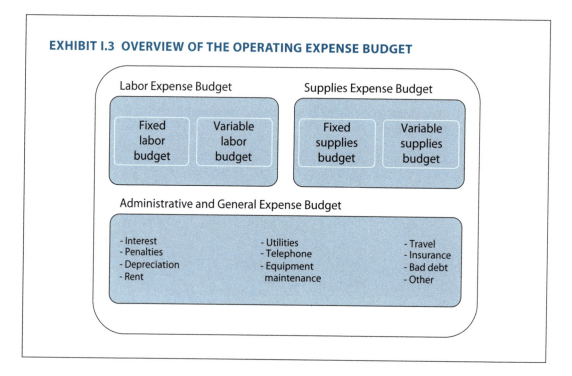

Labor Expense Budget

| Fixed labor budget | Variable labor budget |

Supplies Expense Budget

| Fixed supplies budget | Variable supplies budget |

Administrative and General Expense Budget

- Interest
- Penalties
- Depreciation
- Rent

- Utilities
- Telephone
- Equipment maintenance

- Travel
- Insurance
- Bad debt
- Other

Expense Budget

The second part of the operating budget (see Exhibit 10.10, rows L through V) is the expense budget. The expense budget itself is made up of three other budgets: the labor budget, the supplies budget, and the administrative and general budget (see Exhibit I.3).

Labor Budget

Note that the first item listed under expenses in the operating budget (Exhibit 10.10) is labor, because it consumes the largest amount of the organization's resources. The amount listed for labor expense is developed in the *labor budget* (see Exhibit I.4a), which itself is composed of two budgets: the fixed labor budget and the variable labor budget. The *fixed labor budget* forecasts the costs of salaried personnel; the *variable labor budget* accounts for additional labor costs, which vary as additional part-time personnel or overtime hours are needed. Development of ZMG Hospitalist Practice's labor budget follows.

The fixed labor budget (Exhibit I.4b) consists solely of salaries (Exhibit I.4c) and benefits (Exhibit I.4d), usually presented by position or position category. An example of how the Physician I amounts in the labor budget are calculated for February is presented in Exhibits I.4e and I.4f. Note that ZMG Hospitalist Practice budgets by position, not individual.

Labor Budget
A subset of the expense budget, this budget is composed of the fixed labor budget and the variable labor budget.

Fixed Labor Budget
A subset of the labor budget that forecasts the cost of salaried personnel.

Variable Labor Budget
A subset of the labor budget that forecasts nonsalary labor costs, such as part-time employees and overtime hours.

EXHIBIT I.4a THE LABOR BUDGET

	Jan	Feb	Mar	Apr	May	Jun	Jul	Aug	Sep	Oct	Nov	Dec	Total
Fixed salaries	$383,333	$393,958	$393,958	$393,958	$393,958	$394,333	$401,667	$401,667	$401,667	$401,667	$402,500	$402,500	$4,765,167
Fixed benefits	59,917	61,552	61,552	61,552	61,552	61,646	62,746	62,746	62,746	62,746	62,913	62,913	744,579
Subtotal	443,250	455,510	455,510	455,510	455,510	455,979	464,413	464,413	464,413	464,413	465,413	465,413	5,509,746
Temporary wages		14,356	3,356									18,370	36,081
Bonus[a]												11,712	11,712
Total	$443,250	$469,866	$458,866	$455,510	$455,510	$455,979	$464,413	$464,413	$464,413	$464,413	$465,413	$495,494	$5,557,539

Note: This table illustrates how the labor line item in the operating budget (Exhibit 10.10) was developed.
[a]As bonuses typically might be in the range of 10 to 20 percent of base salary, the small amount noted here warrants further attention to how the bonus program is being implemented.

EXHIBIT I.4b THE FIXED LABOR BUDGET

Position	Jan	Feb	Mar	Apr	May	Jun	Jul	Aug	Sep	Oct	Nov	Dec	Total
Physician I	$230,000	$241,500	$241,500	$241,500	$241,500	$241,500	$241,500	$241,500	$241,500	$241,500	$241,500	$241,500	$2,886,500
Physician II	168,667	168,667	168,667	168,667	168,667	168,667	177,100	177,100	177,100	177,100	177,100	177,100	2,074,600
Physician Assistant	10,000	10,000	10,000	10,000	10,000	10,000	10,000	10,000	10,000	10,000	10,500	10,500	121,000
Nurse Practitioner	10,000	10,000	10,000	10,000	10,000	10,000	10,000	10,000	10,000	10,000	10,500	10,500	121,000
Administrative Director	10,000	10,500	10,500	10,500	10,500	10,500	10,500	10,500	10,500	10,500	10,500	10,500	125,500
Office Staff I	5,208	5,469	5,469	5,469	5,469	5,469	5,469	5,469	5,469	5,469	5,469	5,469	65,365
Office Staff II	9,375	9,375	9,375	9,375	9,375	9,844	9,844	9,844	9,844	9,844	9,844	9,844	115,781
Total	$443,250	$455,510	$455,510	$455,510	$455,510	$455,979	$464,413	$464,413	$464,413	$464,413	$465,413	$465,413	$5,509,746

Note: The totals appearing here are made up of a fixed salary component (Exhibit I.4c) and benefits (Exhibit I.4d).

EXHIBIT I.4c SALARIES SCHEDULE FOR THE FIXED LABOR BUDGET

Position	Jan	Feb	Mar	Apr	May	Jun	Jul	Aug	Sep	Oct	Nov	Dec	Total
Physician I	$200,000	$210,000	$210,000	$210,000	$210,000	$210,000	$210,000	$210,000	$210,000	$210,000	$210,000	$210,000	$2,510,000
Physician II	146,667	146,667	146,667	146,667	146,667	146,667	154,000	154,000	154,000	154,000	154,000	154,000	1,804,000
Physician Assistant	8,333	8,333	8,333	8,333	8,333	8,333	8,333	8,333	8,333	8,333	8,750	8,750	100,833
Nurse Practitioner	8,333	8,333	8,333	8,333	8,333	8,333	8,333	8,333	8,333	8,333	8,750	8,750	100,833
Administrative Director	8,333	8,750	8,750	8,750	8,750	8,750	8,750	8,750	8,750	8,750	8,750	8,750	104,583
Office Staff II	4,167	4,375	4,375	4,375	4,375	4,375	4,375	4,375	4,375	4,375	4,375	4,375	52,292
Office Staff I	7,500	7,500	7,500	7,500	7,500	7,875	7,875	7,875	7,875	7,875	7,875	7,875	92,625
Total	$383,333	$393,958	$393,958	$393,958	$393,958	$394,333	$401,667	$401,667	$401,667	$401,667	$402,500	$402,500	$4,765,167

EXHIBIT I.4d BENEFITS SCHEDULE FOR THE FIXED LABOR BUDGET

Position	Jan	Feb	Mar	Apr	May	Jun	Jul	Aug	Sep	Oct	Nov	Dec	Total
Physician I	$30,000	$31,500	$31,500	$31,500	$31,500	$31,500	$31,500	$31,500	$31,500	$31,500	$31,500	$31,500	$376,500
Physician II	22,000	22,000	22,000	22,000	22,000	22,000	23,100	23,100	23,100	23,100	23,100	23,100	270,600
Physician Assistant	1,667	1,667	1,667	1,667	1,667	1,667	1,667	1,667	1,667	1,667	1,750	1,750	20,167
Nurse Practioner	1,667	1,667	1,667	1,667	1,667	1,667	1,667	1,667	1,667	1,667	1,750	1,750	20,167
Administratve Director	1,667	1,750	1,750	1,750	1,750	1,750	1,750	1,750	1,750	1,750	1,750	1,750	20,917
Office Staff I	1,042	1,094	1,094	1,094	1,094	1,094	1,094	1,094	1,094	1,094	1,094	1,094	13,073
Office Staff II	1,875	1,875	1,875	1,875	1,875	1,969	1,969	1,969	1,969	1,969	1,969	1,969	23,156
Total	$59,917	$61,552	$61,552	$61,552	$61,552	$61,646	$62,746	$62,746	$62,746	$62,746	$62,913	$62,913	$744,579

EXHIBIT I.4e DATA USED TO CONSTRUCT ZMG HOSPITALIST PRACTICE'S FIXED LABOR SALARIES AND BENEFITS

	Number of FTEs	Average Salary	Base Salary	Benefit Percentage	Date of Next Raise	Raise Percentage
Physician I	12	$200,000	$2,400,000	15%	Feb 02	5%
Physician II	8	$220,000	$1,760,000	15%	Jul 02	5%
Physician assistant	1	$100,000	$100,000	20%	Nov 02	5%
Nurse practitioner	1	$100,000	$100,000	20%	Nov 02	5%
Administrative director	1	$100,000	$100,000	20%	Feb 02	5%
Office staff I	1	$50,000	$50,000	25%	Feb 02	5%
Office staff II	3	$30,000	$90,000	25%	Jun 02	5%

Note: All salaries and wages are paid twice monthly in equal amounts. The second payment is made on the last day of each month.

EXHIBIT I.4f HOW FEBRUARY'S SALARIES AND BENEFITS FOR PHYSICIAN I CATEGORY IN EXHIBITS I.4b THROUGH I.4d WERE DEVELOPED

	Item	Source	Annual Amount
A	Annual base salary/month	Exhibit I.4e	$200,000
B	Raise	Exhibit I.4e	5%
C	Salary after raise	$[A \times (1 + B)]$	$210,000
D	Benefits percentage	Exhibit I.4e	15%
E	Benefits after raise	$(C \times D)$	$31,500
F	Salary and benefits	$(C + E)$	$241,500

EXHIBIT I.5a THE VARIABLE LABOR BUDGET

Position	Jan	Feb	Mar	Apr	May	Jun	Jul	Aug	Sep	Oct	Nov	Dec	Total
Variable staffing[a]	$0	$14,356	$3,356	$0	$0	$0	$0	$0	$0	$0	$0	$18,370	$36,081

[a]From Exhibit I.5b, row H. Variable staff for ZMG Hospitalist Practice are all *locum tenens*.

Variable Labor Budget

The second component of the labor budget is the variable labor budget (Exhibit I.5a), which accounts for wages of nonsalaried employees and overtime. Health care organizations are increasingly turning to part-time employees because they can meet flexible demands and may cost less, and often because benefits do not need to be paid to these workers. In the case of ZMG Hospitalist Practice, the variable labor budget can be found in the row titled "variable staffing."

Because part-time and overtime hours per month vary depending on the overall workload, it is not necessary to develop this budget by position as was done for the fixed labor budget. Instead, this budget is developed by (1) estimating how many RVUs will be covered by full-time staff; (2) determining the required RVUs to provide service, based on demand; (3) determining the number of RVUs that cannot be covered by existing staff; (4) determining the number of hours it will take to cover the uncovered RVUs; and (5) determining the cost to hire staff to cover the uncovered RVU demand. In this example, it is assumed that all noncovered hours are filled with temporary staff; individual members of this staff are called *locum tenens*. There is no overtime.

1. The estimate of how many RVUs will be covered by full-time staff is shown in Exhibit I.5b, row A. The development of these estimates involves making a considerable number of estimates, as shown in Exhibit I.5c, which gives an example of how the estimates of RVU capacity for January were made.

2. The estimate of the RVUs required to provide service based on demand (Exhibit I.5b, row B) comes directly from the bottom line of the statistics budget (Exhibit 10.9, Total).

EXHIBIT I.5b CALCULATION OF THE VARIABLE LABOR BUDGET

Position	Jan	Feb	Mar	Apr	May	Jun	Jul	Aug	Sep	Oct	Nov	Dec	Total
Physician I RVU capacity	7,235	6,535	7,235	7,002	7,235	7,002	7,235	7,235	7,002	7,235	7,002	7,235	85,190
Physician II RVU capacity	4,824	4,357	4,824	4,668	4,824	4,668	4,824	4,824	4,668	4,824	4,668	4,824	56,794
Physician assistant RVU capacity	544	491	544	526	544	526	544	544	526	544	526	544	6,403
Nurse practitioner RVU capacity	544	491	544	526	544	526	544	544	526	544	526	544	6,403
A Total RVU productive capacity	13,147	11,874	13,147	12,722	13,147	12,722	13,147	13,147	12,722	13,147	12,722	13,147	154,790
B Required RVUs based on demand	13,140	12,274	13,240	12,298	11,760	12,068	12,330	12,694	12,216	12,922	12,424	13,658	151,024
C Surplus (deficit): required RVUs vs. capacity	7	(400)	(93)	424	1,387	654	817	453	506	225	298	(511)	3,766
D Staffing RVUs per hour at 100% efficiency	4	4	4	4	4	4	4	4	4	4	4	4	48
E Actual efficiency	87%	87%	87%	87%	87%	87%	87%	87%	87%	87%	87%	87%	87%
F Additional hours needed based on uncovered RVUs	0	115	27	0	0	0	0	0	0	0	0	147	289
G Locum tenens MD, PA, or NP avg. hourly rate	$125	$125	$125	$125	$125	$125	$125	$125	$125	$125	$125	$125	$125
H Variable staffing (locum tenens) cost[a]	$0	$14,356	$3,356	$0	$0	$0	$0	$0	$0	$0	$0	$18,370	$36,081

[a]If additional hourly staffing is needed, as shown by a deficit in row C, the formula is F × G. Otherwise, there is surplus capacity, and no extra hourly (locum tenens) staff are needed.

EXHIBIT I.5c CALCULATION OF RVU PRODUCTIVITY CAPACITY IN JANUARY

Givens
Physician Productivity

A	Number of Physician I	12
B	Number of Physician II	8
C	Shifts per year per full-time physician	204
D	Hours per shift per physician	10
E	Minutes per RVU	15
F	RVUs per hour	4
G	Physician efficiency	87%
H	Days in this month	31

PA or NP Productivity

I	Number physician assistants	1
J	Number nurse practitioners	1
K	Shifts per year per full-time PA or NP[a]	230
L	Hours per day per PA or NP	8
M	RVUs per hour	4
N	PA or NP productivity	87%
O	Days in this month	31

	Calculations		**Physician I**	**Physician II**	**Total**
P	Number	(A) and (B)	12	8	
Q	RVUs per physician per year (365 days)	(C × D × F × G)	7,099	7,099	
R	RVUs per day per physician	(Q / 365)	19.4	19.4	
S	Days in this month	(H)	31	31	
T	RVU capacity this month	(P × R × S)	7,235	4,824	12,059

			Physician Assistants	**Nurse Practitioners**	
U	Number	(I) and (J)	1	1	
V	RVUs per PA or NP per year	(K × L × M × N)	6,403	6,403	
W	RVUs per day per PA or NP	(V / 365)	17.5	17.5	
X	Days in this month	(O)	31	31	
Y	RVU capacity this month	(U × W × X)	544	544	1,088

Z	Total RVU capacity this month	(T + Y)			13,147

[a]Assumes 3 weeks of vacation, 1 week of sick leave, and 2 weeks of holidays.

3. To determine the number of RVUs that cannot be covered by existing staff (Exhibit I.5b, row C), the RVU demand (step 2) is subtracted from the RVU capacity of the staff (step 1). If demand is higher than capacity, then temporary staff must be hired. (Remember that in this example there is no overtime.)

4. To determine the cost of hiring temporary staff (step 5), it is first necessary to convert the uncovered RVUs (step 3) to their equivalent in hours (Exhibit I.5b, row F).

In calculating the hourly equivalent, estimates were made of both the number of hours it takes for staff to "do" an RVU if they work at 100 percent efficiency and the hours it takes at the actual efficiency they are expected to have. In this example, the staff are assumed to be working at 87 percent efficiency (Exhibit I.5b, row E). Assumptions like this are often made to take into account such factors as bottlenecks, delays, difficult cases, meetings, and the like.

5. Once the number of temporary staff hours is determined (step 4), finding the cost of those staff is straightforward (Exhibit I.5b, row H). The number of temporary staff hours needed is multiplied by the cost per hour (Exhibit I.5b, rows F and G).

Supplies Budget

Although some organizations have major supplies costs, this is not the case with ZMG Hospitalist Practice, which groups its supplies costs under *other* in the administrative and general expense budget (Exhibits I.6a and I.6b). Organizations that have supplies costs may have a fixed supplies budget and a variable supplies budget. The *fixed supplies budget* covers items such as office supplies, which do not vary with the number of patients seen. The *variable supplies budget* includes those items that do vary with the activities. In a clinical setting, these would include items that vary with RVUs, such as disposable syringes, disposable gloves, and X-ray film. While the fixed supplies budget may be a constant amount each month, the variable supplies budget is likely to change monthly, as the number of RVUs changes.

Often health care organizations want to make sure that they do not run out of supplies in any month and that they begin the next month with a supply inventory. Thus, for any month, in addition to the supplies they start with (*beginning inventory*), they must estimate both the cost of the supplies they are going to use (*cost of goods used*) and the amount of supplies they will need to have on hand at the end of the month (*ending inventory*), which incidentally, becomes the opening inventory for the next

Fixed Supplies Budget
A subset of the supplies budget that covers items that do not vary with volume.

Variable Supplies Budget
A subset of the supplies budget that covers items that vary with volume.

EXHIBIT I.6a ADMINISTRATIVE AND GENERAL EXPENSE BUDGET

	Jan	Feb	Mar	Apr	May	Jun	Jul	Aug	Sep	Oct	Nov	Dec	Total
Interest	$137	$134	$131	$316	$311	$306	$382	$376	$369	$363	$357	$350	$3,533
Depreciation	456	456	456	864	864	864	981	981	981	981	981	981	9,846
Utilities	1,000	1,000	1,000	1,000	1,000	1,000	1,000	1,000	1,000	1,000	1,000	1,000	12,000
Rent	2,500	2,500	2,500	2,500	2,500	2,500	2,500	2,500	2,500	2,500	2,500	2,500	30,000
Cleaning	500	500	500	500	500	500	500	500	500	500	500	500	6,000
Other (phone, supplies, etc.)	600	600	600	600	600	600	600	600	600	600	600	600	7,200
Travel	5,000	5,000	5,000	5,000	5,000	5,000	5,000	5,000	5,000	5,000	5,000	5,000	60,000
Insurance	12,000	12,000	12,000	12,000	12,000	12,000	12,000	12,000	12,000	12,000	12,000	12,000	144,000
Equipment maintenance	300	300	300	300	300	300	300	300	300	300	300	300	3,600
Bad debt expense	4,220	3,942	4,252	3,950	3,777	3,875	3,960	4,076	3,923	4,150	3,991	4,387	48,505
Subtotal	26,713	26,432	26,740	27,030	26,852	26,945	27,223	27,333	27,174	27,395	27,228	27,618	324,684
Add: nonoperating expenses	1300	1750	1750	1750	1300	1300	1300	1300	1300	1300	1300	1300	16,950
Total expenses	$28,013	$28,182	$28,490	$28,780	$28,152	$28,245	$28,523	$28,633	$28,474	$28,695	$28,528	$28,918	$341,634

EXHIBIT I.6b INFORMATION USED TO CONSTRUCT THE ADMINISTRATIVE AND GENERAL EXPENSE BUDGET

Item	Amount	Occurrence and Payment
Interest	Varies	Calculated on an amortization schedule[a]
Depreciation	Varies	Calculated on a depreciation schedule[a]
Utilities	$1,000	Per month, payable each month
Rent	$2,500	Per month, payable on the first day of each month
Cleaning	$500	Per month, payable in advance every three months
Other (phone, supplies, etc.)	$600	Per month, payable each month
Travel	$5,000	Per month, payable each month
Insurance	$12,000	Per month, payable each month
Equipment maintenance	$300	Per month, payable in advance every March
Bad debt expense	Varies	4% of charge-based and 3% of cost-based net patient revenues

[a]Not included; assume the number is a given for this example.

month. The cost of goods used will appear as an expense on the statement of operations whereas the ending inventory will appear on the balance sheet as a current asset. The relationship among these items is shown by the formula:

$$\text{Opening Inventory} + \text{Purchases} - \text{Cost of Goods Used} = \text{Ending Inventory}$$

An example of these calculations is shown in the following table:

Beginning inventory	$5,154	Dollar amount in ending inventory from the month before.
Add: purchases	32,900	Cost of supplies necessary to deliver services this month and still have sufficient ending inventory.
Goods available	38,054	Value of beginning inventory + purchases.
Less: cost of goods used	32,680	Cost of supplies necessary to deliver services this month.
Ending inventory	$5,374	The desired dollar amount of inventory with which to begin the next month; often a percentage of next month's estimated cost of supplies is used.

Key Point The reason that cost of goods used is used in the supplies budget, rather than the cost of goods purchased, is that accrual accounting is being used.

Administrative and General Expense Budget

The last part of the expense section of the operating budget (Exhibit 10.10) is administrative and general (A&G) expenses, which are developed in the general and administrative budget (see Exhibit I.6a). They comprise the day-to-day expenses that are not contained in the labor or supplies budgets. The assumptions for the A&G expenses for ZMG Hospitalist Practice are listed in Exhibit I.6b. Incidentally, some organizations treat interest and penalties as nonoperating expenses.

Cash Budget

As discussed in detail in Chapter Five, the cash budget is developed by determining when payments will be received from others and when payments will be made by the organization. Because it draws on information from the other budgets, the cash budget is the last budget to be developed.

The cash budget (Exhibit 10.11) is organized into two sections. The first section determines how much cash is available before borrowing; the second section compares the cash available with the cash required and then determines whether cash will be needed from other sources (when there is a shortfall) or whether cash will be invested (when there is an excess of cash).

To determine cash available, the cash inflows (revenues) are added, and outflows (expenditures) are subtracted from the beginning balance (Exhibit 10.11, rows A, B, C, and D).

The method to determine these inflows and outflows was discussed in Chapter Five, which shows how accrual data are converted into cash. Here it is illustrated by showing what happens to January's net income from commercial payors. As noted in Exhibit I.2a, ZMG Hospitalist Practice earned $173,828 in January on its commercial payor patients. Under the assumption that 28 percent will be collected in January, 45 percent in February, 14 percent in March, and 10 percent in April and that the remaining 3 percent will be written off, the cash inflow pattern is shown in Exhibit I.7.

The second part of the cash budget (Exhibit 10.11) determines whether the organization has sufficient cash to begin the next month. ZMG Hos-

EXHIBIT I.7 CONVERTING ACCRUAL INFORMATION INTO CASH FLOWS: ZMG
HOSPITALIST PRACTICE'S REVENUES FOR JANUARY

January's Net Revenues Using the Accrual Basis of Accounting: Commercial Patients' Amount Collected in:	Percentage to Be Received by Month	Cash Inflow by Month[a]
January	28%	$48,672
February	45%	$78,222
March	14%	$24,336
April	10%	$17,383
Written off	3%	$5,215
Total	100%	$173,828

[a]Differences due to rounding.

pitalist Practice has decided that it should begin each month with $100,000
cash on hand (Exhibit 10.11, row E). If it does not have $100,000 (Exhibit
10.11, rows I through K), it would either have to obtain such funds from
its own short-term or long-term investments (perhaps with some penalty
for early withdrawal) or else borrow the funds from outside the organization (Exhibit 10.11, row M). Fortunately, ZMG Hospitalist Practice does
not find itself in such a position in January, so it invests the excess $43,975
in short-term investments (Exhibit 10.11, row G). Exhibit I.7 illustrates
how January's net patient service revenues in Exhibit I.2a would be converted into cash flows.

Capital Budget

The capital budget was initially presented in Exhibit 10.12. Although the
budget for ZMG Hospitalist Practice is relatively small, large organizations
may have capital budgets totaling millions of dollars. The items that appear
on the capital budget are likely to have been part of a much larger list of
requests that various departments submitted.

The capital budget presented in Exhibit 10.12 lists financial information only. The term *capital budget* is also used to refer to the process of
requesting large-dollar items. In many organizations, considerable information is requested in addition to summary financial figures to justify a

capital investment. Such information is not limited to the revenue and expense projections discussed in Chapter Seven but also includes potential impact on patients, clinical staff, the organization as a whole, and the community.

Key Point The term *capital budget* is sometimes used to refer to not only summary information about the item being purchased but also potential financial impacts (see Chapter Seven) and impacts on patients, clinical staff, the organization as a whole, and the community.

CHAPTER 11

RESPONSIBILITY ACCOUNTING

Health care organizations have become increasingly complex over the past quarter century. One of the major changes is decentralization, which presents interesting problems when measuring financial performance. Whereas Chapter Four dealt with measuring the financial performance of the organization as a whole, this chapter identifies the types of organizational units *within* a health care organization and measures their financial performance. These units may be as large as subsidiaries or as small as departments. This chapter begins with a discussion of decentralization and then discusses the types of responsibility centers that exist in decentralized organizations. Next, the concepts of responsibility, authority, and accountability are explored. Finally, questions of how to measure the performance of responsibility centers are addressed.

Decentralization

Decentralization is the degree of dispersion of responsibility within an organization. Decentralization may evolve out of working arrangements or may be more formally prescribed in an organization's policies, procedures, and organizational structure. There are various advantages and disadvantages to decentralization, and each organization has to decide what level of decentralization is in its best interest.

Advantages of Decentralization

Selected advantages and disadvantages of decentralization are presented in Exhibit 11.1. The advantages (in no

LEARNING OBJECTIVES

- Define decentralization, and identify its major advantages and disadvantages.

- Identify the major types of responsibility centers found in health care organizations and describe their characteristics.

- Explain the relationship of responsibility, authority, and accountability in the performance measurement of responsibility centers.

- Compute volume and rate variances for revenues.

- Compute volume and cost variances for expenses.

EXHIBIT 11.1 SELECTED ADVANTAGES AND DISADVANTAGES OF DECENTRALIZATION

Advantages	Disadvantages
More efficient use of time	Loss of control
More relevant information	Decreased goal congruence
Higher-quality decisions	Increased need for coordination and formal
Greater speed	communication
Better use of talent	Lack of managerial talent
Increased motivation and allegiance	

---

particular order) include more efficient use of time, more relevant information, higher-quality decisions, greater speed, better use of talent, and increased motivation and allegiance.

More Efficient Use of Time

Decentralization
The dispersion of responsibility within a health care organization.

From the point of view of central management, a major advantage of decentralization is an increase in time available to devote to other tasks. Ideally, decentralization should relieve the central office of day-to-day operational decision making, allowing it to concentrate instead on tactical and strategic-level concerns.

More Relevant Information

When the responsibility for decision making is spread within the organization, the organization moves more toward a *need-to-know* environment where information is filtered at each level, and only the information needed for decision making at higher levels is passed on.

Higher-Quality Decisions

Those closer to a problem may be better suited to understanding the specifics of the problem and may be more responsive to the local context, thus leading to higher-quality decisions.

Greater Speed

Decentralized decision making allows those closest to the problem to respond more quickly by shortening six time-consuming steps in communication. The person who identifies the problem must

- *communicate* the problem *up* the organization
- to those who must *receive* it. Then they
- *become* aware of it,
- *decide on* a course of action, and
- *communicate* their response *down* through the organization,
- where it is ultimately *received* by the person authorized to *respond*.

Better Use of Talent

A health care organization must ensure that it is developing the management capability that will allow it to reach its objectives. Although occasionally it may want to look outside the organization for new blood, this process can become expensive, intrusive, and time consuming. It can also be demoralizing to those within the organization. Decentralization helps the organization to draw on and develop the expertise of existing staff.

Increased Motivation and Allegiance

By delegating responsibility to others, a health care organization can develop increased motivation and allegiance in its members. Increased involvement in the planning, implementation, and control process encourages buy-in by the staff, who may then experience an increased sense of ownership, belonging, and pride in their work.

Disadvantages of Decentralization

In considering what degree of decentralization to have, a health care organization has to balance the advantages of decentralization with its disadvantages, which include loss of control, decreased goal congruence, increased need for coordination and formal communication, and lack of managerial talent.

Loss of Control

When responsibility is spread throughout the organization, upper management loses direct control. For administrators who have an authoritarian style and for organizations that need top-level management's expertise, this can be a significant problem. The specific ramifications of loss of control also appear in the other disadvantages of decentralization, which are all highly interrelated.

Decreased Goal Congruence

To the extent that responsibility is decentralized within the organization, organizational units tend to develop their own goals. To avoid this, considerable effort must be exerted to ensure that each division or unit is making decisions that are consistent with and support the organization's strategic plan and that are in the best interest of the organization as a whole, not just the division.

Increased Need for Coordination and Formal Communication

When responsibility is decentralized within the organization, there is an increased need to coordinate efforts among the various units and divisions. This results in the need for more formal communications, meetings, policies, and procedures.

Lack of Managerial Talent

When an organization decentralizes and does not have the talent available at lower levels to manage the new responsibilities, as a whole it could suffer greatly. This particular problem was all too common during the early stages of managed care development in the United States. Because no one in the managed care organizations had previous experience in running such organizations, people with experience in running other health care entities were put in charge.

Responsibility Center

An organizational unit formally given the responsibility to carry out one or more tasks or achieve one or more outcomes, or both.

Types of Responsibility Centers

When responsibility is formally decentralized into organizational units, rather than informally to specific individuals, these units are called responsibility centers. A *responsibility center* is an organizational unit that has been formally given the responsibility to carry out one or more tasks or to achieve one or more outcomes (or both). The four most common types of responsibility centers in health care are service centers, cost centers, profit centers, and investment centers (Exhibit 11.2).

Service Center

An organizational unit primarily responsible for ensuring that health care–related services are provided to a population in a manner that meets the volume and quality requirements of the organization. It has no direct budgetary control.

Service Centers

Service centers, the most basic type of responsibility center, are primarily responsible for ensuring that services are provided to a population in a manner that meets the volume and quality requirements of the organization. Because service centers have no budgetary control, their main responsibilities revolve around scheduling, directing, and monitoring the staff and providing direct patient care. Although service centers use

---

EXHIBIT 11.2 THE FOUR MAIN TYPES OF RESPONSIBILITY CENTERS AND THEIR MAIN AREAS OF RESPONSIBILITY

	Type of Responsibility Center			
Areas of Responsibility	**Service Centers**	**Cost Centers**	**Profit Centers**	**Investment Centers**
Providing services	☒	☒	☒	☒
Controlling costs		☒	☒	☒
Generating profits			☒	☒
Making investments				☒

---

resources and thus affect costs, the actual budgetary control rests at a higher level in the organization. It is not unusual for nursing units to find themselves defined as service centers. They are responsible for patient care, but the budget is kept at the next higher level in the organization. Patient admitting and patient transportation are also often defined as service centers.

Cost Centers

Cost centers, the most common type of responsibility center in health care organizations, are responsible for providing services and controlling their costs. Ideally, they should be integrally involved in the planning, budgeting, and control process, for they are primarily responsible for resource utilization within the organization. Because payment often cannot be *directly* tied to specific services, under both flat fee (i.e., DRG) and capitated payment systems, a large number of responsibility centers are categorized as cost centers rather than profit centers.

Types of cost centers in health care organizations include production cost centers, clinical cost centers, and administrative cost centers. *Production cost centers* develop or sell products (or both). Certain laboratory and pharmacy activities fall into this category. *Clinical cost centers* are responsible for providing health care–related services to clients, patients, or enrollees. Examples include nursing and physical therapy. *Administrative cost centers* support the clinical cost centers and the organization as a whole. Included in this category are general administration, the business office, information services, quality control, admitting, medical records, and housekeeping. Administrative cost centers are often considered the

Cost Center
An organizational unit responsible for producing products or providing services and controlling its costs.

Production Cost Center
A cost center responsible for producing or selling products (or both).

Clinical Cost Center
A cost center responsible for providing health care–related services to clients, patients, or enrollees.

Administrative Cost Center
A cost center that supports clinical cost centers and the organization as a whole. These centers are often considered the *infrastructure* of the organization.

infrastructure of the organization. As with nursing, units that may be classified as cost centers in one organization may be considered service centers in another.

Profit Centers

Profit Center

An organizational unit responsible for controlling costs and earning revenues.

Although many *profit centers* are responsible for service-related activities, all profit centers are responsible for controlling their costs and earning revenues. In some cases, the costs may be larger than the revenue generated. For example, a pediatric screening program in a health department, which has to be offered, might be charged with earning sufficient revenues to cover just half of its $100,000 cost. Thus, although the pediatric screening program is considered a profit center by the health department, the amount of profit in this case is actually a loss of $50,000. There are three types of profit centers in health care organizations: traditional profit centers, capitated profit centers, and administrative profit centers.

Traditional Profit Centers

Traditional Profit Center

An organizational unit responsible for earning a profit by providing health care services. Revenues are earned either on a fee-for-service or a flat fee basis. Examples include cardiology, women's and children's services, and oncology.

Traditional profit centers are primarily responsible for making a profit selling goods or services. Traditional profit centers have proliferated recently. On the clinical side, much of this growth can be traced back to the emergence of product-line management in health care in the later part of the twentieth century. Common product (or service) lines include cardiology, women's and children's services, and oncology. Traditional profit centers profit through a combination of marking up services and controlling costs in fee-for-service situations, and also through controlling costs in flat fee arrangements such as the DRG payment system.

Capitated Profit Centers

Capitated Profit Center

An organizational unit responsible for earning a profit by agreeing to take care of the defined health care needs of a population for a per member fee (which is not directly tied to services). Examples include HMOs, PPOs, and various managed care organizations.

Capitated profit centers earn revenues by agreeing to take care of the defined health care needs of a population for a per member fee, often regardless of the amount of services needed by any particular patient. Such organizations are commonly called HMOs, PPOs, or managed care organizations. Interestingly enough, many managed care organizations purchase services from traditional profit centers. For example, an HMO may purchase its cardiology services from one health network and many of its oncology services from a different hospital system. Because they receive a set amount to cover the health care needs of a population, providers receiving capitation have considerable incentive to control costs through efficiency (the most service for any level of cost), economy (low costs), and prevention.

Administrative Profit Centers

There are two types of *administrative profit centers*: those that sell inside the organization and those that—although they do not deliver health services—are responsible for generating new revenues from outside the organization. Examples of administrative profit centers that may be required to sell their services inside the organization, as opposed to having their costs absorbed as overhead, are legal services, computer services, and management engineering. The prices for services that are charged internally to other organizational units are called *transfer prices.*

The setting of transfer prices is a delicate matter, and when they are set too high, there are several possible negative consequences. They may encourage potential users to buy these services outside the organization. If internal units (i.e., departments or subsidiary organizations) must use these resources, then they may suboptimize their use to cut costs or use the services but be unhappy about it (causing morale problems).

Examples of administrative profit centers that are responsible for generating new revenues from outside the organization include development offices (whose primary function is to encourage donations and contributions to the organization) and field representatives for HMOs and PPOs (whose primary responsibility is to sign up markets for the organization). Other primary examples are food services, gift shops, parking decks, and motel services. Incidentally, although their effects on profit are difficult to identify, marketing, advertising, and public relations may be considered administrative profit centers in some organizations (others may consider them cost centers).

Administrative Profit Center
An organizational unit that does not provide health care–related services but that is responsible for producing a profit. There are two types: those that sell their services internally, and those whose primary responsibility is to bring revenues into the organization.

Transfer Price
The price for a product or a service that is charged internally to other organizational units.

Investment Centers

In addition to having all the responsibilities of a traditional profit center, *investment centers* are responsible for making a certain return on investment. For example, where a profit center might be content with a simple $100,000 profit, an investment center might find this unacceptable if it does not provide the desired return on investment. An example of this is shown in Exhibit 11.3, where a Surgicenter earns $100,000 in profit, but this is an insufficient amount of revenue to earn a required 15 percent return per year on investment. Perspective 11.1 provides an example of an ambulatory surgery center expanding its service line to increase net income.

Investment centers have proliferated in the past few decades and include all investor-owned health care entities that require their operating units to make a certain return. However, not all investment centers are investor owned, for many not-for-profit health care organizations also

Investment Center
An organizational unit that has all the responsibilities of a traditional profit center and is also responsible for making a certain return on investment.

EXHIBIT 11.3 AN EXAMPLE OF EVALUATING AN INVESTMENT ON ITS PROFIT AND RETURN

A	Investment in new Surgicenter	Given	$1,000,000
B	Desired return on investment (ROI)[a]	Given	15%
C	Desired ROI in dollars[a]	A × B	$150,000
	Actual results		
D	Net revenues	Given	$500,000
E	Expenses	Given	$400,000
F	Net income	D − E	$100,000
G	ROI	F / A	10%

Conclusion: Although the Surgicenter made a profit of $100,000, it did not meet the desired ROI of 15% the first year.

[a]Per year.

PERSPECTIVE 11.1 PHYSICIANS EXPAND SERVICE LINE TO IMPROVE NET INCOME

Ambulatory Surgery Centers (ASCs) are looking to expand their service line by adding spine cases into the service mix. The first reason relates to the increasing market as the baby boomer generation ages: researchers claim that 80 percent of adults, primarily baby boomers, have lower back pain. The second driving force is that health insurers want to lower costs for this condition by moving these cases out of higher-cost hospital settings and into the lower-cost ASCs. The third reason highlights the profitable returns on spine procedures. For example, adding 450 spine cases would almost double the net income of one ASC, which has over 5,000 cases and a net income of $1.8 million.

Before pursuing such a venture, however, ASCs have to consider many factors. ASCs need to determine whether their physicians have conducted an adequate number of cases to ensure quality care, they must determine the capital equipment needs and the amount they will have to invest in this service, and they have to perform a thorough pro forma, return-on-investment analysis.

Source: Adapted from B. Herman, 3 reasons why ASCs should consider implementing spine cases, *Becker's ASC Review*, October 27, 2012, www.beckersasc.com/asc-turnarounds-ideas-to-improve-performance/3-reasons-why-ascs-should-consider-implementing-spine-cases.html.

require various responsibility centers to make a certain return. It is not the ownership status that makes a responsibility center an investment center; it is the requirement that it make a certain return.

Measuring the Performance of Responsibility Centers

The previous section categorized the different types of responsibility centers in terms of their increasing level of financial responsibility. However, measuring the performance of responsibility centers rests on the assumption that a responsibility center should be held accountable only for those things over which it has control. Thus responsibility is only one of three major attributes of a responsibility center. The other two are authority and accountability (Exhibit 11.4).

Responsibility, Authority, and Accountability

The relationship among responsibility, authority, and accountability is straightforward. Ideally, managers should be given the *authority* to carry out their *responsibilities*. To the extent that this occurs, managers should expect to be held *accountable* for the performance of their responsibility centers. Perspective 11.2 highlights the way that many hospitals have altered the salary structures for employed physicians to achieve desired outcomes.

    Responsibility refers to the duties and obligations of a responsibility center, *authority* is the power to carry out these duties and obligations, and

Responsibility
The duties and obligations of a responsibility center.

Authority
The power to carry out a given responsibility.

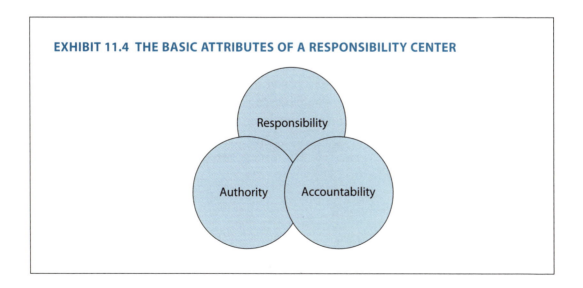

EXHIBIT 11.4 THE BASIC ATTRIBUTES OF A RESPONSIBILITY CENTER

Responsibility

Authority   Accountability

PERSPECTIVE 11.2 USE OF INCENTIVE PAY FOR HOSPITAL-BASED PHYSICIANS

More physicians are considering the security of a guaranteed income that may come with being employed by a hospital. Hospitals' typical compensation packages include a fixed salary coupled with an incentive system based on meeting productivity, quality, and performance measures.

According to one survey of 443 U.S. hospital medicine groups, carried out by the Society of Hospital Medicine (SHM) and the Medical Group Management Association (MGMA), only 21 percent of these groups paid their hospitalists a fully fixed salary, while 56 percent compensated their physicians with a combination of a fixed salary and productivity and/or performance incentives.

The survey also reported that hospitals were more likely to compensate their physicians with fixed salaries than were non-hospital-owned practices. Hospitals, on average, compensated their employed physicians with 82 percent base pay, 12 percent productivity incentives, and 6 percent performance incentives. In contrast, non-hospital-owned practices paid their physicians less in base salary, 69 percent, accompanied by 27 percent in productivity incentives and 4 percent from performance/quality incentives.

Hospitals have implemented various productivity measures based on relative value units, adjusted charges, collections, and volume of encounters. For example, a hospital may pay physicians a fixed dollar amount for each initial consult they perform. Performance-based incentives may relate to quality measures for heart failure, AMI, and pneumonia from the Centers for Medicare and Medicaid Services. Outcomes such as readmission rates and mortality were also used by some hospitals to determine base physician pay, as was timely completion of medical records.

Hospital medicine groups frequently use work relative value units (wRVUs) to measure productivity, but many also incorporate a per diem or shift rate for less busy times, such as night shifts. Other productivity measures cited in the SHM-MGMA survey included gross charges, adjusted charges, collections, number of encounters, and size of a physician's patient panel.

Finally, results from patient and nurse satisfaction surveys were also considered in hospital compensation models. For example, one hospital paid a quarterly productivity bonus of $3,000 for performing above a given patient satisfaction score.

Source: Adapted from J. Bowers, The different ways hospitals pay Incentive compensation aims to improve quality, productivity, *ACP Hospitalist*, October 2010, www.acphospitalist.org/archives/2010/10/money.htm.

accountability is the extent to which there are consequences—positive and/or negative—attached to carrying out responsibilities. Exhibit 11.4 shows that these three attributes do not always coincide, and discrepancies can lead to problems and frustrations. Exhibit 11.5 displays measures often used to evaluate the financial performance of responsibility centers.

Accountability
The extent to which there are consequences, both positive and negative, attached to carrying out responsibilities.

EXHIBIT 11.5 TYPICAL MEASURES USED TO EVALUATE THE FINANCIAL PERFORMANCE OF RESPONSIBILITY CENTERS

Performance Measures	Type of Center			
	Service Centers	Cost Centers	Profit Centers	Investment Centers
Budget variances				
Volume variances	☒	☒	☒	☒
Cost variances		☒	☒	☒
Acuity variances		☒	☒	☒
Revenue variances			☒	☒
Liquidity ratios				
Current ratio			☒	☒
Quick ratio			☒	☒
Days cash on hand			☒	☒
Activity ratios				
Asset turnover			☒	☒
Receivable turnover			☒	☒
Payables turnover			☒	☒
Capitalization ratios				
Debt to equity			☒	☒
Times interest earned			☒	☒
Debt service coverage			☒	☒
Profitability ratios				
Profit			☒	☒
Operating margin			☒	☒
Return on equity				☒
Return on assets				☒

Budget Variances

Budget Variance
The difference between what was planned (budgeted) and what was achieved (actual).

A *budget variance* is the difference between what was budgeted and what actually occurred. Exhibit 11.6 shows an example of a nonlabor budget for an ambulatory care clinic that originally budgeted 1,000 visits during the month but actually provided 1,200 visits. The clinic's expected net income was $35,000, and its actual net income was $47,000. Although it is tempting to assume that the $12,000 increase in net income was due to changes in the number of visits, often more than one factor is responsible for budget variances. The rest of this section presents an approach that systematically explains why a budget variance occurs.

As shown in Exhibit 11.7, it is common for health care organizations to separate their total budget variance (variance in net income) into the

---

EXHIBIT 11.6 REVENUE AND EXPENSE VARIANCE INFORMATION FOR AN AMBULATORY CARE CLINIC

	Givens	Budgeted	Actual	Variance	
A	Visits	1,000	1,200	200	
B	Revenues	$100,000	$117,000	$17,000	Favorable
C	Expenses	$65,000	$70,000	$5,000	Unfavorable
D	Net income	$35,000	$47,000	$12,000	Favorable

EXHIBIT 11.7 COMMON VARIANCES USED BY HEALTH CARE ORGANIZATIONS

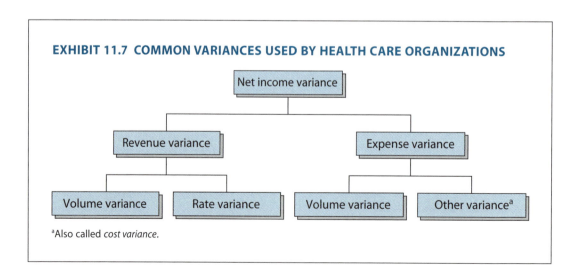

[a]Also called *cost variance*.

portion due to changes in revenue and the portion due to changes in expenses. The revenue variance is then broken down into the portion attributable to volume and the portion attributable to rate differences. The expense variance is subdivided into the portion due to volume and the part due to other factors. This model will now be used to explain the net income variance of $12,000 in Exhibit 11.6.

Revenue Variances

In Exhibit 11.6, both the number of visits and the revenues earned from them increased beyond what was budgeted. This resulted in a positive revenue variance of $17,000. This is called a *favorable* variance because more income was received than was budgeted. Using just this information, it is tempting to conclude that the increase in revenues was due to the increase in employees covered. In fact, a variance analysis of the change in revenues shows that this is only partly the case.

Step 1. Develop the Flexible Budget Estimate for Revenues

In addition to the budgeted estimate and actual results, a variance analysis involves one more piece of information, called a flexible budget estimate. The *flexible budget estimate* adjusts for the actual volume being different from what was planned. The flexible budget estimate is what would have been budgeted had the actual volume been known ahead of time. Determining the flexible budget estimate involves two steps: calculating the budgeted rate and then using this number to determine how much would have been budgeted had the actual volume been known.

Flexible Budget
A budget that accommodates a range or multiple levels of activities.

Step 1A. Determine the Budgeted Revenue per Unit

The budgeted revenues are $100.00 per visit. This is determined by dividing budgeted revenues, $100,000, by the budgeted number of visits, 1,000 (Exhibit 11.8, step 1A).

Step 1B. Develop the Flexible Budget Estimate

The flexible budget estimate is the budgeted revenue per visit multiplied by the actual volume ($100.00 per visit × 1,200 visits = $120,000). This is the amount that would have been budgeted for revenues had it been known when the original budget was made that the actual volume would be 1,200 rather than 1,000 visits (Exhibit 11.8, step 1B).

A flexible budget estimates the revenues or expenses, or both, over a range of volumes to forecast what the revenues and expenses would be at various levels. For example, by multiplying the $100.00 revenue per visit

EXHIBIT 11.8 ANALYSIS OF A REVENUE VARIANCE BY VOLUME AND RATE COMPONENTS

Givens

		Budgeted	Actual		Variance	
1	Visits	1,000	1,200		200	
2	Revenues	$100,000	$117,000		$17,000	Favorable
3	Expenses	$65,000	$70,000		$5,000	Unfavorable
4	Net income	$35,000	$47,000		$12,000	Favorable

Step 1. Develop flexible revenue budget estimate.

Step 1A. Calculate budgeted revenue per unit based on given information.

A	Budgeted revenue per month	Given 2	$100,000
B	Budgeted visits	Given 1	1,000
C	Budgeted revenue per visit	A / B	$100.00

Step 1B. Develop a flexible revenue budget containing the actual volume.

D	Volume (flexible)		1,000	1,100	1,200	1,300	1,400
E	Budgeted revenue per visit	C	$100.00	$100.00	$100.00	$100.00	$100.00
F	Total revenue	D × E	$100,000	$110,000	$120,000	$130,000	$140,000

Step 2. Compare the budgeted amount, the flexible budget at the actual volume, and the actual budget.

			Budgeted Revenues	Flexible Budget	Actual Revenues
G	Visits		1,000	1,200	1,200
H	Revenues		$100,000	$120,000	$117,000
I	Rate	H / G	$100.00	$100.00	$97.50

J	$20,000	($3,000)
	Volume variance[a]	Rate variance[b]
	(Favorable)	(Unfavorable)

[a]Volume Variance = (Actual Volume − Budgeted Volume) × Budgeted Rate = (1,200 − 1,000) × $100.00 = $20,000
[b]Rate Variance = (Actual Rate − Budgeted Rate) × Actual Volume = ($97.50 − $100.00) × 1,200 = −$3,000
Note: Of the $17,000 total revenue variance to be explained, the $20,000 increase is due to an increase in visits from 1,000 budgeted to 1,200 actual, and the $3,000 decrease is due to a decrease in the rate from $100.00 budgeted to $97.50 actual.

by a range of visits from 1,000 through 1,400, the clinic could develop a range of revenue estimates at selected levels (Exhibit 11.8, rows D through F).

Both the range of volume estimates and the gap between each estimate are open to judgment. However, the range should include both the budgeted and actual volumes. Using this approach, the clinic just as easily could have estimated the results for a range of 800 to 1,500 using steps of

100. Either way, at 1,200 visits the budget estimate would have been $120,000.

Step 2. Calculate the Revenue Variance Due to Changes in Volume and Rate

This step begins by laying out, side by side, the three revenue budget figures: budgeted amount, flexible budget, and actual revenues (Exhibit 11.8, rows G through I).

All that remains is to compare these three figures. The difference between the original budget, $100,000, and the flexible budget, $120,000, shows how much of the revenue variance is due to volume: $20,000 (Exhibit 11.8, row J). The difference between the flexible budget, $120,000, and actual results, $117,000, is the amount of the revenue variance that is due to a change in rate: −$3,000.

These differences can also be derived in another way. Looking at the volume variance, because the rate is held constant at $100.00 per visit, the only difference between the original budget and the flexible budget is volume (1,000 rather than 1,200 visits). Thus, using the formula

Revenue Volume Variance = (Actual Volume − Budgeted Volume) × Budgeted Rate

the *revenue volume variance* is $20,000 [(1,200 − 1,000) × $100.00]. That is, because volume increased by 200 at $100.00 per visit, $20,000 extra was earned.

The −$3,000 rate variance can be analyzed similarly. Because the flexible budgeted revenue per visit was $100.00 and the actual revenue is $97.50 per visit ($117,000 / 1,200), there has been a rate decrease of $2.50 per visit. Using the formula

Revenue Rate Variance = (Actual Rate − Budgeted Rate) × Actual Volume

the *revenue rate variance* is −$3,000: [($97.50 − $100.00) × 1,200]. Thus, because the organization earned $2.50 less per visit than was budgeted, and it provided 1,200 visits, the variance due to a change in rate is −$3,000.

The procedure to calculate revenue volume and rate variances is summarized in Exhibit 11.9.

Expense Variances

This section explains why the ambulatory clinic was $5,000 over its budgeted expenses ($65,000 − $70,000). As shown in Exhibit 11.10, analyzing expense variances is similar to analyzing revenue variances.

Revenue Volume Variance
The portion of total variance in revenues due to the actual volume being either higher or lower than the budgeted volume. It is the difference between the revenues forecast in the original budget and those in the flexible budget. It can be computed using the formula (Actual Volume − Budgeted Volume) × Budgeted Rate.

Revenue Rate Variance
The amount of the total revenue variance that occurs because the actual average rate charged varies from the one originally budgeted. It is the difference between the revenues forecast in the flexible budget and those actually earned. It can be calculated using the formula (Actual Rate − Budgeted Rate) × Actual Volume.

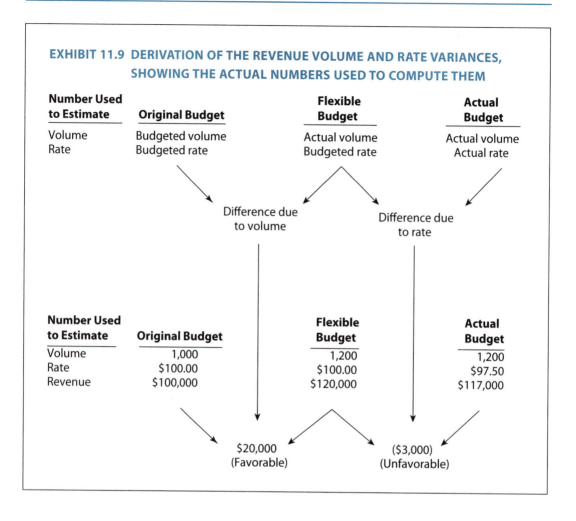

EXHIBIT 11.9 DERIVATION OF THE REVENUE VOLUME AND RATE VARIANCES, SHOWING THE ACTUAL NUMBERS USED TO COMPUTE THEM

Step 1. Identify the Amount of Variance Due to Fixed Costs

Although variable costs are directly affected by volume, fixed costs should not be. There are a number of reasons why fixed costs might have been incurred beyond what was budgeted. For example, additional depreciation might be taken on the purchase of new equipment, unanticipated raises given, or new employees hired. (Consider also that volume might go beyond the relevant range into a higher step of step-fixed costs.) This example assumes that fixed expenses increased because additional equipment had to be leased for $1,000 per month.

Original expense variance (Exhibit 11.6, row C)	$5,000
Amount explained by fixed expenses (Exhibit 11.10, row B)	1,000
Amount of expense variance still unexplained	$4,000

EXHIBIT 11.10 BREAKING DOWN THE EXPENSE VARIANCE INTO FIXED, VOLUME, AND COST VARIANCES

Step 1. Identify the amount of variance due to nonvariable expenses.

		Budgeted	Actual	Variance	
A	Volume	1,000	1,200	200	
B	Nonvariable expenses	$0	$1,000	$1,000	Unfavorable
C	Variable expenses	$65,000	$69,000	$4,000	Unfavorable
D	Total expenses	$65,000	$70,000	$5,000	Unfavorable

Step 2. Develop flexible expense budget estimate.

Step 2A. Calculate budgeted expense per unit based on information in step 1.

E	Budgeted total variable expenses	C	$65,000
F	Budgeted visits	A	1,000
G	Budgeted variable expenses	E / F	$65.00 Per visit

Step 2B. Develop a flexible expense budget using budgeted expense per unit.

H	Volume (flexible)		1,000	1,100	1,200	1,300	1,400
I	Budgeted variable expenses per visit	G	$65	$65	$65	$65	$65
J	Total variable expenses	H × I	$65,000	$71,500	$78,000	$84,500	$91,000

Step 3. Compare the budgeted expenses, the flexible budget at the actual volume, and actual expenses.

			Budgeted Expenses	Flexible Budget	Actual Expenses
K	Volume	A	1,000	1,200	1,200
L	Total variable expenses	C	$65,000	$78,000	$69,000
M	Expense per visit	L / K	$65.00	$65.00	$57.50

N	$13,000 Volume variance[a] (Unfavorable)	($9,000) Other variance[b] (Favorable)

Summary

Visits	1,200
Total variance to be explained	$5,000
Nonvariable variance	$1,000
Volume variance	$13,000
Variance due to other factors	($9,000)
Total unexplained variance	$0

[a]Volume Variance = (Actual Volume − Budgeted Volume) × Budgeted Rate = (1,200 − 1,000) × $65.00 = $13,000.
[b]Cost Variance = (Actual Cost − Budgeted Cost) × Actual Volume = ($57.50 − $65.00) × 1,200 = −$9,000.
Note: The $13,000 increase in expenses was due to an increase in visits from the 1,000 that were budgeted to 1,200, and also due to $1,000 from an increase in fixed costs from the amount budgeted. However, $9,000 in other savings were gained due to a decrease in per visit variable cost from the $65.00 budgeted to $57.50 actual.

This explains $1,000 of the $5,000 expense variance. The following steps explain the remaining $4,000 unfavorable expense variance due to variable expenses.

Step 2. Develop a Flexible Expense Budget

This step involves developing a flexible budget to determine how much would have been budgeted had it been known at the time the budget was prepared that the actual number of visits would be 1,200 and not 1,000.

Step 2A. Determine the Budgeted Cost per Unit

The budgeted cost per unit in the example is calculated by dividing the $65,000 in budgeted expenses by the 1,000 budgeted visits (Exhibit 11.10, rows E and F). Thus the budgeted cost per visit is $65.00 (Exhibit 11.10, row G).

Step 2B. Develop the Flexible Budget Estimate

The flexible expense budget estimate is the budgeted cost per unit multiplied by the actual volume ($65.00 × 1,200 = $78,000). This is the amount that would have been budgeted for expenses had it been known when the original budget was made that the actual volume would be 1,200 rather than 1,000 visits (Exhibit 11.10, rows H through J).

Step 3. Calculate the Expense Variance Due to Changes in Volume and Other Factors

As in step 2 of the revenue variance analysis presented earlier (Exhibit 11.8), this step begins by laying out side by side the three expense budget figures: budgeted, flexible, and actual expenses. As shown in Exhibit 11.10, step 3, the difference between the original budget, $65,000, and the flexible budget, $78,000, is the amount of the variance due to volume, $13,000 (rows L and N). The difference between the actual results and the flexible budget ($69,000 − $78,000 = −$9,000) is due to a change in costs per unit (also rows L and N). Note that this is a cost saving and is therefore considered *favorable*. Variable costs actually decreased from what was expected.

As with the revenue variances, expense variances can also be derived a different way. In regard to the volume variance, because the cost per unit is held constant ($65.00 per visit), the only difference between the original budget and the flexible budget is volume (1,200 rather than 1,000 visits). Thus, using the formula

Expense Volume Variance = (Actual Volume − Budgeted Volume) × Budgeted Cost per Unit the *expense volume variance* is $13,000: [(1,200 − 1,000) × $65.00]. This is because there were 200 more visits than budgeted at a cost of $65 per visit. The expense volume variance is the portion of total variance in variable expenses that is due to the actual volume being either higher or lower than the budgeted volume. It is the difference between the expenses forecast in the original budget and those in the flexible budget. It can be computed using the formula (Actual Volume − Budgeted Volume) × Budgeted Cost per Unit.

The $9,000 savings shown in the remaining variance, called a cost variance, can be analyzed similarly. Because the flexible budgeted cost per visit was $65.00 and the actual cost per visit is $57.50 ($69,000 / 1,200), there is a decrease in the cost per visit of $7.50. Using the formula

$$\text{Expense Cost Variance} = (\text{Actual Cost per Unit} - \text{Budgeted Cost per Unit}) \times \text{Actual Volume}$$

the *expense cost variance* is −$9,000. Thus, because the organization spent $7.50 less per visit than had been budgeted, and it provided 1,200 visits, the variance due to a change in cost per visit is −$9,000 (−$7.50 × 1,200). The procedure to calculate expense volume and cost variances is summarized in Exhibit 11.11.

Although the amount of the cost variance was calculated, the reason for it remains unclear in this example. The cost variance could be due to a variety of factors, including changes in quality, case mix, intensity of services, efficiency, and wages. Although it is possible to decompose the cost variance into other variances, that methodology is beyond the scope of this text.

 Key Point In the formula for expense volume variance, the sign of the answer is crucial. A negative answer indicates a decrease in volume, but this is considered a *favorable variance* because it leads to a decrease in costs. A positive answer indicates an increase in volume, and this is considered an *unfavorable variance* because it leads to an increase in costs.

Summary of the Example

When considering both revenues and expenses, the total variance was $12,000. Of this, on the one hand, a change in volume resulted in increased revenues of $20,000 and increased costs of $13,000. On the other hand, the

---

Expense Volume Variance
The portion of total variance in expenses that is due to the actual volume being either higher or lower than the budgeted volume. It is the difference between the expenses forecast in the original budget and those in the flexible budget. It can be computed using the formula (Actual Volume − Budgeted Volume) × Budgeted Cost per Unit.

Expense Cost Variance
The amount of the variable expense variance that occurs because the actual cost per unit varies from that originally budgeted. It is the difference between the variable expenses forecast in the flexible budget and those actually incurred. It can be calculated using the formula (Actual Cost per Unit − Budgeted Cost per Unit) × Actual Volume.

EXHIBIT 11.11 DERIVATION OF THE EXPENSE VOLUME AND COST PER UNIT VARIANCES, SHOWING THE ACTUAL NUMBERS USED TO COMPUTE THEM

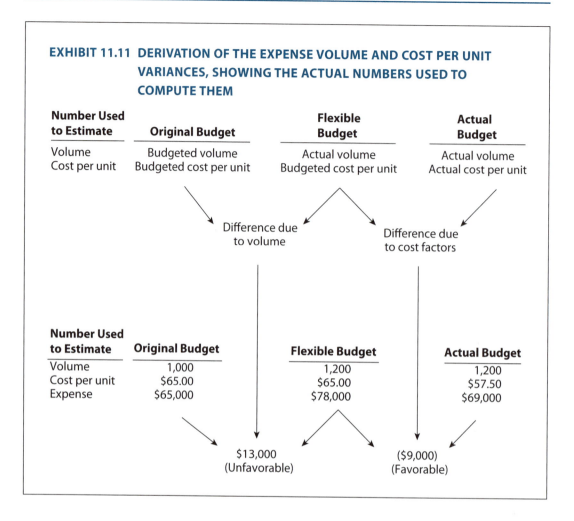

change in rate from $100.00 to $97.50 decreased revenue by $3,000, and the change in cost per unit from $65.00 to $57.50 accounted for $9,000 in savings from what was budgeted. Futhermore, an additional fixed cost was incurred by leasing equipment at $1,000 per month.

Increase in visits from 1,000 to 1,200 (revenues)	$20,000
Increase in visits from 1,000 to 1,200 (expenses)	(13,000)
Decrease in rates from $100.00 to $97.50 per visit	(3,000)
Decrease in cost per visit from $65.00 to $57.50 per visit	9,000
Increase in fixed costs from leasing additional equipment	(1,000)
Total variance explained	$12,000

Key Point In the formula for expense cost variance, the sign of the answer is crucial. A negative answer indicates a decrease in variable cost per unit, and this is considered a *favorable variance* because it leads to decreased costs. A positive answer indicates an increase in variable cost per unit, and this is considered an *unfavorable variance* because it leads to increased costs.

Beyond Variances

Budget variances are usually associated with the operating budget, which focuses on short-term *revenue attainment* (earning the amount of revenue budgeted) and *cost containment* (not spending more than budgeted). A longer-term focus is necessary to effect major efficiencies in the organization. Measures must be implemented to promote *revenue enhancement* (finding new sources of revenue) and *cost avoidance* (finding new ways to operate the business that eliminate certain classes of costs) in the long term. For instance, just-in-time (JIT) inventory methods deliver supplies "automatically" to the organization as needed, and they avoid many of the traditional costs of ordering, storing, and keeping track of inventories that flow through health care organizations. If only short-term measures were used, the initial costs might discourage an administrator from installing such a system; however, long-term measures might encourage such a decision.

Revenue Attainment
Earning the amount of revenue budgeted.

Cost Containment
Not spending more than is budgeted in the expense budget.

Revenue Enhancement
Finding supplemental sources of revenue.

Cost Avoidance
Finding ways to operate an organization that eliminate certain classes of costs.

Other Financial Performance Measures

Although budget variances are the most commonly used financial measures, various ratios are increasingly being used as financial performance measures for profit and investment centers. Although the use of these indicators is basically the same for profit centers and investment centers as it is for the organization as a whole, some complications arise when using these measures to judge the financial performance of divisions within the organization. The most common complications are these:

- They may promote a lack of goal congruence; that is, they may encourage the organizational unit to make decisions that are in its own best interest but not in the best interest of the organization as a whole.

- They may introduce complicated measurement problems. For instance, when two organizational units share the same assets, it is difficult to partition the assets between the two units when calculating such measures as return on assets.

- They may promote short-term thinking.

Compensation Systems

The responsibility, accountability, and authority components of responsibility centers do not operate in isolation and may be highly intertwined with the employee compensation system. Although these systems can be extremely complex, they can be thought of as falling into three major categories: salary-based, at-risk, and mixed systems (see Exhibit 11.12 and Perspective 11.2).

Salary-Based Compensation System

As the name implies, the fundamental attribute of a salary-based compensation system is that employees receive a guaranteed salary. Salaried employees know what they will get paid, and employers know what their salary expense will be over a given period of time. Such payments are based on employees "doing their job," and as such, provide no financial incentives to reward individual performance and promote group and organizational goals. Organizations may not provide rewards because it is felt they are not necessary or because the structure or infrastructure is not there to support them.

EXHIBIT 11.12 MAJOR EMPLOYEE COMPENSATION MODELS

Model	Major Attribute	Key Advantages	Key Disadvantages
Salary-based	Guaranteed salary.	Income predictability.	No financial incentives to reward individual performance and promote organizational goals.
At-risk	Amount of compensation is based totally on meeting performance goals.	Financial incentives to reward individual performance and promote organizational goals.	Income is not necessarily predictable and may be contingent on noncontrollable forces.
Mixed	Only a portion of salary is guaranteed, and remainder is based on meeting performance goals.	Combines a level of salary predictability with rewards for performance.	Depending on base and at-risk distribution, may have the disadvantages of both systems.

At-Risk Compensation System

In a full at-risk system, compensation is based totally on achieving certain targets, called *performance goals*. A major advantage of at-risk systems is that they financially reward performance and, when structured appropriately, can incentivize not only individual and group performance but also participation in activities that help the organization as a whole (such as assisting other departments to achieve their goals or serving on committees). A major disadvantage of total at-risk systems is that participants' revenues are uncertain, as are a portion of the organization's expenses. This can be especially problematic to the extent that noncontrollable forces (e.g., the economy) interfere with performance.

Mixed Compensation System

In a mixed system, a portion of compensation is at risk. When well designed, a mixed system can provide a base of certainty for part of individuals' compensation while also providing performance incentives. However, when not well structured, it may have the disadvantages of each of the other systems (see Exhibit 11.12).

Compensation System Design

In designing compensation systems, a number of factors should be considered, including the goals of the system, which can generally be categorized into goals pertaining to productivity and quality, financial viability, and general characteristics. In addressing each of these areas, both employers and employees have relatively specific concerns, which are presented in Exhibit 11.13.

EXHIBIT 11.13 KEY GOALS OF MAJOR EMPLOYEE COMPENSATION MODELS

Model	Productivity and Quality	Financial Viability	Basic Characteristics of Compensation System
Key employer concerns	Promotes *mission-*related goals	Promotes *margin-*related goals	Ease of implementation
Key employee concerns	Promotes personal work-life balance goals	Promotes financial goals	Fair, ease of understanding, ease of participating, and consistently applied
Focus of incentives	Productivity and quality	Revenue generation, resource use, and profitability	Sufficiently motivating to each party's goals

Summary

A growing trend in the structure of health care organizations is decentralization, which presents some interesting problems in the measurement of financial performance of organizational units. Decentralization is the degree of dispersion of responsibility within an organization.

The advantages of decentralization include more efficient use of time, more relevant information, higher-quality decisions, greater speed, better use of talent, and increased motivation and allegiance. The disadvantages include loss of control, decreased goal congruence, increased need for coordination and formal communication, and lack of managerial talent.

A responsibility center is an organizational unit that has been formally assigned the responsibility to carry out one or more tasks or to achieve one or more outcomes. There are four major types of responsibility centers:

- Service centers are responsible for ensuring that health care–related services are provided to a population in a manner that meets the volume and quality requirements of the organization. They have no direct budgetary control.

- Cost centers are responsible for providing services and controlling their costs. They are the primary level in the organization with direct budget control. The three types of cost centers in health care organizations are production, clinical, and administrative cost centers. Production cost centers develop and/or sell products. Clinical cost centers provide health care–related services to clients, patients, or enrollees. Administrative cost centers provide support to the clinical cost centers and the organization as a whole. Often included in this category are general administration, the business office, information services, admitting, medical records, and housekeeping.

- Profit centers are responsible for controlling costs and earning revenues. The three types of profit centers are traditional profit centers, capitated profit centers, and administrative profit centers.

- Investment centers are responsible for attaining a return on investment.

The relationship among responsibility, accountability, and authority is straightforward. Ideally, managers should be given the authority to carry out their responsibilities. To the extent that this occurs, managers are held accountable for the performance of their responsibility centers. Responsibility refers to the duties and obligations of a responsibility center; authority is the power to carry out a given responsibility; and accountability means there are consequences, both positive and/or negative, attached to carrying out responsibilities.

Cost, profit, and investment centers are held accountable for increasing levels of financial responsibility. (Service centers have no direct financial responsibilities.) Budget variances are the most universal measure of financial performance. A budget variance is the difference between what was budgeted and what actually occurred. It is common for health care organizations to separate their total budget variance (variance in net income) into revenue variances and expense variances. The revenue variance is broken down into volume and rate variances. The expense variance is separated into volume variance and other factors.

The revenue volume variance is the portion of total variance in revenues due to the actual volume being either higher or lower than the budgeted volume. It is the difference between the revenues forecast in the original budget and those in the flexible budget. It can be computed using the formula (Actual Volume − Budgeted Volume) × Budgeted Rate. The rate variance is the amount of the total revenue variance that occurs because the actual average rate received varies from that originally budgeted. It is the difference between the revenues forecast in the flexible budget and those actually earned. It can be calculated using the formula (Actual Rate − Budgeted Rate) × Actual Volume.

The expense volume variance is the portion of total variance in variable expenses due to the actual volume being either higher or lower than the budgeted volume. It is the difference between the expenses forecast in the original budget and those in the flexible budget. It can be computed using the formula (Actual Volume − Budgeted Volume) × Budgeted Cost per Unit.

The expense cost variance is the amount of the variable expense variance that occurs because the actual cost per visit varies from that originally budgeted. It is the difference between the variable expenses forecast in the flexible budget and those actually incurred. It can be calculated by the formula (Actual Cost per Unit − Budgeted Cost per Unit) × Actual Volume. Cost variance may be due to a variety of factors, including changes in quality, case mix, intensity of service, efficiency, and wages.

In addition to variances, which tend to focus on operational concerns, organizations may also be concerned with longer-term goals of revenue enhancement and cost avoidance. To attain operational as well as strategic goals, employers may often use financial and nonfinancial ratios and may use compensation systems designed to achieve various goals.

KEY TERMS

a.   Accountability

b.   Administrative cost center

c.   Administrative profit center

d.   Authority

e.   Budget variance

f.   Capitated profit center

g.   Clinical cost center

h.   Cost avoidance

i.   Cost center

j.   Cost containment

k.   Decentralization

l.   Expense cost variance

m.   Expense volume variance

n.   Flexible budget

o.   Investment center

p.   Production cost center

q.   Profit center

r.   Responsibility

s.   Responsibility center

t.   Revenue attainment

u.   Revenue enhancement

v.   Revenue rate variance

w.   Revenue volume variance

x.   Service center

y.   Traditional profit center

z.   Transfer price

Key Equations

*   Expense cost variance:

$$(\text{Actual Cost per Unit} - \text{Budgeted Cost per Unit}) \times \text{Actual Volume}$$

*   Expense volume variance:

$$(\text{Actual Volume} - \text{Budgeted Volume}) \times \text{Budgeted Cost per Unit}$$

*   Revenue rate variance:

$$(\text{Actual Rate} - \text{Budgeted Rate}) \times \text{Actual Volume}$$

*   Revenue volume variance:

$$(\text{Actual Volume} - \text{Budgeted Volume}) \times \text{Budgeted Rate}$$

REVIEW QUESTIONS AND PROBLEMS

1. **Definitions**. Define the key terms listed above.

2. **Advantages of decentralization**. List and discuss the advantages associated with decentralization.

3. **Disadvantages of decentralization**. List and discuss the disadvantages of decentralization.

4. **Types of responsibility centers**. What are the four types of responsibility centers? Describe the characteristics of each of them.

5. **Responsibility centers**.

   a. What is the most common type of responsibility center?

   b. What is the most basic type of responsibility center?

6. **Identifying responsibility centers**. Identify each responsibility center in the list below as either a service center, cost center (clinical or administrative), profit center (capitated or administrative), or investment center. Explain your choices:

   a. Radiology department that must control its own costs.

   b. Admitting department of a hospital.

   c. HMO.

   d. Stand-alone outpatient clinic that must earn a 10 percent ROI.

   e. Volunteer department with no budget.

   f. Development office.

7. **Relationship among accountability, responsibility, and authority**. What is the relationship among accountability, responsibility, and authority with respect to a responsibility center?

8. **Transfer prices**. What are transfer prices? Discuss their major disadvantages.

9. **Performance measures**. What is the most commonly used financial performance measure?

10. **Performance measures**. Name two financial measures that are used to judge the performance of investment centers and not used to measure the financial performance of profit centers.

11. **Performance measures**. What are major disadvantages of using traditional performance measures?

12. **Variance analysis**. What does the term *variance analysis* mean when applied to financial performance of health care organizations?

13. **Budget variances.** What are the most common types of budget variances found in health care organizations?

14. **Cost variances.** What occurrences can account for cost variances?

15. **ROI for an investment center.** An outpatient clinic invests $3,300,000. The desired ROI is 12 percent. In the first year, revenues are $1,750,000 and expenses are $1,270,000. Does the clinic meet its ROI requirement that year?

16. **ROI for an investment center.** A new cardiac catheterization lab was constructed at Have a Heart Hospital. The investment in this lab was $950,000 in equipment costs and $50,000 in renovation costs. A desired return on investment is 12 percent. Once the lab was operating, 7,000 patients were served in the first year and were charged $640 for each procedure. The annual fixed cost for the catheterization lab is $2 million, and the variable cost is $329 per procedure. What was the catheterization lab's profit? Did this profit meet its desired ROI?

17. **Detailed variance analysis.** The following are the planned and actual revenues for Cutting Edge Surgery Center. Because it is one of four surgery centers in the community, the administrator is concerned about its rates in relation to the rates of its competitors.

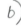

Givens

	Planned	Actual
Surgical volume	2,500	2,700
Gift shop revenues	$19,000	$20,000
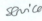 Surgery revenues	$600,500	$850,750
Parking revenues	$16,000	$18,000

a. Determine the total variance between the planned and actual budgets.

b. Determine the service-related revenues and calculate service-related variance still unexplained.

c. Prepare a flexible budget estimate. Present side by side the budget, flexible budget estimate, and actual surgical revenues (and related volumes).

d. Determine what variance is due to change in volume and what variance is due to change in rates.

e. Determine the volume variance and rate variance based on per unit rates.

18. **Detailed variance analysis.** The administrator of Break-a-Leg Hospital is aware of the need to keep costs down because he has just negotiated a new capitated arrangement with a large insurance company. The following are selected planned and actual expenses for the previous month.

Givens

	Planned	Actual
Patient days	27,000	26,000
gerille Pharmacy	$120,000	$160,000
Miscellaneous supplies	$66,000	$77,500
Fixed overhead costs	$808,000	$880,000

a. Determine the total variance associated with the planned and actual expenses.

b. Calculate the amount of service-related variance.

c. Prepare a flexible expense estimate for variable costs. Compare budgeted amount, flexible budget, and actual amount (show related volumes).

d. Determine what variance is due to change in volume and what variance is due to change in rates.

e. Determine the volume variance and rate variance based on per unit rates.

19. **Detailed variance analysis.** A dermatology clinic expects to contract with an HMO for an estimated 100,000 enrollees. The HMO expects one in four of its enrolled members to use the dermatology services per month. At the end of the year, the dermatology clinic's business manager looked at her monthly figures and saw that the number of enrolled members had increased by 5 percent over the budgeted amount and that one in three of the total HMO members had used the dermatology services per month. Net monthly revenues of the dermatology clinic were budgeted at $360,000 but were actually $550,000. Monthly expenses for the clinic were budgeted at $300,000 but were actually $370,000.

a. Prepare a monthly revenue and expense variance report for the clinic.

b. Are these variances favorable or unfavorable? Why?

20. **Detailed variance analysis.** The controller of the Conrad Aiken Surgical Center was reviewing monthly financial reports and noted some differences. The center had fallen 8 short of its plan to perform 450 procedures during the month. Despite that shortfall, surgical revenue exceeded the $830,250 budget, coming in at $848,640.

a. What was the total revenue per procedure projected in the flexible budget estimate?

b. Calculate the revenue volume variance and revenue rate variance. Was each favorable or unfavorable?

c. Calculate the total variance. Was it favorable or unfavorable?

21. **Detailed variance analysis.** The student clinic at Schumpeter University is run as a profit center. The dean of student services was reviewing the expenses on last month's financial report for the clinic, which also treated nonstudents on a fee-for-service basis. During the

month the building's furnace needed to be replaced, and the nonstudent department of the clinic was charged $400 for its share in addition to its normal fixed overhead assessment, which was usually $800. The dean was concerned because actual departmental expenses exceeded budget, but then noticed that 250 nonstudent patients had been treated, compared to a budget estimate of 150. And costs to serve the patients per unit were 10 percent below the $85.00 budgeted.

a. How much was the total expense variance? Was it favorable or unfavorable?

b. What was the variance for the variable costs? Was it favorable or unfavorable?

c. What was the flexible budget estimate?

d. What was the volume variance for the patient costs? The cost variance for patient costs?

22. Thor County Hospital is the only medical facility serving an area with a population of 8,400. In 20X1, the Radiology Department purchased a used CAT scanner from a larger hospital for $50,000. The purchase had not been anticipated when the department's 20X1 budget was drawn up, and the repair costs for the machine were $7,300 more than the expected $40,300. There were 680 scans performed rather than the 600 budgeted, and revenue was $300 less per scan than the $2,600 expected. During that period, additional temporary staff had to be used, which increased the variable costs per scan from $275 budgeted to an unexpected $475 per scan. Nonvariable expenses were budgeted at $40,300, and the repairs were the only variance.

a. Is the nonvariable expense variance favorable or unfavorable? What is the amount?

b. What is the unexplained cost-related variance?

c. Create a flexible budget for revenue.

d. What is the revenue rate variance? Is it favorable or unfavorable? What is the volume variance? Is it favorable or unfavorable?

e. Create a flexible budget for the variable cost.

f. What is the cost variance? Is it favorable or unfavorable? What is the volume variance due to cost? Is it favorable or unfavorable?

CHAPTER 12

PROVIDER COST-FINDING METHODS

Finding the costs to serve various populations (e.g., the elderly, Medicare patients, rehabilitation patients), to produce various goods and services, and to work with various payors (e.g., Medicaid, insurance companies) is an important activity for most health care providers. A *cost object* is anything for which costs are being estimated, such as a population, a test, a visit, a patient, or a patient day. This chapter discusses the three most commonly used approaches to find costs for various cost objects: the cost-to-charge ratio, the step-down method, and activity-based costing.

Cost-to-Charge Ratio

Historically, the *cost-to-charge ratio* (CCR) is one of the most common methods used by dentists and physicians to estimate costs. It is based on an assumed relationship of costs to charges, usually determined by industry norms or special studies. CCR begins with charges (or reimbursements) and assumes that costs are a certain percentage of this amount. For example, a group planning a dental office might use the rule of thumb that all nondirect labor expenses amounted to 22 percent of charges.

The main advantage of this approach is simplicity. The disadvantages include the following:

- Though the ratio used may be typical for the industry or a segment of the industry, it may not apply as well to any particular organization.

- When the ratio has been determined by a study, to the extent that actual volume or service mix deviates from the figures used in the study, the CCR may be inaccurate.

LEARNING OBJECTIVES

- Identify three methods to estimate costs.

- Calculate costs using the step-down method.

- Calculate costs using activity-based costing.

- Understand the major advantages and disadvantages of activity-based costing.

Cost Object
Anything for which a cost is being estimated, such as a population, a test, a visit, a patient, or a patient day.

Cost-to-Charge Ratio
A method to estimate costs that assumes costs are a certain percentage of charges (or reimbursements).

- To the extent that the fixed or variable cost composition has changed, the ratio may provide an inaccurate measurement.

- To the extent that an overall ratio is used for all procedures, the CCR may underestimate or overestimate the cost of individual procedures.

Although the CCR is relatively simple to implement, more complex health care organizations usually use a step-down or an activity-based costing approach, either of which is commonly thought to be more accurate but also more difficult to calculate.

Step-Down Method

A cost-finding method based on allocating costs that are not directly paid for to products or services to which payment is attached. The method derives its name from the stair-step pattern that results from allocating costs.

Step-Down Method

The *step-down method* is a cost-finding method based on allocating costs that are not directly paid for (indirect costs) to products or services that are directly paid for (direct costs). The example in Exhibit 12.1 shows three responsibility centers to which payment is not attached (utilities, administration, and laboratory) and three to which revenues are attached (walk-in services, pediatric services, and adolescent services). The goal of the step-down method is to allocate the costs of the support centers (utilities, administration, and laboratory) fairly among each of the three patient services. The full step-down allocation is shown in Exhibit 12.2.

EXHIBIT 12.1 EXAMPLE OF COSTS TO WHICH PAYMENT IS NOT DIRECTLY ATTACHED AND COSTS TO WHICH PAYMENT IS DIRECTLY ATTACHED

	Indirect Costs	
Utilities	$50,000	These costs, which are
Administration	100,000	← not paid for directly . . .
Laboratory	175,000	
	Direct Costs	
Walk-in clinic services	200,000	must be folded into
Pediatric services	200,000	← these services, to which
Adolescent clinic services	300,000	payment is attached.
Total costs	$1,025,000	

EXHIBIT 12.2 THE STEP-DOWN METHOD OF ALLOCATING COSTS

	Step 1. Compile Basic Statistics			Step 2. Compute Converted Statistics		
	A	B	C	D	E	F
	Square Feet	Dept. Costs	Lab Tests	Square Feet	Dept. Costs	Lab Tests
Utilities		$50,000				
Administration	1,000	$100,000		1,000		
Laboratory	2,000	$175,000		2,000	$175,000	
Walk-in services	2,000	$200,000	250	2,000	$200,000	250
Pediatric services	2,500	$200,000	450	2,500	$200,000	450
Adolescent services	2,500	$300,000	300	2,500	$300,000	300
Total	10,000	$1,025,000	1,000	10,000	$875,000	1,000

Step 3. Compute Allocation %

	G	H	I
	Utilities	Administration	Laboratory
	(Square Feet)	(Dept. Costs)	(Tests)
Utilities			
Administration	10%		
Laboratory	20%	20.0%	
Walk-in services	20%	22.9%	25%
Pediatric services	25%	22.9%	45%
Adolescent services	25%	34.3%	30%
Total	100%	100%	100%

Step 4. Allocate Costs[a]

	J	K	L	M	N
	Direct Costs	Utilities	Administration	Laboratory	Total
Utilities	$50,000	($50,000)			
Administration	$100,000	$5,000	($105,000)		
Laboratory	$175,000	$10,000	$21,000	($206,000)	
Walk-in services	$200,000	$10,000	$24,000	$51,500	$285,500
Pediatric services	$200,000	$12,500	$24,000	$92,700	$329,200
Adolescent services	$300,000	$12,500	$36,000	$61,800	$410,300
Total	$1,025,000	$0	$0	$0	$1,025,000

[a]Differences due to rounding.

There are four steps in allocating indirect costs to services for which payment is attached:

- Determine an allocation base and compile basic statistics.
- Convert basic statistics for the step-down approach.
- Calculate allocation percentages.
- Allocate costs from each support center to each of the centers below it (thus the *down* in *step-down*).

These steps will now be followed to allocate utilities, administration, and laboratory costs, respectively.

Allocating Utilities

Allocation Base

A statistic (e.g., square feet, number of full-time employees) used to allocate costs because it is assumed to be related to why the costs occurred.

An *allocation base* is a statistic used to allocate costs because it is related to why the costs occurred. Some common allocation bases are listed in Exhibit 12.3. The better the cause-and-effect relationship between the cost occurrence and the allocation basis, the more accurate the cost allocation. Because of their causal relationship to costs, allocation bases are also called *cost drivers* (discussed in more detail below). For instance, a common base for allocating utilities is square footage, on the assumption that actual utility usage is proportional to the size of the space a service occupies.

EXHIBIT 12.3 SOME COMMON ALLOCATION BASES

Costs to Be Allocated	Allocation Basis
Billing office	Number of bills
General administration	Costs of department
	Number of FTEs[a]
Laboratory[b]	Weighted average costs of tests
	Number of tests
Medical records	Number of records "pulled"
Nursing[b]	Nursing hours
	Acuity-weighted hours
Purchasing	Number of purchase orders
Rent, utilities, cleaning	Square feet

[a]Full-time equivalent employees.
[b]Laboratory and nursing are frequently charged directly to patients, rather than being allocated.

EXHIBIT 12.4 STEPS IN THE STEP-DOWN PROCESS RELEVANT TO THE ALLOCATION OF UTILITY COSTS

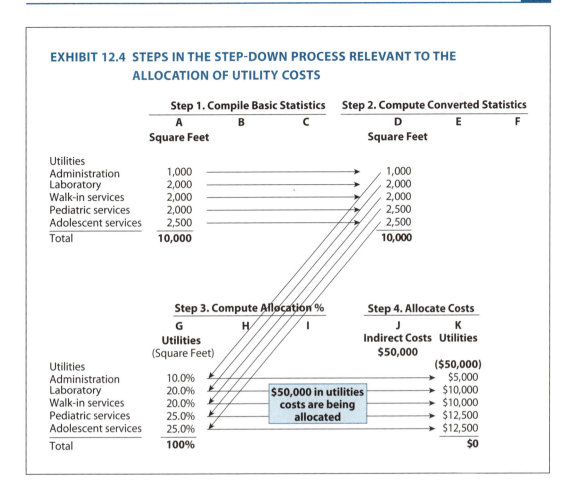

Exhibit 12.4 highlights those parts of Exhibit 12.2 relevant to allocating utilities. Because administration occupies 1,000 of the 10,000 square feet of the facility (Exhibit 12.4, columns A and D), it is allocated 10 percent (column G) of the $50,000 indirect cost of utilities, which is $5,000 (column K). Similarly, because the laboratory and the walk-in services each occupy 2,000 of the 10,000 square feet (columns A and D), each is allocated 20 percent (column G), which is $10,000 (column K). Finally, because the pediatric and adolescent services each occupy 2,500 square feet (columns A and D), each is allocated 25 percent (column G), which is $12,500 (column K).

Allocating Administrative Costs

Exhibit 12.5 highlights those parts of Exhibit 12.2 relevant to allocating administrative costs. Note that instead of allocating just the $100,000 in administrative costs that were there at the beginning of the allocation (column J), $105,000 is now being allocated from administration: $100,000 in original administrative costs, and the additional $5,000 that has been allocated to administration from utilities.

The allocation base used to allocate administration is direct costs of the responsibility centers (see Exhibit 12.5, column E), based on the assumption that administrative costs are incurred by each of the other responsibility centers in the same proportion as are their direct costs. Another allocation base sometimes used to allocate administrative costs is the number of FTEs (full-time equivalent employees) in each responsibility

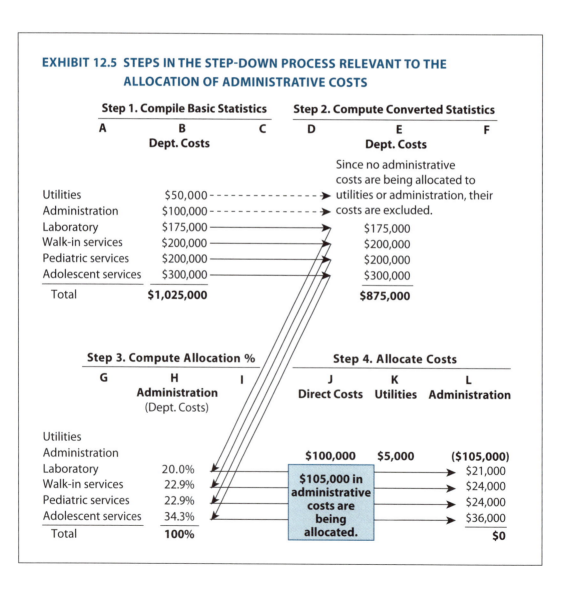

EXHIBIT 12.5 STEPS IN THE STEP-DOWN PROCESS RELEVANT TO THE ALLOCATION OF ADMINISTRATIVE COSTS

Step 1. Compile Basic Statistics

A	B	C
	Dept. Costs	
Utilities	$50,000	
Administration	$100,000	
Laboratory	$175,000	
Walk-in services	$200,000	
Pediatric services	$200,000	
Adolescent services	$300,000	
Total	$1,025,000	

Step 2. Compute Converted Statistics

D	E	F
	Dept. Costs	
	Since no administrative costs are being allocated to utilities or administration, their costs are excluded.	
	$175,000	
	$200,000	
	$200,000	
	$300,000	
	$875,000	

Step 3. Compute Allocation %

G	H	I
	Administration (Dept. Costs)	
Utilities		
Administration		
Laboratory	20.0%	
Walk-in services	22.9%	
Pediatric services	22.9%	
Adolescent services	34.3%	
Total	100%	

Step 4. Allocate Costs

J	K	L
Direct Costs	Utilities	Administration
$100,000	$5,000	($105,000)
$105,000 in administrative costs are being allocated.		$21,000
		$24,000
		$24,000
		$36,000
		$0

center. This assumes that administrative costs are incurred in proportion to the number of employees working in each responsibility center.

Although the procedure here is similar to allocating utilities, there is one major difference. Note that in column B of Exhibit 12.5, there is $1,025,000 in costs, including $50,000 in utilities and $100,000 in administrative costs, whereas in column E there is only $875,000 in costs because utilities and administrative costs have been omitted. This is done for two reasons: First, by convention, the step-down allocation method always proceeds downward from one responsibility center to those below it. Thus, no administrative costs are allocated (upward) to utilities. Therefore, the $50,000 in utilities cost is excluded (column E) when determining the proportional share of administration to be allocated on the basis of direct costs. Second, because administration is fully allocated to the services below it, it cannot give any of its cost to itself. Therefore, in using direct costs as the basis to determine what percentage of the administrative costs being allocated go to the services below it, the $100,000 in administrative indirect costs are omitted (column E).

Without the $150,000 of utilities and administration, there is $875,000 in costs over which to allocate administration. Laboratory has $175,000 in costs (column E), and thus it receives $175,000 / $875,000, or 20 percent (column H), of the $105,000 in administration being allocated, which is $21,000 (column L). The walk-in services clinic has $200,000 of direct costs (column E), so it receives $200,000 / $875,000, or 22.9 percent (column H), of the $105,000 in administrative costs being allocated, which is $24,000 (column L). The remaining administrative costs are allocated to the pediatric and adolescent services in a similar manner (column L).

Allocating Laboratory Costs

The only costs that have not yet been allocated are those of the laboratory. Note that in Exhibit 12.2, instead of the original $175,000 in indirect laboratory costs, $206,000 is being allocated (column M). That is because, in addition to its own costs, laboratory also includes $10,000 in costs allocated from utilities and $21,000 in costs allocated from administration.

Laboratory costs are allocated on the basis of lab tests under the assumption that the fair share of the laboratory costs due to each of the three services is in proportion to the number of tests each service ordered (see Exhibit 12.2, column C). Using lab tests as a basis, the walk-in services clinic is allocated 25 percent (column I) of the $206,000 (column M), which is $51,500 (column M). The pediatric services and the adolescent services clinics are allocated 45 percent and 30 percent, respectively (column I), of the $206,000 (column M), which are $92,700 and $61,800, respectively (column M).

Fully Allocated Cost

Fully Allocated Cost

The cost of a cost object that includes both its direct costs and all other costs allocated to it.

After all the indirect costs of the support services that are not directly paid for have been allocated to those services that are paid for, the totals are summed (see Exhibit 12.2, column N). Rather than the $200,000 it costs to deliver walk-in services when only direct costs are considered, the *fully allocated costs* are $285,500. Similarly, pediatric services changed from $200,000 to $329,200, and adolescent services changed from $300,000 to $410,300 when allocated costs are included. Thus, the fully allocated cost reflects both the original direct costs and all allocated indirect costs, but the total cost, $1,025,000, remains the same as before.

Here are some final comments regarding the step-down allocation method:

- To the extent that services use different allocation bases, the *order* in which the services are allocated makes a difference in the final costs. For example, if administration were placed ahead of utilities in the allocation order, the costs of walk-in, pediatric, and adolescent services would be different from those in the example. There are two sometimes conflicting rules of thumb to help with choosing a reasonable order: first, rank-order the centers being allocated from highest dollar amount to lowest dollar amount (according to this rule, in the example, laboratory and then administration should have been listed ahead of utilities); or second, list the centers from highest to lowest in an order that reflects the number of other centers they affect. It was for this reason that the centers were ordered as they were in the example, with laboratory being last.

- The *allocation basis* used to allocate costs makes a difference in the final costs. If instead of direct costs, the number of FTEs were the allocation basis for administration, and if there were a low correlation between the two, then the costs of walk-in, pediatric, and adolescent services would be different.

- The number of centers to which costs are allocated makes a difference. For example, if there were four services instead of three, then the costs allocated to the original three services (walk-in, pediatric, and adolescent) would be different (probably less).

- Although the step-down method is the most widely used, because it has been associated with Medicare reporting, there are several other related methods available to providers to calculate costs. These are the direct method, the double apportionment method, and the reciprocal method. Because they are used relatively infrequently, they are not discussed here.

• The step-down method is useful for pricing and reimbursement-related decisions but is less useful for controlling costs. There are other methods, including activity-based costing, that are better for cost control.

Most inpatient facilities use the step-down method to report their Medicare costs. However, as shown in Perspective 12.1, network integration has added to the complexity of cost-finding methodologies as services are being offered across a variety of settings. Perspective 12.2 illustrates problems that may arise in using a cost report as the basis for calculating a cost-to-charge ratio.

Activity-Based Costing

Although the step-down method of cost allocation is widely used to find the cost of services for pricing and reimbursement purposes, a newer

PERSPECTIVE 12.1 STEP-DOWN APPROACH MAY BE OUTDATED WITH CONTINUUM OF CARE FROM PROVIDERS

The movement to bundle systems based on episode of care across a continuum of providers is making the historical, step-down cost allocation models less effective in assessing true cost of care. This movement toward provision and coordination of care across a multitude of providers requires managers to not only analyze the location of the care but also to demonstrate how to reduce cost in the provision of care away from the hospital setting. Now health care managers need to investigate whether the various types of costs—fixed versus variable, direct versus indirect—possess a common definition across providers. For example, if a hospital has contracted with a rehab unit and a home health agency to provide post-acute care services, managers must measure whether these providers have implemented costing systems that can measure costs for each unit of service. If these providers have not implemented a cost accounting system, managers will need to develop a proxy measure for each unit of care. Finally, electronic health records and payment systems will help these providers and health care systems to maintain timely standards of costs based on monthly data rather than prior year fiscal-year data.

Source: Adapted from J. Glaser and A. Sett, Using technology to reveal true costs, *Healthcare Financial Management*, 2012;66(2):44–49.

PERSPECTIVE 12.2 COST-TO-CHARGE RATIO: QUICK APPROACH TO MEASURE DEPARTMENTAL PERFORMANCE

Can departmental managers assess their performance utilizing their hospital's Medicare cost report? Yes, this report is a quick and readily available assessment tool for a hospital's costs and a department's performance. For ancillary departments such as laboratory, radiology, operating room, and so forth, a health care manager can identify those departments with a ratio of costs to charges of less than 1.00, for profitable departments, and a ratio of greater than 1.00, for unprofitable areas. A ratio value greater than 1.00 indicates that a department's total costs exceed its gross charges and it is losing money, while a ratio value less than 1.00 means the hospital department is profitable. For unprofitable departments, health care managers can take action by lowering costs, raising charges, and/or eliminating the department. Typically, hospital ancillary departments, such as a skilled nursing facility (SNF), home health agency, clinic, or hospice, have values less than 1.00, to be certain their charges exceed the fully allocated costs, which include both direct costs of the department and allocated overhead expenses such as laundry and maintenance. Since departmental managers are unable to directly manage allocated expenses, top management may consider assessing the performance of departmental managers on the costs they can control, specifically the direct cost-to-charge ratio.

Source: Adapted from K. J. LaBrake and H. S. Pokrandt, Using the Medicare cost report to improve financial performance, *Healthcare Financial Management*, 2010;64(10):72–78.

Activity-Based Costing
A method of estimating the costs of a service or product by measuring the costs of the activities it takes to produce that service or product.

cost-finding method, called *activity-based costing* (ABC), is receiving increased attention from health care providers. ABC is based on the paradigm that activities consume resources and products consume activities (Exhibit 12.6). Therefore, if activities or processes are controlled, then costs will be controlled. Similarly, if the resources an activity uses can be measured, a more accurate picture of the actual costs of services can be found, as compared with traditional cost allocation.

Traditional cost allocation is called a top-down approach because it begins with all costs and allocates them downward into various services for which payment will be received (Exhibit 12.7a). ABC, conversely, is called a bottom-up approach because it finds the cost of each service at the lowest level, the point at which resources are used, and aggregates them upward into products (Exhibit 12.7b).

For example, in Exhibit 12.8, the service "Normal Delivery" comprises three intermediate products (or processes): prenatal visit, labor and delivery, and postpartum care. Each of these intermediate products encompasses a number of activities. For example, the prenatal visit includes a urinalysis,

EXHIBIT 12.6 PRODUCTS RESULT FROM ACTIVITIES AND PROCESSES, WHICH RESULT FROM THE UTILIZATION OF RESOURCES

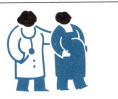

Healthier Patient

Products

  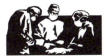

Admitting   Screening   Surgery   Rehabilitation

Activities and Processes

Supplies   Labor   Equipment

Resources

EXHIBIT 12.7a TRADITIONAL COSTING

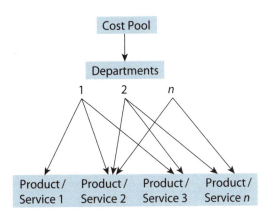

Cost Pool

Departments

1   2   n

Product / Service 1   Product / Service 2   Product / Service 3   Product / Service n

- Costs (e.g., *labor, supplies, facilities*) of various kinds of functions (e.g., purchasing, setup, monitoring, delivery of services)

- Organizational units that deliver or support the delivery of services

- Various services (e.g., lab tests, CBC, physical exam)

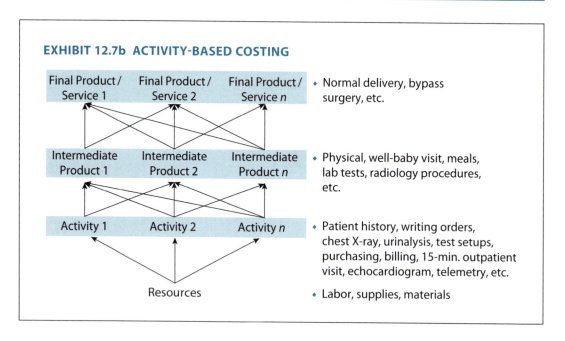

EXHIBIT 12.7b ACTIVITY-BASED COSTING

Final Product/ Service 1	Final Product/ Service 2	Final Product/ Service n	• Normal delivery, bypass surgery, etc.
Intermediate Product 1	Intermediate Product 2	Intermediate Product n	• Physical, well-baby visit, meals, lab tests, radiology procedures, etc.
Activity 1	Activity 2	Activity n	• Patient history, writing orders, chest X-ray, urinalysis, test setups, purchasing, billing, 15-min. outpatient visit, echocardiogram, telemetry, etc.
	Resources		• Labor, supplies, materials

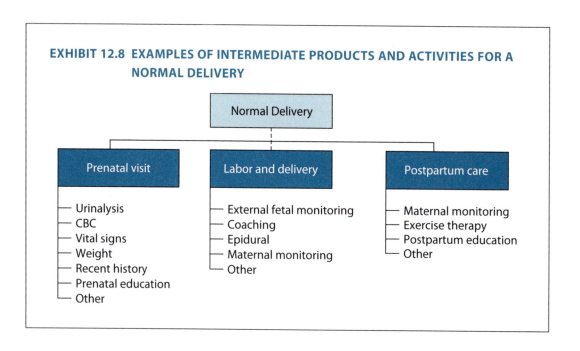

EXHIBIT 12.8 EXAMPLES OF INTERMEDIATE PRODUCTS AND ACTIVITIES FOR A NORMAL DELIVERY

Normal Delivery

Prenatal visit
- Urinalysis
- CBC
- Vital signs
- Weight
- Recent history
- Prenatal education
- Other

Labor and delivery
- External fetal monitoring
- Coaching
- Epidural
- Maternal monitoring
- Other

Postpartum care
- Maternal monitoring
- Exercise therapy
- Postpartum education
- Other

a complete blood count (CBC), vital signs, recent history, and so forth. Each of these activities might also include a portion of what are usually considered indirect costs, such as those associated with ordering supplies, updating medical records, or providing financial counseling.

Costing Terminology

Before continuing, it is important to understand three key terms: direct costs, indirect costs, and cost drivers. *Direct costs* are costs (e.g., nursing costs) that an organization can trace to a particular cost object (e.g., a patient). *Indirect costs* are costs that an organization is not able to trace directly to a particular cost object. For example, many health care organizations have great difficulty tracing to a particular patient or service such items as the cost of the billing clerk, rent, or information systems. Thus, a cost is not direct or indirect by its nature but by the ability or inability of the organization to trace it to a cost object.

An important difference between traditional cost allocation and activity-based costing is how each handles indirect costs. Traditional cost allocation methods usually deal with indirect costs by allocating them to cost objects using relatively gross cause-and-effect relationships, as described earlier. ABC attempts to overcome this problem by more directly tracing costs to their cost objects or by finding more precise cost drivers. *Cost drivers* are things that cause a change in the cost of an activity.

For example, under traditional step-down costing, purchasing costs might be bundled with other administrative costs and allocated to a service based on the relative size of its budget. Under ABC, it is more likely that the costs of purchasing would be allocated to that service more precisely on the basis of the number of purchase orders emanating from that service or even more precisely by measuring the number of minutes spent processing purchase orders from that department.

Direct Costs
Costs (e.g., nursing costs) that an organization can trace to a particular cost object (e.g., a patient).

Indirect Costs
Costs that cannot be traced to a particular cost object. Common indirect costs are billing, rent, utilities, information services, and overhead. Typically, these costs are allocated to cost objects according to an accepted methodology (e.g., the step-down method).

Cost Driver
That which causes a change in the cost of an activity.

An Example

Exhibit 12.9 compares the results of a traditional cost allocation approach with the results of an ABC approach. In this example, the organization is offering three outpatient services: an initial visit, a routine regular visit, and an intensive visit. It is assumed that labor and materials can be directly traced to each type of visit and therefore that labor and materials costs do not vary between the two cost-finding approaches. Thus, the main difference between the two approaches (as is often the case in practice) is in the allocation of overhead. As explained below, the traditional approach, on the one hand, uses a single cost driver, visits, and thus assigns the same

EXHIBIT 12.9 A COMPARISON OF THE RESULTS OF USING A CONVENTIONAL VERSUS AN ABC APPROACH TO COSTING THREE SERVICES

	Conventional Cost Method Visit Type			Activity-Based Costing Visit Type		
Per visit costs	**A** Initial	**B** Regular	**C** Intensive	**D** Initial	**E** Regular	**F** Intensive
1 Direct materials (etc.)	$2.50	$3.00	$10.00	$2.50	$3.00	$10.00
2 Direct labor	$45.00	$27.00	$75.00	$45.00	$27.00	$75.00
3 Estimated overhead	$17.50	$17.50	$17.50	$34.56	$11.73	$15.75
4 Total cost per visit	$65.00	$47.50	$102.50	$82.06	$41.73	$100.75
Total visit costs						
5 Direct materials (etc.)	$5,000	$15,000	$30,000	$5,000	$15,000	$30,000
6 Direct labor	$90,000	$135,000	$225,000	$90,000	$135,000	$225,000
7 Estimated overhead	$35,000	$87,500	$52,500	$69,125	$58,625	$47,250
8 Total costs	$130,000	$237,500	$307,500	$164,125	$208,625	$302,250

Difference in Cost Estimates
(ABC – Traditional)
Visit Type

	G Initial	**H** Regular	**I** Intensive
Per visit costs			
1 Direct materials (etc.)	$0.00	$0.00	$0.00
2 Direct labor	$0.00	$0.00	$0.00
3 Estimated overhead	$17.06	($5.78)	($1.75)
4 Total cost per visit	$17.06	($5.78)	($1.75)
Total visit costs			
5 Direct materials (etc.)	$0.00	$0.00	$0.00
6 Direct labor	$0.00	$0.00	$0.00
7 Estimated overhead	$34,125	($28,875)	($5,250)
8 Total costs	$34,125	($28,875)	($5,250)

overhead cost per visit ($17.50) to all three services (row 3, columns A, B, and C). The ABC approach, on the other hand, uses three cost drivers and derives an overhead cost per visit of $34.56 for an initial visit, $11.73 for a regular visit, and $15.75 for an intensive visit (row 3, columns D, E, and F). Thus, relative to the traditional approach, the ABC approach estimates overhead cost to be $17.06 higher than the average $17.50 for an initial visit, and $5.78 and $1.75 lower for a regular and intensive visit, respectively (row 3, columns G, H, and I).

When spread across all 10,000 visits, these unit cost differences result in considerably different estimates of the total cost for each type of visit. Using the $17.50 estimate for overhead costs for each visit, the conventional method estimates the total costs of an initial, regular, and intensive visit to be, respectively, $130,000, $237,500, and $307,500 (row 8, columns A, B, and C). On the other hand, the ABC approach estimates the total costs of initial, regular, and intensive visits to be, respectively, $164,125, $208,625, and $302,250 (row 8, columns D, E, and F). Thus, the ABC approach estimates the initial visit cost as $34,125 more than what was estimated using a conventional approach, and the regular and intensive visits costs as $28,875 and $5,250 less, respectively, than the conventional approach's estimate (row 8, columns G, H, and I). Such differences can be highly significant when making decisions. In the case of the initial visits, the cost estimate differed by more than 26 percent ($34,125 / $130,000 = 0.2625). Exhibit 12.10 illustrates more closely how the numbers in Exhibit 12.9 were derived.

In Exhibit 12.10, the total overhead cost is $175,000 (row 4, column D). Under the conventional method, it is assumed that all overhead costs are driven by visits. Thus, the $175,000 in overhead is divided by the 10,000 visits made during the year to calculate the average cost per visit for each type of visit, $17.50 (row 4, columns E, F, G, and H).

Rather than assuming that overhead costs are driven solely by the number of visits, the ABC approach assumes multiple cost drivers. In this case, the ABC approach breaks down overhead costs into four categories and looks more closely at what may be driving the $175,000 overhead cost. The four categories are the intake process, medical records, billing, and other (see rows 6 through 9). The intake process occurs when background information is gathered and an account is set up for each new patient. It is assumed that these costs occur each time a new-patient visit occurs; thus, the cost driver is a new-patient visit (row 6, column J). Assuming that the total salaries and benefits of all the employees engaged in this process are $26,250 (row 6, column I) and there are 2,500 visits a year (row 6, column K), the intake process costs the organization

EXHIBIT 12.10 A COMPARISON OF A CONVENTIONAL AND AN ABC APPROACH TO COSTING THREE SERVICES

Givens: overall percentages and totals

	GA	GB	GC	GD	GE	GF	GG
			Visit Type				
	Initial	Regular	Intensive	Row Total	Overhead Total	Total	Annual Hours
Number of visits	20%	50%	30%	100%		10,000	
Number of new visits	80%	10%	10%	100%		2,500	
Direct materials (etc.)	10%	30%	60%	100%		$50,000	
Direct labor	20%	30%	50%	100%		$450,000	
Intake or referral	70%	10%	20%	100%	15%		2,040
Medical records	30%	40%	30%	100%	15%		2,040
Billing	50%	20%	30%	100%	30%		4,080
Other	33%	33%	33%	100%	40%		
Total overhead					100%	$175,000	

Basic data and calculation of unit costs using a conventional approach

	Basic Data: Total Cost by Visit Type				Calculation of Cost: Unit by Visit Type			
	A	**B**	**C**	**D**	**E**	**F**	**G**	**H**
	Initial	Regular	Intensive	Total	Initial	Regular	Intensive	Cost per Unit Formula
	(Given)	(Given)	(Given)	(A + B + C)				
1 Number of visits	2,000	5,000	3,000	10,000				
2 Direct materials (etc.)	$5,000	$15,000	$30,000	$50,000	$2.50	$3.00	$10.00	(Row 2 / Row 1)
3 Direct labor	$90,000	$135,000	$225,000	$450,000	$45.00	$27.00	$75.00	(Row 3 / Row 1)
4 Estimated overhead (total is a given)				$175,000	$17.50	$17.50	$17.50	(D4 / D1)
5 Cost per visit: conventional method					$65.00	$47.50	$102.50	(Sum: Rows 2–4)

EXHIBIT 12.10 (CONTINUED)

(1) Annual projections of overhead costs by activity and cost driver; (2) Unit cost calculations for these overhead activities

Cost and Cost Driver Information

	I Cost (Given)	J Driver (Given)	K Units (Given)	L Unit Cost (I / K)
Activity				
6 Intake	$26,250	New visits	2,500 new visits	$10.50 per new visit
7 Medical records	$26,250	Hours spent	2,040 hours	$12.87 per hour
8 Billing	$52,500	Hours spent	4,080 hours	$12.87 per hour
9 Other	$70,000	Visits	10,000 visits	$7.00 per visit
10 Total	$175,000			

(3) Basic data: actual annual operating results of cost drivers to be used in assigning ABC overhead cost

Visit Type

	M Initial (Given)	N Regular (Given)	O Intensive (Given)	P Total (M + N + O)
11 New visits	2,000	250	250	2,500
12 Medical records	612	816	612	2,040
13 Billing	2,040	816	1,224	4,080
14 Other	2,000	5,000	3,000	10,000

(Continued)

Additional basic data

EXHIBIT 12.10 (CONTINUED)

Calculation of total and per visit overhead costs using ABC

	Q	R	S	T	U
		Visit Type			
	Initial	**Regular**	**Intensive**	**Total**	**Formula**
15 New visits	$21,000	$2,625	$2,625	$26,250	(L6 × Row 11)
16 Medical records	$7,875	$10,500	$7,875	$26,250	(L7 × Row 12)
17 Billing	$26,250	$10,500	$15,750	$52,500	(L8 × Row 13)
18 Other	$14,000	$35,000	$21,000	$70,000	(L9 × Row 14)
19 Total	$69,125	$58,625	$47,250	$175,000	(Sum: Rows 15–18)
20 Per visit	$34.56	$11.73	$15.75	$17.50	(Row 19 / Row 1)

Unit cost estimates using ABC

	V	W	X	Y
		Visit Type		
ABC	**Initial**	**Regular**	**Intensive**	**Formula**
21 Direct materials	$2.50	$3.00	$10.00	(Row 2, cols. E, F, G)
22 Direct labor	$45.00	$27.00	$75.00	(Row 3, cols. E, F, G)
23 Overhead	$34.56	$11.73	$15.75	(Row 20)
24 Total using ABC	$82.06	$41.73	$100.75	(Sum: Rows 21–23)

EXHIBIT 12.10 (CONTINUED)

Comparison of unit costs: ABC versus conventional

		Visit Type				
	Z Initial	AA Regular	AB Intensive	AC		AD Formula
25 Total conventional	$65.00	$47.50	$102.50			(Row 5, cols. E, F, G)
26 **Amount ABC estimate is more (less) than conventional**	$17.06	($5.78)	($1.75)			(Row 24 − Row 25)

Comparison of total costs: ABC versus conventional

		Visit Type		Total		
	AE Initial	AF Regular	AG Intensive	AH (AE + AF + AG)		AI Formula
Activity-based costing method						
27 Number of visits	2,000	5,000	3,000	10,000		(Row 1)
28 Direct materials	$5,000	$15,000	$30,000	$50,000		(Row 2)
29 Direct labor	$90,000	$135,000	$225,000	$450,000		(Row 3)
30 Overhead	$69,125	$58,625	$47,250	$175,000		(Row 27 × Row 23)
31 **Total ABC**	**$164,125**	**$208,625**	**$302,250**	**$675,000**		(Sum: Rows 28–30)
Conventional method						
32 Direct materials	$5,000	$15,000	$30,000	$50,000		(Row 2)
33 Direct labor	$90,000	$135,000	$225,000	$450,000		(Row 3)
34 Overhead	$35,000	$87,500	$52,500	$175,000		(Row 27 × Row 5, E,F,G)
35 **Total conventional**	**$130,000**	**$237,500**	**$307,500**	**$675,000**		(Sum: Rows 32–34)
36 **Amount ABC estimate is more (less) than conventional**	$34,125	($28,875)	($5,250)	$0		(Row 31 − Row 35)

$10.50 ($26,250 /$2,500) for each new patient (row 6, column L). Because there were 2,000 new patients making initial visits, 250 new patients each making a regular visit (referrals), and 250 patients making an intensive visit (row 11, columns M, N, O, and P), it costs $21,000 for the intake process for these new patients ($10.50 / patient × 2,000 new patients) and $2,625 each ($10.50 / patient × 250 patients) for regular and intensive visits, respectively (row 15, columns Q, R, S, T, and U).

The second category, medical records, refers to the process of coding and charting the visit onto the medical records (row 7). Because it is assumed that these costs are driven by the time spent coding and charting, the cost driver is hours spent (row 7, column J). Because the salary and benefit costs associated with medical records are $26,250 and there are 2,040 hours devoted to this activity, the cost per hour is $12.87 (row 7, columns I, J, K, and L). The medical records staff estimate that they spent 30 percent, 40 percent, and 30 percent of their time with initial, regular, and intensive visit records, respectively ("Givens" section, columns GA, GB, and GC). This equates to 612, 816, and 612 hours for each of the respective types of visits (row 12, columns M, N, O, and P). At $12.87 per hour, the initial visits medical record cost is $7,875 ($12.87 / hour × 612 hours), whereas the regular and intensive visit medical record cost is $10,500 ($12.87 / hour × 816 hours) and $7,875 ($12.87 / hour × 612 hours), respectively (row 16, columns Q, R, S, T, and U; differences due to rounding).

The billing costs and other costs are derived in a similar manner to those just discussed. When this process is completed, the estimated total overhead cost of initial visits is $69,125, and the overhead costs for regular and intensive visits are $58,625 and $47,250, respectively (row 19, columns Q, R, and S). Dividing these numbers by the number of visits in their respective categories (rows 1, 19, and 20) results in the per visit cost estimates of $34.56 ($69,125 / 2,000 visits) for initial visits, $11.73 ($58,625 / 5,000 visits) for regular visits, and $15.75 ($47,250 / 3,000 visits) for intensive visits. As can be seen, these numbers are different from the $17.50 overhead cost per visit estimated using the conventional approach, though the overall average is the same (column T).

The various parts are now in place to compare costs using a conventional approach and an ABC approach. Under the ABC approach, the per visit costs for an initial, regular, and intensive visit, respectively, are $82.06, $41.73, and $100.75 (row 24, columns V, W, and X). Under the conventional method, they are $65.00, $47.50, and $102.50, respectively, for these same types of visits (row 25, columns Z, AA, and AB). Thus, on a comparative basis, the ABC approach estimates that the cost of an initial visit is

$17.06 higher than that calculated using the conventional approach, and the costs of a regular and an intensive visit are $5.78 and $1.75 lower, respectively (row 26, columns Z, AA, and AB).

The differences between the cost per visit estimates using ABC and a conventional approach are due totally to how the overhead is handled. The conventional approach used a single cost driver, total visits, to derive a $17.50 per visit overhead rate (row 4, columns E, F, and G). As stated above, the ABC approach decomposed overhead into four separate categories of activities. It then determined the unit cost of each type of activity based on what was driving these costs. Thus the ABC approach more closely matched the actual usage of resources by each type of visit.

The importance of having the more accurate cost estimates from ABC cannot be overemphasized. For example, assume that a practice decided to charge $75.00 per visit for initial visits, thinking its costs were $65.00, as derived by the conventional method, but its costs were really $82.06 (as shown by using ABC). It would be pricing at a loss, when it thought it was making a profit.

Caution: Though more precise, ABC costs are still average costs. As noted in Chapter Nine, incremental costs should be used in make-or-buy types of decisions.

There are a number of other differences between the traditional step-down and ABC methods, but a discussion of these is beyond the scope of this text. The important issue here is that in many cases these two methods are likely to yield vastly different estimates of cost. Although the step-down method is relatively inexpensive to implement and may provide an adequate estimate in some cases, those using ABC feel it provides several advantages, including increased accuracy and insights on how to control processes and thus costs. In the future, the management of most health care facilities will be faced with weighing the relatively low costs of the step-down method against the added costs, greater precision, and cost-control uses of ABC. In an increasingly cost-driven health care system, it is likely that activity-based costing will gain greater prominence.

Summary

Because providers are assuming more risk, they must be able to measure their costs accurately. Providers generally use one of three approaches: the cost-to-charge ratio, the step-down method, or activity-based costing. The step-down method finds costs by allocating those costs that are not directly paid for into products or services to which payment is attached. It is a top-down approach because it begins with all costs and allocates them downward into various services for which payment will be received. As a result of methodological idiosyncrasies, those performing a step-down cost finding must pay considerable attention to the order of allocation, the allocation basis, and the number of cost centers. The step-down method is useful for pricing and reimbursement-related decisions but should not be used to control costs.

Activity-based costing not only finds costs but also helps to control them. ABC is a bottom-up approach because it finds the cost of each service at the point at which resources are used and then aggregates them upward into products. ABC is based on the paradigm that activities consume resources and processes consume activities. Therefore, because the use of resources is what causes cost (by definition), if activities or processes are controlled, then costs will be controlled. Similarly, if the resource use of an activity can be measured, then a more accurate picture of the actual costs of services can be determined.

KEY TERMS

a. Activity-based costing

b. Allocation base

c. Cost driver

d. Cost object

e. Cost-to-charge ratio

f. Direct costs

g. Fully allocated cost

h. Indirect costs

i. Step-down method

REVIEW QUESTIONS AND PROBLEMS

1. **Definitions**. Define the key terms listed above.

2. **Cost-to-charge ratio**. What is the basic concept of the cost-to-charge ratio method of estimating costs? Give an example.

3. **Cost-to-charge ratio**. What are the four major concerns with using the cost-to-charge ratio method?

4. **Step-down method**. How did the step-down method of cost allocation acquire its name?

5. **Cost allocation and cost drivers**. What is the relationship between the concept of the cost allocation basis, used in the step-down method, and the concept of the cost driver, used in activity-based costing (ABC)?

6. **Fully allocated costs**. What is the difference between a cost object's direct cost and its fully allocated cost? Give an example.

7. **Step-down method**. Identify and discuss four points that must be considered when using the step-down method of cost allocation.

8. **ABC and step-down methods**. What are the advantages and disadvantages of ABC relative to the step-down method of cost allocation?

9. **Activity-based costing**. Referring to Exhibit 12.10, suppose that instead of 2,000, 5,000, and 3,000 visits for an initial, regular, and intensive visit, respectively, the number of visits was 3,000, 5,000, and 2,000. Assume that the costs associated with intake, new visits, medical records, and billing do not change in number or distribution.

   a. Would there be a change in the overhead cost *per visit* of an initial visit using either the conventional or ABC methods?

   b. Would there be a change in the *total* overhead cost of initial visits using either the conventional or ABC methods?

10. **Activity-based costing**. Referring to Exhibit 12.10, suppose that instead of 2,000, 5,000, and 3,000 visits for an initial, regular, and intensive visit, respectively, the number of visits was 2,500, 6,000, and 1,500. Assume that the costs associated with intake, new visits, medical records, and billing do not change in number or distribution.

   a. Would there be a change in the overhead cost per visit of an initial visit using either the conventional or ABC methods?

   b. Would there be a change in the total overhead cost of initial visits using either the conventional or ABC methods?

11. **Cost allocation**. Use the information in Exhibit 12.11 to answer these questions.

   a. Louis Clark, the new administrator for the surgical clinic, was trying to figure out how to allocate his indirect expenses. His staff were complaining that the current method of taking a percentage of revenues was unfair. He decided to try to allocate utilities expense based on square footage for each department, to allocate administration expense based on direct costs, and to allocate laboratory expense based on tests. What would the results be?

   b. Carol West, the nurse manager of the cystoscopy suite, was given approval to add more space to her current area by converting 500 square feet of administrative space into another cystoscopy bay. What will her new fully allocated expenses be? (Assume that there are no new additional costs incurred by adding the 500 square feet.)

EXHIBIT 12.11 BASIC STATISTICS FOR COST ALLOCATION IN A SURGERY CLINIC, FOR PROBLEM 11

	A Square Feet	B Dept. Costs	C Lab Tests
Utilities		$400,000	
Administration	4,000	$700,000	
Laboratory	2,000	$750,000	
Day-op suite	4,000	$2,500,000	6,000
Cystoscopy	2,000	$575,000	2,000
Endoscopy	1,000	$300,000	1,500
Total	**13,000**	**$5,225,000**	**9,500**

c.   Bobbie Jones, the manager of the endoscopy suite, is concerned about adding more space. She contends that if the cystoscopy and endoscopy units were combined, fewer staff would be needed, and direct costs could be reduced by $50,000 ($25,000 in each unit). She also feels that the day-op area is underutilized, and that 500 square feet could be used by a combined unit when excess capacity was needed. Assuming that the 500 square feet were to be allocated equally between the endoscopy and cystoscopy suites, in addition to the renovations as described in part b, what would the total allocated costs for each of these two services be under this scenario?

12. **Cost allocation.** Use the information in Exhibit 12.12 to answer these questions.

a.   Dick Clark, the new administrator for the surgical clinic, was trying to figure out how to allocate his indirect expenses. He decided to try to allocate utilities based on square footage of each department, to allocate administration based on direct costs, and to allocate laboratory based on tests. How would indirect costs be distributed as a result?

b.   Joe Ryan, the director of laboratories, was given approval to add 250 square feet of space to the lab by expanding into the day-op suite, which lost the space. What will his new fully allocated expenses be? (Assume that there are no new additional costs incurred by adding the 250 square feet.)

c.   Mary Jones, the manager of the endoscopy suite, is concerned about adding more space. She contends that if the cystoscopy and endoscopy units were combined,

EXHIBIT 12.12 BASIC STATISTICS FOR COST ALLOCATION IN A SURGERY CLINIC, FOR PROBLEM 12

	A Square Feet	B Dept. Costs	C Lab Tests
Utilities		$300,000	
Administration	3,000	$700,000	
Laboratory	4,000	$800,000	
Day-op suite	5,000	$1,800,000	6,000
Cystoscopy	2,000	$600,000	2,000
Endoscopy	2,500	$650,000	2,000
Total	**16,500**	**$4,850,000**	**10,000**

fewer staff would be needed, and direct costs could be reduced by $40,000 ($20,000 in each unit). She also feels that the day-op area is underutilized and that 200 square feet could be used by a combined unit when excess capacity was needed. Assuming that the 200 square feet were to be allocated equally between the endoscopy and cystoscopy suites, in addition to the renovations as described in part b, what would the total allocated costs for each of these two services be under this scenario?

13. **Traditional and activity-based costing.** Use the information in Exhibit 12.13 to answer these questions.

   a. What is the per unit cost of an initial, regular, and intensive visit using the conventional and ABC approaches?

   b. What is the total cost of initial, regular, and intensive visits using the conventional and ABC approaches?

14. **Traditional and activity-based costing.** Use the information in Exhibit 12.14 to answer these questions.

   a. What is the per unit cost of an initial, regular, and intensive visit using the conventional and ABC approaches?

   b. What is the total cost of initial, regular, and intensive visits using the conventional and ABC approaches?

EXHIBIT 12.13 DATA FOR TRADITIONAL AND ABC COST ALLOCATION, FOR PROBLEM 13

Basic data and calculation of unit costs using a conventional approach

		Total Cost by Visit Type Basic Data			
		A Initial (Given)	B Regular (Given)	C Intensive (Given)	D Total (A + B + C)
1	Number of visits	6,000	24,000	7,600	37,600
2	Direct materials (etc.)	$30,000	$25,000	$45,000	$100,000
3	Direct labor	$90,000	$90,000	$270,000	$450,000
4	Estimated overhead (total is a given)				$200,000
5	Cost per visit: conventional method				

Additional basic data

(1) Basic data: annual projections of overhead costs by activity

		Cost Driver Information		
	Activity	I Cost (Given)	J Driver (Given)	K Units (Given)
6	Intake	$32,500	New visits	3,150 new visits
7	Medical records	$32,500	Time spent	2,090 hours
8	Billing	$55,000	Time spent	5,080 hours
9	Other	$80,000	Visits	37,600 visits
10	Total	$200,000		

(2) Basic data: actual annual operating results of cost drivers to be used to assign ABC overhead cost

		Visit Type			
	*	M Initial (Given)	N Regular (Given)	O Intensive (Given)	P Total (M + N + O)
11	New visits	2,200	800	150	3,150
12	Medical records	500	540	1,050	2,090
13	Billing	3,040	916	1,124	5,080
14	Other	6,000	24,000	7,600	37,600

EXHIBIT 12.14 DATA FOR TRADITIONAL AND ABC COST ALLOCATION, FOR PROBLEM 14

Basic data and calculation of unit costs using a conventional approach

		Total Cost by Visit Type Basic Data			
		A Initial (Given)	B Regular (Given)	C Intensive (Given)	D Total (A + B + C)
1	Number of visits	8,000	26,000	8,600	42,600
2	Direct materials (etc.)	$40,000	$50,000	$65,000	$155,000
3	Direct labor	$100,000	$120,000	$280,000	$500,000
4	Estimated overhead (total is a given)				$229,000
5	Cost per visit: conventional method				

Additional basic data

(1) Basic data: annual projections of overhead costs by activity

		Cost Driver Information		
	Activity	I Cost (Given)	J Driver (Given)	K Units (Given)
6	Intake	$34,000	New visits	3,550 new visits
7	Medical records	$35,000	Time spent	2,390 hours
8	Billing	$65,000	Time spent	5,400 hours
9	Other	$95,000	Visits	42,600 visits
10	Total	$229,000		

(2) Basic data: actual annual operating results of cost drivers to be used to assign ABC overhead cost

		Visit Type			
		M Initial (Given)	N Regular (Given)	O Intensive (Given)	P Total (M + N + O)
11	New visits	2,500	700	350	3,550
12	Medical records	600	640	1,150	2,390
13	Billing	3,200	1,000	1,200	5,400
14	Other	8,000	26,000	8,600	42,600

CHAPTER 13

PROVIDER PAYMENT SYSTEMS

This chapter provides an overview of the development of the *health care payment system* in the United States and some of the basic methods currently used to determine health care payments. The evolution of the payment system will be emphasized in light of the ongoing public policy debate about the roles, responsibilities, and effects of the payment system on various stakeholders (Exhibit 13.1), including

- Patients
- Providers—including physicians, institutional providers, and ancillary providers (e.g., physical therapists, laboratories, hospices, and home care providers)
- Employers
- Payors—including various levels of governmental agencies and managed care organizations
- Regulators—including governmental (e.g., Medicare and Medicaid) and private agencies (e.g., the Joint Commission on Accreditation of Healthcare Organizations [JCAHO] and the National Committee for Quality Assurance [NCQA])

Simply put, this debate has been over, Who gets paid?, How much?, By whom?, For what types of services?, and, With what consequences?

The U.S. health care system attempts to balance cost, quality, and access. Over the years, each of these three facets has received more or less emphasis as policymakers questioned the incentives-based health care system and as value-based payment mechanisms emerged. The questions now may be, Do these programs really improve quality?, and, Is the payment focus a return to the managed

LEARNING OBJECTIVES

- Identify the history, theory, and characteristics of the major types of payment systems.

- Identify the tactics payors and providers use to reduce their financial risk.

- Determine the cost per member per month for specific procedures.

- Understand the new wave of innovations in health care payment systems.

Payor
An entity responsible for paying for the services of a health care provider; it may be an insurance company or a governmental agency. In addition, many larger employers have elected to self-fund insurance for their employees and use insurers such as BlueCross as third-party administrators.

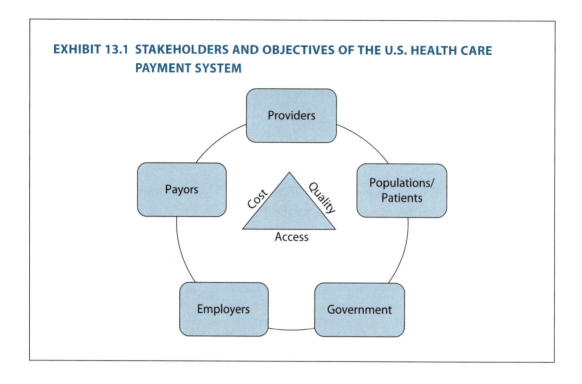

EXHIBIT 13.1 STAKEHOLDERS AND OBJECTIVES OF THE U.S. HEALTH CARE PAYMENT SYSTEM

care mechanism of the 1990s which was viewed as rationing care? (See Perspective 13.1.)

Managed Care

Any of a number of arrangements designed to control health care costs through monitoring and prescribing or proscribing the provision of health care to a patient or population.

While in the past the debate focused on the roles of governmental entities, payors, and providers, now individual consumers have become significant participants in the conversation. Not only are individual consumers more educated and able to obtain information on health and health issues, but also the onus is more on patients for payment. Today's emphasis on care will result in focusing on the patient holistically rather than on episodes of care delivered and procedures performed. And, with these new developments, as was discussed in Chapter One, health care providers are on the front line every day, trying to balance their missions and their margins, walking a fine line between the art of healing, the science of medicine, and the business of health care.

Key Point By convention, the terms *payor* and *payer* are used interchangeably in the health care field.

To truly understand the current health care payment system, it is important to have insight into how it has evolved. Before the late 1920s and early 1930s, health care was funded primarily by patients. The growth

PERSPECTIVE 13.1 DO PAY-FOR-PERFORMANCE (P4P) SYSTEMS IMPROVE QUALITY?

Policymakers have been concerned for many years that the health care system contains incentives to increase cost to the system. The more services provided, the higher the compensation to the provider. Although prospective payment has served to limit reimbursement by bundling services into DRGs and APCs, until recently the system has done little to penalize for readmissions and has even paid for remediation of medical errors. Studies performed by the Institute of Medicine and others have highlighted serious deficiencies in the quality of health care in the United States, leading policymakers to conclude that more care doesn't mean better quality.

Pay-for-performance (P4P) emerged as a payment mechanism around the year 2000. The mechanism is intended to focus on quality, with the expectation that in the long run this would also reduce costs. Pay-for-performance is the term given to financial initiatives (e.g., shared savings, value-based purchasing, and accountable care organizations) that link reimbursement to improved quality, efficiency, and value of the care provided. At the outset quality is measured by improved adherence to protocols grounded in evidence-based medicine and patient satisfaction. As P4P programs mature, the intent is that goals will become more outcome-based. The Patient Protection and Affordable Care Act (ACA) expands the use of these approaches in Medicare, and CMS initiative programs are encouraging providers to identify the P4P designs and programs that are most effective.

Pay-for-performance programs, in general, provide a bonus to providers if they meet or exceed agreed-upon quality or performance measures. Many of the measures relate to processes of care, but some relate to patient satisfaction outcomes, such as reductions in hemoglobin A1c in diabetic patients.

The Inpatient Prospective Payment System (IPPS) rule for fiscal year 2013 provides for a 1 percent cut in payments for inpatient stays. Note that those hospitals that do not report quality measures are also subject to a 2 percent reduction in payments.

However, studies related to the effects of pay-for-performance have found mixed results. A study of the Premier Hospital Quality Incentive Demonstration project found that hospitals in the demonstration initially showed improvements in quality compared to a control group. But unfortunately, after the fifth year of the demonstration, there were no significant differences in performance scores between participating hospitals and a comparison group of hospitals not in the project [see Exhibit 13.2]. The study admits it is possible that performance was improving across all hospitals, since many hospitals were worried about the consequences if they displayed poor performance. Hospitals have been required to report on quality measures in order to receive their full Medicare update, and scores are publicly available on a website, "Hospital Compare."

No matter the initial results, payors including insurance companies and policymakers still view the pay-for-performance initiatives as positive and are optimistic about their eventual result. As value-based purchasing is rolled out for fiscal year 2013 and beyond, it will be interesting to see if quality continues to improve and how much the Medicare program will realize in terms of savings.

Source: Adapted from J. James, *Pay-for-Performance: New Payment Systems Reward Doctors and Hospitals for Improving the Quality of Care, but Studies to Date Show Mixed Results*, Health Policy Brief, October 11, 2012, Health Affairs/Robert Wood Johnson Foundation, healthaffairs.org/healthpolicybriefs/brief_pdfs/healthpolicybrief_78 .pdf.

EXHIBIT 13.2 LESSONS LEARNED FROM MEDICARE'S VALUE-BASED PAYMENT DEMONSTRATIONS

	Premier Hospital Quality Demonstration	Physician Group Practice Demonstration	Medicare Home Health Pay-for-Performance Demonstration
Estimated effect on Medicare expenditures	Little or no effect.	No effect.	Little or no effect on expenditures in year 1.
Estimated effect on quality of care	Little or no effect on patient outcomes in the first year.	Small improvement in processes of care.	Little or no effect on patient outcomes.
Payment approach	Hospital received bonus for meeting quality of care targets.	Group practices received bonuses if total Medicare spending was reduced. Bonuses were dependent on number of quality care targets met.	For each region, estimated savings were distributed to home health agencies that had the highest quality scores or greatest improvement in quality scores.
Participating organizations	278 hospitals.	10 physician practices.	556 home health agencies in 7 states.

Source: L. Nelson, *Lessons from Medicare's Demonstration on Value Based Payments*, Congressional Budget Office Report, February 2012, and Centers for Medicare & Medicaid Services, *Roadmap for Implementing Value-Driven Health Care in the Traditional Medicare Fee-for-Service Program*, http://www.cms.gov/Medicare/Quality-Initiatives -Patient-Assessment-Instruments/QualityInitiativesGenInfo/index.html.

of the country's population, however, brought additional costs in the form of more doctors and more health care facilities. The burden of paying for health care shifted to employers and later to government. A summary of key events in this evolution follows, ending with some future trends.

Caution: The issues surrounding health care payment systems in the United States are extremely complicated and ever-changing, and this chapter provides only a basic introduction. The following websites are recommended for more details and updates:

- The Centers for Medicare and Medicaid Services: www.cms.gov/index.html
- Agency for Healthcare Research and Quality: www.ahrq.gov
- The Kaiser Family Foundations: www.kff.org
- PriceWaterhouseCoopers: Health Research Institute: healthcare.pwc.com
- MedPAC: www.medpac.gov
- American Health Systems Annual Survey: www.aha.org/research/reports/index.shtml

Evolution of the Payment System

From 1929 through the advent of Medicare and Medicaid in the mid 1960s, the health care payment system was largely a combination of *charge-based payment*, *fee-for-service*, and *employer-based indemnity insurance*. Even when an employer paid for all or a portion of the services, the provider was the price setter. Despite the massive amount of governmental funding created for facility development, there was relatively little involvement of the federal government or state governments as payors.

Blue Cross Blue Shield (BCBS) got its start in 1929 when Justin Kimball, an official at Baylor University, introduced a plan to guarantee teachers twenty-one days of hospital care a year for $6. Other employee groups joined the plan, which was then known as the Baylor Plan. The idea gained national attention and the Blue Cross symbol was adopted by a commission of the American Hospital Association as the national emblem for plans that met certain criteria. Blue Shield was developed as a medical plan for physician services. These plans have since come to be offered together and have evolved into health insurance companies offering not only underwritten products but also administrative services to self-insured employer groups and others.

Evidence-Based Medicine
Health care based on the best evidence currently available from both individual clinical expertise and research-based clinical findings.

Shared Savings
A payment strategy used by CMS that encourages providers to reduce health care spending for a defined patient population by offering them a percentage of the net savings realized as a result of their efforts.

Fee-for-Service
A method of reimbursement based on payment for services rendered, with a specific fee correlated with each specific service. An insurance company, the patient, or a governmental program such as Medicare or Medicaid may make the payments.

Price Setter
The entity that controls the amount paid for a health care service.

Premium

A monthly payment made by a person or an employer, or both, to an insurer that makes the covered individuals eligible for a defined level of health care for a given period of time.

Community Rating

A rating method used by indemnity and HMO insurers that guarantees that equivalent amounts will be collected from members of a specific group, without regard to demographics such as age, sex, size of covered group, and industry type.

The first prepaid health plan was established by the Western Clinic in Tacoma, Washington, providing care to lumber company employees. Other examples were plans offered by the Ross-Loos Medical Group and the Group Health Association. Perhaps one of the most significant providers of health care plans is Kaiser Foundation Health Plans, which was founded in 1945 as a way to finance and deliver care to Henry Kaiser's steel mill employees. From the 1940s to 1970, Kaiser grew significantly, becoming responsible for the majority of prepaid health plan enrollees in the United States. Over time Kaiser expanded to cover individuals and employer groups.

In 1965, the Medicare program was enacted as a federal social program, under Title XVIII of the Social Security Act, to provide insurance primarily to the population aged sixty-five and older, who found coverage almost impossible to obtain. The Medicaid program was enacted a short while later as a state program partially funded with federal dollars, under Title XIX of the Social Security Act, to provide coverage for low-income individuals, particularly children, pregnant women, and the elderly. When these programs were established, no one could foresee the growth in governmental expenditures that would occur. According to the National Health Statistics Group of the Centers for Medicare and Medicaid Services (CMS), governmental expenditure on health care as a percentage of total health care expenditures was projected to be 36.6 percent and is expected to grow to 41.1 percent by 2021.[1]

By 1970, however, there was an increased focus on the rapidly rising cost of health care. The payment mechanisms for providers at the time were primarily fee-for-service for physicians and cost-based reimbursement for hospitals. Coverage expanded, but with it costs did too, and so federal health policy turned away from its emphasis on access to an emphasis on cost containment. At this time many believed that the prepaid health plan would be the "answer" to cost containment.

Health Maintenance Organization (HMO)

A legally incorporated organization that offers health insurance and medical care. HMOs typically offer a range of health care services at a fixed price. Two types of HMOs are the staff model and the group model.

The name *health maintenance organization* (HMO) has been attributed to Paul Ellwood, an advisor to the federal government. The term became institutionalized in 1973 with the HMO Act, enacted in an effort to expand the number of HMOs and which required employers with more than twenty-five employees to offer an HMO in addition to other insurance options. The act did as intended, and the number of HMOs expanded; however, there were some unintended consequences, and many of the newly created HMOs subsequently went out of business, leading to poor publicity. As discussed below, other issues also tarnished the HMO name, which had evolved to *managed care organization*, such as the assumption that care was not only managed but rationed.

Eventually this caused another change in the term of reference, to *health plan*.

During the 1960s and throughout the 1970s, employers played a relatively passive role in the health care discussion. But as the cost of care continued to grow, employers, paying for a majority of employee health care costs, became increasingly concerned about how these costs were affecting profitability. To address the escalating cost of care, Medicare implemented prospective payment systems for hospitals and fee schedules for physicians. Private insurers also introduced capitation, which fixes a limit on payouts to providers by reimbursing them *per capita* and not by the actual services provided.

Capitation, however, was a two-edged sword. Whereas on the one hand providers did not have to worry about the amount they would earn from insurers in total and had flexibility to provide the care needed without restriction, on the other hand providers felt that they had to accept the rate offered to them, because if they did not their competition would. So even when providers felt the offered rate seemed too low, they had concerns about losing patients. In addition, some providers really did not understand what it cost to provide the care and were unable to judge the adequacy of the rate. This is one reason why capitation failed as a cost containment strategy in the 1990s.

On the surface, capitation also appeared to many to incentivize delivering less care in order to achieve more profit. Capitation works best when there is a critical mass of subscribers over which to spread the risk of loss, and so while used extensively in many populous parts of California, Minnesota, and New York, it did not catch on in other parts of the country, such as Georgia and North Carolina.

In addition, consumers were not ready for managed care and resisted the lack of provider choice. Employers demanded more control over benefits and plan design. Though the HMO form of delivery remains today, new forms of plan design have emerged, including the *point of service product*, whereby plan members could, for an additional cost, go *out of network*.

Prospective payment systems began in the early 1980s, and since that time there has been a movement away from the provider as a price-setter, since the government was setting the prices that the Medicare and Medicaid programs would pay, and many providers did not have the size and clout to negotiate with insurers, including HMOs.

The Hill-Burton Act of 1946, enacted to improve access in rural areas, achieved its purpose by catalyzing the construction of new hospitals. However, paying for the care provided at these new and improved facilities (and the new technology associated with them) became increasingly expensive. While being employed was one way to access health care coverage, there was a growing concern about the ability to pay for care among the unemployed, the underinsured (perhaps self-employed or employed by an employer not offering an insurance benefit, for example), the poor, the young, the elderly, and the disabled. Therefore, during the 1990s and into the mid-2000s much of the national debate focused on the issue of access to care. Today, access to care, as discussed in Chapter One, is important, but there is also a significant focus on integrating quality with cost for a more balanced cost-access-quality triangle (Exhibit 13.1).

Quest for Quality: Population-Based Payment Mechanisms Emerge

The following section discusses value-based and population-based payment mechanisms initiated by CMS to improve value and at the same time lower cost for Medicare patients. Although this chapter looks at these mechanisms from the Medicare point of view, they are in use for Medicaid and commercial populations as well. Where Medicare goes, others seem to follow.

Value-Based Purchasing

Health care providers have always espoused a desire to provide the best quality of care. However, an intense focus on quality began in the late 1990s and took shape for hospitals in 2005 with the advent of *value-based purchasing* (VBP) programs. The Deficit Reduction Act of 2005 authorized CMS to develop a plan for VBP for Medicare hospital services beginning in fiscal year 2009, and the ACA provided the implementation plan.[2]

The VBP rule released in April of 2011 by CMS has two facets: the hospital inpatient VBP program, and the hospital readmission reduction program.

Payments under the VBP program are characterized as rewards or incentive payments for hospitals on their achievement and improvement over time on specific measures related to national benchmarks. The fiscal year 2013 payment determination is based on an initial set of twelve care measures and eight patient satisfaction measures. Beginning in fiscal year 2014, hospitals will be judged on their outcome (mortality) measures. Perspective 13.2 provides additional detail on value-based purchasing and the future implications for inpatient stay services.

There are two aspects to the care measures: how well did the hospital perform on each measure, and how much did the hospital improve its

---

Centers for Medicare and Medicaid Services (CMS)

The U.S. government agency that oversees the provision of and payment for health care supplied under federal entitlement programs (Medicare and Medicaid); CMS replaced the Health Care Financing Administration (HCFA).

Value-Based Purchasing (VBP)

A payment methodology designed to provide incentives to providers for delivering quality health care at a lower cost. The financial rewards come from funds being withheld by the payor; these funds are then redistributed on providers' achievement of and improvement on specific performance measures, including patient satisfaction. The goal of VBP is to encourage quality of care in multiple care settings (e.g., physicians' offices, hospitals, etc.).

PERSPECTIVE 13.2 FUTURE IMPLICATIONS FOR VALUE-BASED PURCHASING

The Inpatient Prospective Payment System (IPPS) final rule for 2013 provides details on operating payments for 2013 as well as some further details on the Hospital VBP Program and Hospital Readmissions Reduction Program.

1. The rule leaves little doubt that contingent payments are here to stay. The pay-for-performance programs made possible by the ACA are mandatory and link inpatient payments to certain measures of quality, outcomes, and patient satisfaction.

2. The 1 percent reimbursement reduction for 2013 will grow over time to 2 percent. CMS expects the VBP program to reallocate approximately $956 million to those providers meeting or exceeding targets (see Appendix J at the end of this chapter for a description of this payment mechanism). Other penalties on the horizon are for readmissions. CMS expects those penalties to be approximately $300 million.

3. The number and types of measures will grow over time. The focus is moving from process to outcomes. In fiscal year 2015, Medicare will add a measure for Medicare spending per beneficiary. This will hold providers accountable for Part A and B spending per episode of care. This is how CMS will duplicate the performance standards of voluntary, episode-based, bundled payments. But under the VBP program, this approach will be mandatory.

4. Hospital measures will evolve to system measures in the coming years. As CMS collects information on readmissions, mortality, and spending per episode, these will become the benchmarks for system-level quality and efficiency. Coordination of care strategies will become even more important.

5. Medicaid and commercial payors have tended to follow Medicare's lead in reimbursement schemes. The Hospital VBP and Hospital Readmissions Reduction Programs will drive performance risk. Only time will tell if other payors will make performance risk a component of their reimbursement contracts.

Source: Adapted from R. Lazerow, Exploring the future of Medicare pay-for-performance programs, Health Care Advisory Board, May 3, 2012.

performance on each measure compared to its performance in the baseline period?[3] Achievement points are awarded by comparing the individual hospital's rates with all hospitals' rates (benchmark) from the baseline period, as follows:

• Hospital at or above the benchmark: 10 points

• Hospital below the achievement threshold (minimum): 0 points

- Hospital with a rate equal to or above the achievement threshold but less than the benchmark: 1 to 9 points

Improvement points are awarded as follows:

- Hospital at or above benchmark: 9 points
- Hospital at or below the baseline period rate: 0 points
- Hospital with a rate between baseline and the benchmark: 0 to 9 improvement points

Exhibit 13.3 illustrates the scoring methodology for one *process of care* measure and one *patient experience of care* measure. The scores of the measures that apply to a hospital are summed and weighted. Seventy percent of the total performance score is awarded for the process of care component and 30 percent is awarded for the patient's experience of care component. For 2014, a consistency score will be added.

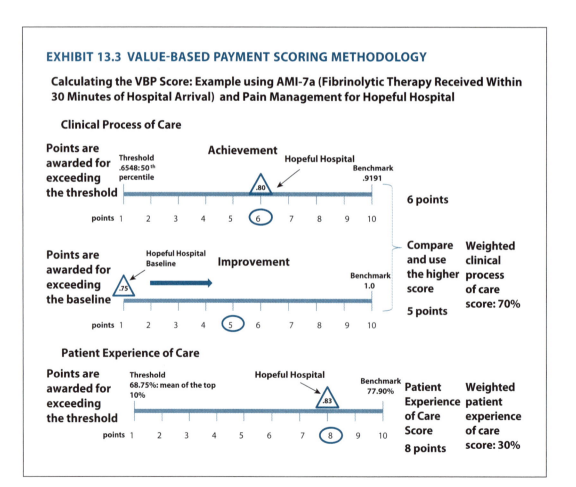

EXHIBIT 13.3 VALUE-BASED PAYMENT SCORING METHODOLOGY

Calculating the VBP Score: Example using AMI-7a (Fibrinolytic Therapy Received Within 30 Minutes of Hospital Arrival) and Pain Management for Hopeful Hospital

The fiscal year 2013 incentive payments were based on performance data collected from July 2011 to March 2012. The period used for outcome measures ran from July 2011 through June 2012. CMS will continue to add performance measures over the next several years.

CMS intends this initiative to be budget neutral, by having the incentive payments come from reimbursement that is withheld from other providers. The initial payment withheld gradually increases from 1 percent in fiscal year 2013 to 2 percent in fiscal year 2017 (0.25% a year). CMS has finalized a linear exchange function to translate the performance scores earned by hospitals into value-based incentive payments.

Psychiatric, rehabilitation, long-term care, and children's and cancer hospitals are excluded from the program, as are those hospitals that have failed to submit either clinical process of care surveys or HCAHPS (Hospital Consumer Assessment of Healthcare Providers and Systems) patient satisfaction surveys.

Hospital Readmissions Reduction and Never Events

Until the 1990s, accreditation organizations such as JCAHO (primarily for hospitals) and NCQA (primarily for health plans) and, of course, the medical profession were largely in charge of ensuring quality. But various occurrences and published reports, such as a study from HealthGrades, a Colorado health care ratings organization, led the government, watchdog groups, and consumers to be concerned about the quality of health care. The 2010 HealthGrades study documented more than 900,000 patient safety incidents between 2006 and 2008, and 99,000 mortalities related to patient safety occurrences during that same period.

Some of the issues identified were hospital-acquired conditions such as surgical site infections obtained while in the hospital, traumas and falls, surgical items left in the body, and wrong site amputations. According to the Centers for Disease Control, these *never events* cost CMS approximately $4.5 billion a year, to say nothing of the harm inflicted on the patients.

In addition, according to a study published in the *New England Journal of Medicine*,[4] readmissions to hospitals, which may occur because of premature hospital discharge or poor follow-up care, cost CMS approximately $15 billion each year. Both of these patient safety issues are indicative of poor quality. Accordingly, the health policy movement supporting *value-based purchasing* emerged.

The Deficit Reduction Act of 2005 began the journey toward no longer paying for never events, and the number of such events for which Medicare will no longer pay has grown since then to twenty-nine events

Never Events
Adverse patient outcomes due to provider negligence that are not ever supposed to happen and that therefore are typically not reimbursed.

in six categories. Other payors have taken Medicare's lead and are also no longer paying for them. It is interesting to note that the 2012 HealthGrades study documented approximately 254,000 patient safety incidents between 2008 and 2010 and 56,000 mortalities related to patient safety occurrences during that period, a dramatic improvement.

The ACA established the Hospital Readmissions Reduction Program, whereby Inpatient Prospective Payment System (IPPS) payments to hospitals for readmissions deemed to be excessive would be reclaimed beginning on or after October 1, 2012. A readmission is an admission to a hospital within thirty days of discharge from that same hospital or another part of the system containing that hospital. The estimate of excess payments for readmissions of Medicare patients for 2010 was over $17.5 billion. *Kaiser Health News* reported that 2,217 hospitals would be penalized, and of those, 307 would be penalized the maximum amount, 1 percent of Medicare reimbursements.[5]

This program has become controversial because many see it as penalizing those hospitals that serve the lower-income and sicker patients, and hospitals believe that Medicare is not doing an adequate job of distinguishing between the necessary and planned readmissions and those that are unnecessary. But this program has caused hospitals to institute improvements in coordinating care after the patient leaves the hospital, improvements that include home health nurse visits and other mechanisms to help to ensure patient compliance with discharge instructions, including taking medications.

Accountable Care Organizations

The ACA established policies that permit various providers to join together to provide seamless, high-quality care to members of the Medicare population. An *accountable care organization* (ACO) is a patient-centered, population-based health care organization made up of various providers (most notably hospitals, primary care physicians, and specialists) and suppliers of services covered by Medicare. The CMS final rule says that all Medicare providers can participate in an ACO but only certain providers can sponsor an ACO. Physician group practices, networks of individual practitioners, and hospitals partnering with or employing eligible physicians, nurse practitioners, physician assistants, and specialists are qualified to sponsor ACOs. Rural Health Clinics and Federally Qualified Health Centers may participate in the program by becoming ACOs or participating with others in an ACO.

ACOs are part of the traditional Medicare fee-for-service program, and although aligned with an ACO, Medicare beneficiaries may choose the providers they want to see. Beneficiaries are notified by the ACO of their alignment. A beneficiary aligns with an ACO based on where that person is already receiving his or her primary care services, unless the person receives less than 10 percent of his or her care from a primary care provider. In the latter case, the person is aligned with the specialist who delivers the majority of the care. An ACO with a Medicare contract must be responsible for a minimum of 5,000 aligned beneficiaries for three years. An ACO's governing board must include health care providers and Medicare beneficiaries.

In simple terms, even though the provider organization agrees to a set budget for serving all the needs of its aligned population, including long-term care, payments are made on a fee-for-service basis using prospective payment mechanisms.

There are two ACO models: one is a shared savings model (a one-sided model), while the other is a model in which both savings and risk are shared (a two-sided model). In this shared savings and risk model, when costs exceed the budget the ACO shares in the losses, and when the costs are lower the ACO shares in the profits. The ACO can receive up to 60 percent of the savings it generates in the two-sided model. Those participating in the shared savings model (the one-sided model) can receive up to 50 percent of the savings. Because the experience of patients can vary from year to year, there are minimum savings and loss rates.[6]

Payments are also linked to quality measures. Medicare will assess an ACO's quality in addition to its financial performance each year. Performance will be measured on

- Quality standards (patient experience)
- Care coordination and patient safety
- Preventive health care
- Care of at-risk populations (populations with diabetes, hypertension, ischemic vascular disease, heart failure, and/or coronary artery disease)

ACOs are not just a Medicare phenomenon. The concept has caught on for commercial populations as well as with private insurers.[7]

Provider Payment Mechanisms

This section explores the different mechanisms used to pay providers. As mentioned earlier, although this chapter focuses primarily on the mechanisms used by Medicare, other payors, such as Medicaid and private insurers, generally follow Medicare's lead.

Key Point Much of the current health care payment system in the United States is driven by the government's role in that system. A more detailed history of Medicare and Medicaid can be found at http://understandingmymedicare.com/history-of-medicare/.

Origins of Provider Payment Systems

At its inception, Medicare based its payment policies on the mechanism used by Blue Cross and Blue Shield to pay hospitals and physicians: it paid the customary amounts charged for these providers' services. This *cost-based reimbursement* was paid on a *retrospective* basis. Hospitals and certain other providers (skilled nursing facilities, Federally Qualified Health Centers and Rural Health Clinics, home health agencies, hospices, and renal dialysis clinics) filed a *Medicare cost report*, detailing all the costs associated with the provision of Medicare services throughout a set period. The government, in turn, scrutinized the costs being claimed and would allow or disallow costs on the basis of standards and settle with the provider. Over the years, most Medicare reimbursement has evolved into a prospective payment system and, as was previously discussed, is continuing to evolve into a payment system based in part on value rather than on the quantity of services performed. Medicare cost reports are still filed today by the providers noted above, although their significance has changed and they are now seen primarily as a reporting and evaluation mechanism. As noted in Exhibits 13.4 and 13.5, government is now responsible for paying a significant amount of the cost of health care in the United States. In 2011, the amount surpassed $882 billion.

Medicare

A nationwide, federally financed health insurance program for people aged sixty-five and older. It also covers certain people younger than sixty-five who are disabled or have chronic kidney (end-stage renal) disease. Medicare Part A is the hospital inpatient insurance program; Part B covers physician and outpatient services. Part C allows beneficiaries to receive benefits through private health plans, and Part D covers prescription drug benefit plans.

Medicaid

A federally mandated program operated and partially funded by individual states (in conjunction with the federal government) to provide medical benefits to certain low-income people. The state, under broad federal guidelines, determines what benefits are covered, who is eligible, and how much providers will be paid.

Adding Precision to Reimbursement

In order to add precision to payment for services, International Classification of Disease, 9th Revision, Clinical Modification (ICD-9-CM) codes are assigned to diagnoses and treatments when they are reported, and Healthcare Common Procedure Coding System (HCPCS) codes are assigned to services and supplies provided relative to those diagnoses and treatments. HCPCS codes are also assigned to outpatient treatments and physician services. The ICD-9 and HCPCS codes are then grouped into the payment mechanisms discussed below, known as diagnosis related groups (DRGs) and ambulatory payment classifications (APCs). These were mandated by the Medicare Catastrophic Coverage Act of 1988.

The ICD-9 has three major functions for reimbursement purposes:

- Provides justification of procedures and services provided by the physician

EXHIBIT 13.4 MEDICARE AND MEDICAID ENTITLEMENT PROGRAMS

	Medicare	Medicaid
Who pays for program?	Federal tax on income	Federal and state tax on income (federal government pays larger share; share is based on state's per capita income)
Who is covered?	People aged 65 and older Some people with disabilities under age 65 People with end-stage renal disease	People with disabilities The poor Needy women and children Childless adults (health reform)
How many are covered?	1980: 28.5 million 1990: 34.2 million 2000: 39 million 2007: 41 million 2011: 48 million 2012: 50 million	1981: 20.2 million 1990: 23.9 million 2000: 33.6 million 2005: 45.6 million 2009: 62.5 million 2010: 66.0 million
How much are expenditures?	1980: $36 billion 1990: $108 billion 2000: $221 billion 2007: $431 billion 2009: $471 billion 2012: $574 billion	1980: $24.7 billion 1990: $71.2 billion 2000: $205 billion 2006: $314 billion 2010: $389 billion

Source: Data from Kaiser Family Foundation, State Health Facts: Medicaid & CHIP, www.statehealthfacts .org/comparecat.jsp?cat=4&rgn=6&rgn=1; Centers for Medicare and Medicaid Services, Medicare & Medicaid Statistical Supplement: 2013 Edition, www.cms.gov/Research-Statistics-Data-and-Systems/Statistics-Trends-and -Reports/MedicareMedicaidStatSupp/2013.html; Centers for Medicare and Medicaid Services, [Medicare] Trust-ees Report and Trust Funds, www.cms.gov/Research-Statistics-Data-and-Systems/Statistics-Trends-and-Reports/ ReportsTrustFunds/index.html; and Medicaid and CHIP Payment and Access Commission (MACPAC), MACStats, www.macpac.gov/macstats.

EXHIBIT 13.5 NATIONAL EXPENDITURES BY SERVICE AND PAYOR TYPE

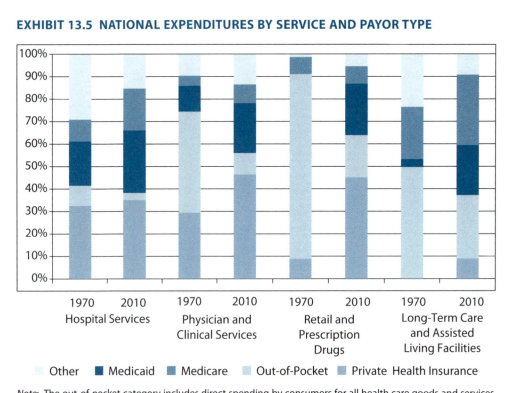

Note: The out-of-pocket category includes direct spending by consumers for all health care goods and services not covered by insurance, except for health care premiums. The private health insurance category includes premiums paid to health insurance plans and the net cost of private health insurance (administrative costs, reserves, taxes, and profits or losses).

Source: Data from Centers for Medicare and Medicaid Services, National Health Statistics Group, National health expenditure data, www.cms.gov/NationalHealthExpendData.

Prospective Payment System

A payment method that establishes rates, prices, or budgets before services are rendered and costs are incurred. Providers retain or absorb at least a portion of the difference between established revenues and actual costs.

- Assists in establishing medical necessity for services and procedures performed

- Serves as an indicator in measuring the quality of health care delivered

The Department of Health and Human Services (HHS) has mandated the replacement of the ICD-9 code sets used by medical coders and billers to report health care diagnoses and procedures with ICD-10 code sets, effective October 1, 2014. While ICD-9 contains 17,000 codes, ICD-10 contains more than 141,000 codes and accommodates a host of new diagnoses and procedures. The number of diagnostic codes under ICD-10-CM will increase from 13,500 to 69,000. For inpatient procedures, the number increases from 4,000 codes to 71,000 codes.

The HCPCS code system consists of Common Procedural Terminology (CPT) and national codes to identify procedures, supplies, and medications, except for vaccines and equipment. The CPT codes are numeric codes published by the American Medical Association (AMA) for services and procedures performed by providers.

Hospital Billing

Hospitals are reimbursed by Medicare for services primarily in these ways:

* Medicare severity-adjusted diagnosis related groups (MS-DRGs)

* Ambulatory payment classifications (APC)

* Per diem (psychiatric hospitals)

* Cost (critical access hospitals)

* Case rates

The Medicare severity-adjusted diagnosis related groups (MS-DRGs) are built on major diagnostic categories (MDCs), which are grouped by body systems (see Exhibit 12.7 for examples of MS-DRGs). There are twenty-five MDCs. From those MDCs come 999 MS-DRGs (only 751 of these MS-DRGs were used in 2013). Each MS-DRG carries a unique weight, and those weights are multiplied by a base. DRGs are assigned by grouper software and are driven by the principal diagnosis and the location of discharge. The ICD-9-CM is the code set required by Medicare for inpatient reporting. The HCPCS code set is required to report supplies, procedures, and services. HCPCS includes the coding classifications of CPT.

The DRG classifications have evolved over time with changes in disease states, technology, and types of procedures. For example, the DRGs of the 1980s were modified over the 1990s and early 2000s until a new level of sophistication was needed to reflect new complications and comorbidities, including major illnesses that utilize more resources. The Medicare severity-adjusted DRG (MS-DRG) system was then created; it became effective in fiscal year 2008, replacing the existing 538 DRGs.

Exhibit 13.6 illustrates the mechanism by which inpatient services are paid by Medicare. These inpatient payments provide approximately 20 percent of the average hospital's revenue. Medicare paid approximately $116 billion for inpatient services in 2011. Each MS-DRG is assigned a relative weight that correlates to the expected cost of the patient stay given local market conditions, and that also pays for the capital involved. For fiscal year 2013, the operating base rate was $5,349 and the capital rate was $425. Graduate medical education and organ acquisition costs, if

Cost-Based Reimbursement
A payment method that uses the provider's cost of providing services (i.e., supplies, staff salaries, space costs, etc.) as the basis for reimbursement. By 2012, very little cost-based reimbursement remained. Critical access hospitals still receive reimbursement at 101 percent of reasonable cost.

Medicare Severity-Adjusted Diagnostic Related Groups (MS-DRGs)
The CMS payment system that replaced the DRG payment system and is designed to better correlate payments with patient severity. (See Exhibit 13.7.) To find out more about this change and MS-DRGs, see the fact sheet "Medicare Policy Changes for the Fiscal Year (FY) 2009 Hospital Inpatient Prospective Payment System" (www.cms.gov/ Newsroom/MediaRelease Database/Fact-Sheets/ 2008-Fact-Sheets -Items/2008-08-04 .html).

EXHIBIT 13.6 MEDICARE INPATIENT PAYMENT SYSTEM

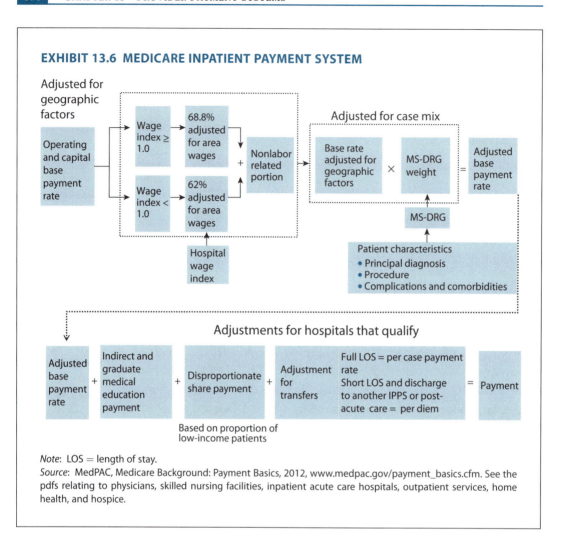

Note: LOS = length of stay.
Source: MedPAC, Medicare Background: Payment Basics, 2012, www.medpac.gov/payment_basics.cfm. See the pdfs relating to physicians, skilled nursing facilities, inpatient acute care hospitals, outpatient services, home health, and hospice.

applicable, are not included. The operating and capital base payments are adjusted to reflect the differences in the local market for labor. If the wage index is greater than 1.0 (more costly markets), then 68.8 percent of the payment is adjusted. If less than 1.0, 62 percent of the payment is adjusted for the index. CMS publishes the hospital wage index.

Certain hospitals have a disproportionate share of Medicare and Medicaid patients and receive additional payments for those patients. In addition, special payments are made to rural hospitals considered to be sole community hospitals and Medicare dependent hospitals. For fiscal years 2012 and 2013, hospitals received additional payments if they were considered low-volume facilities, and for fiscal year 2013 they were required to be at least twenty-five miles from the nearest like hospital to qualify.

EXHIBIT 13.7 EXAMPLES OF MS-DRGS

DRG	Description	A Relative Weight (Given)	B Geographic Adjustment[a] (Given)	C Average Payment per Weighted Unit (Given)	D Total MS-DRG Payment (A × B × C)
592	Skin ulcers with MCC[b]	1.4632	0.97	$5,349	$7,592
175	Pulmonary embolism with MCC[b]	1.5870	0.97	$5,349	$8,234
1	Heart transplant	24.2794	0.97	$5,349	$125,974

[a]Geographic adjustment varies by area.
[b]MCC = major complications and comorbidity.
Source: Data from Centers for Medicare and Medicaid Services, FY 2013 Final Rule Tables, www.cms.gov/Medicare/Medicare-Fee-for-Service-Payment/AcuteInpatientPPS/FY-2013-IPPS-Final-Rule-Home-Page-Items/FY2013-Final-Rule-Tables.html.

Outlier payments are given for extremely costly cases. The national fixed loss amount for fiscal year 2013 was $21,821. Payments are made for amounts above that threshold at 80 percent of cost.

At times when hospitals transfer patients to other hospitals, the transferring facilities are paid a per diem rate (which is higher for the first day) for each day of the period before the transfer, up to the amount of the MS-DRG.

Ambulatory Payment Classifications (APCs)

Similar to MS-DRGs, APCs are a prospective payment mechanism for outpatient services delivered at a hospital. They reflect the compensation for the bundle of outpatient services. APCs were introduced in 2000 as a way to reduce and stabilize the amount of reimbursement hospitals receive for outpatient care, and to shift the financial risk of care to the hospital. The development of this system came in response to the exponential growth of the cost and volume of outpatient medicine, since hospitals had converted many procedures from inpatient to outpatient with the advent of the DRGs.

As noted in Exhibit 13.8, more patients are receiving their care on an outpatient rather than an inpatient basis. This rise in outpatient visits drove up outpatient expenses and resulted in the development and implementation of APCs. (Although APCs apply primarily to hospital outpatient services, they have no relationship with professional fees to physicians,

Ambulatory Payment Classifications (APCs)
The basis of a flat fee, prospective payment system instituted by CMS to shift the financial risk of care to the provider in the provision of outpatient services for Medicare recipients. APCs apply primarily to hospital outpatient services.

which will be discussed below.) Medicare paid approximately $32 billion for outpatient services in 2011.

As discussed above, outpatient services are identified by HCPCS codes. These codes are classified into APCs on the basis of clinical and cost similarity, and each service within an APC receives the same rate. As with the MS-DRGs, there is a standard rate, which for APCs is called a *conversion factor*. For calendar year 2013, the proposed factor was $71.537. APCs are adjusted for geographic factors but are not dependent on the level of the wage index. Sixty percent of the payment is adjusted for area wages.

There is a 7.1 percent add-on payment for rural sole community hospitals (SCHs). Children's and cancer hospitals are held harmless in the event that the prospective payments are lower than they would have received under previous CMS policies. Sole community and rural hospitals with 1,000 or fewer beds receive 85 percent of the full hold harmless payment. Hospitals receive outlier payments for services that cost 1.75 times the APC payment rate and exceed it by at least $1,900. In 2012, outlier payments were limited to 1 percent of the total Outpatient

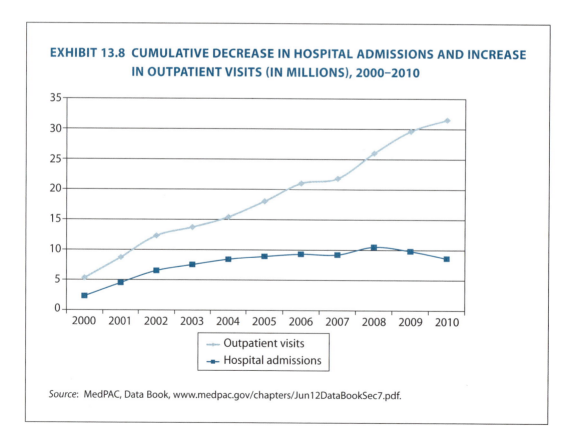

EXHIBIT 13.8 CUMULATIVE DECREASE IN HOSPITAL ADMISSIONS AND INCREASE IN OUTPATIENT VISITS (IN MILLIONS), 2000–2010

Legend: Outpatient visits; Hospital admissions

Source: MedPAC, Data Book, www.medpac.gov/chapters/Jun12DataBookSec7.pdf.

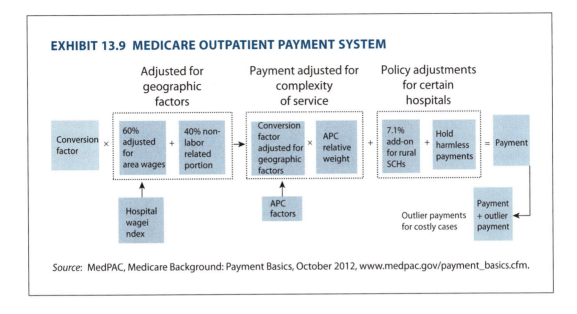

EXHIBIT 13.9 MEDICARE OUTPATIENT PAYMENT SYSTEM

Source: MedPAC, Medicare Background: Payment Basics, October 2012, www.medpac.gov/payment_basics.cfm.

Prospective Payment System (OPPS) payment. Exhibit 13.9 illustrates the APC payment mechanism.

Reimbursement to Physicians for Professional Services

Medicare reimburses physicians and other health professionals (nurse practitioners, physician assistants, and physical therapists) through a fee schedule known as the *resource-based relative value scale* (RBRVS), which was enacted through the Omnibus Budget Reconciliation Act of 1989. This system assigns a relative value to more than seven thousand professional services (including pathology and radiology) and establishes a flat fee for each service based on its relative weight compared with a standard *relative value unit* (RVU) of 1.00. The fee schedule covers services delivered by health professionals in physicians' offices and in other settings, such as hospitals, ambulatory surgical centers, skilled nursing facilities, outpatient dialysis facilities, clinical laboratories, patient homes, and hospices. In 2011, Medicare spent approximately $68 billion on these services.

Although it might appear as if the unit of payment is an office visit or procedure, in many cases it is a bundle of services associated with a specific procedure. For example, a surgery is bundled with pre- and post-operative visits. As described above, an HCPCS code is assigned to each service or bundle of services, and as illustrated in Exhibits 13.10 and 13.11, each service is also assigned three RVU weights.

Resource-Based Relative Value Scale (RBRVS)
A system of paying physicians based on the relative value of the services rendered. Helpful discussions of RBRVS are available from the American Medical Association (http://www .ama-assn.org/ama/pub/ physician-resources/ solutions-managing -your-practice/ coding-billing-insurance/ medicare/the-resource -based-relative-value -scale/overview-of-rbrvs .page) and the American Academy of Pediatrics (www.aap.org/visit/ codingrbrvs.htm).

EXHIBIT 13.10 RVUS USED IN COMPUTING PHYSICIAN PAYMENT

RVU	What It Reflects	Adjusted for Geographic Differences
Work RVU	Time, skill, and stress level related to the service provided	Yes
Practice expense RVU	Rent; supplies; nonphysician clinical and administrative staff; equipment	Yes
Professional liability RVU	Malpractice insurance premiums	Yes

EXHIBIT 13.11 MEDICARE PHYSICIAN AND OTHER HEALTH PROFESSIONALS PAYMENT SYSTEM

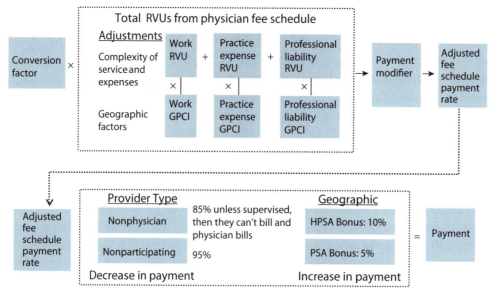

Note: GPCI = geographic practice cost index.
Source: MedPAC, Medicare Background: Payment Basics, October 2012, www.medpac.gov/payment_basics.cfm.

The payment for each service could also be adjusted through payment modifiers. For example, if a physician assists in a surgery, the payment for the assistant is 16 percent of the fee schedule amount for the primary surgeon. Other factors, as illustrated in Exhibit 13.11, are negative adjustments to reflect services furnished by other practitioners or when nonphysicians perform services under the supervision of a physician. Physicians who do not choose to participate in the Medicare program are compensated at 95 percent of the fee schedule. Physicians in areas where there is a shortage of health professionals receive a 10 percent additional payment. Payment to physicians is net of 20 percent coinsurance.

CMS updates the physician fee schedule every year with input from the American Medical Association and other physician groups. These annual updates are based on the sustainable growth rate (SGR) formula, created to maintain a level of spending in the national economy. However, if the SGR had actually been put into effect in the updates over the last ten years, it would have resulted in a negative adjustment for many of those years. For example, the adjustment proposed for the fiscal year beginning January 1, 2013, was 29.5 percent. Fortunately, Congress specified an update outside the formula, so the conversion factor for 2012 was $34.04. It was unchanged for 2013. (See Perspective 13.3.)

Exhibit 13.12 illustrates how RVUs and the geographic practice cost index (GPCI) are used to calculate the payment for a visit in the physician's office for an established patient.

Copayments and Deductibles

Copayments and deductibles are a mechanism whereby the patient absorbs some of the cost of services provided. With *copayments*, insured patients are required to pay part of the cost of the service at the point of service. For instance, if the fee for an office visit is $90, the patient may have to pay either a preestablished amount (e.g., $25) or a certain percentage of the fee for the service (e.g., 20 percent for Medicare beneficiaries receiving physician services), and the insurer pays the remainder of the allowable reimbursement, up to the remaining $65.

With *deductibles*, the insured patient is responsible for paying a certain base amount before coverage begins. For example, a patient may be required to pay for the first $500 of services in the calendar year before an insurer pays any of the bill. Exhibit 13.13 provides examples of coinsurance, deductible, and base amounts for various services for a sample of providers. Exhibit 13.14 illustrates how a health care plan uses copayments and deductibles.

Relative Value Unit (RVU)
A standardized weighting that is assigned to each encounter, procedure, or surgery and that reflects resources consumed. Although discussed in this chapter as a Medicare metric used to compensate physicians for services, it is also widely used by hospitals to evaluate the amount of resources required to perform various services in a single department or across departments. RVUs are determined by assigning weights to such factors as the personnel time, level of skill, and sophistication of equipment used to deliver patient services. RVUs are also an input used in bonus plans when rewarding physicians based partially on productivity.

Copayment (Coinsurance)
A payment the patient is required to make to cover part of the cost of a health care service, such as an office visit. These payments may be a fixed amount or a percentage of the charge.

Deductible
A base amount the patient is responsible for paying before insurance coverage begins.

PERSPECTIVE 13.3 HISTORY OF THE SUSTAINABLE GROWTH RATE

When prospective payment was introduced for hospitals, the growth in payments to physicians was limited by the Medicare Economic Index. It appeared, however, that physician fees were not the only factor behind the rise in expense for the government: volume of services also posed a problem. In the 1990s, a volume performance standard (VPS) was used to limit spending and update the physician fee schedule, but it was found to produce updates that were not reliable. The VPS was replaced with the sustainable growth rate (SGR) in 1997, through the Balanced Budget Act. It was a much more aggressive measure to control spending because it tied the allowable increase in the physician schedule to the GDP per capita growth rate (in 2004 a ten-year moving average GDP was used). But in every year since 2003, Congress has stepped in to prevent the decrease in payments to physicians that would have resulted had the SGR been used. Congress was concerned that it would limit Medicare beneficiaries' access to physician care.

Several short-term fixes to the SGR are under consideration. One is to have multiple SGRs to curb the spending growth of specialists, and to use multispecialty SGRs to encourage the development of more multispecialty groups. Another is to decrease the RBRVS values for services that have experienced significant increases in productivity, and to use better data to update estimates of practice expense.

This will not affect the behavior of individual physicians, and it would be difficult to link physician updates at this level. The ACA sets forth a value-based modifier, but it represents a very small portion of physician reimbursement. Policies to encourage the development of medical homes and bundled payments may also be helpful. However, there is no easy fix, and CMS needs to devote the time needed to correct this issue. Relatively little attention was given to physician payment in the ACA because, on a relative basis, the amounts paid to physicians are not a significant part of the health care dollar.

Physicians were again facing a cut (of 27 percent) beginning January 1, 2013.

Source: Adapted from G. Wilensky, *Medicare Physician Payments: Where We've Been: Where We Need to Go*, Presentation to the Finance Round Table, United States Senate, May 10, 2012.

The Many Parts of Medicare

As illustrated in Exhibit 13.15, Medicare has four parts. Part A covers inpatient services and Part B covers physician and outpatient services. In 2003, Congress passed the Medicare Modernization Act, which added prescription drug coverage, known as Medicare Part D, for program beneficiaries. In addition, this law enhanced the compensation for health plans that give Medicare beneficiaries the option to enroll in a private health plan

EXHIBIT 13.12 EXAMPLE OF PAYMENT CALCULATED USING THE MEDICARE PHYSICIAN FEE SCHEDULE, 2012

Office or outpatient visits for established patients

A	B	C	D	E	F	G	H	I	J	K	L	M	N
HCPCS Code	Evaluation and Management Level	Work RVUs	GPCI (Alabama)	(C × D)	Practice Expense RVUs	GPCI (Alabama)	(F × G)	Professional Liability RVUs	GPCI (Alabama)	(I × J)	Total (E + H + K)	Conversion Factor	Payment (L × M)
99211	1	0.180	1.0000	0.1800	0.390	0.8780	0.3424	0.010	0.4740	0.0047	0.5272	$34.04	$17.94
99212	2	0.480	1.0000	0.4800	0.730	0.8780	0.6409	0.040	0.4740	0.0190	1.1399	$34.04	$38.80
99213	3	0.970	1.0000	0.9700	1.030	0.8780	0.9043	0.070	0.4740	0.0332	1.9075	$34.04	$64.93
99214	4	1.500	1.0000	1.5000	1.460	0.8780	1.2819	0.100	0.4740	0.0474	2.8293	$34.04	$96.31
99215	5	2.110	1.0000	2.1100	1.860	0.8780	1.6331	0.140	0.4740	0.0664	3.8094	$34.04	$129.67

Evaluation and Management Codes

A set of CPT codes used to classify services by physicians, nurse practitioners (where permitted), certified nurse midwives, physician assistants, and clinical nurse specialists offered in physicians' offices, outpatient facilities, inpatient facilities, emergency departments, and nursing facilities on one of five levels, depending on the complexity of the patient's problem. For a summary of level characteristics, see www.cms.gov/Outreach-and-Education/Medicare-Learning-Network-MLN/MLNProducts/downloads/eval_mgmt_serv_guide-ICN006764.pdf.

EXHIBIT 13.13 COINSURANCE, DEDUCTIBLE, AND BASE RATES FOR SELECTED PROVIDERS, 2012

Payment System	Payment Category	Base Amount	Patient Coinsurance	Patient Deductible
Physicians and other health professionals		$34.04	20%	
Outpatient hospital services			20%	
Hospital acute inpatient services	Operating	$5,349.00	$289 per day after day 60	$1,156.00
	Capital	$425.00		
Ambulatory surgical center		$42.63	20%	
Skilled nursing facility services (daily)	Urban: Nursing	$163.58	$144.50 per day after day 20	
	Therapy	$123.22		
	Other	$83.48		
	Rural: Nursing	$156.28		
	Therapy	$142.08		
	Other	$85.03		
Home health care	60-day episode	$2,137.73		
Hospice (daily)[a]	Routine home care (RHC)	$153.00	(5% up to $5) per drug	
	Continuous home care (CHC)	$896.00	(5% up to $5) per drug	
	Inpatient respite care (IRC)	$159.00	5% up to $1,156	
	General inpatient care (GIC)	$683.00		

[a]RHC is home care provided on a typical day; CHC is home care provided during periods of patient crisis; IRC is inpatient care for a short period to provide respite for primary caregiver; GIC is inpatient care to treat symptoms that cannot be managed in another setting.

EXHIBIT 13.14 EXAMPLE OF AN INSURANCE PLAN USING COPAYMENTS AND DEDUCTIBLES

	Plan Coverage	
Service	**Participating Provider**	**Nonparticipating Provider**
Physician's office visit	100% after copayment	70% after copayment
Emergency room visit	100%	100%
Inpatient stay	100% after deductible	70% after deductible
Prescription drugs	100% after copayment	70% after copayment

	Employee Responsibility	
Service	**Participating Provider**	**Nonparticipating Provider**
Physician's office visit	$25 copayment per visit	$35 copayment per visit
Emergency room visit	Subject to plan approval	Subject to plan approval
Inpatient stay	$200 deductible per stay; $1,000 maximum per year	$200 deductible per stay; $1,000 maximum per year
Prescription drugs	$20 copayment per prescription	$30 copayment per prescription

instead of the traditional fee-for-service Medicare program. These Medicare Advantage (MA) plans, known as Medicare Part C, offer more benefits than the traditional Medicare program does. Since their inception, enrollment in these MA plans has continued to increase, providing care for approximately 27 percent of Medicare beneficiaries in 2012.

Other Payment Mechanisms

Per Diem

Another method of payment is a *per diem* ("per day") rate. In a per diem arrangement, a payor negotiates an amount that it will pay for one day of care. For example, Medicare pays psychiatric hospitals on a per diem basis. This amount covers all services associated with the day (including nursing care, supplies, medications, etc.). Hospice providers are paid for much of the care provided to hospice patients through per diem arrangements. As

Per Diem

The amount a payor will pay for one day of care, covering all services associated with the inpatient day (including nursing care, surgeries, medications, etc.).

EXHIBIT 13.15 THE MANY PARTS OF MEDICARE

	Part A	Part B	Part C	Part D
Who is covered	Covered program; based on age and disability.	Voluntary program; Medicare beneficiaries who enroll pay a monthly premium ($99.90 in 2012).	Voluntary program; Medicare beneficiaries who participate enroll in private plans (HMOs, PPOs, or private fee-for-service plans). Medicare pays a capitated rate for the beneficiaries enrolled in Medicare Advantage plans.	Voluntary program; Medicare beneficiaries who participate enroll in prescription drug benefit plans.
Services	Hospital inpatient care Short-term skilled nursing care Postinstitutional home care Hospice care	Physician (and other practitioner) services Hospital outpatient services Home health services (not covered under Part A) Durable medical equipment Ambulance services Limited preventive services Outpatient prescription drugs	Part A and Part B services Part D benefits may be received through these plans. Other benefits may be available depending on the plan.	Outpatient prescription drugs not covered under Part B. All Part D plans must cover the same services, but the cost-sharing requirements may be different as long as they are actuarially equivalent to the traditional plan.

illustrated in the following example, a hospice is paid more for a day of continuous care than for a day of routine care.

Assume a hospice patient spent twenty-three days in hospice care during a given month. Eighteen of the days were considered routine care days. The other five days were considered continuous care days. Medicare paid the hospice the following:

$$18 \text{ days} @ \$153 = \$2,754$$

$$+ 5 \text{ days} @ \$896 = \$4,480$$

$$\text{Total} = \$7,234$$

Medicare also pays skilled nursing facilities on a per diem rate. State Medicaid agencies and commercial insurers may pay hospitals on a per diem basis.

Case Rate

The *case rate* is a popular payment mechanism used by insurers. For example, a hospital may negotiate a case rate that is inclusive of everything that it provides during the entire inpatient stay. In this instance, the insurer and the provider agree to a fixed rate, which limits the liability of the payor and shifts some of the financial risk to the provider.

> **Case Rate**
> A rate that covers everything a hospital provides during an entire inpatient stay.

More specifically, a hospital might agree to accept a case rate of $30,000 for a patient who needs a coronary artery bypass graft (CABG). In setting case rates, providers must understand the cost of cases, especially those that are complicated, as there is always the possibility that a case may be an *outlier* that costs far more than the negotiated rate. Providers may want to consider negotiating provisions for outliers into their contract. Additionally, they may want to consider insurance with a *stop-loss* limit, which means that the provider will be compensated for costs that exceed the limit.

> **Stop-Loss**
> The insurance providers use to limit their exposure when a possibility exists that charges will go far beyond negotiated rates; a level of charges for which the provider is no longer totally liable.

For example, in the case just described, a hospital and insurer might agree that the insurer will pay 80 percent of any amount of charges incurred (using the provider's charge master system) over $50,000 in providing care related to the CABG. In the illustration in Exhibit 13.16, the charges exceeded $50,000 by $25,000. But because of the stop-loss coverage, the provider was compensated for 80 percent of the excess in costs, or an additional $20,000, bringing payment for the case up to $50,000. Therefore the provider lost only $25,000 on the case.

EXHIBIT 13.16 ILLUSTRATION OF HOW STOP-LOSS INSURANCE WORKS WHEN USING A CASE RATE

A	Total charges		$75,000
B	Negotiated case rate payment		30,000
C	Balance	A – B	45,000
D	Stop-loss amount (given)		50,000
E	Amount over stop-loss	A – D	25,000
F	Additional payment from insurer (@ 80%)	$0.8 \times E$	20,000
G	Negotiated case rate payment	B	30,000
H	Total insurance payment	F + G	50,000
I	Uncompensated charges (amount for which provider is at risk)	A – B – F	$25,000

Risk Sharing and the Principles of Insurance

The concept of health insurance goes back to the 1860s when companies sold policies to people who wanted coverage in the event of accidents. These single benefit plans expanded to more comprehensive insurance benefits over time, and in the 1930s and 1940s, life insurance companies began to offer health insurance plans. Blue Cross Blue Shield was the first insurer to negotiate contracts with hospitals and physicians at discounted rates. The group insurance market expanded when employers began offering health insurance to attract employees during World War II, when the government had imposed a wage freeze. In addition, unions began bargaining to have health insurance included in benefit packages for their members.

The largest insurer today, however, is the government. The federal and state governments provide health coverage to the elderly and disabled (Medicare) and to poor adults and children (Medicaid). And as discussed above and in Chapter One, health care costs have been rising for some time.

The concept of health care insurance includes the ideas that a premium will be charged for coverage; that an array of benefits will be offered, depending on the plan document; and today, that beneficiaries will generally be expected to use some form of provider network. The goal of the insurer is to set the premium at a rate that will be attractive to those buying the product and at the same time will adequately compensate hospitals, physicians, and other providers for the care they give to the enrollee; pay for the administrative expenses, fees, and taxes; and make a profit for the insurer.

Since the advent of the HMO (discussed earlier), many traditional insurance carriers have added HMO and HMO-like products, such as the *point of service* (POS) product, to their offerings. And although HMOs still have their traditional gatekeeper-driven, in-network products, they have added other less restrictive products in response to market demand. The lines between HMOs and insurance companies have blurred, and where the word HMO was once used to describe an organization, it is now used to describe one product that a health plan offers. The term *health plan* is now used to refer to most health insurers, HMOs like Kaiser Permanente, and employer self-funded benefit plans such as the North Carolina State Health Plan. Although most people do not think of them in this manner, Medicare and Medicaid are also health plans in that they cover an array of services to beneficiaries.

The health plan takes on risk because the premiums received must cover the cost of care and pay other expenses. In order to manage the cost of care, the plan uses various techniques including deductibles, coinsurance, stop-loss insurance (also referred to as *reinsurance*), and provider payment mechanisms. (Due to space constraints this chapter discusses only the payment mechanisms.) However, those trained in the health care field need to understand insurance principles, which have taken on additional significance with the ACA. Population-based payment arrangements such as capitation, bundled payments, and shared savings programs will be used extensively by payors in the coming years to compensate ACOs, other providers, and provider groups.

Steerage

Steerage is a technique designed to influence a population. It is used in benefit plan design by self-insured and other health plans to influence, or steer, enrollees toward using in-network providers by offering savings in the form of lower or no copayments and deductibles. And today, certain health plans may also give incentives to their members to have procedures performed in less costly settings, such as overseas.

Steerage also increases volume to participating providers. The provider accepts a reduced fee (discount) from the payor in exchange for the payor's agreement to employ mechanisms that direct patients to the participating provider. One example is the *center of excellence* designation used by insurers. Typically, a provider with this designation has distinguished itself as a

Point of Service Product/Plan (POS)
A hybrid arrangement between an HMO and a PPO in which patients are given an incentive to see providers participating in a defined network but may see non-network providers as well, though usually at some additional cost.

Preferred Provider Organization (PPO)
A network of independent providers selected by the payor to provide a specific service or range of services at predetermined (usually discounted) rates to the payor's covered members.

Participating Provider
A provider who has contracted with a health plan to provide medical services to covered members at predetermined rates.

Steerage
The influencing of patients to use a particular set of providers; an entity (often an employer or payor) may receive a discount for doing this.

high-quality provider of one or more services by meeting or exceeding predetermined criteria.

Bundled Payments

Medicare has been moving to a *bundled payment* strategy since beginning a prospective payment system in the early 1980s. Over time this approach has been applied to outpatient care, home care, and nursing home care. Medicare Advantage plans are the ultimate in bundled services because they cover most of or all the needs of the enrolled population.

Since 2012, CMS has been testing a bundled payment initiative in which physicians and hospitals work together to provide inpatient and postdischarge care to Medicare patients. The coordination of care should improve efficiency and lower cost. Physicians and hospitals will have to submit a bid to participate. There are two bundled payment models that focus solely on inpatient services: one model that focuses on postdischarge care only, and another that combines inpatient and postdischarge care. The bids will propose target prices for an episode of care, such as for a hip fracture. The hospitals and physicians would share the savings generated for Medicare, but if the cost were higher than the target bid, then they would also share in the loss.

Capitation

Capitation is a form of payment that compensates the provider a certain amount per capita for a defined set of services. In a health plan, this may be for primary care services only, certain specialists only, hospital services only, or a combination of services.

This is similar to the premium paid to the insurer in that the provider who takes this form of reimbursement assumes the risk that it will be able to deliver the services in the contract to the population designated for the contracted prepaid fee. The unit of analysis is the amount paid per member (or enrollee or subscriber) per month or per year. The philosophy is that this payment system will encourage prudent medical management and preventive care, which will prevent more expensive services in the future, such as inpatient care.

Although capitation lost favor in the 1990s, it is once again poised to replace a significant portion of the fee-for-service payment in the country for government and commercial payors. One expectation is that in the future, as ACOs gain experience, the shared savings model could diminish, and ACOs could begin receiving global capitation payments.[8] These would cover the full array of services along the continuum of care required by the

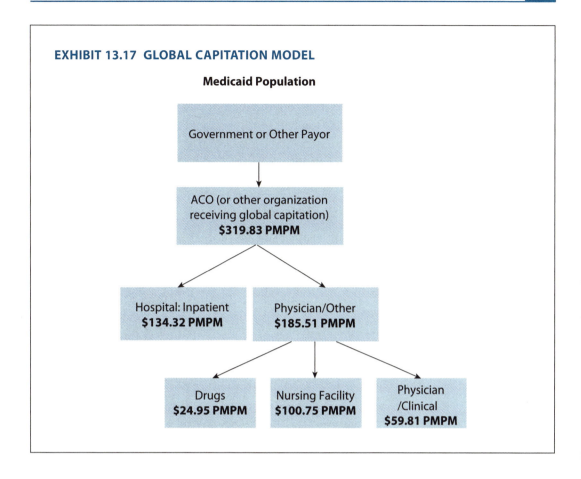

EXHIBIT 13.17 GLOBAL CAPITATION MODEL

Medicaid Population

Government or Other Payor

ACO (or other organization receiving global capitation)
$319.83 PMPM

Hospital: Inpatient
$134.32 PMPM

Physician/Other
$185.51 PMPM

Drugs
$24.95 PMPM

Nursing Facility
$100.75 PMPM

Physician /Clinical
$59.81 PMPM

contract. An ACO, in turn, would be expected to share risk with its providers, which could take the form of subcapitation. Exhibit 13.17 is an example of a global capitation model for a Medicaid population.

Inherent in capitation, however, is that the very act of providing services in any form causes the provider to incur a cost that would not have been incurred had the service not been provided. In short, a perverse incentive exists in the short run to provide a minimum level of care or *not* to provide care at all: to withhold care, to settle for a less expensive but also less effective course of treatment, or to create obstacles for patients in accessing care (e.g., having appointments available only weeks or months in advance so as to discourage unnecessary utilization). In the instance of hospitals, patients have allegedly been discharged prematurely or, again, have not received a more expensive course of treatment when a cheaper Band-Aid approach would suffice. In short, although capitation initially was intended to force a new level of fiscal accountability on providers— forcing them to understand the costs of medical care and to use only the

Per Member per Month (PMPM)
A metric generally used by health plans and their medical providers when evaluating revenue, expenses, or utilization of services. Using this metric takes volume variance out of the evaluation.

most cost-effective treatments—it has become a controversial payment form because of the temptation it presents to focus more on the short-term financial aspects of medical care than on patient care itself.

These assumptions, erroneous or not, are in part responsible for the backlash against the capitation method. It may be that in the early 1990s, when the method first came into use, there was insufficient monitoring of quality. Today, there is an intense focus on quality, and so many believe that this payment mechanism will now be successful.

Premium-Setting Methods

Techniques used by health plans to set premiums are actuarially based (see Exhibit 13.17). Accurate cost data that include the lag period from the date of service to the date of receipt of claim are vital to the calculation of the cost of medical services. Since receipt of medical claims from providers occurs later than the date of service, this information is necessary to forecast the amount of claims incurred but not reported (IBNR), which is added to the expense of the claims currently known by the health plan.[9]

Experience Rating

A method of setting group premium rates that are based on the actual health care costs of individuals in a group or groups.

There are two basic methods that payors use when developing premiums: *community rating* and *experience rating*. The difference is that community rating evaluates the health risk of a population as a whole, whereas experience rating focuses on assessing the potential medical expenditures of individuals in a group and then aggregates this information in order to calculate a group premium.

Self-insured health plans can apply experience rating while health plans offering individual and small-group policies (at-risk health plans) must apply community rating. The regulation for community rating limits the adjustment of health insurance premium rates to the following factors: family size, age, geographic location, and tobacco use. In terms of age adjustment, premiums for older policyholders can be no more than three times those charged younger adults. In sum, community rating prevents the adjustment of premium rates on the basis of previous health care claims or health status.[10]

Exhibit 13.18 illustrates a simple actuarial model that could be used to set an insurance premium or a global capitation rate. Premium development starts with the collection of accurate data on the population, with each medical service category defined. In this simple example, the inpatient cost (representing the cost to the health plan, which is different from the rate the provider charges) is defined by DRG. The physician cost is grouped by CPT code. In this example, the primary care physicians are identified

EXHIBIT 13.18 ILLUSTRATION OF PREMIUM DEVELOPMENT FOR A COMMERCIAL POPULATION

	A	B	C	D	E	F	G
	Annual Utilization per 1,000 Members (Given)	Average Cost per Service (Given)	Cost per Member [(A × B) / 1,000]	Cost PMPM (C / 12)	Copay (Given)	Cost Sharing PMPM [(A × E) / 1,000 / 12]	PMPM Net Claim Costs (D − F)
Hospital inpatient							
Medical/surgical (days)	229	$2,400.31	$549.67	$45.81			$45.81
Psychiatric/substance abuse (days)	14	1,235.74	17.30	1.44			1.44
Extended care (days)	5	470.00	2.35	0.20			0.20
Subtotal	319	$4,106.05	$569.32	$47.44		$0.00	$47.44
Hospital outpatient							
Emergency room (visits)	245	$300.78	$73.69	$6.14	$50.00	$1.02	$5.12
Surgery (visits)	89	2,204.22	196.18	16.35			16.35
Other (services)	612	281.12	172.04	14.34			14.34
Subtotal		$2,786.12	$441.91	$36.83		$1.02	$35.81
Primary care							
Office and inpatient visits	2,354	$80.41	$189.28	$15.77	$25.00	$4.90	$10.87
Immunizations and injections	175	32.22	5.64	0.47			0.47
Subtotal		$112.63	$194.92	$16.24		$4.90	$11.34
Specialists							
Surgery (procedures)	445	$501.26	$223.06	$18.59			$18.59
Anesthesia (procedures)	78	1,081.71	84.37	7.03			7.03
Office and inpatient visits	1,035	86.07	89.08	7.42	$25.00	2.16	5.27
Other (services)	3,458	141.00	487.58	40.63			40.63
Subtotal		$1,810.05	$884.09	$73.67		$2.16	$71.52
Other							
Prescription drugs (scripts)	5,651	$77.40	$437.39	$36.45	$25.00	$11.77	$24.68
Home health care (visits)	35	429.03	15.02	1.25			1.25
Ambulance (runs)	14	606.17	8.49	0.71			0.71
Durable medical equipment (units)	30	506.74	15.20	1.27			1.27
Subtotal		$1,619.34	$476.09	$39.67		$11.77	$27.90
Total medical costs PMPM				$213.86		$19.85	$194.01
Retention load PMPM (14% of premium)							27.16
Required rate PMPM							**$221.17**

Note: All amounts are rounded to two decimal places.

Subcapitation

The payment by a main provider (such as a primary care physician) of a portion of the total capitated dollars received to another provider (i.e., a specialist).

Incurred But Not Reported (IBNR)

A term that describes medical claims that have been incurred but have not yet been reported to the health plan. Since the time it takes for claims to be reported varies, data must include the date of service as well as the date of receipt. Only in this way can an actuary factor in how much expense has been incurred in a given period that is not yet in the general ledger. The actuary makes an estimate of IBNR using claims lag tables and adjusts the data for anomalies and for any known or forecast but unreported high-dollar claims outstanding. The IBNR is then added in to give the health plan its expense number for the year.

separately from the specialists to permit development of specific subcapitation rates for those services. The data are expressed in utilization per 1,000 members per year. To calculate the rate for one member per month (PMPM), the *cost per service* is divided by 1,000 and then by 12 (columns A through D). The *retention load* is the amount of administrative cost that must be recouped by the organization. As noted in Chapter One, the ACA requires rebates to be paid to health plan members when the amount spent on medical services (medical loss ratio) is less than 80 to 85 percent of premium revenues, depending on the plan.

Evolving Issues

Payment systems will continue to evolve in reaction to external forces, such as pressure to disclose quality-of-care information and to connect it with payment pricing, consumer choice in health care, and demands for health care reform. Hospitals generate more than half of their patient revenues from Medicare and Medicaid. Policymakers expect declining payment rates for Medicare and Medicaid to slow the growth of governmental spending. Recently, Medicare and other payors have pressured health care providers to accept a linkage between quality-of-care criteria and payment levels. Two approaches that link quality with payment are *pay-for-performance* measures and *pay-for-reporting* measures. Underlying the drive to have quality data reported and to link these data to payment were the needs to provide reliable and valid data so that health care consumers could make informed decisions about quality and price when selecting a hospital, and to create an incentive for hospitals to report these data.

Technology

Employers and providers now have a much greater awareness of the power of health care data and information technology. While they may have once thought health care data were a nonessential by-product of simple claims payment, today they face a strong, even urgent, need for information that is timely, informative, and in a usable format. The health care industry has a constant need and desire to employ technology in manners never explored before. The information services arena has evolved from an accounting-based, relatively basic means of analyzing charge and payment data into an integral part of modern health care delivery, payment, and even quality improvement (see Perspectives 13.4 and 13.5).

PERSPECTIVE 13.4 REALIZING THE FULL POTENTIAL OF HEALTH INFORMATION TECHNOLOGY

In a speech given to the President's Council of Advisors on Science and Technology in December 2010, Secretary of Health and Human Services Kathleen Sebelius said, "In industry after industry, we've seen the power of information technology to bring down costs and improve customers' experience. Imagine going back to the days when you had to wait at the grocery store while a cashier punched in all the hand-written price tags. Or wait for the bank to open every time you wanted to get cash. We'd never accept that. Health care shouldn't be any different."

She also commented on the use of electronic health records and the positive force they have on reducing errors, lowering costs, and increasing patient and physician satisfaction. This is an important impetus behind HHS's commitment to and historic investments of Recovery Act funds in furthering the use of information technology, not only by sophisticated health care systems but also by those providers who are currently lagging in the use of technology.

In addition to providing funding for information technology (IT) to be used in health care, HHS has created Regional Extension Centers to help providers with the technical support needed to set up and run their health IT systems. It also provided grants to states so that they could create mechanisms for doctors and hospitals to exchange information with full protections on patient privacy.

The most important component of the effort provided incentive payments for adopting electronic health records (EHRs), which would be used to improve the quality of patient care.

Two years later, in early 2012, Sebelius announced major progress in both physician and hospital use of health information technology reporting, and said that the number of hospitals using health information technology (IT) had more than doubled in the last two years. She noted that nearly 2,000 hospitals and more than 41,000 doctors had received $3.1 billion in incentive payments to ensure meaningful use of health IT, particularly certified electronic health records.

This IT effort has not been without controversy, as some providers have stated they would rather incur the penalties associated with *not* using EHRs, penalties directed to occur by 2015.

EHRs have a significant impact on quality but are also necessary if health care providers are to achieve the type of clinical integration necessary to participate in ACOs and other CMS programs.

Source: K. Sebelius, Raising healthcare quality & lowering costs through health IT, President's Council of Advisors on Science and Technology (PCAST) Release Health Information Technology Report, www.hhs.gov/news/imagelibrary/video/2010-12-08_press.html; and HHS Secretary Kathleen Sebelius announces major progress in doctors, hospital use of health information, News release, technologywww.hhs.gov/news/press/2012pres/02/20120217a.html.

PERSPECTIVE 13.5 FINANCIAL BENEFITS FROM IT

Investment in IT is considered a driving factor in improving patient care; the critical question asked by CEOs, CFOs, and board members is whether hospitals achieve a financial return from their IT investments. The inability to measure and account for financial benefits from IT investments has led some hospital administrators to avoid making these types of capital investments that can provide more efficient, higher-quality care and also improve patient and provider satisfaction.

One health care system that decided to make this investment is Banner Health, which implemented an IT system at its newest hospital, Banner Estrella Medical Center in Phoenix, Arizona. By investing in IT and receiving input from physicians, pharmacists, nurses, informaticists, and other clinicians, the hospital was able to design new work flows and establish evidence-based order sets. The improved IT design and standard order sets were implemented across departmental functions such as care management, clinical documentation, computerized provider order entry (CPOE), nursing order management, and medication administration and scheduling, and also across processes in departments such as health information management, emergency services, obstetrics, pediatrics, pharmacy, and surgery. This IT investment resulted in a $2.6 million cost savings from greater retention of nurses, which lowered the costs of recruiting, hiring, and training new nurses, and from reducing accounts receivable billing by one day, which resulted in faster payment; decreasing the incidence of adverse drug events, length of stay, and pharmacy costs; decreasing overtime expenses for nurses as a result of improving their efficiency in charting and shifting tasks; and reducing forms costs because information was digitized.

Source: Adapted from J. Hensing, D. Dahlen, M. Warden, J. V. Norman, B. C. Wilson, and S. Kisiel, Measuring the benefits of IT-enabled care transformation, *Healthcare Financial Management*, 2008;62(2):74–80.

Summary

The provision of health care services has evolved to meet the growth in the American population and rising costs. Different payment methods have been attempted in an effort to find a reasonable balance among costs, quality, and access. Health care payment in the United States has remained a "living experiment" from the early days of private, cash-based exchanges through the exponential growth of costs and numerous efforts to curb that growth. The system continues to evolve, with an increased focus on quality, value, and access, and it is still testing different payment methods and structures of care delivery.

KEY TERMS

a. Allowable costs

b. Ambulatory payment classifications (APCs)

c. Capitation

d. Case rate

e. Centers for Medicare and Medicaid Services (CMS)

f. Charge-based payment

g. Common Procedural Terminology (CPT)

h. Community rating

i. Conversion factor

j. Copayment

k. Cost-based reimbursement

l. Cost shifting

m. Deductible

n. Diagnosis related groups (DRGs)

o. Evaluation and management codes

p. Evidence-based medicine

q. Experience rating

r. Fee-for-service

s. Financial requirements

t. Flat fee

u. Gatekeeper

v. Healthcare Common Procedure Coding System (HCPCS)

w. Health maintenance organization (HMO)

x. Incurred but not reported (IBNR)

y. Managed care

z. Medicaid

aa. Medicare

bb. Medicare severity-adjusted diagnosis related groups (MS-DRGs)

cc. Members

dd. Never events

ee. Participating provider

ff. Payor

gg. Per diem

hh. Per member per month (PMPM)

ii. Point-of-service (POS)

jj. Preferred provider organization (PPO)

kk. Premium

ll. Price setter

mm. Primary care provider

nn. Prospective payment system (PPS)

oo. Relative value unit (RVU)

pp. Resource-based relative value scale (RBRVS)

qq. Shared savings

rr. Steerage

ss. Stop-loss

tt. Subcapitation

uu. Value-based purchasing

QUESTIONS AND PROBLEMS

1. **Definitions**. Define the key terms listed above.

(2.) **Stakeholders and objectives**. Exhibit 13.1 illustrates the stakeholders and objectives of the U.S. health care payment system. What are the biggest changes over the last five years?

(3.) **Value-based payment**. What were the major events and trends that caused CMS to institute a value-based payment structure for Medicare?

(4.) **Hospital Readmissions Reduction Program**. What is the rationale behind Medicare's refusal to pay for certain readmissions? What is the risk?

(5.) **ACOs**. In what ways do ACOs resemble insurers?

(6.) **Copayments and deductibles**. What is the purpose of copayments and deductibles?

(7.) **Steerage**. Name the uses of steerage.

(8.) **Diagnosis related groups.** What are DRGs? Why was the DRG system developed?

(9.) **Ambulatory payment classifications**. What are APCs? Why was the APC system developed?

(10.) **Health plans**. How do insurers determine their premiums?

11. **Health plan premium**. If a health plan covers 150,000 lives, expects 25 myocardial infarctions (MIs) to occur each year within the covered lives, expects a length of stay of 4.5 days for each MI, and has to pay an average of $950 per day for each day the MI patient is in the hospital, what is the PMPM cost to the health plan? What would have to be charged to the patient or employer if the health plan has administrative costs equaling 10 percent of its costs and it wants a profit margin of 7 percent?

12. **Health plan premium**. Given the same scenario as in question 11, what if the health plan's stockholders demand a 9 percent profit margin? What would the premium be in that case?

13. **Health plan premium**. In question 12, what if the employer or patient refuses to pay the new premium? What could the health plan offer to pay the hospital for an inpatient day? (*Hint*: Try lowering the per diem rate until the PMPM charge with a 9 percent profit margin equals the PMPM charge with the 7 percent in question 11.)

14. **Health plan premium**. In question 13, what if the hospital refuses to take the new rate, an employer refuses to pay the new premium, and that employer decides to take its employees (10,000) to another health plan? Also, suppose these departing employees/health plan members represent 6 percent of the total MI cases. What would the new PMPM premium be for the 140,000 remaining members? (*Hint*: revert back to the question 11 information, except for the changes in the numbers of employees and MI cases.)

15. **Capitation systems**. Who bears the financial risk in a capitated payment sy

16. **Capitation systems**. Why might a provider be willing to accept a globa payment?

17. **Cost-based payment**. What are four factors to consider when developing charges in a charge-based system? (*Hint*: see Appendix J.)

18. **Cost-based payment**. What charge method uses primarily the market price to establish a charge? (*Hint*: see Appendix J.)

19. **Cost-based payment**. What charge method relies on the case mix, volume, and financial requirements of the institution? (*Hint*: see Appendix J.)

20. **Cost-based payment**. What is the difference between determining charges on an average-cost basis and determining charges on a weighted-cost basis? (*Hint*: see Appendix J.)

21. **Cost-based payment**. What are the steps in determining weighted-average costs? (*Hint*: see Appendix J.)

22. **Cost-based payment**. Describe the two margin-based approaches to developing charges. (*Hint*: see Appendix J.)

Appendix J: Cost-Based Payment Systems

Reasonable and Allowable Costs

In establishing cost-based payment systems, the natural tension that exists between providers and payors revolves around five issues: reasonableness, case mix, service mix, staff mix, and efficiency.

- *Reasonableness* issues are concerned with the cost of one provider versus others. Payors often set boundaries to establish what is usual, customary, and reasonable. For instance, a payor may pay only up to 85 percent of the cost of a procedure, based on an analysis of all providers who have submitted cost reports.

- *Case mix* issues revolve around patient eligibility. For example, although a hospital may incur legitimate costs treating a patient who has a deviated septum, a payor may decide not to pay for this surgery because the patient failed to receive the necessary preadmission certification. Similarly, if a health department treats a pregnant woman who resides outside its county, the county's prenatal care program may not pay for the treatment because the patient lives outside the health department's eligibility area.

- *Service mix* issues focus on the appropriateness of care. For instance, in treating stroke patients, the provider may feel that recreational therapy is an important part of treatment. Though the treatment may be useful, the payor may not pay for it because the payor does not consider the treatment necessary within its guidelines.

- *Staff mix* issues pertain to the appropriateness of the person who provides the service. In the mental health field, for example, although a payor may agree that a patient needs psychological services, it might not pay for care provided by a pastoral counselor who is not a licensed psychologist.

- *Efficiency* issues address the appropriateness of the cost of service per unit rendered. A hospital with a low volume may have high unit costs, or a radiology center with old equipment may have to take several X-rays to get one good image. In such instances, although the payor may agree to pay for some level of the service, it will not pay for what it feels are inefficiencies.

Under any of these five conditions, if the payor denies payment and the service has already been rendered, the provider has two choices: absorb the cost, or transfer the cost to another payor. This latter technique is called *cost shifting* or *cross-subsidization*. Under this system, overpayment, or reimbursement in excess of total costs, for one service helps to cover the costs associated with underpayment, or reimbursement that falls below total costs, for another service. This technique has been one of the major reasons for the rise in the number of alternatives to cost-based systems.

Cost Shifting

Charging one group of patients more to make up for underpayment by another group.. Most commonly, charging some privately insured patients more to make up for underpayment by Medicaid or Medicare.

Unit-Based Payment Systems

Two key issues that arise in cost-based payment systems are, What is the unit of service to which payments are attached?, and, What are reasonable and allowable costs? Cost-based payors pay providers on the basis of a variety of units of care, including

- Per procedure
- Per inpatient day
- Per admission
- Per discharge
- Per diagnosis

Unfortunately for many providers, little consistency exists among third parties with respect to the unit of service on which payment is made. It is not unusual for a single provider to receive payments from Medicare on the basis of DRGs, from private insurance companies on the basis of reasonable charges, and from managed care organizations in the form of capitation. Although it is relatively straightforward to have a cost-finding system that establishes the costs for any one of these payment schemes, it takes a complicated information system to find costs along several of these bases at once.

Charge-Based Systems

A charge-based system is based in large part on the assumption that a provider is entitled to a reasonable return for its efforts. It relies heavily on the market to ensure that profits are not excessive. Although it would seem that charge-based payment systems are *reactionary* from the payor perspective (because the providers establish the charges on the front end and seemingly dictate the level of payment), the dynamic is not that simple. What follows is the reasoning that underlies the establishment of provider charges.

In setting charges, a provider must consider a wide range of costs that must be covered. These fall into the same categories discussed in the working capital chapter (operations, opportunities, contingencies, and return on investment). Together, these constitute the organization's *financial requirements.*

Allowable Costs
Costs that are allowable under the principles of reimbursement of governmental (Medicaid, Medicare) and other payors.

Financial Requirements
For health care providers, a combination of revenue and expense issues in the areas of operations, opportunities, contingencies, and return on investment.

- *Operations.* This category includes all operating costs, now and into the future. Thus, operating charges must cover costs associated with supplies, equipment, labor, and working capital and have a sufficient margin to ensure that staff remain current and that technology and facilities can be kept sufficiently up-to-date.

- *Opportunities.* Providers must build a reasonable markup into their charges so they can take advantage of opportunities to hold onto or expand into existing markets, serve new markets, or exit existing markets.

- *Contingencies.* The changing health care environment presents not only various positive opportunities but also the possibility of such difficult events as evolving payment systems, labor shortages, and uncovered catastrophic events. Therefore, charges must build in a reasonable margin for contingencies that siphon off the organization's capital.

- *Return on investment.* For for-profit providers, charges must also sufficiently compensate the organization and its owners for their investment.

Although all these cost-based methods have been employed, they all present a common concern from the point of view of payors: are they reasonable? Two ways of dealing with this problem have been to limit payments to that part of the charge considered reasonable or to employ another basis of payment altogether.

Historical, Market, or Payor Method

The *historical, market,* or *payor* payment method is extremely simple: charges are established through a process that identifies what the organization has traditionally charged, what similar organizations charge, and what payors will pay. This approach to establishing charges is only loosely related to costs, but it is widely used, especially in ambulatory care settings.

Weighted-Average Method

The *weighted-average method* sets charges as a function of the number and type of procedures an organization performs and the financial requirements of the organization. For example, assume a small health care clinic expects 10,000 visits and anticipates having $1 million in financial requirements next year (see Exhibit J.1). If visit type is ignored, the clinic could set its price by charging the same price for each visit, $100 ($1,000,000 / 10,000). However, charging each visit an average price of $100 overlooks questions of equity. Because each visit does not consume the same resources, some patients would pay more than their fair share while others would pay less.

An alternative to charging the same amount for each visit is to take into account the type of visit and to weight the visit types by the relative amount of resources they consume. This is accomplished through the following steps:

- Step 1. Categorize visits by resource consumption. Exhibit J.1 assumes there are three types of visits: brief, routine, and complex. It further assumes that 60 percent (6,000) of the 10,000 visits are brief, 30 percent (3,000) routine, and 10 percent (1,000) complex (row D).

- Step 2. Convert visits by category into weighted visit units by category. Exhibit J.1 also assumes that routine visits consume twice the resources and complex visits consume four times the resources as brief visits do (row E). Because the 3,000 routine visits consume twice the resources as brief visits do, they count the same as if they were 6,000 brief visits (3,000 × 2, row G). Similarly, because the complex visits consume four times the resources as brief visits do, the 1,000 complex visits count as

EXHIBIT J.1 ILLUSTRATION OF THE WEIGHTED-AVERAGE METHOD OF SETTING CHARGES

Givens

A	Number of procedures	a	10,000
B	Financial requirements	b	$1,000,000
C	Average charge per visit	B / A	$100

			Type of Visit[a]			
			Brief	**Routine**	**Complex**	**Total**
D	Distribution of visit by type, %	a	60%	30%	10%	100%
E	Relative weight of visit by type	a	1	2	4	
F	Number of visits	A × D	6,000	3,000	1,000	10,000
G	Number of weighted visits	E × F	6,000	6,000	4,000	16,000
H	Charge per weighted visit	c	$62.50	$62.50	$62.50	$62.50
I	Total charges	G × H	$375,000	$375,000	$250,000	$1,000,000
J	Charges using average charge	C × F	$600,000	$300,000	$100,000	$1,000,000
K	Overcharge or undercharge compared with weighted average charge	I – J	($225,000)	$75,000	$150,000	$0

[a]Given.
[b]Includes all financial requirements of the organization, not just ongoing operating costs.
[c]B / Total Number of Weighted Visits (16,000, row G).

if they were 4,000 brief visits (1,000 × 4). In this way, the 10,000 undifferentiated visits are converted to 16,000 weighted visit units (6,000 Brief Visits + 6,000 Routine Visits + 4,000 Complex Visits, row G).

- Step 3: Determine charge per weighted visit unit and apply charges to categories. Rather than spreading the $1 million in financial requirements over 10,000 visits and charging $100, the $1 million now can be spread over 16,000 weighted visit units and the charge is reduced to $62.50 ($1,000,000 / 16,000) per weighted visit unit. For instance, although there are 3,000 routine visits, they equal 6,000 weighted units. At $62.50 per unit, they will raise $375,000 (row I).

Note in row K that there is a considerable difference between charging the average price ($100) for all visits and charging by taking into account the amount of resources used. After the weighting for resource consumption, those making a brief visit pay $225,000 less, and those making routine and complex visits pay, respectively, $75,000 and $150,000 more than they would under the undifferentiated system. Some would argue that this is more equitable. This is the logic Medicare used to establish the RBRVS system currently in use in ambulatory care reimbursement along with APCs.

Margin Approaches

There are two margin-based approaches to setting charges: cost plus and coverage. The *cost-plus approach* starts with cost and adds a margin for profit. For instance, assume a free-standing radiology center desires to make a 10 percent profit over and above its cost. If it has determined that

---

EXHIBIT J.2 ILLUSTRATION OF THE COVERAGE APPROACH TO SETTING CHARGES

Given

A	Variable cost per unit: $20

B	C	D	E	F	G	H	I
Volume (Given)	Charge (D / B)	Total Charges (E)	Financial Requirements (F + G + H + I)	Direct Fixed Costs (Given)	Direct Variable Costs (A × B)	Other Costs (Given)	Desired Profit (Given]
5,000	$48	$240,000	$240,000	$100,000	$100,000	$20,000	$20,000
5,500	$45	$247,500	$250,000	$100,000	$110,000	$20,000	$20,000
6,000	$43	$258,000	$260,000	$100,000	$120,000	$20,000	$20,000
6,500	$42	$273,000	$270,000	$100,000	$130,000	$20,000	$20,000
7,000	$40	$280,000	$280,000	$100,000	$140,000	$20,000	$20,000
7,500	$39	$292,500	$290,000	$100,000	$150,000	$20,000	$20,000
8,000	$38	$304,000	$300,000	$100,000	$160,000	$20,000	$20,000
8,500	$36	$306,000	$310,000	$100,000	$170,000	$20,000	$20,000
9,000	$36	$324,000	$320,000	$100,000	$180,000	$20,000	$20,000
9,500	$35	$332,500	$330,000	$100,000	$190,000	$20,000	$20,000
10,000	$34	$340,000	$340,000	$100,000	$200,000	$20,000	$20,000

the cost of performing a certain radiological procedure is $125, then it adds a 10 percent surcharge of $12.50, creating a final charge of $137.50. The cost-plus approach is most often used with ancillary services, such as radiology, pharmacy, and laboratory services.

The *coverage approach* essentially sets charges using a break-even formula. Once the organization's cost structure, desired profit, and projected volume are known, charges can be set. Notice in Exhibit J.2 that the charge changes with volume. If the organization thought that 5,000 visits could be expected, it would establish a charge of $48 per visit, whereas if volume were forecast at 7,500 visits, it would establish a charge of $39 per visit.

Notes

1. Centers for Medicare and Medicaid Services, Office of the Actuary, National Health Statistics Group, *National Health Expenditure Projections 2011–2021*, retrieved August 7, 2013, from www.cms.gov/Research-Statistics-Data-and -Systems/Statistics-Trends-and-Reports/NationalHealthExpendData/ Downloads/Proj2011PDF.pdf.

2. U.S. Department of Health & Human Services, *Medicare Hospital Value-Based Purchasing Plan Development*, Issue Paper, 1st Public Listening Session, January 17, 2007, www.cms.gov/AcuteInpatientPPS/downloads/hospital _VBP_plan_issues_paper.pdf.

3. Health Care Advisory Board, *Medicare Payment Strategy: Dissecting CMS's Hospital Inpatient Value Based Purchasing and Readmissions Programs*, The Advisory Board Company, 2011.

4. S. F. Jencks, M. V. Williams, and E. A. Coleman, Rehospitalizations among patients in the Medicare fee-for-service program, *New England Journal of Medicine*, 2009;360:1418–1428.

5. J. Rau, Medicare revises hospitals' readmissions penalties, *Kaiser Health News*, October 2, 2012, www.kaiserhealthnews.org/Stories/2012/October/03/ medicare-revises-hospitals-readmissions-penalties.aspx.

6. *Next Steps for ACOs*, Health Policy Brief, January 31, 2012, Health Affairs/ Robert Wood Johnson Foundation, healthaffairs.org/healthpolicybriefs/brief _pdfs/healthpolicybrief_61.pdf.

7. C. Vestal, Accountable care explained: an experiment in state health policy, *Kaiser Health News*, October 18, 2012, www.kaiserhealthnews.org/stories/ 2012/october/18/aco-accountable-care-organization-states-medicaid.aspx.

8. J. W. Pearce, "The return of capitation: preparing for population based health care," *Healthcare Financial Management*, 2012;66(7):50–57.

9. P. R. Kongstvedt, *Essentials of Managed Health Care*, 6th ed. (Burlington, MA: Jones & Bartlett, 2013).

10. Kongstvedt, *Essentials of Managed Health Care*.

ACCOUNTABILITY The extent to which there are consequences, both positive and negative, attached to carrying out responsibilities.

ACCOUNTABLE CARE ORGANIZATION (ACO) A group of health care providers who provide coordinated care to target patient populations, with the intent of tying financial incentives to quality outcomes and lowered costs.

ACCRUAL BASIS OF ACCOUNTING An accounting method that aligns the flow of resources and the revenues those resources helped to generate. It records revenues when earned and resources when used, regardless of the flow of cash in or out of the organization. This is the standard method in use today.

ACCUMULATED DEPRECIATION The total amount of depreciation taken on an asset since it was put into use.

ACTIVITY-BASED COSTING (ABC) A method of estimating the costs of a service or product by measuring the costs of the activities it takes to produce that service or product.

ADMINISTRATIVE COST CENTER A cost center that supports clinical cost centers and the organization as a whole. These centers are often considered the infrastructure of the organization.

ADMINISTRATIVE PROFIT CENTER An organizational unit that does not provide health care–related services but is responsible for producing a profit. There are two types: those that sell their services internally and those whose primary responsibility is to bring revenues into the organization.

AGING SCHEDULE A table that shows the percentage of receivables outstanding by the month they were incurred.

ALLOCATION BASE A statistic (e.g., square feet, number of full-time employees) used to allocate costs because it is assumed to be related to why the costs occurred.

ALLOWABLE COSTS Costs that are allowable under the reimbursement rules of governmental (Medicaid and Medicare) and other payors.

AMBULATORY PAYMENT CLASSIFICATIONS (APCS) The basis of a flat fee, prospective payment system instituted by CMS to shift the financial risk of care to the provider in the provision of outpatient services to Medicare recipients. APCs apply primarily to hospital outpatient services.

AMORTIZATION (1) The allocation of the acquisition cost of debt to the period that it benefits. (2) The gradual process of paying off debt through a series of equal periodic payments. Each payment covers a portion of the principal plus current interest. The periodic payments are equal over the lifetime of the loan, but the proportion going toward the principal gradually increases. The amount of a payment can be determined by using the formula to calculate the present value of an annuity.

ANNUITY A series of equal payments made or received at regular time intervals.

ANNUITY DUE A series of equal annuity payments made or received at the beginning of each period.

APC See *ambulatory payment classification*.

APPROXIMATE INTEREST RATE The interest rate incurred by not taking advantage of a supplier's discount offer on bills paid early.

ASSET MIX The amount of working capital an organization keeps on hand relative to its potential working capital obligations.

ASSETS Probable future economic benefits obtained or controlled by a particular entity as a result of past transactions or events. In many instances assets represent resources that the entity owns. Assets are recorded at their cost, unless donated. In these latter cases they are recorded at fair value at the date of donation.

AUTHORITARIAN APPROACH Budgeting and decision making done by relatively few people concentrated in the highest level of the organizational structure (opposite of the *participatory approach*).

AUTHORITY The power to carry out a given responsibility.

AVAILABLE FOR SALE SECURITY A security is considered available for sale when it is not held for trading.

AVOIDABLE FIXED COST A fixed cost that will be avoided if a service is not provided: for example, full-time nursing costs that would be saved if a service were to be closed.

BANK-QUALIFIED LOAN A variable rate loan arranged by the health care provider directly with a bank, with a typical term of twenty-five years (also called a *private placement loan*).

BASIC ACCOUNTING EQUATION Assets = Liabilities + Net Assets (or Stockholders' Equity).

BETA Measures the risk of an individual stock return relative to the return of the overall stock market, which is measured by a market index such as Standard & Poor's 500 index.

BOND A form of long-term financing whereby an issuer receives cash from a lender (an investor) and in return issues a promissory note (a bond) agreeing to make principal or interest payments or both on specific dates.

BOND INSURANCE Insurance that protects against default and helps a hospital borrower to lower its cost of debt and improve bond marketability.

BOND ISSUANCE A lengthy six-step process that a health care organization goes through to sell bonds in the open public market, starting with initial preparations and ending with receipt of cash.

BREAK-EVEN ANALYSIS A technique to analyze the relationship among revenues, costs, and volume (also called *cost-volume-profit analysis*, or *CVP analysis*).

BREAK-EVEN POINT The point where total revenues equal total costs.

BUDGET VARIANCE The difference between what was planned (budgeted) and what was achieved (actual).

CANNIBALIZATION What occurs when a new service or product decreases the revenues from other established services or product lines; this result is considered a cash outflow.

CAPITAL APPRECIATION A gain that occurs when an asset is worth more when sold than when purchased.

CAPITAL ASSET PRICING MODEL (CAPM) This model measures a company's cost of equity by summing the return of the risk-free rate and the return for the equity market premium, which is risk adjusted by beta for the company's stock.

CAPITAL BUDGET One of the four major types of budgets, it summarizes the anticipated purchases for the year. Typically, to be included in this budget, an item must have a minimum purchase price, such as $500.

CAPITAL INVESTMENT A large-dollar, multiyear investment expected to achieve long-term benefits.

CAPITAL INVESTMENT DECISION A decision involving a high-dollar investment expected to achieve long-term benefits for an organization.

CAPITAL LEASE A lease that lasts for an extended period, up to the life of the leased asset. This type of lease cannot be canceled without penalty, and at the end of the lease period, the lessee may have the option to purchase the asset (also called a *financial lease*).

CAPITATED PROFIT CENTER An organizational unit responsible for earning a profit by agreeing to take care of the defined health care needs of a population for a per member fee (which is not directly tied to services); examples include HMOs, PPOs, and various managed care organizations.

CAPITATION A system that pays providers a specific amount in advance to care for the health care needs of a population over a specific time period. Providers are usually paid on per member per month (PMPM) basis. The provider then assumes the risk that the cost of caring for the population may exceed the aggregate PMPM amount received.

CARE MAPPING A process that specifies in advance the preferred treatment regimen for patients with particular diagnoses. This is also referred to as a clinical pathway, clinical protocol, or practice guideline.

CASE RATE A rate that covers everything a hospital provides during an entire inpatient stay.

CASH BASIS OF ACCOUNTING An accounting method that tracks when cash was received and when cash was expended, regardless of when services were provided or resources were used.

CASH BUDGET One of the four major types of budgets, it displays all of the organization's projected cash inflows and outflows. The bottom line for this budget is the amount of cash available at the end of the period.

CENTERS FOR MEDICARE AND MEDICAID SERVICES (CMS) The U.S. government agency that oversees the provision of and payment for health care supplied under federal entitlement programs (Medicare and Medicaid); CMS replaced the Healthcare Financing Administration (HFCA).

CHARGE-BASED PAYMENT A method of payment based on the charge made by the provider.

CHARITY CARE DISCOUNTS Discounts from gross patient accounts receivable given to patients who cannot pay their bills and who meet the entity's charity care policy.

CLAIMS SCRUBBING The process of ensuring that billing claims contain all information required by an insurer before it will submit payment.

CLASSIFIED BALANCE SHEET A balance sheet that presents current and noncurrent assets and liabilities.

CLINICAL COST CENTER A cost center responsible for providing health care–related services to clients, patients, or enrollees.

COLLATERAL (1) A tangible asset that is pledged as a promise to repay a loan. If the loan is not paid, the lending institution may, as a legal recourse, seize the pledged asset. (2) An asset with clear value (such as land or buildings) that is pledged against a loan to reduce risk to the lender. If the loan is not paid off satisfactorily, the lender has a legal claim to seize the pledged asset.

COLLECTION FLOAT The time between the issuance of a bill and the monies being available for use.

COMMITMENT FEE A percentage of the unused portion of a credit line that is charged to the potential borrower.

COMMON COSTS Costs that benefit a number of services shared by all: for example, rent, utilities, and billing (also called *joint costs*).

COMMON PROCEDURAL TERMINOLOGY (CPT) CPT codes are numeric codes, published by the American Medical Association (AMA), for services and procedures performed by providers.

COMMUNITY RATING A rating method used by indemnity and HMO insurers that guarantees that equivalent amounts will be collected from members of a specific group, without regard to demographics such as age, sex, size of covered group, and industry type.

COMPARATIVE FINANCIAL STATEMENT A statement that presents financial information as of more than one date (for the balance sheet) or covering more than one time period (for other financial statements).

COMPENSATING BALANCE A designated dollar amount on deposit with a bank that a borrower is required to maintain.

COMPLIANCE The process of abiding by governmental regulations, whether in the provision of care, billing, privacy, accounting standards, security, or any other regulated area.

COMPOUND INTEREST METHOD A method in which interest is calculated on both the original principal and on all interest accumulated since the beginning of the investment time period.

COMPOUNDING Converting a present value into its future value, taking into account the time value of money; also see *compound interest method*. It is the opposite of discounting.

CONTRA-ASSET An asset that when increased decreases the value of a related asset on the books. Two primary examples are accumulated depreciation, which is the contra-asset to properties and equipment, and the allowance for uncollectibles, which is the contra-asset to accounts receivable.

CONTRIBUTION MARGIN PER UNIT Per unit revenue minus per unit variable cost. If all other costs (fixed costs, overhead, etc.) remain the same, it is the amount of profit made on each additional unit produced (also see *total contribution margin*).

CONTRIBUTION MARGIN RULE If the contribution margin per unit is positive and no other additional costs will be incurred, then it is in the best financial interest of the organization to continue to provide additional units of that service, even if the organization is not fully covering all of its other costs, *ceteris paribus* ("all else being the same"). Conversely, if the contribution margin is negative, it is not in the best interest of the organization to continue to provide additional units of service, *ceteris paribus*.

CONTROLLING ACTIVITIES Activities that provide guidance and feedback to keep the organization within its budget once that budget has been approved and is being implemented.

CONVERSION FACTOR An actuarially based formula developed to adjust rates to allow for differences in population demographics.

COPAYMENT A payment the patient is required to make to cover part of the cost of a health care service, such as an office visit. These payments may be a fixed amount or a percentage of the charge (also called *coinsurance*).

CORPORATE COMPLIANCE Acting in accordance with the legislation and regulations bestowed on health care institutions to ensure fairness, accuracy, honesty, and quality in the provision of and billing for health care services.

COST AVOIDANCE Finding ways to operate an organization that eliminate certain classes of costs.

COST-BASED REIMBURSEMENT A payment method that uses the provider's cost of providing services (i.e., supplies, staff salaries, space costs, etc.) as the basis for reimbursement. By 2012, very little cost-based reimbursement remained. Critical access hospitals still receive reimbursement at 101 percent of reasonable cost.

COST CENTER An organizational unit responsible for producing products or providing services and controlling their costs.

COST CONTAINMENT Not spending more than is budgeted in the expense budget.

COST DRIVER That which causes a change in the cost of an activity.

COST OBJECT Anything for which a cost is being estimated, such as a population, a test, a visit, a patient, or a patient day.

COST OF CAPITAL The rate of return required to undertake a project; the cost of capital accounts for both the time value of money and risk (also called the *hurdle rate* or *discount rate*).

COST SHIFTING Charging one group of patients more in order to make up for underpayment by another group. Most commonly, charging some privately insured patients more to make up for underpayment by Medicaid or Medicare.

COST-TO-CHARGE RATIO (CCR) A method to estimate costs that assumes costs are a certain percentage of charges (or reimbursements).

CURRENT ASSETS Assets that will be used or consumed within one year.

CURRENT LIABILITIES Financial obligations due within one year.

DEBT CAPACITY The amount of total debt that an organization can be reasonably expected to take on and pay off in a timely manner.

DECENTRALIZATION The dispersion of responsibility within a health care organization.

DEDUCTIBLE A base amount the patient is responsible for paying before insurance coverage begins.

DEFERRED REVENUE Payment that has been received in advance and that confers an obligation to provide or deliver goods or services.

DEPRECIATION A measure of the extent to which a tangible asset (such as plant or equipment) has been used up or consumed.

DIAGNOSIS RELATED GROUPS (DRGS) A system for classifying inpatients based on their diagnoses. In the most pervasive system, which is used by Medicare, there are approximately 751 diagnostic groups (also see *Medicare severity-adjusted related groups*).

DIRECT COSTS Costs (e.g., nursing costs) that an organization can trace to a particular cost object (e.g., a patient).

DISBURSEMENT FLOAT An organization's practice of delaying payment as long as possible to its creditors without causing ill will.

DISCOUNT When the market rate is higher than the coupon rate, a bond is said to be selling at a discount from its par value (compare *premium*).

DISCOUNT RATE See *cost of capital* and *internal rate of return*.

DISCOUNTED CASH FLOWS Cash flows adjusted to account for the cost of capital.

DISCOUNTING Converting future cash flows into their present value, taking into account the time value of money. It is the opposite of compounding.

DIVIDEND The portion of profit that an organization distributes to equity investors.

EFFECTIVE INTEREST RATE The true interest rate that a borrower pays. This actual rate earned or charged is affected by the number of compounding periods during the year.

ELECTRONIC HEALTH RECORD (EHR) Also called an *electronic medical record* (EMR), this online version of patients' charts can include patient demographics, insurance information, dictations and notes, medication and immunization histories, ancillary test results, and the like. Under strict security permissions, the information can be accessed either in-house or in private office settings.

ELECTRONIC MEDICAL RECORD (EMR) See *electronic health record*.

EVALUATION AND MANAGEMENT CODES A set of CPT codes used to classify services by physicians, nurse practitioners (where permitted), certified nurse midwives, physician assistants, and clinical nurse specialists offered in physicians' offices, outpatient facilities, inpatient facilities, emergency departments, and nursing facilities on one of five levels, depending on the complexity of the patient's problem.

EVIDENCE-BASED MEDICINE Health care based on the best evidence currently available from both individual clinical expertise and research-based clinical findings.

EXPANSION DECISION A capital investment decision designed to increase the operational capability of a health care organization.

EXPENSE BUDGET A subset of the operating budget that is a forecast of the operating expenses that will be incurred during the current budget period.

EXPENSE COST VARIANCE The amount of the variable expense variance that occurs because the actual cost per visit varies from that originally budgeted. It is the difference between the variable expenses forecast in the flexible budget and those actually incurred. It can be calculated using the formula: (Actual Cost per Unit − Budgeted Cost per Unit) × Actual Volume.

EXPENSE VOLUME VARIANCE The portion of total variance in variable expenses that is due to the actual volume being either higher or lower than the budgeted volume. It is the difference between the expenses forecast in the original budget and those in the flexible budget. It can be computed using the formula: (Actual Volume − Budgeted Volume) × Budgeted Cost per Unit.

EXPERIENCE RATING A method of setting group premium rates that are based on the actual health care costs of individuals in a group or groups.

FACTORING Selling accounts receivable at a discount, usually to a financial institution. The latter then assumes the role of trying to collect on the outstanding payment obligations.

FAIR VALUE The amount for which an investment could currently be sold in the market.

FEASIBILITY STUDY A preliminary study undertaken by an organization and compiled by a third party to determine and document a project's financial viability.

FEE-FOR-SERVICE A method of reimbursement based on payment for services rendered, with a specific fee correlated with each specific service. An insurance company, the patient, or a governmental program such as Medicare or Medicaid may make the payments.

FINANCIAL LEASE See *capital lease.*

FINANCIAL LEVERAGE The degree to which an organization is financed by debt.

FINANCIAL REQUIREMENTS For health care providers, a combination of revenue and expense issues in the areas of operations, opportunities, contingencies, and return on investment.

FINANCING MIX How an organization chooses to finance its working capital needs.

FIXED COSTS Costs that stay the same in total over the relevant range but change inversely on a per unit basis as activity changes.

FIXED INCOME SECURITY A bond that pays fixed amounts of interest at regular periodic intervals, usually semiannually.

FIXED LABOR BUDGET A subset of the labor budget that forecasts the cost of salaried personnel.

FIXED SUPPLIES BUDGET A subset of the supplies budget that covers items that do not vary with volume.

FLEXIBLE BUDGET A budget that accommodates a range or multiple levels of activities.

FLAT FEE A predefined amount of money paid to a provider for a unit of service.

FLOAT The time delay between the process of assembling a bill and depositing the payment in the bank and making subsequent payments to creditors.

FULLY ALLOCATED COST The cost of a cost object that includes both its direct costs and all other costs allocated to it.

FUND BALANCE A term used until 1996 for owners' equity by not-for-profit health care organizations. It was replaced with the present term, *net assets*, for nongovernmental not-for-profit organizations.

FUTURE VALUE (FV) What an amount invested today (or a series of payments made over time) will be worth at a given time in the future using the compound interest method, which accounts for the time value of money; also see *present value*.

FUTURE VALUE FACTOR The factor used to compound a present amount to its future worth. It is the reciprocal of the present value factor and is calculated using the formula $(1 + i)^n$.

FUTURE VALUE FACTOR OF AN ANNUITY (FVFA) A factor that when multiplied by a stream of equal payments equals the future value of that stream; also see *present value factor of an annuity*. A factor that when multiplied by a stream of equal payments equals the future value of that stream.

FUTURE VALUE OF AN ANNUITY What an equal series of payments will be worth at some future date, using compound interest; also see *future value factor of an annuity* and *present value of an annuity*.

FUTURE VALUE OF AN ANNUITY TABLE Table of factors that shows the future value of equal flows at the end of each period, given a particular interest rate.

FUTURE VALUE TABLE Table of factors that shows the future value of a single investment at a given interest rate.

GATEKEEPER A provider (typically the primary care provider) who must preapprove specified types of care received by a patient, such as a visit to a specialist. Gatekeepers are used in most POS and HMO plans.

GOODWILL The value of intangible factors such as brand reputation, customer or supplier relationships, employee competencies, and the like that are expected to affect an entity's future earning power. An acquiring entity may pay cash and assume liabilities in excess of the fair value of the assets acquired in order to account for this value. Goodwill is no longer amortized. However, it must be evaluated for impairment every year.

GROSS CHARGES The full amount an organization bills its patients for rendered services (compare *net charges*).

GROUP PURCHASING ORGANIZATION (GPO) A network of health care organizations and a third-party vendor who are able to acquire large volumes of supplies from manufacturers at negotiated discounted rates owing to economies of scale.

HEALTHCARE COMMON PROCEDURE CODING SYSTEM (HCPCS) A system of codes used for services and supplies provided relative to a diagnosis.

HEALTH INSURANCE EXCHANGE A state-level, competitive insurance marketplace, authorized by the ACA. In each state, there will be one for individuals and one for small businesses needing insurance.

HEALTH INSURANCE PORTABILITY AND ACCOUNTABILITY ACT OF 1996 (HIPAA) A set of federal compliance regulations enacted in 1996 to ensure standardization of billing, privacy, and reporting practices as institutions convert to electronic systems.

HEALTH MAINTENANCE ORGANIZATION (HMO) A legally incorporated organization that offers health insurance and medical care. HMOs typically offer a range of health care services at a fixed price. Two types of HMOs are the staff model and the group model.

HEDGING The art of offsetting high variable rate debt payments with returns from variable rate investments.

HELD TO MATURITY SECURITY A debt security that the entity intends to hold until maturity; it is reported at amortized cost.

HORIZONTAL ANALYSIS A method of analyzing financial statements that looks at the percentage change in a line item from one year to the next. It is computed by the formula (Subsequent Year − Previous Year) / Previous Year.

HURDLE RATE See *required rate of return*.

ICD-10 The World Health Organization's International Statistical Classification of Diseases and Related Health Problems (ICD) is a coding system for diseases that is used in the United States for health insurance claim reimbursement. Currently, the United States uses the ninth version of these codes. Other countries use the tenth version, ICD-10. U.S. implementation of ICD-10 has been delayed until October 1, 2014.

INCREMENTAL CASH FLOWS Cash flows that occur solely as a result of a particular action, such as undertaking a project.

INCREMENTAL COSTS Additional costs incurred solely as a result of an action or activity or a particular set of actions or activities.

INCREMENTAL-DECREMENTAL APPROACH A method of budgeting that starts with an existing budget to plan future budgets.

INCURRED BUT NOT REPORTED (IBNR) A term that describes medical claims incurred but not yet been reported to the health plan. Since the time it takes for claims to be reported varies, data must include the date of service as well as the date of receipt. Only in this way can an actuary factor in how much expense has been incurred in a given period that is not yet in the general ledger. The actuary makes an estimate of IBNR using claims lag tables and adjusts the data for anomalies and for any known or forecast but unreported high-dollar claims outstanding. The IBNR is then added in to give the health plan its expense number for the year.

INDIRECT COSTS Costs that cannot be directly traced to a particular cost object. Common indirect costs are billing, rent, utilities, information services, and overhead. Typically, these costs are allocated to cost objects according to an accepted methodology (e.g., the step-down method).

INTEREST A payment to creditors, those who have loaned the organization funds or otherwise extended credit.

INTEREST RATE RISK The risk associated with holding variable rate bonds since the interest rate can change over the life of the bond.

INTEREST RATE SWAP An exchange, or swap, of interest rates (from fixed to variable rate or from variable to fixed rate) between a hospital borrower and another party, typically a bank or investment banking firm, with the intent of securing a more favorable rate.

INTERNAL RATE OF RETURN The rate of return on an investment that makes the net present value equal to $0 after all cash flows have been discounted at the same rate. It is also the discount rate at which the discounted cash flows over the life of the project exactly equal the initial investment.

INTERNAL RATE OF RETURN METHOD A method to evaluate the financial feasibility of an investment decision by comparing the investment's rate of return with the return required by the organization.

INVESTMENT CENTER An organizational unit that has all the responsibilities of a traditional profit center and is also responsible for making a certain return on investment.

JOINT COSTS See *common costs.*

LABOR BUDGET A subset of the expense budget, it is composed of the fixed labor budget and the variable labor budget.

LESSEE An entity that negotiates the use of another's asset via a lease.

LESSOR An entity that owns an asset that is then leased out.

LETTER OF CREDIT Offered through a bank, this instrument can enhance the creditworthiness of an institution and, hence, a bond's rating, and can also be used to pay off a bond.

LIABILITIES The financial obligations (e.g., debts) of an organization.

LIABILITY UNDER LEASE The liability account for a leased asset, which represents the outstanding obligation to pay the remaining balance on the leased asset.

LINE-ITEM BUDGET The least-detailed budget, showing only revenues and expenses by category, such as labor or supplies.

LIQUIDITY A measure of how quickly an asset can be converted into cash.

LOCKBOX A post office box located near a Federal Reserve bank or branch that, for a fee, will pick up and process checks quickly.

LONG-LIVED ASSET The resources of the entity that will be used or consumed over periods longer than one year. Also known as *noncurrent assets*.

MALPRACTICE REFORM The ACA addresses medical liability in two ways: (1) extension of federal malpractice protections to nonmedical personnel working in free clinics, and (2) authorization of $50 million over the next five years for HHS to award demonstration project grants. These grants would be provided to states to develop, implement, institute, and evaluate alternatives to the present system used in the United States to resolve charges against physicians and other health care providers of wrongdoing to patients.

MANAGED CARE Any of a number of arrangements designed to control health care costs through monitoring and prescribing or proscribing the provision of health care to a patient or population.

MARKET VALUE What a bond would sell for in today's open market.

MEDICAID A federally mandated program operated and partially funded by individual states (in conjunction with the federal government) to provide medical benefits to certain low-income people. The state, under broad federal guidelines, determines what benefits are covered, who is eligible, and how much providers will be paid.

MEDICAL TOURISM Travel to a foreign country to obtain normally expensive medical services at a steep discount. Even with a family member escorting the patient (and getting the added benefit of foreign travel), the total cost is typically less than it would be at home.

MEDICARE A nationwide, federally financed health insurance program for people aged sixty-five and older. It also covers certain people younger than sixty-five who are disabled or have chronic kidney (end-stage renal) disease. Medicare Part A is the inpatient hospital insurance program; Part B covers physician and outpatient services. Part C allows beneficiaries to receive benefits through private health plans, and Part D covers prescription drug benefit plans.

MEDICARE SEVERITY-ADJUSTED DIAGNOSIS RELATED GROUPS (MS-DRGS) The basis for the CMS payment system that replaced the DRG payment system and is designed to better correlate payments with patient severity. See *diagnosis related groups (DRGs)*.

MEMBERS The people who are covered by a health care plan (also called *enrollees*). Typically, the member or the employer of the member (or both) pays a premium to the plan for the privilege of being covered.

MISSION STATEMENT A statement that guides the organization by identifying the unique attributes of the organization, why it exists, and what it hopes to achieve. Some organizations divide these attributes between a vision statement and a mission statement.

MULTIYEAR BUDGET A budget that is forecast multiple years out, rather than just for the upcoming year.

NET ASSETS (OR EQUITY) The assets of an entity that remain after deducting its liabilities (also called residual interest). In a business enterprise, the equity is the ownership interest. In a not-for-profit organization, which has no ownership interest, net assets is divided into three classes based on the presence or absence of donor-imposed restrictions—permanently restricted, temporarily restricted, and unrestricted net assets.

NET CHARGES The amount an organization expects to receive after accounting for discounts and allowances (compare *gross charges*).

NET INCOME Equivalent to *excess of revenue over expenses* for a not-for-profit entity.

NET PRESENT VALUE (NPV) The present value of future cash flows from an investment net (less) the cost of the initial investment. It represents the difference between the initial amount paid for an investment and the future cash inflows that the investment will bring in, after adjusting for the cost of capital.

NET PRESENT VALUE METHOD A method to evaluate the financial feasibility of an investment decision solely on the basis of net present value. It uses a specific discount rate that may not be equal to the organization's required rate of return.

NET PROCEEDS FROM A BOND ISSUANCE Gross proceeds less the underwriters' and others' issuance fees.

NET WORKING CAPITAL The difference between current assets and current liabilities.

NEVER EVENTS Adverse patient outcomes due to provider negligence that are not ever supposed to happen and that therefore are typically not reimbursed.

NOMINAL INTEREST RATE The stated annual interest rate of a loan, which does not account for compounding within the year.

NONAVOIDABLE FIXED COST A fixed cost that will remain even if a particular service is discontinued: for example, full-time nursing costs in a hospital that will continue even after one of several services is dropped.

NONCONTROLLING INTEREST The amount of a partially owned subsidiary entity that the parent does not own. In the not-for-profit parent's consolidated financial statement, this noncontrolling interest is reported as a separate component of the appropriate class of net assets. This distinguishes it from the other components of the net assets of the parent.

NONCURRENT ASSETS The resources of the organization that will be used or consumed over periods longer than one year. Also known as *long-lived assets*.

NONCURRENT LIABILITIES The financial obligations not due within one year.

NONREGULAR CASH FLOWS Cash flows that occur sporadically or on an irregular basis. A common nonregular cash flow is salvage value, receipt of funds following a one-time sale of an asset at the end of its useful life.

NORMAL LINE OF CREDIT An agreement established by a bank and a borrower that establishes the maximum amount of funds that may be borrowed, and the bank may loan the funds at its own discretion.

NOTES TO THE FINANCIAL STATEMENTS Footnotes that provide information about all the financial statements and explain in more detail the significant elements. They are placed following all the statements.

OFF BALANCE SHEET FINANCING Reporting an operating lease on the income statement as an operating expense, rather than on the balance sheet under long-term debt.

OPERATING BUDGET One of the four major types of budgets, it comprises the revenue budget and the expense budget. The bottom line for this budget is net income.

OPERATING CASH FLOWS Cash flows that occur on a regular basis, often following implementation of a project (also called *regular cash flows*).

OPERATING INCOME Income derived from the entity's main line of business.

OPERATING LEASE A lease for a period shorter than the useful life of the leased asset, typically one year or less. This type of leasing arrangement can be canceled at any time without penalty, but there is no option to purchase the asset once the lease has expired.

OPPORTUNITY COST Proceeds lost by forgoing other opportunities.

ORDINARY ANNUITY A series of equal annuity payments made or received at the end of each period.

OUTSTANDING BOND ISSUE A bond that trades in the marketplace.

OWNER'S EQUITY In for-profit institutions, the difference between assets and liabilities (Assets − Liabilities).

PAR VALUE The face value amount of a bond; it is the amount the bond-holder is paid at maturity, and it does not include any coupon payments.

PARTICIPATING PROVIDER A provider who has contracted with a health plan to provide medical services to covered members at predetermined rates.

PARTICIPATORY APPROACH A method of budgeting in which the roles and responsibilities of putting together a budget are diffused throughout the organization, typically originating at the department level. There are guide-lines to follow, and top-management approval must be secured (opposite of the *authoritarian approach*).

PATIENT-CENTERED MEDICAL HOME (PCMH) A partnership between primary care providers (PCPs), the patients, and patients' families to deliver coordinated and comprehensive care over the long term in a variety of settings.

PATIENT PROTECTION AND AFFORDABLE CARE ACT (ACA) A U.S. federal statute requiring individuals to obtain health insurance coverage (the "indi-vidual mandate") or pay a penalty based upon their financial means. The goal of the ACA is to provide mechanisms to expand access to care, improve quality, and control costs. It also extends insurance coverage to preexisting conditions.

PAY FOR PERFORMANCE (P4P) A recent alternative payment arrangement that makes a portion of provider reimbursement dependent on adherence to predefined standards for quality of care and/or creates additional reim-bursement incentives for providers based on such adherence. Indicators include various patient outcomes and the frequency and types of tests ordered and services performed.

PAY FOR REPORTING (P4R) Before value-based purchasing was instituted, CMS was requiring hospitals to submit Hospital Quality Data for their adult inpatient populations, reporting on a variety of clinical performance measures, in order to avoid a 2 percent reduction in their Medicare payments.

PAYBACK METHOD A method to evaluate the feasibility of an investment by determining how long it would take to recover the initial investment, disregarding the time value of money.

PAYOR An entity responsible for paying for the services of a health care provider; it may be an insurance company or a governmental agency. In addition, many larger employers have elected to self-fund insurance for their employees and use insurers such as BlueCross as third-party administrators. By convention, the terms *payor* and *payer* are used interchangeably in the health care field.

PER DIEM The amount a payor will pay for one day of care, which includes all services associated with the inpatient day (including nursing care, surgeries, medications, etc.).

PER MEMBER PER MONTH (PMPM) A metric generally used by health plans and their medical providers when evaluating revenue, expenses, or utilization of services. Using this metric takes volume variance out of the evaluation.

PERFORMANCE BUDGET An extension of the program budget that also lays out performance objectives.

PERFORMANCE INDICATOR The FASB requires not-for-profit health care entities to include a performance indicator in their statement of operations. The FASB defines it as an intermediate level that reports the results of operations. Note that *operations* includes both operating and nonoperating items. It is analogous to income from continuing operations or net income in an investor-owned entity.

PERPETUITY An annuity for an infinite period of time, also called a *perpetual annuity*.

PLANNING The process of identifying goals, objectives, tasks, activities, and resources necessary to carry out the strategic plan of an organization over the next time period, typically one year.

POINT OF SERVICE PRODUCT/PLAN (POS) A hybrid arrangement between a HMO and a PPO product in which patients are given an incentive to see providers participating in a defined network but may see non-network providers as well, though usually at some additional cost.

PREDETERMINED RATE A set fee paid to a provider for an inpatient episode of care.

PREFERRED PROVIDER ORGANIZATION (PPO) A network of independent providers selected by the payor to provide a specific service or range of services at predetermined (usually discounted) rates to the payor's covered members.

PRELIMINARY OFFICIAL STATEMENT A statement offered to prospective buyers of a bond by the underwriters to help determine a fair market price for the bond (also called a *red herring*).

PREMIUM (1) A monthly payment made by a person or an employer, or both, to an insurer that makes the covered individuals eligible for a defined level of health care for a given period of time. (2) When the market rate is lower than the coupon rate, a bond is said to be selling at a premium (compare *discount*).

PRESENT VALUE (PV) The value today of a payment (or series of payments) to be received in the future, taking into account the cost of capital.

PRESENT VALUE FACTOR The factor used to discount a future amount to its current worth. It is the reciprocal of the future value factor and is calculated using the formula $1 / (1 + i)^n$.

PRESENT VALUE FACTOR OF AN ANNUITY (PVFA) A factor that when multiplied by a stream of equal payments equals the present value of that stream.

PRESENT VALUE OF AN ANNUITY What a series of equal payments in the future is worth today, taking into account the time value of money.

PRESENT VALUE OF AN ANNUITY TABLE Table of factors that shows the value today of equal flows at the end of each future period, given a particular interest rate.

PRESENT VALUE TABLE Table of factors that shows what a single amount to be received in the future is worth today, at a given interest rate.

PRICE SETTER The entity that controls the amount paid for a health care service.

PRIMARY CARE PROVIDER A physician (typically a family medicine, internal medicine, pediatric, or sometimes an obstetrics and gynecology provider) who is the primary caregiver for a patient.

PRO FORMA A simplified table of categorized line items with volumes and associated revenues and expenses that are used to estimate overall financial performance.

PRODUCT MARGIN Total Contribution Margin − Avoidable Fixed Costs. It represents the amount that a service contributes toward covering all other costs after it has covered the costs that are there solely because the service is offered (its total variable cost and avoidable fixed costs) and that would not be there if the service were dropped.

PRODUCT MARGIN DECISION RULE If a service's product margin is positive, the organization will be better off financially if it continues with the service, *ceteris paribus* ("all else being the same"). Conversely, if a service's product margin is negative, the organization will be better off financially if it discontinues the service, *ceteris paribus*.

PRODUCTION COST CENTER A cost center responsible for producing or selling products (or both).

PROFIT CENTER An organizational unit responsible for controlling costs and earning revenues.

PROGRAM BUDGET An extension of the line-item budget that shows revenues and expenses by program or service lines.

PROSPECTIVE PAYMENT SYSTEM (PPS) A payment system used by Medicare to reimburse providers a predetermined amount; rates, prices, or budgets are established before services are rendered and costs are incurred. Several payment methods fall under the PPS umbrella, including methods based on DRGs (for inpatient admissions), APCs (for outpatient visits), a resource-based relative value scale (RBRVS) (for professional services), and resource utilization groups (RUGs) (for skilled nursing home care). Use of DRGs was the first method that fell under this type of predetermined payment arrangement. Providers retain or absorb at least a portion of the difference between established revenues and actual costs.

PUT RISK The risk associated with variable rate bonds because the bondholder can sell back the bond, typically within a thirty-day period.

RATING OF BOND A rating by a bond rating agency, which measures the credit default risk of a bond by assessing its financial, operational, and market conditions.

RATIO An expression of the relationship between two numbers as a single number.

RECOVERY AUDIT CONTRACTOR (RAC) PROGRAM A program created under the Medicare Modernization Act of 2003 to identify and recover improper Medicare payments to health care providers.

RED HERRING See *preliminary official statement.*

REGULAR CASH FLOWS See *operating cash flows.*

RELATIVE VALUE UNIT (RVU) A standardized weighting that is assigned to each encounter, procedure, or surgery and that reflects resources consumed. It is also widely used by hospitals in evaluating the amounts of resources required to perform various services in a single department or across departments. RVUs are determined by assigning weights to such factors as the personnel time, level of skill, and sophistication of equipment used to deliver patient services. RVUs are also an input used in bonus plans when rewarding physicians based partially on productivity.

RELEVANT RANGE The range of activity over which total fixed costs or per unit variable cost (or both) do not vary.

REMARKETING RISK Risk associated with variable rate bonds because the bondholder can sell back its bond and the remarketing agent may be unable to sell the bond again.

REPLACEMENT DECISION A capital investment decision designed to replace older assets with newer (often cost-saving) ones.

REQUIRED CASH BALANCE The amount of cash an organization must have on hand at the end of the current period to ensure that it has enough cash to cover the expected outflows during the next forecasting period.

REQUIRED MARKET RATE The market interest rate on bonds of similar risk.

REQUIRED RATE OF RETURN The minimal *internal rate of return* on any investment that will justify that investment (also called *cost of capital* or *hurdle rate*).

RESIDUAL VALUE See *salvage value.*

RESOURCE-BASED RELATIVE VALUE SCALE (RBRVS) A system of paying physicians based on the relative value of the services rendered.

RESPONSIBILITY The duties and obligations of a responsibility center.

RESPONSIBILITY CENTER An organizational unit formally given the responsibility to carry out one or more tasks or achieve one or more outcomes (or both).

RETAIL HEALTH CARE Walk-in medical services for basic preventive health care provided in a retail outlet, such as a pharmacy, by a licensed care provider.

RETAINED EARNINGS A second type of benefit to an investor. The portion of profits the organization keeps for itself to use for growth and in support of its mission.

REVENUE ATTAINMENT Earning the amount of revenue budgeted.

REVENUE BUDGET A subset of the operating budget that is a forecast of the operating revenues that will be earned during the current budget period.

REVENUE CYCLE MANAGEMENT A set of management techniques focused on the goals, roles and responsibilities, and procedures to be used at various stages in the billing process.

REVENUE ENHANCEMENT Finding supplemental sources of revenue.

REVENUE RATE VARIANCE The amount of the total revenue variance that occurs because the actual average rate charged varies from the one originally budgeted. It is the difference between the revenues forecast in the flexible budget and those actually earned. It can be calculated using the formula (Actual Rate − Budgeted Rate) × Actual Volume.

REVENUE VOLUME VARIANCE The portion of total variance in revenues due to the actual volume being either higher or lower than the budgeted volume. It is the difference between the revenues forecast in the original budget and those in the flexible budget. It can be computed using the formula (Actual Volume − Budgeted Volume) × Budgeted Rate.

REVOLVING LINE OF CREDIT An agreement established by a bank and a borrower that legally requires the bank to loan money to the borrower at any time requested, up to a prenegotiated limit.

RIGHT OF USE ASSET The recorded value of a leased asset, which is equal to the present value of the lease payments.

ROLLING BUDGET A multiyear budget that is updated more frequently than annually, such as semiannually or quarterly.

RVU See *relative value unit.*

SALE AND LEASEBACK ARRANGEMENT A type of capital lease whereby an institution sells an owned asset and simultaneously leases it back from the purchaser. The selling institution retains the right to use the asset and also benefits from the immediate acquisition of cash from the sale.

SALVAGE VALUE The amount of cash to be received when an asset is sold, usually at the end of its useful life; also called *terminal value, residual value,* or *scrap value.*

SCRAP VALUE See *salvage value.*

SERVICE CENTER An organizational unit primarily responsible for ensuring that health care–related services are provided to a population in a manner that meets the volume and quality requirements of the organization. It has no direct budgetary control.

SHARED SAVINGS A payment strategy that encourages providers to reduce health care spending for a defined patient population by offering them a percentage of the net savings realized as a result of their efforts.

SHORT-TERM PLANS Plans that identify an organization's short-term goals and objectives in detail, primarily in regard to organizational marketing, production, control, and financing.

SIMPLE INTEREST METHOD A method in which interest is calculated only on the original principal. The principal is the amount invested.

SINKING FUND A fund in which monies are set aside each year to ensure that a bond can be liquidated at maturity.

STATIC BUDGET A budget that uses a single or fixed level of activity.

STATISTICS BUDGET The first budget to be prepared; one of the four major types of budgets. It identifies the amount of services that will be provided, typically categorized by payor type.

STEERAGE The influencing of patients to use a particular set of providers; an entity (often an employer or payor) may receive a discount for doing this.

STEP-DOWN METHOD A cost-finding method based on allocating costs that are not directly paid for to products or services to which payment is attached. The method derives its name from the stair-step pattern that results from allocating costs.

STEP-FIXED COSTS Costs that increase in total over wide, discrete steps.

STOCKHOLDERS' EQUITY In an investor-owned entity, the residual interest in the assets of the entity that remain after deducting its liabilities.

STOP-LOSS The insurance providers use to limit their exposure when a possibility exists that charges will go far beyond negotiated rates; a level of charges for which the provider is no longer totally liable.

STRAIGHT-LINE DEPRECIATION A depreciation method that depreciates an asset an equal amount each year until it reaches its salvage value at the end of its useful life.

STRATEGIC DECISION A capital investment decision designed to increase a health care organization's strategic (long-term) position.

STRATEGIC PLANNING The process of identifying an organization's mission, goals, and strategy for best positioning itself for the future.

SUBCAPITATION The payment by a main provider (such as a primary care physician) of a portion of the total capitated dollars received to another provider (i.e., a specialist).

SUNK COSTS Costs incurred in the past. (They should not be included in NPV-type analyses.)

SUPPLY CHAIN The entities involved in distributing finished goods from the manufacturer to the end consumer, oftentimes including a third-party vendor, or middleman (also see *supply chain management*).

SUPPLY CHAIN MANAGEMENT The oversight of the supply chain process, up to and including storage and consumption by the end users (also see *supply chain*).

TARGET COSTING Controlling costs or decreasing profit margins (or both) to meet or beat a predetermined price or reimbursement rate.

TAX SHIELD An investment for a for-profit entity that reduces the amount of income tax to be paid, often because interest and depreciation expenses are tax deductible.

TERM LOAN A loan, typically issued by a bank, that has a maturity of one to ten years.

TERMINAL VALUE See *salvage value.*

THIRD-PARTY PAYORS Commonly referred to as *third parties*, these are entities that pay on behalf of patients.

TIME VALUE OF MONEY The concept that a dollar received today is worth more than a dollar received in the future.

TOP-DOWN BUDGETING See *authoritarian approach.*

TOP-DOWN-BOTTOM-UP APPROACH See *participatory approach.*

TOTAL CONTRIBUTION MARGIN Total revenues minus total variable costs.

TRADE CREDIT Short-term credit offered by the supplier of a good or service to the purchaser.

TRADE PAYABLES Short-term debt that results from supplies purchased on credit for a given length of time.

TRADING SECURITY Investments in equity securities with readily determinable fair values and all investments in debt securities (except those intended to be held to maturity) are measured at fair value and are classified as trading securities.

TRADITIONAL PROFIT CENTER An organizational unit responsible for earning a profit by providing health care services. Revenues are earned on either a fee-for-service or flat fee basis. Examples include cardiology, women's and children's services, and oncology.

TRANSACTION NOTE A short-term, unsecured loan made for some specific purpose.

TRANSFER PRICE The price for a product or service that is charged internally to other organizational units.

TREND ANALYSIS A type of horizontal analysis that looks at changes in line items compared with a base year. It is calculated by the formula (Any Subsequent Year – Base Year) / Base Year.

TRUSTEE An agent for bondholders who ensures that the health care facility is making timely principal and interest payments to the bondholders and complies with legal covenants of the bond.

VALUE-BASED PURCHASING (VBP) A payment methodology designed to provide incentives to providers for delivering quality health care at a lower cost. The financial rewards come from funds being withheld by the payor; these funds are then redistributed on providers' achievement of and improvement on specific performance measures, including patient satisfaction.

VARIABLE COSTS Costs that stay the same per unit but change directly in total with a change in activity over the relevant range: Total Variable Cost = Variable Cost per Unit × Number of Units of Activity.

VARIABLE LABOR BUDGET A subset of the labor budget that forecasts nonsalary labor costs, such as part-time employees and overtime hours.

VARIABLE SUPPLIES BUDGET A subset of the supplies budget that covers items that vary with volume.

VERTICAL ANALYSIS A method of analyzing financial statements that answers the general question, what percentage of one line item is another line item? Also called *common-size analysis* because it converts every line item to a percentage, thus allowing comparisons among the financial statements of different organizations.

WEIGHTED AVERAGE COST OF CAPITAL (WACC) A hospital's cost of capital calculated as a combination of both its cost of debt (*Kd*) and cost of equity (*Ke*), which are weighted by the respective proportions of debt and equity it possesses.

WORKING CAPITAL Measures current asset accounts of the health care entity (also see *net working capital*).

WORKING CAPITAL STRATEGY The amount of working capital an organization determines it must keep as a cushion to protect against unforeseen expenditures.

YIELD TO MATURITY The rate at which the market value of a bond is equal to the bond's present value of future coupon payments plus par value.

ZERO-BASED BUDGETING (ZBB) An approach to budgeting that continually questions both the need for existing programs and their level of funding, as well as the need for new programs (often referred to as ZBB).

Websites

1. American Hospital Association (AHA) trend data

   Link: www.aha.org/research/index.shtml or go to the AHA website and click on "Research and Trends."

   > Website: (a) A freely available resource. (b) These reports are released by the American Hospital Association annually. The data are compiled from various sources and provide information on health and hospital trends. Other reports available here provide insights into issues like workforce shortages, disaster preparedness, and health care costs.

2. Healthcare Financial Management Association (HFMA)

   Link: www.hfma.org/ or go to the HFMA website.

   > Website: (a) Paid website. Free information is available only about HFMA; however, there are selected contents area, (e.g., Health Reform) that are free. (b) HFMA is an association that is considered a leader in information on top trends and issues facing the health care industry. It is a membership organization for health care financial management executives and leaders and currently consists of more than 34,000 members. It publishes many magazines on various topics. Each magazine is available to nonmembers for an annual subscription fee. Members receive these publications for free, but there is an annual fee for membership.

3. National Association of Rural Health Clinics (NARHC)

   Link: www.narhc.org/or go to the NARHC website and click on "Resources."

   > Website: (a) Free resources plus paid membership. (b) NARHC is the only national organization dedicated exclusively to improving the delivery of quality, cost-effective health care in rural, underserved areas through the Rural Health Clinics Program (RHC Program). NARHC is a vital link between health clinics and federal legislators and regulators as it brings the real-world experience of

rural health clinic practice to policymaking and policymakers. NARHC works with Congress and other federal agencies. NARHC members pay a membership fee. However, NARHC makes some reports and information resources available for free at the link above. Most of the site's information about RHCs is freely available through this link.

4. American Hospital Directory (AHD)

Link: www.ahd.com

Website: (a) Some free information plus detailed information for paid subscribers. (b) The AHD provides online data for over 6,000 hospitals. Its database of information about hospitals is built from both public and private sources, including Medicare claims data, hospital cost reports, and other files obtained from the federal Centers for Medicare and Medicaid Services. The directory also includes AHA annual survey data, licensed from Health Forum, an AHA company. AHD also makes available some free hospital information, especially state and national statistics. However, more detailed information is available for paid subscribers.

5. U.S. Department of Health and Human Services (HHS)

Link: healthmeasures.aspe.hhs.gov or from here choose links to any HHS area or agency of interest.

Website: (a) Free resource center. (b) This link from HHS tracks government data on critical U.S. health system indicators. The website presents national trend data as well as detailed views broken out by population characteristics such as age, sex, income level, and insurance coverage status.

6. Centers for Medicare and Medicaid Services (CMS) statistics, trends, and reports

Link: www.cms.hhs.gov/home/rsds.asp or go to the CMS website and click on "Research, Statistics, Data and Systems."

Website: (a) Free resource center. (b) This website offers research, statistics, trends, and reports related to Medicare and Medicaid and made available for free by the CMS.

7. Healthcare Finance Group (HFG)

Link: www.hfgusa.com

Website: (a) This is the homepage of HFG, a specialty finance company, investing exclusively in the health care industry. (b) HFG provides secured revolving lines of credit, term loans, real estate loans, and letters of credit from $5 million to $100 million to health care service providers who are HFG clients, and these services are described on its website. Clients include acute care hospitals, skilled nursing facilities, home health agencies, large physician groups, pharmacy services; LTAC and rehab hospitals, behavioral health centers, and diagnostic imaging centers.

8. North Carolina Healthcare Information and Communications Alliance (NCHICA)

   Link: www.nchica.org

   Website: (a) This homepage offers partially free resources and paid NCHICA memberships (full-time students at an accredited institution of higher learning are charged $25 annually to become nonvoting members. (b) NCHICA, a nationally recognized nonprofit organization, is a consortium that serves as an open and effective forum for health information technology (HIT) initiatives in North Carolina. It is dedicated to improving health care through information technology and secure communications. It offers resources relating to HIPAA, privacy, electronic data interchange (EDI), and the like.

9. *Wall Street Journal (WSJ)*

   Link: online.wsj.com/public/us or from this homepage go to "news by industry."

   Website: The *WSJ* provides news by industry, including articles on the health care industry and health care finance. However, users must become subscribers to gain online access to all the information provided on this website. A student subscription is available for a subsidized rate of $49.95 for fifteen weeks.

10. Hospital and health care system financial statements from bond issues

    Links: Muni-OS, www.munios.com (homepage), and Electronic Municipal Market Access, www.emma.msrb.org

    Website: (a) The Muni-OS website requires registration, which is free. Both websites allow one to download the financial statements of hospitals and health care systems that have issued municipal bonds (download the "Official Statement" of the bond issue to get the financial statement). (b) These sites also provide detailed information about the bond issuance, specifically the amount of the issue, bond issuer, underwriter of the bond, and so forth. They also define how the proceeds of the bond issue will be used.

11. Kaiser Family Foundation (KFF)

Link: www.kff.org/

Website: This website provides the latest information on the topics of health reform, Medicaid, Medicare, insurance, the uninsured, and state policies. Each topic area offers issue briefs, slides, charts, and reports.

12. American Medical Association (AMA)

Link: www.ama-assn.org/amednews

Website: This website has drop boxes for finding information on governmental, professional, and business issues. The business section provides news and feature stories in the following topic areas: accountable care organizations, billing, economy, health industry, hospitals, meaningful use, and practice management.

13. Agency for Healthcare Research and Quality (AHRQ)

Link: www.ahrq.gov/data/dataresources.htm

Website: The AHRQ website provides a range of data sources for researchers, clinician, and policymakers. These data sources include information on access to care, ambulatory surgeries, emergency visits, health care quality, and more

14. Hospital Compare and quality of care data

Link: www.hospitalcompare.hhs.gov

Website: Hospital Compare is a website that lets consumers compare the quality of hospital outpatient services. Hospital Compare displays rates for process of care measures that show how often hospitals provide particular types of care that are recommended for patients with a heart attack, heart failure, pneumonia, surgery, or children's asthma. Information is also provided on patient outcomes and the patients' experiences at the hospital.

15. Health care reform and health insurance regulation

Link: http://www.cms.gov/CCIIO/

Website: (a) CMS provides information on health care reform law with respect to changes in commercial insurance. (b) The website section titled Data Resources provides specific medical loss ratio information, which reveals the percentage of premium dollars spent on medical expenses, for health insurers across the United States as well as health insurers undergoing an insurance rates review. It also provides information on rate increases by health insurers.

Health Policy APPs for iPad and iPhone from the Apple iTunes Store

1. California Healthline is an app that provides information on health policy nationally as well as health issues for the state of California. The app is funded by the California Healthcare Foundation.

2. *Health Affairs*, a health policy journal, offers an app (www.healthaffairs .org/iPad.php) for reading and learning about timely health policy issues as well as health care blogs from Washington DC. Some of the content accessed with the app is free, but there is a fee for *Health Affairs* articles unless one is a *Health Affairs* subscriber.